Addiction Medicine: Neuroscientific Approaches and Therapeutical Implications

Addiction Medicine: Neuroscientific Approaches and Therapeutical Implications

Edited by Lois Rivera

hayle medical

New York

Hayle Medical,
750 Third Avenue, 9th Floor,
New York, NY 10017, USA

Visit us on the World Wide Web at:
www.haylemedical.com

ISBN: 978-1-64647-549-0

Cataloging-in-Publication Data

Addiction medicine : neuroscientific approaches and therapeutical implications / edited by Lois Rivera.
p. cm.
Includes bibliographical references and index.
ISBN 978-1-64647-549-0
1. Substance abuse--Treatment. 2. Neurosciences--Therapeutic use. 3. Addicts--Medical care.
4. Psychology, Pathological. I. Rivera, Lois.
RC564 .A33 2023
362.29--dc23

Table of Contents

Preface

This book has been a concerted effort by a group of academicians, researchers and scientists, who have contributed their research works for the realization of the book. This book has materialized in the wake of emerging advancements and innovations in this field. Therefore, the need of the hour was to compile all the required researches and disseminate the knowledge to a broad spectrum of people comprising of students, researchers and specialists of the field.

Addiction is defined as the inability to stop utilizing a substance or engaging in an activity despite the fact that doing so is harmful to the physical and mental health of a person. Exhaustion, declining physical health and irritation are all common signs of addiction. Addiction medicine is a specialized branch of medicine primarily concerned with the evaluation, diagnosis, recovery, prevention and treatment of addiction related disorders. Substance-related and addictive disorders and people who exhibit unhealthy use of substances like prescription drugs, nicotine, alcohol and other illicit and licit drugs are all treated under this area of medical science. Addiction medicine involves the study of drug cravings from different perspectives such as brain states, regional, small-scale networks, and large-scale networks. It also encompasses craving management through cognitive, behavioral, psychosocial, environmental and neural perspectives. This book provides significant information to help develop a good understanding of addiction medicine, its neuroscientific approaches and therapeutical implications. Those in search of information to further their knowledge will be greatly assisted by it.

At the end of the preface, I would like to thank the authors for their brilliant chapters and the publisher for guiding us all-through the making of the book till its final stage. Also, I would like to thank my family for providing the support and encouragement throughout my academic career and research projects.

Editor

1

Forging Neuroimaging Targets for Recovery in Opioid use Disorder

Jennifer L. Stewart[1,2]*, *April C. May*[3], *Robin L. Aupperle*[1,2] *and Jerzy Bodurka*[1]

[1] *Laureate Institute for Brain Research, Tulsa, OK, United States,* [2] *Department of Community Medicine, University of Tulsa, Tulsa, OK, United States,* [3] *Joint Doctoral Program in Clinical Psychology, San Diego State University, University of California, San Diego, San Diego, CA, United States*

***Correspondence:**
Jennifer L. Stewart
jstewart@laureateinstitute.org

The United States is in the midst of an opioid epidemic and lacks a range of successful interventions to reduce this public health burden. Many individuals with opioid use disorder (OUD) consume drugs to relieve physical and/or emotional pain, a pattern that may increasingly result in death. The field of addiction research lacks a comprehensive understanding of physiological and neural mechanisms instantiating this cycle of *Negative Reinforcement* in OUD, resulting in limited interventions that successfully promote abstinence and recovery. Given the urgency of the opioid crisis, the present review highlights faulty brain circuitry and processes associated with OUD within the context of the *Three-Stage Model of Addiction* (1). This model underscores *Negative Reinforcement* processes as crucial to the maintenance and exacerbation of chronic substance use together with *Binge/Intoxication* and *Preoccupation/Anticipation* processes. This review focuses on cross-sectional as well as longitudinal studies of relapse and treatment outcome that employ magnetic resonance imaging (MRI), functional near-infrared spectroscopy (fNIRs), brain stimulation methods, and/or electroencephalography (EEG) explored in frequency and time domains (the latter measured by event-related potentials, or ERPs). We discuss strengths and limitations of this neuroimaging work with respect to study design and individual differences that may influence interpretation of findings (e.g., opioid use chronicity/recency, comorbid symptoms, and biological sex). Lastly, we translate gaps in the OUD literature, particularly with respect to *Negative Reinforcement* processes, into future research directions involving operant and classical conditioning involving aversion/stress. Overall, opioid-related stimuli may lessen their hold on frontocingulate mechanisms implicated in *Preoccupation/Anticipation* as a function of prolonged abstinence and that degree of frontocingulate impairment may predict treatment outcome. In addition, longitudinal studies suggest that brain stimulation/drug treatments and prolonged abstinence can change brain responses during *Negative Reinforcement* and *Preoccupation/Anticipation* to reduce salience of drug cues, which may attenuate further craving and relapse. Incorporating this neuroscience-derived knowledge with the *Three-Stage Model of Addiction* may offer a useful plan for delineating specific neurobiological targets for OUD treatment.

Keywords: opioid use disorder, neuroimaging, magnetic resonance imaging, electroencephalography, event related potentials, recovery, abstinence

THE DEVASTATION OF OPIOID USE DISORDER

Opioid use disorder (OUD) is a chronic, relapsing condition, associated with a staggering $75 billion public health burden and millions of years of premature mortality, attributable to a 350% increase in opioid-related deaths over the past two decades (2, 3). In 2016, more than 60 million patients had used and misused opioid-based anti-pain medication despite growing awareness of negative consequences and reduced effectiveness of long-term use (4). It is estimated that 20–30% of opioid-related overdoses are actually intentional suicide attempts, as opposed to accidents (5). It is not surprising that OUD-related suicide risk is over six times the national average, as individuals with OUD are struggling with disproportionate amounts of aversive mood states (anhedonia, dysphoria, suicidal ideation, irritability, anger, guilt, and shame) that are associated with heightened stress and drug craving (5–10). Moreover, the longer the temporary abstinence from drug use, the greater attention users devote to bodily sensations signaling a homeostatic imbalance. The process of attending to these sensations in an attempt to restore homeostasis, also known as allostasis (11), contributes to increased craving and withdrawal (9). Users actively attempt to avoid withdrawal comprised of agonizing physiological states (e.g., sweating, racing heartbeat, fever, nausea/vomiting, stomach cramps, diarrhea, generalized pain, depression, and anxiety) starting within hours of last use and lasting for days (12, 13). Opioid consumption relieves symptoms of negative affect as well as craving/urges in individuals with OUD (14), thereby increasing the likelihood of future drug use in the presence of negative affective and physical states, a process known as negative reinforcement. In short, individuals with OUD consume drugs to relieve emotional and/or physical pain. A *Three-Stage Model of Addiction* based on substantial animal and human studies highlights the importance of negative reinforcement, as well as binging and anticipation processes, to the exacerbation and maintenance of chronic substance use (1, 15). This model can be applied to various substance use disorders and further expanded to elucidate processes unfolding as a function of prolonged abstinence from use. At this point in time, however, we lack a comprehensive understanding of the underlying physiological and neural mechanisms involved in allostasis and negative reinforcement processes. As a result, we possess limited interventions to promote recovery and abstinence, and are left treating symptoms rather than underlying biological systems contributing to OUD.

Successful overdose-reversal and OUD treatment interventions are urgently needed to reduce mortality, increase quality of life, and lessen economic burden to society and healthcare systems. Modern neuroimaging technology advanced our ability to measure and quantify structural abnormalities and disrupted functionalities of brain circuitry. Neuroimaging research can be particularly beneficial for identifying brain circuitry and systems underlying allostasis and aversive states within OUD, thus leading to identification of targets for pharmacological and behavioral interventions to aid in addiction recovery. The goals of the present review are to: (1) highlight faulty brain circuitry and processes associated with OUD within the context of a *Three-Stage Model of Addiction* (1, 15); (2) discuss strengths and limitations of this imaging work with respect to study design and when available, individual differences such as opioid use chronicity/recency, comorbid symptoms, and biological sex that may influence interpretation of findings; and (3) translate gaps in the OUD literature into future research directions to lead toward a neuroscience-informed understanding of individual differences and potential points for intervention.

FRAMING OUD RESEARCH WITHIN THE NEUROCIRCUITRY OF ADDICTION

It is argued that three stages of motivational dysregulation instantiate and maintain the chronic cycle or stages of addiction: *Binge/Intoxication, Negative Reinforcement,* and *Preoccupation/Anticipation* (1, 15, 16). Within this model, these stages, which are likely not entirely separable from each other, are linked to aberrant patterns of activity within/between brain regions involved in reward processing [ventral striatum (VS)], cognitive control [frontocingulate regions including inferior frontal gyrus (IFG) and anterior cingulate cortex (ACC)], aversive emotional states [amygdala (AMG)], and a sense of the internal body state, known as interoception [insula (INS)]. **Figure 1** illustrates psychological and neurobiological processes associated with each stage.

Whereas the *Binge/Intoxication* stage lays the groundwork for initial transition to addiction, the latter two stages act to drive drug relapse. *Binge/Intoxication* reflects positive reinforcement processes that begin with recreational drug use, wherein rewarding consequences of drug use (e.g., euphoria, high), accompanied by increased VS (nucleus accumbens, globus pallidus) activity and dopamine release, increase the likelihood of future drug consumption. This cycle eventually leads to impulsive, intensified use that is difficult to control. Both animal and human research demonstrate that *Binge/Intoxication* initially weakens the brain's response to natural rewards while increasing drug tolerance by remapping striatal circuitry (consisting of decreased VS activity paired with increased dorsal striatum responses) to prioritize habitual drug rewards, a process termed incentive sensitization (17–20).

The *Negative Reinforcement* stage is thought to strengthen the likelihood of future drug use by reducing aversive mood, stress, and withdrawal states exacerbated by lack of recent drug administration. It is argued that a compulsive, habitual cycle persists: heightened anxiety and stress are briefly reduced as a result of drug use, but then build up over time, leading to obsessions about future drug-taking until the drug is used again (21). The extended AMG (comprised of AMG central nucleus, bed nucleus of the stria terminalis, and posterior nucleus accumbens shell) interacts with hypothalamic regions involved in neurochemical stress reactions and is also linked to aversive emotional reactions in humans (21). The stria terminalis, in particular, is implicated in norepinephrine hyperactivity associated with opioid withdrawal (22). Researchers theorize that

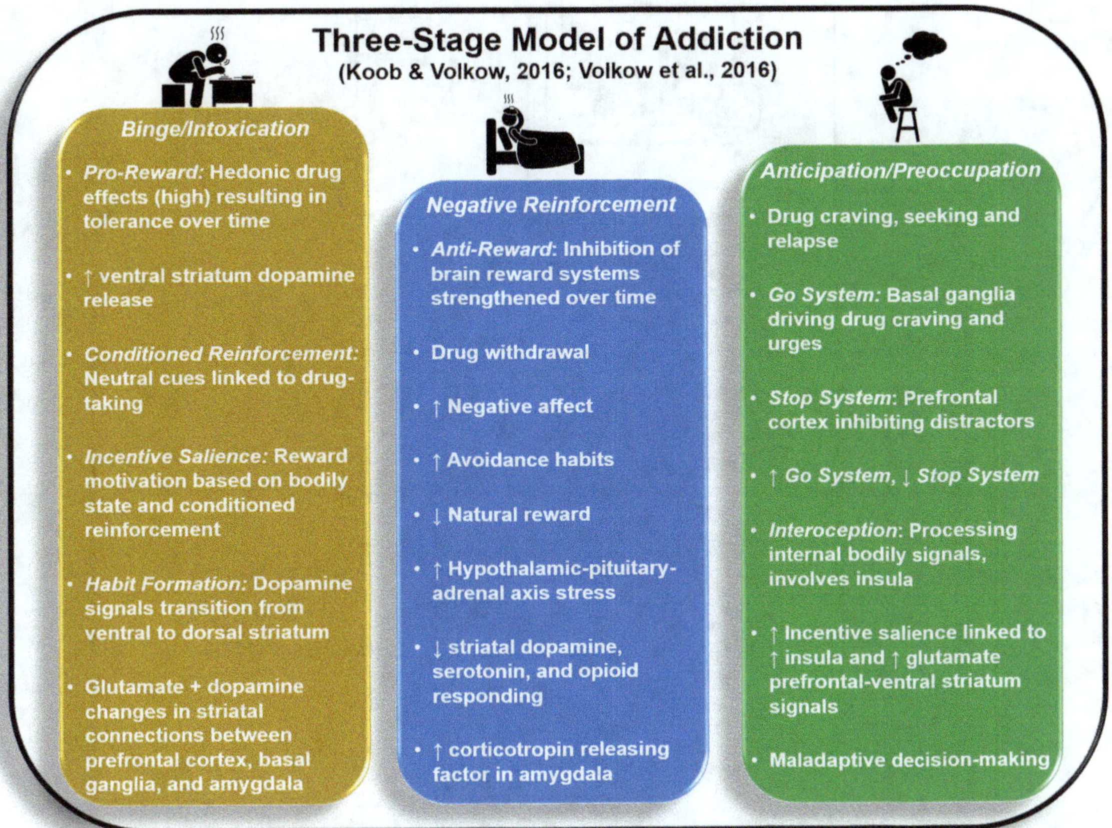

FIGURE 1 | Key psychological and neurobiological processes reflected in the *Three-Stage Model of Addiction* (1, 15).

stress-related brain systems/circuitry are activated first during the *Binge/Intoxication* stage to counteract excessive dopamine release; over time, neurochemical stress signals are thought to suppress dopaminergic responsivity to drug reward (23).

It is argued that the *Preoccupation/Anticipation* stage involves obsessive thoughts about future drug-taking that are prioritized over other goals, paired with weakened inhibitory control over drug craving/urges (1). Substantial evidence implicates INS in drug craving and aversive feeling states linked to withdrawal and short-term abstinence (24–26). In addition, heightened prefrontal cortex (PFC) and ACC activities evident within the context of drug cue-elicited craving theoretically drive increased preoccupation with and motivated actions toward drug-taking (25). While drug cues are often associated with exaggerated INS, ACC, and PFC responses (27), decision-making involving non-drug stimuli reflects attenuation in these regions as a function of addiction (28–30). With respect to recovery from drug addiction, however, it is still unclear how brain mechanisms implicated in *Preoccupation/Anticipation* and *Negative Reinforcement* stages change as a function of detoxification, early abstinence (e.g., 1–3 months sober), and prolonged abstinence (e.g., greater than 1 year sober), particularly within the same individuals over time, and whether brain changes parallel reductions in wanting to use drugs. As we review neuroimaging studies below, whenever possible we couch findings within the context of participant abstinence duration to develop predictions for what functions might improve with sobriety.

Taken together, neuroimaging studies provide compelling evidence that striatal, frontocingulate, AMG, and/or INS structure, function, and/or connections are disrupted in OUD. What do these disruptions mean with respect to specific impairments in OUD? Research findings indicate that the meaning of INS dysfunction depends on the particular location that is affected. Anterior INS, connected to IFG and dorsal striatum, is implicated in awareness of bodily feeling states as well as the learning and implementation of goal-directed actions that can be conceptually linked to cognitive control processes, whereas ventral INS is more strongly connected to AMG and VS and is thought to be involved in emotional salience and affective feeling states. In contrast, middle and posterior INS are connected with somatosensory regions (sensory and parietal cortices) associated with the processing of bodily feeling states, including pain signals (31, 32). Dorsolateral PFC is thought to work with ACC to regulate goal-directed behavior, wherein it is argued that dorsal ACC processes the value and difficulty of behavior change via its connections with dorsolateral

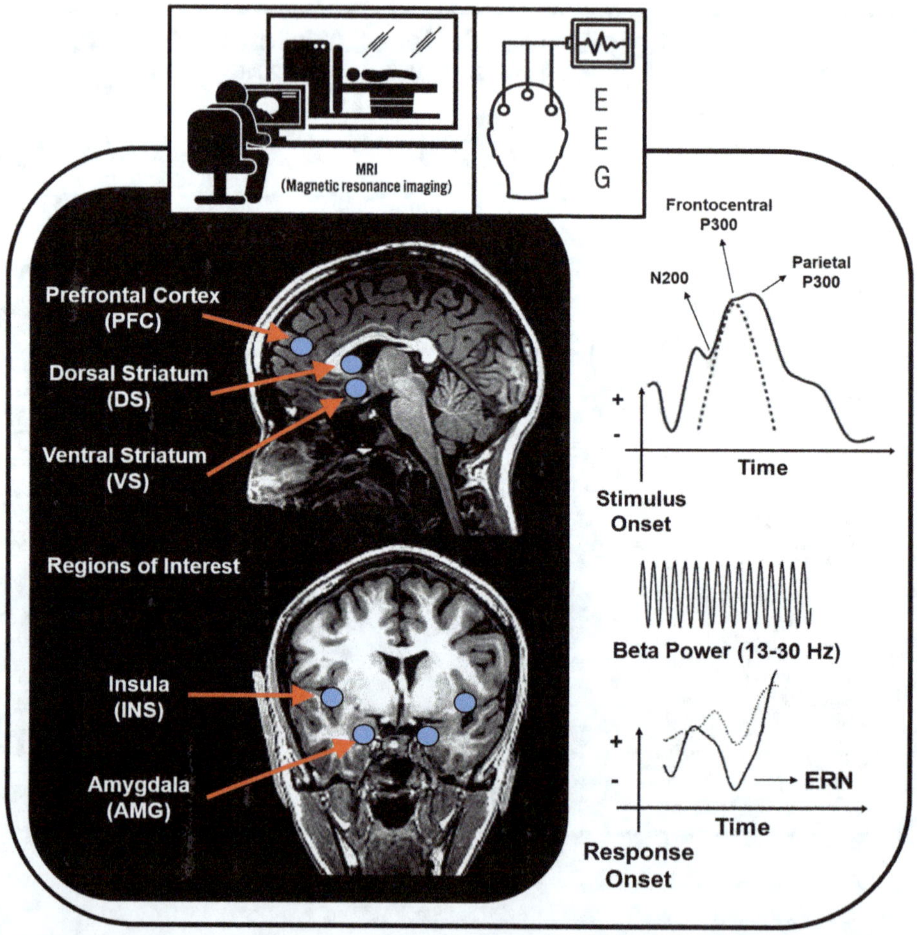

FIGURE 2 | Brain regions and processes that potentially map onto *Negative Reinforcement* and *Anticipation/Preoccupation* stages of the *Three-Stage Model of Addiction* (1, 15). EEG, electroencephalography; ERN, error related negativity.

PFC as well as AMG, dorsal striatum, and primary motor cortex (33). Within the context of stress, cognitive control functions in frontocingulate and anterior INS regions are argued to be hijacked by AMG connections. For example, although the dorsolateral PFC is thought to play an active role in pain suppression (34), within the context of aversive events, heightened AMG signals activate neurochemical stress reactions that serve to downregulate dorsolateral PFC in favor of salience-driven habitual, impulsive responses instantiated via dorsal striatum (35). Moreover, greater functional and structural links between basolateral AMG and anterior INS are associated with higher state and trait anxiety (36), instantiating aversive feeling states accompanying stress.

Deficits in the brain circuitry outlined above are present in conjunction with aberrant timing and allocation of neural resources to drug and non-drug related stimuli, consistent with the *Three-Stage Model of Addiction*. In the following sections, specific neuroimaging tools related to magnetic resonance imaging (MRI), functional near-infrared spectroscopy (fNIRs), electroencephalography (EEG), event related potentials (ERP), repetitive transcranial magnetic stimulation (rTMS) and deep brain stimulation (DBS) are briefly explained and cross-sectional and longitudinal OUD-relevant literature is summarized for each technique. **Figure 2** illustrates brain regions and processes of interest that are described in more detail below. Next, **Figures 3** and **4** summarize brain findings that appear to map onto *Negative Reinforcement* and *Anticipation/Preoccupation* stages. To compile research articles for this review, combinations of the following search terms were entered in Google Scholar: "opioid," "heroin," "MRI," "EEG," "rTMS," "fNIRs," "DBS," "ERP," "prescription opiate," "methadone," "naltrexone," "therapy," "abstinence," "relapse," "resting state fMRI," and "buprenorphine."

Structural MRI (sMRI)

With its high spatial resolution (typically in order of 1 mm^3), sMRI offers ways to differentiate different brain tissues, such as gray and white matter, and to quantify gray and white matter volume within various brain regions. Gray matter consists of cell bodies, dendrites, unmyelinated axons, and synapses that facilitate specialized information processing in cortical and subcortical regions, whereas white matter consists of myelinated axons that relay signals from one brain region to another. Studies employing sMRI demonstrate that OUD is characterized

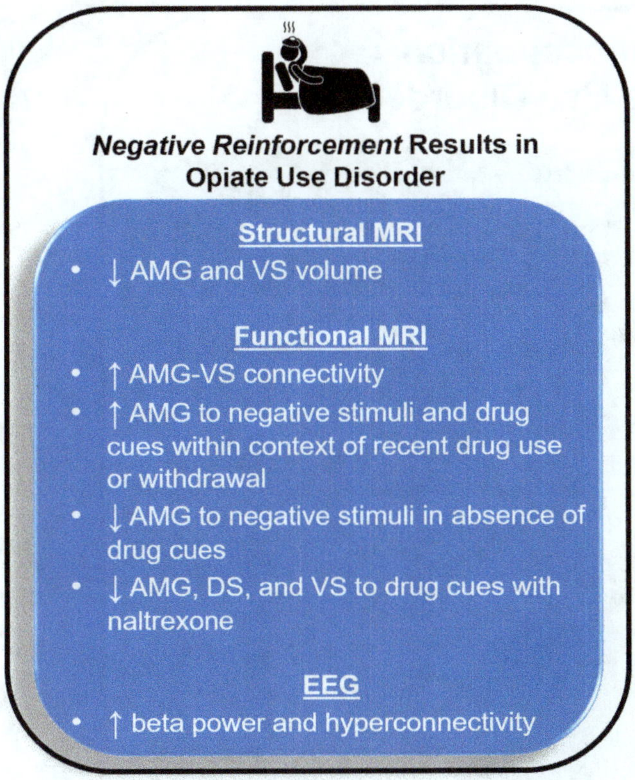

FIGURE 3 | Magnetic resonance imaging (MRI) and electroencephalography (EEG) results for opioid use disorder that may map onto the *Negative Reinforcement* stage of the *Three-Stage Model of Addiction* (1, 15). AMG, amygdala; VS, ventral striatum; DS, dorsal striatum.

by attenuated gray matter volume and white matter integrity in/surrounding striatum, frontocingulate regions (including IFG), AMG, and INS, with higher opioid use chronicity, use recency, and depression symptoms linked to greater reductions in specific regions (37–41). For instance, greater opioid use chronicity is associated with lower frontocingulate and/or INS cortical thickness in active as well as abstinent OUD users (37, 42, 43) in addition to decreased VS gray matter volume (44). Moreover, within individuals on opioid maintenance treatment for OUD, lower VS volume is associated with higher depression symptoms, whereas lower AMG volume is linked to greater daily opioid dose (40). Gray matter reductions within orbito-medial prefrontal cortex and bilateral globus pallidus are also associated with increased cognitive impulsivity among individuals on opioid maintenance treatment (45). With respect to abstinence, higher compulsive behavior reported by sober individuals with OUD is linked to lower white matter surrounding VS and rostral ACC when compared to that of active OUD users and healthy controls (44). In summary, brain regions implicated in *Binge/Intoxication* (VS), *Negative Reinforcement* (AMG), and *Preoccupation/Anticipation* stages (PFC, ACC, and INS) show structural attenuations, ostensibly contributing to various information processing impairments that may have a stronger impact when users are attempting to resist using opioids. For instance, VS attenuation may reflect the capacity for heightened drug tolerance and reduced euphoric effects of drug consumption. Additionally, PFC, ACC, and anterior INS volume reductions could manifest in impairments in adaptive goal-directed behavior, whereas diminished AMG structure might manifest in dysregulated stress and salience signaling in the presence/absence of drugs.

Functional MRI (fMRI)

fMRI offers good spatial resolution (typically in order of a few mm^3) to detect and measure temporal changes in blood flow, volume, and blood oxygenation (e.g., blood oxygenation level dependent, or BOLD contrast) while individuals are resting or performing various tasks. Active neurons in the brain require oxygenated blood to replenish energy; BOLD fMRI is affected by the differences in magnetic susceptibility between deoxygenated and oxygenated blood, and by local increases in blood flow and volume, signaling brain regions that are more active during one particular condition, stimulus, response, or timeframe vs. another. Researchers often quantify brain changes by computing the percent signal change between an active condition and a baseline condition. It is argued that the characterization of spontaneous (or intrinsic) brain signals during a resting state (e.g., without any particular task involved) are just as worthy of study as brain signals evoked by a particular stimulus and/or response because these spontaneous measurements reflect degree of energy consumption required to maintain default functioning in the absence of particular task demands (46, 47). Most fMRI research in OUD focuses on either drug-cue valuation processes compared to neutral cues and/or natural rewards (food, sex, social interactions, money), or decision-making in the absence of emotional, reward, or drug-related cues. Only a few studies have examined brain mechanisms involved in responses to negative stimuli, limiting interpretability.

Resting-State fMRI

Studies of spontaneous fMRI often focus on coherence (or connectivity) of signals across multiple spatially distinct cortical and subcortical brain regions. OUD is associated with weak frontocingulate functional connectivity with subcortical regions, but strong functional connectivity within subcortical regions such as striatum and AMG (48), findings consistent with a reward-control imbalance in OUD [stronger reward-stress connectivity paired with weaker cognitive control connectivity; (49)]. Multiple fMRI studies report weakened INS connectivity to IFG, striatum, and AMG, with those testing positive for opioids or reporting greater opioid use chronicity exhibiting the greatest dysfunction, findings in line with the *Preoccupation/Anticipation* stage (41, 49, 50). Finally, research indicates that individuals with OUD exhibit attenuated ACC activity and reduced connectivity with PFC and striatal regions; moreover, lower ACC signal within this context is linked to greater drug cue-induced craving (51, 52).

Task-Based fMRI: Cue Reactivity and Non-drug Rewards

OUD is marked by frontocingulate and striatal hyperactivation to drug cues, particularly within active users (up to a few hours sober), with degree of response decreasing as a function of longer

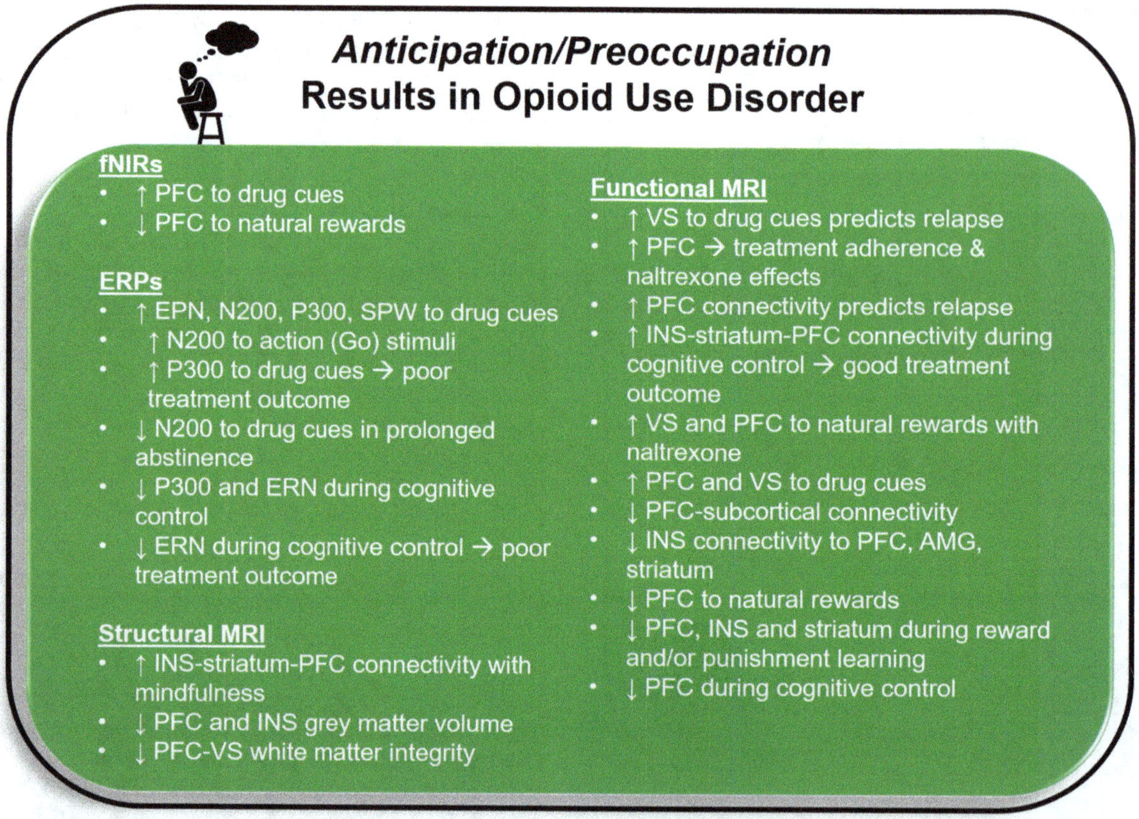

FIGURE 4 | Functional near-infrared spectroscopy (fNIRs), event related potential (ERP), and magnetic resonance imaging (MRI) results for opioid use disorder that may map onto the *Anticipation/Preoccupation* stage of the *Three-Stage Model of Addiction* (1, 15). PFC, prefrontal cortex, including anterior cingulate cortex; EPN, early positive negativity; SPW, slow positive wave; ERN, error related negativity; INS, insula; VS, ventral striatum; AMG, amygdala.

abstinence (i.e., 6–14 months as opposed to 1 month), findings consistent with the *Preoccupation/Anticipation* stage of addiction (53–62). Compared to non-substance using individuals, those with OUD show frontal attenuation to pleasant non-drug stimuli such as food, pornography, and interactive social situations (54, 63), although this pattern may dissipate as a function of abstinence [3 years; (54)]. With respect to reward sensitivity, users with OUD exhibit difficulty distinguishing between non-drug win and no-win outcomes in striatal brain regions (64); moreover, individuals with OUD show INS, ACC, and IFG attenuation during win/loss anticipation and feedback (65) in line with the *Preoccupation/Anticipation* stage of addiction.

Task-Based fMRI: Cognitive Control

OUD is associated with frontocingulate hypoactivation during tasks requiring sustained attention, working memory, and/or cognitive/behavioral inhibition compatible with the *Anticipation/Preoccupation* stage of addiction, with fMRI studies reporting this pattern regardless of abstinence duration or presence of opioid-replacement treatment (66–69). One study demonstrates no difference in ACC activation between users with OUD on opioid replacement therapy (buprenorphine or methadone) and non-users during behavioral control. However, users do not show a positive correlation between ACC activation and behavioral performance as seen in non-users, indicating a notable discrepancy between brain signaling and behavior (70); these findings suggest that even when recruited, these regions may not function as effectively for OUD. Some evidence suggests that cognitive control functions involving IFG and ACC may improve as a function of prolonged abstinence in OUD, given that former opioid users abstinent for at least 6 months perform similarly to healthy individuals and/or better than users on opioid replacement therapy during cognitive control tasks. However, the literature is far from conclusive and mixed results may be due, in part, to variability in opiate use chronicity and recency across studies (39).

Task-Based fMRI: Aversive Stimuli

On the whole, very limited research suggests that OUD is characterized by blunted brain responses to negatively valenced stimuli as well as punishing outcomes in the absence of drug cues. Two fMRI studies report hypoactive AMG responses to negative and positive as opposed to neutral stimuli in OUD individuals who are abstinent 2–5 months (71) as well as current users with OUD; it is important to note that these results are based on samples with comorbid borderline personality disorder who are also on opioid replacement therapy (72). Thus, findings may not easily generalize to other OUD samples. These reports of blunted AMG signals are the opposite of what would be predicted by the *Negative Reinforcement* stage, which suggests that AMG responses should be intensified as a function of aversive cues. In contrast, two fMRI studies demonstrate that drug cues evoke AMG hyperactivation in individuals with OUD who are expecting to consume opioids or have recently withdrawn from opioids, potentially reflecting exaggerated salience associated with drug cues and/or bodily signals that in the past have signaled opioid withdrawal. More specifically, when active OUD users are administered saline as opposed to opioids, they display greater AMG activation than healthy individuals to fearful faces, a pattern that is linked to elevated state anxiety (73). Similarly, newly detoxified individuals with OUD exhibit hyperactive AMG responses to drug as opposed to neutral films, a pattern correlated with heightened craving (74). Furthermore, OUD patients on methadone replacement exhibit greater INS and AMG activation to opioid cues before as opposed to after ingestion of their daily methadone dose (75). Drug cues in abstinent individuals with OUD also appear to act as salient stimuli, linked to heightened anxiety, other negative emotions, and physiological blood pressure/heart rate increases (76). On the whole, these findings are accordant with the *Negative Reinforcement* stage.

Non-imaging data indicate that active OUD is associated with exaggerated self-reported arousal to negative non-drug images (77), suggesting that additional brain-behavior research is needed to determine whether patterns of AMG response to emotional stimuli change as a function of abstinence. Greater negative affect induced by film clips still increases drug craving in OUD users without the presence of drug cues, congruent with the *Negative Reinforcement* stage of addiction; furthermore, this relationship is stronger for users with high as opposed to low anxiety sensitivity (78). Moderation by anxiety sensitivity points to the importance of measuring individual differences in users' perceptions and awareness of bodily sensations, as these may intensify stress responses that hijack abstinence efforts.

Lastly, OUD is linked to difficulty differentiating punishing vs. non-punishing feedback within striatum (64). Behavioral studies indicate that individuals with active and/or former OUD show difficulties avoiding punishment (79–81) and demonstrate heightened risk-taking following punishment (82). This pattern of impaired decision-making in the face of punishment may be more relevant to the *Preoccupation/Anticipation* than the *Negative Reinforcement* stage, as a meta-analysis implicates INS in the implementation of punishment-related prediction errors and ACC and PFC regions in reinforcement-based decision making more generally (83).

Functional Near-Infrared Spectroscopy (fNIRs)

The fNIRs technology employs near-infrared light attenuation to quantify concentration of oxy- and deoxy-hemoglobin. fNIRs can differentiate skin, skull, and cortical surface tissue, and produce a BOLD contrast similar to fMRI, however without the ability to measure whole brain responses. Studies using this technology indicate that OUD patients recently detoxified from opioids show: (1) greater right dorsolateral PFC activation to opioid cues than individuals with OUD abstinent for at least 2 months (84); and (2) higher anhedonia symptoms paired with lower rostral and/or ventrolateral PFC to appetitive food and positive social interactions than healthy individuals (63). These results point to greater attentional resources being devoted to drug cues than other types of rewards, consistent with the *Preoccupation/Anticipation* stage of addiction.

Electroencephalography (EEG)

EEG Time and Frequency Domains

EEG, the continuous recording of ongoing brain electrical activity via scalp electrodes, possesses high temporal resolution (order of milliseconds) (85). Resting state EEG recordings measure the brain's pseudo-periodic oscillatory activity due to coherent activity from many neurons synchronized in time and space. For EEG signal frequency analyses, a Fast Fourier Transform (FFT) technique decomposes the EEG time series into a frequency spectrum by voltage (a measure of signal magnitude, or amplitude) matrix; this information can then be segmented as a function of specific frequency "bands" that are associated with various mental processes. Frequencies most studied in OUD samples include those segmented within theta, alpha, beta, and gamma bands. Theta band (4–7 Hz) activity is implicated in cognitive control processes including working memory and error monitoring (86–88). Decreases in alpha band (8–13 Hz) activity are associated with increases in active information processing involving attention (89), whereas beta band (13–30 Hz) decreases signal an impending voluntary motor action (90). Finally, gamma band (30–100 Hz) activity is theorized to reflect the comparison of a stimulus with information held in memory to determine a match or mismatch (91). EEG power (the square of the EEG magnitude of the signal amplitude within a particular band) is often calculated to compare between clinical groups or conditions. In addition, EEG coherence metrics are calculated to reflect how strongly oscillations between two or more measuring electrodes reflecting and mapping into synchronized brain regions activities within a particular frequency band.

Although EEG frequencies can be measured within the context of a particular task, resting-state EEG studies investigating frequency band differences as a function of OUD are the norm. On the whole, this literature indicates that EEG power and coherence are disrupted in chronic OUD users compared to healthy individuals, although findings are inconsistent as to directionality (which group is higher or lower) as well as which frequency band, hemisphere, or specific brain region is affected and whether these patterns normalize as a function of abstinence or methadone maintenance (92, 93). However, EEG frequency studies of OUD are atheoretical with respect to how findings map onto stages of addiction or cognitive/emotional functioning, and low spatial resolution of most EEG recording montages limit spatial (brain) localization of frequency signals within OUD samples.

The most consistent finding is that individuals with OUD (whether actively using, maintained on methadone for at least 6 months, or in the early stages of abstinence) exhibit greater beta power than healthy individuals [91–93). With respect to longer abstinence duration, one study reports no difference in beta power between healthy controls and OUD users abstinent 1–6 months, whereas another study indicates that beta power decreases as a function of longer OUD abstinence (94). As beta power increases are thought to reflect decreased need for future motor actions, these results suggest that active opioid users can be characterized by reduced behavioral activation, at least during intrinsic processing. Additional research probing beta power changes during reward and stress states in opioid users may contribute to our understanding of *Binge/Intoxication*, *Negative Reinforcement*, and *Preoccupation/Anticipation* stages within the context of OUD. Perhaps beta power changes as a function of prolonged abstinence can track stages of recovery, although longitudinal studies are warranted to test this hypothesis.

In contrast to beta band results, findings for the alpha band are somewhat mixed, with: (1) active OUD users exhibiting either higher (93) or lower (95) power than healthy comparison subjects; (2) OUD users maintained on methadone for 6+ months displaying lower (96) or higher (93) power than non-users; and (3) abstinent OUD users showing similar levels of power as healthy individuals (97) or increasing alpha power as a function of sobriety duration (94). For theta band activity, active OUD users either exhibit lower (95) or higher (93) power than healthy individuals. However, OUD users abstinent 1–6 months display similar theta power as control subjects (97), findings suggestive of a state-like change in theta power as a function of current drug use. Time frequency analysis of short duration EEG frequency band distribution (as opposed to averaging frequency bands across the entire length of EEG recording) indicate that active OUD users exhibit higher occurrence of alpha and beta rhythms but lower occurrence of theta rhythms than comparison subjects; moreover, OUD users show greater occurrence of these rhythms in the right than the left hemisphere (98); these findings could be consistent with fMRI data suggesting weakened right frontal processing in OUD that could reflect inhibitory impairments associated with faulty IFG/ACC signaling, consistent with the *Preoccupation/Anticipation* stage of addiction.

With regard to EEG coherence within and across regions of the brain, active OUD exhibit local hyperconnectivity in alpha and beta frequency bands, a pattern that does not change as a function of early (2-week) abstinence. However, remote alpha and beta hypoconnectivity evident in active OUD users does appear to normalize during the early stages of sobriety (99, 100). Finally, gamma band findings indicate that active OUD as well as OUD on prolonged methadone treatment display greater gamma power than healthy individuals (50), and OUD abstinent at least 2 weeks exhibit greater fronto-occipital gamma band coherence within the left hemisphere than CTL, although the significance of this greater coherence is not well-understood (101).

EEG Event Related Potentials (ERPs)

ERPs are averaged periods of EEG recordings interpreted within the time domain that are elicited by a particular stimulus or a response. ERPs allow researchers to understand the onset and/or duration of perceptual, attentive, and other cognitive and emotional processes (85). Unlike fMRI studies suggesting that faulty cognitive control circuitry may normalize as a function of OUD abstinence, ERP studies provide mixed results, suggesting that this may not be the case (95, 102–110), although greater opioid use chronicity does appear to be associated with greater frontocingulate reductions (103). Temporal resolution differences between ERPs (milliseconds) and fMRI (seconds) suggest that aspects of early stimulus evaluation (measured by multiple ERP amplitude/latency components) are still disrupted in OUD at various stages of abstinence accordant with the Preoccupation/Anticipation stage of addiction.

ERP components

Details regarding timing and proposed function of various ERP components, including early posterior negativity (EPN), N200, P300, slow positive wave (SPW) and error related negativity (ERN), are provided below within the context of various paradigms, including cognitive control, cue reactivity, working memory, attention and emotion tasks.

EPN

The EPN is a positive ERP deflection occurring 200 ms post-stimulus, thought to reflect and associate with early perceptual processing in temporal/occipital brain regions (111). During an emotional Stroop task involving positive, negative, neutral, and opioid images, OUD users abstinent an average of 9 months show larger EPN amplitude to opioid images than healthy participants in the absence of behavioral differences between groups (109). These results indicate that even with prolonged sobriety, perception of drug cues is prioritized.

N200

N200 is a negative ERP deflection occurring 200–350 ms after a stimulus, thought to reflect and associate with conflict monitoring processes (112, 113). During a go/nogo task, individuals with OUD (abstinent for 4 months) show larger frontocentral N200 amplitudes to go (action) trials than healthy controls, but groups do not differ on N200 amplitudes to nogo (inhibition) trials (110); findings imply that neural resources are overly devoted to action tendencies, perhaps related to impulsivity. In contrast, however, former OUD and cocaine users display no N200 differences from non-users during response inhibition tasks involving neutral and emotional stimuli (114). OUD users abstinent at least 1 month show greater N200 amplitude to opioid images during a dot probe task than controls (115), in contrast, OUD users abstinent 8–24 months exhibit smaller N200 to opioid images than healthy subjects (108). These results suggest that addicted individuals experience inhibitory difficulties in the presence of drug cues as represented by the *Preoccupation/Anticipation* stage of addiction that may change as a function of prolonged recovery.

P300

P300 is a positive ERP deflection occurring 300–600 ms after a stimulus thought to reflect and associate with attention allocation, motivational salience, and/or updating of short-term memory, depending on the paradigm used (85). Among current OUD, findings point to exaggerated salience of opioid cues at the expense of other stimuli, accordant with the *Preoccupation/Anticipation* stage of addiction. Chronic users with OUD display smaller P300 amplitude and longer P300 latency than healthy individuals during digit span and auditory oddball tasks, but larger P300 amplitude to opioid images during a cue reactivity task (95). P300 responsivity has also been examined among substance users with varying lengths of remission. For example, substance users in residential treatment with a history of addiction (cocaine use disorder with/without alcohol use disorder and OUD) exhibit lower P300 amplitude across the entire cortex than healthy individuals to targets during a visual continuous performance test; furthermore, across the three user groups, shorter abstinence is associated with smaller P300 amplitude (102). Similarly, individuals with OUD who are recently detoxified or on opioid replacement therapy exhibit greater P300 amplitude to opioid images than positive, negative, or neutral images, with larger opioid-related P300 amplitude linked to greater self-reported craving; however, OUD subjects do not differ in P300 amplitude from healthy individuals across conditions (116). Moreover, OUD users abstinent for at least 6 months show smaller P300 amplitudes during a working memory task than healthy individuals and current OUD users in frontal regions (105, 106). However, OUD users, their first-degree relatives, and healthy controls do not differ in P300 amplitude to auditory oddball targets (107). Overall, findings among recently abstinent and treatment-seeking individuals are inconsistent as to whether neural resources devoted to attention/salience of non-drug cues improve as a function of abstinence.

SPW

The SPW is a positive frontal ERP deflection that onsets at least 600 ms post-stimulus and lasts for several 100 ms, reflecting and associated with sensitivity to emotional valence as well as motivational salience (117, 118). OUD users abstinent for a minimum of 2 weeks show greater SPW amplitude to opioid than neutral images, whereas healthy individuals show no difference between opioid and neutral pictures; moreover, within users, greater central SPW amplitudes are associated with heightened arousal to opioid cues (101). These results are in line with SPN and P300 findings for opioid cues, indicating heightened resources devoted to drug cues in active or early-abstinent users with OUD.

ERN

The ERN is a negative ERP deflection occurring approximately 50 ms after an individual makes an error; the ERN is localized to anterior cingulate cortex and thought to reflect and associate with error monitoring processes (119). During an Eriksen flanker task, individuals with OUD exhibit faster reaction time to correct and incorrect trials than healthy controls, paired with smaller ERN amplitudes and faster latencies in frontocentral regions, suggestive of impairments related to impulsivity (103).

Repetitive Transcranial Magnetic Stimulation (rTMS)

rTMS utilizes a handheld coil placed against the scalp, transmitting transient electric current to produce a changing magnetic field. This magnetic field can painlessly penetrate the skull and deliver a magnetic pulse to stimulate nerve cells in the brain. The TMS coil can be positioned to selectively target a region of the brain and excite or inhibit cortical neurons. rTMS studies are more common among other substance use disorders including alcohol, nicotine, and stimulants. However, one study employed rTMS within a sample of 20 men with OUD. This randomized, sham-controlled crossover study demonstrated that active but not sham 10 Hz rTMS over left dorsolateral PFC reduced craving induced by viewing videos of opioid use. Continued rTMS treatment for an additional 4 days further reduced cue-induced craving (120). These results are consistent with the *Preoccupation/Anticipation* stage of addiction wherein overactivation of frontal regions in response to cue-elicited craving drives preoccupation with drug-taking, suggesting that targeted rTMS stimulation of frontal regions may be a potential avenue for recovery in OUD.

Deep Brain Stimulation (DBS)

In contrast to non-invasive rTMS, DBS is a invasive neuromodulation procedure administered via electrodes surgically implanted in subcortical brain areas. High frequency electrical stimulation is delivered to inhibit neural activity in targeted regions of the brain (121). DBS is used to treat movement disorders such as Parkinson's disease, and double-blind control trials show promise for its use in the treatment of refractory depression and obsessive compulsive disorder (122). Recently, DBS has been explored as an experimental treatment for patients with refractory substance use disorders, including OUD.

Among patients with OUD, DBS has been used to modulate activity in reward-network regions such as nucleus accumbens. Thus far, findings suggest that DBS is associated with partial to full remission and few side effects. For instance, within a small sample of chronic, treatment-resistant opioid users, DBS of the anterior limb of the internal capsule and nucleus accumbens resulted in prolonged sobriety greater than 2 years paired with reduced drug craving (123). Positron emission tomography scans also revealed increased glucose metabolism within bilateral IFG from pre- to post-DBS within these patients. Similarly, a case report demonstrated that an individual with a 5-year opioid use history underwent rapid detoxification and received DBS to bilateral nucleus accumbens for over 2 years. He subsequently maintained complete abstinence for the 6-year follow-up period after the electrode implantation surgery (121). Similarly, nucleus accumbens DBS in two chronic OUD patients resulted in decreased depression and anxiety paired with prolonged abstinence from opioids (124). However, an alternative case report of nucleus accumbens DBS stimulation in a man with 17 years of opioid use was unsuccessful in alleviating cravings 2 months post-DBS initiation. He relapsed eight times within the following 2 months and eventually overdosed within 5 months of DBS onset (122).

Abstinence following DBS treatment targeting reward-network regions is consistent with the *Binge/Intoxication* stage of addiction. DBS may reduce the reward response to drug use thereby interrupting the cycle that typically results in increased dopamine release and future drug use. While initial binge/intoxication may lead to incentive sensitization by weakening the brain's response to natural rewards in favor of drug rewards, use of DBS may interrupt the reward response, thereby reversing this process and allowing the brain to return to its initial preference for natural rewards (123, 125).

Longitudinal Studies of Relapse and Treatment Outcome

Extant longitudinal neuroimaging studies of OUD combine imaging data with treatment to examine changes with treatment or baseline neural predictors of response. This research primarily concentrates on brain responses to drug cues, which within the context of abstinent individuals can be construed as appetitive and/or aversive. ERP results indicate that larger P300 amplitudes to opioid than pleasant images predicts greater opioid use frequency 6 months later (126), whereas lower frontal P300 amplitudes to non-drug distractors (127) and smaller ERN amplitudes during cognitive control (128) predict future treatment discontinuation. These findings point to executive function deficits within the *Preoccupation/Anticipation* stage that discount goals other than drug-seeking. Studies of fMRI prediction show that greater VS response (paired with higher self-reported craving) to opioid cues predicts relapse within 3 months (129), whereas higher medial PFC activation to opioid cues at baseline predicts more successful naloxone adherence (93) Additionally, functional connectivity fMRI studies demonstrate that although higher resting-state connectivity between ACC and medial PFC predicts relapse within 3 months (130), greater functional connectivity between INS, striatum, and ACC during a go/nogo task predicts successful 12-week substance use treatment (131). On the whole, these findings indicate that heightened salience of drug cues (particularly in striatal and frontal regions) forecasts difficulty maintaining sobriety, data congruent with the *Preoccupation/Anticipation* stage. Divergent task conditions across studies (cognitive control, resting-state, cue reactivity) may account for inconsistent findings; it would be helpful for future research to assess patterns of brain function across multiple paradigms to determine whether exaggerated or attenuated regions reflect global or context-dependent predictions.

Neuroimaging studies of OUD recorded at multiple timepoints demonstrate that naltrexone treatment: (1) decreases AMG and dorsal striatum signals while increasing medial PFC responses to opioid cues (132); (2) reduces VS and orbitofrontal responses to opioid cues as well as self- and clinician-reported withdrawal symptoms (133); and (3) increases VS activation to natural rewards (pictures of cute infants) (134). In contrast, a recent study shows that methadone maintenance treatment (>3 months) does not change frontocingulate mechanisms implicated in cognitive control during go/nogo task performance (135). These results convey that naltrexone shows promise in reducing appetitive (and perhaps aversive) salience of drug-related stimuli related to *Preoccupation/Anticipation* and *Negative Reinforcement* stages of addiction. Additional studies are warranted to replicate and extend these findings beyond naltrexone to buprenorphine and various therapy interventions. With respect to sMRI findings, OUD users completing 4 weeks of mindfulness-based treatment display improved striatum-INS and frontocingulate structural network strength than OUD users who received treatment as usual (136).

Limitations and Gaps in Knowledge

Several gaps in the neuroimaging literature preclude development of accurate targets to identify and track treatment in OUD. First, inconsistent results are reported cross-sectionally for individuals with former OUD at various stages of recovery (from weeks to months) who also show wide variability in opioid use chronicity. Although testing interactions between drug use recency and chronicity may clarify inconsistent findings, this analysis has rarely been attempted (39). Longitudinal within-subjects designs provide increased statistical power to detect dynamic brain signal changes as a function of prolonged abstinence within each individual; however, few longitudinal neuroimaging studies tracking both brain and behavior change within OUD individuals exist, particularly accounting for both opioid use chronicity and recency. In addition, longitudinal designs can track changes in psychological symptoms related to negative mood states (e.g., depression and anxiety) that in conjunction with brain changes may distinguish OUD who relapse vs. those who are able to remain abstinent. Second, small sample sizes limit statistical power to detect potentially meaningful differences as a function of OUD status, and the majority of OUD studies are comprised of male participants [e.g., (50, 55, 57, 72, 74, 95, 101, 103, 107–109, 126)], limiting generalizability. Although more men use opioids than women, heroin use is increasing at a faster rate and prescription opioid use is decreasing at a slower rate among women than men, contributing significantly to the OUD crisis (137). In addition, research suggests that stress predicts opioid use in women but not men, pointing to the idea that *Negative Reinforcement* processes may be more crucial to target in women's recovery programs (138). Third, only a few OUD studies integrate neuroimaging methods with high temporal (EEG, ERPs) and spatial (sMRI, fMRI) resolution, limiting conclusions that can be drawn regarding precisely when and where brain processes change with abstinence. Longitudinal multimodal (EEG/ERP paired with sMRI, fMRI, and/or fNIRs) neuroimaging studies of OUD recovery are warranted to map temporal and spatial brain changes as a function of early vs. late stages of opiate abstinence and treatment outcome, while mapping changes in individual differences in psychological symptoms [e.g., depression and anxiety; (12, 13)] and co-use of other substances (e.g., alcohol, nicotine) (139). Lastly, despite the fact that processing during the *Negative Reinforcement* stage of addiction is theorized to drive users to relapse (140), few neuroimaging studies of OUD have evaluated how aversive or stressful stimuli, alone or in conjunction with opioid cues, transform brain circuitry to hijack intended abstinence efforts and drive relentless capitulation to drug use despite increasingly dire consequences. The following sections highlight two promising avenues of research that can evaluate aversive sensitization in individuals with OUD.

Operant Conditioning and Interoception

Interoception, the perception and awareness of bodily signals, is thought to be dysregulated as a function of addiction, contributing to drug craving and urges (26, 141–144), but only two studies have examined interoceptive processing in OUD, demonstrating impaired interoceptive awareness as measured by heartbeat tracking accuracy (145), and greater stress-related physiological arousal and craving in response to paired pain-opioid stimuli as a function of pain-driven opioid misuse (146). However, no neuroimaging studies have probed the integrity of brain circuitry implicated in aversive interoceptive processing in OUD. Work by our research team demonstrates that, within the context of an aversive interoceptive manipulation (inspiratory breathing load), stimulant use disorder is characterized by exaggerated trait anxiety paired with attenuated striatum, INS, IFG, and ACC responses during decision-making (147–149). These findings point to increased arousal mismatched with blunted processing of bodily signals in the absence of drug-related stimuli, a pattern that could translate into impaired awareness of or attention to negative consequences during real-world decision-making consistent with the *Preoccupation/Anticipation* and *Negative Reinforcement* stages of addiction. Future studies could attempt to replicate this brain-based pattern of blunted aversive interoceptive processing in OUD and then extend this work by pairing aversive interoception with the presence vs. absence of drug cues to test the role of opioids in aversive sensitization.

Classical Conditioning and Extinction

Fear conditioning is a process where individuals learn which cues are associated with aversive outcomes (shocks, sounds, odors). With repetitive cue-outcome pairings, the cue alone can trigger the same response as the aversive outcome (conditioned fear). A recent meta-analysis demonstrates that fear-conditioned cues consistently elicit greater INS, striatum, and frontocingulate responses than unconditioned cues (150). Heightened AMG signaling for fear-conditioned cues is present across several studies, but may vary across tasks as a function of stimulus duration, predictability, and presentation modality [e.g., (151–156)]. Exaggerated physiological arousal during fear conditioning is specifically associated with AMG-INS signaling and connectivity (157, 158). Fear extinction, in contrast to conditioning, is the process wherein individuals learn to dissociate cues from their previously paired aversive outcomes, involving INS and ACC across studies (159) as well as AMG, particularly within early extinction (153, 160, 161). No studies have examined whether brain mechanisms of classical conditioning and extinction are intact in OUD within the context of aversive stimuli, but given behavioral impairments in decision-making as a function of punishment in OUD (64, 79–82), it is possible that associative learning and unlearning involving negative stimuli is disrupted in opioid users. Future research could identify whether brain circuitry impairments to fear-conditioned and extinguished-stimuli characterizes OUD in the presence vs. absence of drug cues.

SUMMARY AND CONCLUSIONS

Delineating neuroimaging targets for recovery from OUD is a difficult task, given that the majority of studies investigating abstinence are cross-sectional, comprised of opiate users with heterogeneous patterns of use chronicity and recency that may complicate results. In particular, methadone maintained individuals with OUD show brain impairments that are more similar to active illicit opioid users than individuals abstinent from opioids altogether. However, longitudinal studies show some promise that other treatments (e.g., rTMS, DBS, and naltrexone) or prolonged abstinence can change brain signals implicated in *Negative Reinforcement* and *Preoccupation/Anticipation* to reduce salience of drug cues, which may attenuate craving and anguish driving individuals to resume opioid use. The pairing of cue-reactive stimuli with established paradigms targeting cognitive control (e.g., flanker, go/nogo, stop signal) and/or emotion regulation [cognitive reappraisal of negative stimuli; e.g., (162)] may be beneficial for tracking the degree of brain resources that continue to be captured by drug cues over the course of recovery. Many more longitudinal investigations, particularly with males and females and within the context of aversive or stress-related stimuli, are warranted to develop individual-difference prediction models of recovery in OUD.

AUTHOR CONTRIBUTIONS

JS wrote the first draft of the manuscript with AM's input and created the figures. AM, RA, and JB provided revisions to further manuscript drafts. AM formatted the manuscript for publication.

ACKNOWLEDGMENTS

The authors wish to thank The William K. Warren Foundation for financial support of this work.

REFERENCES

1. Koob GF, Volkow ND. Neurobiology of addiction: a neurocircuitry analysis. *Lancet Psychiatry.* (2016) 3:760–73. doi: 10.1016/S2215-0366(16)00104-8
2. Florence C, Luo F, Xu L, Zhou C. The economic burden of prescription opioid overdose, abuse and dependence in the United States, 2013. *Med Care.* (2016) 54:901–6. doi: 10.1097/MLR.0000000000000625
3. Gomes T, Tadrous M, Mamdani MM, Paterson JM, Juurlink DN. The Burden of opioid-related mortality in the United States. *JAMA Network Open.* (2018) 1:e180217. doi: 10.1001/jamanetworkopen.2018.0217
4. Hagemeier NE. Introduction to the opioid epidemic: the economic burden on the healthcare system and impact on quality of life. *Am J Manag Care.* (2018) 24:S200–6.
5. Oquendo MA, Volkow ND. Suicide: a silent contributor to opioid-overdose deaths. *N Engl J Med.* (2018) 378:1567–9. doi: 10.1056/NEJMp1801417
6. Garfield JB, Cotton SM, Allen NB, Cheetham A, Kras M, Yücel M, et al. Evidence that anhedonia is a symptom of opioid dependence associated with recent use. *Drug Alcohol Depend.* (2017) 177:29–38. doi: 10.1016/j.drugalcdep.2017.03.012
7. Huhn AS, Harris J, Cleveland HH, Lydon DM, Stankoski D, Cleveland MJ, et al. Ecological momentary assessment of affect and craving in patients

in treatment for prescription opioid dependence. *Brain Res Bull.* (2016a) 123:94–101. doi: 10.1016/j.brainresbull.2016.01.012

8. Neale J, Pickering L, Nettleton S. *The Everyday Lives of Recovering Heroin Users*. London: Royal Society of Arts. (2012)
9. Nettleton S, Neale J, Pickering L. 'I don't think there's much of a rational mind in a drug addict when they are in the thick of it': towards an embodied analysis of recovering heroin users. *Sociol Health Illn.* (2011) 33:341–55. doi: 10.1111/j.1467-9566.2010.01278.x
10. Preston KL, Epstein DH. Stress in the daily lives of cocaine and heroin users: relationship to mood, craving, relapse triggers, and cocaine use. *Psychopharmacology.* (2011) 218:29–37. doi: 10.1007/s00213-011-2183-x
11. Koob GF, Le Moal M. Drug addiction, dysregulation of reward, and allostasis. *Neuropsychopharmacology.* (2001) 24:97–129. doi: 10.1016/S0893-133X(00)00195-0
12. Mars SG, Bourgois P, Karandinos G, Montero F, Ciccarone D. "Every 'never' I ever said came true": Transitions from opioid pills to heroin injecting. *Int J Drug Policy.* (2014) 25:257–66. doi: 10.1016/j.drugpo.2013.10.004
13. Schuckit MA. Treatment of opioid-use disorders. *N Engl J Med.* (2016) 375:357–68. doi: 10.1056/NEJMra1604339
14. Blum J, Gerber H, Gerhard U, Schmid O, Petitjean S, Riecher-Rössler A, et al. Acute effects of heroin on emotions in heroin-dependent patients. *Am J Addict.* (2013) 22, 598–604. doi: 10.1111/j.1521-0391.2013.12025.x
15. Volkow ND, Koob GF, McLellan AT. Neurobiologic advances from the brain disease model of addiction. *N Engl J Med.* (2016) 374:363–71. doi: 10.1056/NEJMra1511480
16. Koob GF. Negative reinforcement in drug addiction: the darkness within. *Curr Opin Neurobiol.* (2013) 23:559–63. doi: 10.1016/j.conb.2013.03.011
17. Everitt BJ, Robbins TW. Neural systems of reinforcement for drug addiction: from actions to habits to compulsion. *Nat Neurosci.* (2005) 8:1481–9. doi: 10.1038/nn1579
18. Robinson TE, Berridge KC. The neural basis of drug craving: an incentive-sensitization theory of addiction. *Brain Res Rev.* (1993) 18:247–91. doi: 10.1016/0165-0173(93)90013-P
19. Robinson TE, Berridge KC. The psychology and neurobiology of addiction: an incentive–sensitization view. *Addiction.* (2000) 95:91–117. doi: 10.1046/j.1360-0443.95.8s2.19.x
20. Berridge KC, Robinson TE. Liking, wanting, and the incentive-sensitization theory of addiction. *Am Psychol.* (2016) 71:670–9. doi: 10.1037/amp0000059
21. Kwako LE, Koob GF. Neuroclinical framework for the role of stress in addiction. *Chronic Stress.* (2017) 1:1–14. doi: 10.1177/2470547017698140
22. Aston-Jones G, Delfs JM, Druhan J, Zhu Y. The bed nucleus of the stria terminalis: a target site for noradrenergic actions in opiate withdrawal. *Ann N Y Acad Sci.* (1999) 877:486–98. doi: 10.1111/j.1749-6632.1999.tb09284.x
23. Koob GF, Buck CL, Cohen A, Edwards S, Park PE, Schlosburg JE, et al. Addiction as a stress surfeit disorder. *Neuropharmacology.* (2014) 76:370–82. doi: 10.1016/j.neuropharm.2013.05.024
24. Garavan H. Insula and drug cravings. *Brain Struct Funct.* (2010) 214:593–601. doi: 10.1007/s00429-010-0259-8
25. George O, Koob GF. Individual differences in the neuropsychopathology of addiction. *Dialog Clin Neurosci.* (2017) 19:217–29.
26. Naqvi NH, Bechara A. The INS and drug addiction: an interoceptive view of pleasure, urges, and decision-making. *Brain Struct Funct.* (2010) 214:435–50. doi: 10.1007/s00429-010-0268-7
27. Jasinska AJ, Stein EA, Kaiser J, Naumer MJ, Yalachkov Y. Factors modulating neural reactivity to drug cues in addiction: a survey of human neuroimaging studies. *Neurosci Biobehav Rev.* (2014) 38:1–16. doi: 10.1016/j.neubiorev.2013.10.013
28. Droutman V, Read SJ, Bechara A. Revisiting the role of the insula in addiction. *Trends Cogn Sci.* (2015) 19:414–20. doi: 10.1016/j.tics.2015.05.005
29. Goldstein RZ, Volkow ND. Dysfunction of the prefrontal cortex in addiction: neuroimaging findings and clinical implications. *Nat Rev Neurosci.* (2011) 12:652–69. doi: 10.1038/nrn3119
30. Volkow ND, Wang GJ, Fowler JS, Tomasi D, Telang F. Addiction: beyond dopamine reward circuitry. *Proc Natl Acad Sci.* (2011) 108:15037–42. doi: 10.1073/pnas.1010654108
31. Nomi JS, Farrant K, Damaraju E, Rachakonda S, Calhoun VD, Uddin LQ. Dynamic functional network connectivity reveals unique and overlapping profiles of INS subdivisions. *Hum Brain Mapp.* (2016) 37:1770–87. doi: 10.1002/hbm.23135
32. Wager TD, Barrett LF. From affect to control: functional specialization of the insula in motivation and regulation. *bioRxiv*. (2017). doi: 10.1101/102368
33. Kolling N, Wittmann MK, Behrens TE, Boorman ED, Mars RB, Rushworth MF. Value, search, persistence and model updating in anterior cingulate cortex. *Nat Neurosci.* (2016) 19:1280–5. doi: 10.1038/nn.4382
34. Seminowicz DA, Moayedi M. The dorsolateral prefrontal cortex in acute and chronic pain. *J Pain.* (2017) 18:1027–35. doi: 10.1016/j.jpain.2017.03.008
35. Arnsten AF. Stress signalling pathways that impair prefrontal cortex structure and function. *Nat Rev Neurosci.* (2009) 10:410–22. doi: 10.1038/nrn2648
36. Baur V, Hänggi J, Langer N, Jäncke L. Resting-state functional and structural connectivity within an INS–amygdala route specifically index state and trait anxiety. *Biol Psychiatry.* (2013) 73:85–92. doi: 10.1016/j.biopsych.2012.06.003
37. Li M, Tian J, Zhang R, Qiu Y, Wen X, Ma X, et al. Abnormal cortical thickness in heroin-dependent individuals. *Neuroimage.* (2014) 88:295–307. doi: 10.1016/j.neuroimage.2013.10.021
38. Liu H, Hao Y, Kaneko Y, Ouyang X, Zhang Y, Xu L, et al. Frontal and cingulate gray matter volume reduction in heroin dependence: optimized voxel-based morphometry. *Psychiatry Clin Neurosci.* (2009) 63:563–8. doi: 10.1111/j.1440-1819.2009.01989.x
39. Schmidt A, Walter M, Borgwardt S. Impaired cognition control and inferior frontal cortex modulation in heroin addiction. In: Preedy VR, editor. *Neuropathology of Drug Addictions and Substance Misuse*. Cambridge, MA: Academic Press (2016), p. 1037–47.
40. Seifert CL, Magon S, Sprenger T, Lang UE, Huber CG, Denier N, et al. Reduced volume of the nucleus accumbens in heroin addiction. *Eur Arch Psychiatry Clin Neurosci.* (2015) 265:637–45. doi: 10.1007/s00406-014-0564-y
41. Upadhyay J, Maleki N, Potter J, Elman I, Rudrauf D, Knudsen J, et al. Alterations in brain structure and functional connectivity in prescription opioid-dependent patients. *Brain.* (2010) 133:2098–114. doi: 10.1093/brain/awq138
42. Yuan Y, Zhu Z, Shi J, Zou Z, Yuan F, Liu Y, et al. Gray matter density negatively correlates with duration of heroin use in young lifetime heroin-dependent individuals. *Brain Cogn.* (2009) 71:223–8. doi: 10.1016/j.bandc.2009.08.014
43. Yuan K, Qin W, Dong M, Liu J, Sun J, Liu P, et al. Gray matter deficits and resting-state abnormalities in abstinent heroin-dependent individuals. *Neurosci Lett.* (2010) 482:101–5. doi: 10.1016/j.neulet.2010.07.005
44. Tolomeo S, Matthews K, Steele D, Baldacchino A. Compulsivity in opioid dependence. *Prog Neuro-Psychopharmacol Biol Psychiatry.* (2018) 81:333–9. doi: 10.1016/j.pnpbp.2017.09.007
45. Tolomeo S, Gray S, Matthews K, Steele JD, Baldacchino A. Multifaceted impairments in impulsivity and brain structural abnormalities in opioid dependence and abstinence. *Psychol med.* (2016). 46:2841–2853. doi: 10.1017/S0033291716001513
46. Raichle ME. A paradigm shift in functional brain imaging. *J Neurosci.* (2009) 29:12729–34. doi: 10.1523/JNEUROSCI.4366-09.2009
47. Snyder AZ, Raichle ME. A brief history of the resting state: the Washington University perspective. *Neuroimage.* (2012) 62:902–10. doi: 10.1016/j.neuroimage.2012.01.044
48. Fareed A, Kim J, Ketchen B, Kwak WJ, Wang D, Shongo-Hiango H, et al. Effect of heroin use on changes of brain functions as measured by functional magnetic resonance imaging, a systematic review. *J Addict Dis.* (2017) 36:105–16. doi: 10.1080/10550887.2017.1280898
49. Xie C, Shao Y, Ma L, Zhai T, Ye E, Fu L, et al. Imbalanced functional link between valuation networks in abstinent heroin-dependent subjects. *Mol Psychiatry.* (2014) 19:10–2. doi: 10.1038/mp.2012.169
50. Wang PW, Lin HC, Liu GC, Yang YHC, Ko CH, Yen CF. Abnormal interhemispheric resting state functional connectivity of the INS in heroin users under methadone maintenance treatment. *Psychiatry Res Neuroimaging.* (2016) 255:9–14. doi: 10.1016/j.pscychresns.2016.07.009
51. Jiang GH, Qiu YW, Zhang XL, Han LJ, Lv XF, Li LM, et al. Amplitude low-frequency oscillation abnormalities in the heroin users: a resting state fMRI study. *Neuroimage.* (2011) 57:149–54. doi: 10.1016/j.neuroimage.2011.04.004
52. Liu J, Qin W, Yuan K, Li J, Wang W, Li Q, et al. Interaction between dysfunctional connectivity at rest and heroin cues-induced brain responses

in male abstinent heroin-dependent individuals. *PLoS ONE.* (2011) 6:e23098. doi: 10.1371/journal.pone.0023098

53. Hassani-Abharian P, Ganjgahi H, Tabatabaei-Jafari H, Oghabian MA, Mokri A, Ekhtiari H. Exploring neural correlates of different dimensions in drug craving self-reports among heroin dependents. *Basic Clin Neurosci.* (2015) 6:271–84.
54. Jiang YL, Tian W, Lu G, Rudd JA, Lai KF, Yeung LY, et al. Patterns of cortical activation following motor tasks and psychological-inducing movie cues in heroin users: an fMRI study. *Int J Psychiatry Med.* (2014) 47:25–40. doi: 10.2190/PM.47.1.c
55. Li Q, Wang Y, Zhang Y, Li W, Yang W, Zhu J, et al. Craving correlates with mesolimbic responses to heroin-related cues in short-term abstinence from heroin: an event-related fMRI study. *Brain Res.* (2012) 1469:63–72. doi: 10.1016/j.brainres.2012.06.024
56. Li Q, Wang Y, Zhang Y, Li W, Zhu J, Zheng Y, et al. Assessing cue-induced brain response as a function of abstinence duration in heroin-dependent individuals: an event-related fMRI study. *PLoS ONE.* (2013) 8:e62911. doi: 10.1371/journal.pone.0062911
57. Lou M, Wang E, Shen Y, Wang J. Cue-elicited craving in heroin addicts at different abstinent time: an fMRI pilot study. *Subst Use Misuse.* (2012) 47:631–9. doi: 10.3109/10826084.2011.646381
58. Tabatabaei-Jafari H, Ekhtiari H, Ganjgahi H, Hassani-Abharian P, Oghabian MA, Moradi A, et al. Patterns of brain activation during craving in heroin dependents successfully treated by methadone maintenance and abstinence-based treatments. *J Addict Med.* (2014) 8:123–9. doi: 10.1097/ADM.0000000000000022
59. Walter M, Denier N, Gerber H, Schmid O, Lanz C, Brenneisen R, et al. Orbitofrontal response to drug-related stimuli after heroin administration. *Addict Biol.* (2015) 20:570–9. doi: 10.1111/adb.12145
60. Wang W, Li Q, Wang Y, Tian J, Yang W, Li W, et al. Brain fMRI and craving response to heroin-related cues in patients on methadone maintenance treatment. *Am J Drug Alcohol Abuse.* (2011) 37:123–30. doi: 10.3109/00952990.2010.543997
61. Xiao Z, Lee T, Zhang JX, Wu Q, Wu R, Weng X, et al. Thirsty heroin addicts show different fMRI activations when exposed to water-related and drug-related cues. *Drug Alcohol Depend.* (2006) 83:157–62. doi: 10.1016/j.drugalcdep.2005.11.012
62. Yang Z, Xie J, Shao YC, Xie CM, Fu LP, Li DJ, et al. Dynamic neural responses to cue-reactivity paradigms in heroin-dependent users: An fMRI study. *Hum Brain Mapp.* (2009) 30:766–75. doi: 10.1002/hbm.20542
63. Huhn AS, Meyer RE, Harris JD, Ayaz H, Deneke E, Stankoski DM, et al. Evidence of anhedonia and differential reward processing in prefrontal cortex among post-withdrawal patients with prescription opiate dependence. *Brain Res Bull.* (2016b) 123:102–9. doi: 10.1016/j.brainresbull.2015.12.004
64. Gradin VB, Baldacchino A, Balfour D, Matthews K, Steele JD. Abnormal brain activity during a reward and loss task in opiate-dependent patients receiving methadone maintenance therapy. *Neuropsychopharmacology.* (2014) 39:885–94. doi: 10.1038/npp.2013.289
65. Zhao Q, Li H, Hu B, Wu H, Liu Q. Abstinent heroin addicts tend to take risks: ERP and source localization. *Front Neurosci.* (2017) 11:681. doi: 10.3389/fnins.2017.00681
66. Forman SD, Dougherty GG, Casey BJ, Siegle GJ, Braver TS, Barch DM, et al. Opiate addicts lack error-dependent activation of rostral anterior cingulate. *Biol Psychiatry.* (2004) 55:531–7. doi: 10.1016/j.biopsych.2003.09.011
67. Fu LP, Bi GH, Zou ZT, Wang Y, Ye EM, Ma L, et al. Impaired response inhibition function in abstinent heroin dependents: an fMRI study. *Neurosci Lett.* (2008) 438:322–6. doi: 10.1016/j.neulet.2008.04.033
68. Lee TM, Zhou WH, Luo XJ, Yuen KS, Ruan XZ, Weng XC. Neural activity associated with cognitive regulation in heroin users: a fMRI study. *Neurosci Lett.* (2005) 382:211–6. doi: 10.1016/j.neulet.2005.03.053
69. Schmidt A, Walter M, Gerber H, Schmid O, Smieskova R, Bendfeldt K, et al. Inferior frontal cortex modulation with an acute dose of heroin during cognitive control. *Neuropsychopharmacology.* (2013) 38:2231–9. doi: 10.1038/npp.2013.123
70. Yücel M, Lubman DI, Harrison BJ, Fornito A, Allen NB, Wellard RM, et al. A combined spectroscopic and functional MRI investigation of the dorsal anterior cingulate region in opiate addiction. *Mol Psychiatry.* (2007) 12:691–702. doi: 10.1038/sj.mp.4001955
71. Wang ZX, Zhang JX, Wu QL, Liu N, Hu XP, Chan RC, et al. Alterations in the processing of non-drug-related affective stimuli in abstinent heroin addicts. *Neuroimage.* (2010) 49:971–6. doi: 10.1016/j.neuroimage.2009.08.020
72. Smoski MJ, Salsman N, Wang L, Smith V, Lynch TR, Dager SR, et al. Functional imaging of emotion reactivity in opiate-dependent borderline personality disorder. *Person Disord Theory Res Treat.* (2011) 2:230–41. doi: 10.1037/a0022228
73. Schmidt A, Borgwardt S, Gerber H, Wiesbeck GA, Schmid O, Riecher-Rössler A, et al. Acute effects of heroin on negative emotional processing: relation of amygdala activity and stress-related responses. *Biol Psychiatry.* (2014) 76:289–96. doi: 10.1016/j.biopsych.2013.10.019
74. Murphy A, Lubman DI, McKie S, Bijral PS, Peters LA, Faiz Q, et al. Time-dependent neuronal changes associated with craving in opioid dependence: An fMRI study. *Addict Biol.* (2017) 23:1168–78. doi: 10.1111/adb.12554
75. Langleben DD, Ruparel K, Elman I, Busch-Winokur S, Pratiwadi R, Loughead J, et al. Acute effect of methadone maintenance dose on brain FMRI response to heroin-related cues. *Am J Psychiatry.* (2008) 165:390–4. doi: 10.1176/appi.ajp.2007.07010070
76. Yu J, Zhang S, Epstein DH, Fang Y, Shi J, Qin H, et al. Gender and stimulus difference in cue-induced responses in abstinent heroin users. *Pharmacol Biochem Behav.* (2007) 86:485–92. doi: 10.1016/j.pbb.2007.01.008
77. de Arcos FA, Verdejo-García A, Ceverino A, Montañez-Pareja M, López-Juárez E, Sánchez-Barrera M, et al. Dysregulation of emotional response in current and abstinent heroin users: negative heightening and positive blunting. *Psychopharmacology.* (2008) 198:159–66. doi: 10.1007/s00213-008-1110-2
78. Stathopoulou G, Pollack MH, Otto MW. Anxiety sensitivity moderates drug cravings in response to induced negative affect in opioid dependent outpatients. *Addict Behav.* (2018) 84:75–8. doi: 10.1016/j.addbeh.2018.03.020
79. Ahn WY, Vasilev G, Lee SH, Busemeyer JR, Kruschke JK, Bechara A, et al. Decision-making in stimulant and opiate addicts in protracted abstinence: evidence from computational modeling with pure users. *Front Psychol.* (2014) 5:849. doi: 10.3389/fpsyg.2014.00849
80. Hou Y, Zhao L, Yao Q, Ding L. Altered economic decision-making in abstinent heroin addicts: evidence from the ultimatum game. *Neurosci Lett.* (2016) 627:148–54. doi: 10.1016/j.neulet.2016.06.002
81. Myers CE, Rego J, Haber P, Morley K, Beck KD, Hogarth L, et al. Learning and generalization from reward and punishment in opioid addiction. *Behav Brain Res.* (2017) 317:122–31. doi: 10.1016/j.bbr.2016.09.033
82. Ersche KD, Roiser JP, Clark L, London M, Robbins TW, Sahakian BJ. Punishment induces risky decision-making in methadone-maintained opiate users but not in heroin users or healthy volunteers. *Neuropsychopharmacology.* (2005) 30:2115–24. doi: 10.1038/sj.npp.1300812
83. Garrison J, Erdeniz B, Done J. Prediction error in reinforcement learning: a meta-analysis of neuroimaging studies. *Neurosci Biobehav Rev.* (2013) 37:1297–310. doi: 10.1016/j.neubiorev.2013.03.023
84. Bunce SC, Harris JD, Bixler EO, Taylor M, Muelly E, Deneke E, et al. Possible evidence for re-regulation of HPA axis and brain reward systems over time in treatment in prescription opioid-dependent patients. *J Addict Med.* (2015) 9:53–60. doi: 10.1097/ADM.0000000000000087
85. Fabiani M, Gratton G, Coles M. Event-related brain potentials: methods, theory, and applications. In: JT Cacioppo, LG Tassinary, editors. *Handbook of Psychophysiology,* 2nd ed. Cambridge, UK: Cambridge University Press (2000). p. 53–84.
86. Sauseng P, Klimesch W, Schabus M, Doppelmayr M. Fronto-parietal EEG coherence in theta and upper alpha reflect central executive functions of working memory. *Int J Psychophysiol.* (2005) 57:97–103. doi: 10.1016/j.ijpsycho.2005.03.018
87. Sauseng P, Griesmayr B, Freunberger R, Klimesch W. Control mechanisms in working memory: a possible function of EEG theta oscillations. *Neurosci Biobehav Rev.* (2010) 34:1015–22. doi: 10.1016/j.neubiorev.2009.12.006
88. Trujillo LT, Allen JJ. Theta EEG dynamics of the error-related negativity. *Clin Neurophysiol.* (2007) 118:645–68. doi: 10.1016/j.clinph.2006.11.009
89. Klimesch W, Sauseng P, Hanslmayr S. EEG alpha oscillations: the inhibition–timing hypothesis. *Brain Res Rev.* (2007) 53:63–88. doi: 10.1016/j.brainresrev.2006.06.003
90. Jenkinson N, Brown P. New insights into the relationship between dopamine, beta oscillations and motor function. *Trends Neurosci.* (2011) 34:611–8. doi: 10.1016/j.tins.2011.09.003

91. Herrmann CS, Munk MH, Engel AK. Cognitive functions of gamma-band activity: memory match and utilization. *Trends Cogn Sci.* (2004) 8:347–55. doi: 10.1016/j.tics.2004.06.006
92. Ieong HFH, Yuan Z. Abnormal resting-state functional connectivity in the orbitofrontal cortex of heroin users and its relationship with anxiety: a pilot fNIRS study. *Sci Rep.* (2017) 7:46522. doi: 10.1038/srep46522
93. Wang AL, Elman I, Lowen SB, Blady SJ, Lynch KG, Hyatt JM, et al. Neural correlates of adherence to extended-release naltrexone pharmacotherapy in heroin dependence. *Transl Psychiatry.* (2015) 5:e531. doi: 10.1038/tp.2015.20
94. Polunina AG, Davydov DM. EEG spectral power and mean frequencies in early heroin abstinence. *Prog Neuro-Psychopharmacol Biol Psychiatry.* (2004) 28:73–82. doi: 10.1016/j.pnpbp.2003.09.022
95. Motlagh F, Ibrahim F, Rashid R, Seghatoleslam T, Habil H. Investigation of brain electrophysiological properties among heroin addicts: quantitative EEG and event-related potentials. *J Neurosci Res.* (2017) 95:1633–46. doi: 10.1002/jnr.23988
96. Gorricho MD, Usón JRV. QEEG mapping and methadone. *Euro J Psychiatry.* (2008) 22:29–37.
97. Costa L, Bauer, L. Quantitative electroencephalographic differences associated with alcohol, cocaine, heroin and dual-substance dependence. *Drug alcohol depend.* (1997). 46:87–93. doi: 10.1016/S0376-8716(97)00058-6
98. Fingelkurts AA, Fingelkurts AA, Kivisaari R, Autti T, Borisov S, Puuskari V, et al. Increased local and decreased remote functional connectivity at EEG alpha and beta frequency bands in opioid-dependent patients. *Psychopharmacology.* (2006a) 188:42–52. doi: 10.1007/s00213-006-0474-4
99. Fingelkurts AA, Fingelkurts AA, Kivisaari R, Autti T, Borisov S, Puuskari V, et al. Reorganization of the composition of brain oscillations and their temporal characteristics in opioid dependent patients. *Prog Neuro-Psychopharmacol Biol Psychiatry.* (2006) 30:1453–65. doi: 10.1016/j.pnpbp.2006.06.005
100. Fingelkurts AA, Fingelkurts AA, Kivisaari R, Autti T, Borisov S, Puuskari V, et al. Opioid withdrawal results in an increased local and remote functional connectivity at EEG alpha and beta frequency bands. *Neurosci Res.* (2007) 58:40–9. doi: 10.1016/j.neures.2007.01.011
101. Franken IH, Stam CJ, Hendriks VM, van den Brink W. Neurophysiological evidence for abnormal cognitive processing of drug cues in heroin dependence. *Psychopharmacology.* (2003) 170:205–12. doi: 10.1007/s00213-003-1542-7
102. Bauer LO. CNS recovery from cocaine, cocaine and alcohol, or opioid dependence: a P300 study. *Clin Neurophysiol.* (2001) 112:1508–15. doi: 10.1016/S1388-2457(01)00583-1
103. Chen H, Jiang H, Guo Q, Du J, Wang J, Zhao M. Case-control study of error-related negativity among males with heroin dependence undergoing rehabilitation. *Shanghai Arch Psychiatry.* (2013) 25:141–8. doi: 10.3969/j.issn.1002-0829.2013.03.003
104. Papageorgiou C, Liappas I, Asvestas P, Vasios C, Matsopoulos GK, Nikolaou C, et al. Abnormal P600 in heroin addicts with prolonged abstinence elicited during a working memory test. *Neuroreport.* (2001) 12:1773–8. doi: 10.1097/00001756-200106130-00051
105. Papageorgiou C, Rabavilas A, Liappas I, Stefanis C. Do obsessive-compulsive patients and abstinent heroin addicts share a common psychophysiological mechanism? *Neuropsychobiology.* (2003) 47:1–11. doi: 10.1159/000068868
106. Papageorgiou CC, Liappas IA, Ventouras EM, Nikolaou CC, Kitsonas EN, Uzunoglu NK, et al. Long-term abstinence syndrome in heroin addicts: indices of P300 alterations associated with a short memory task. *Prog Neuro-Psychopharmacol Biol Psychiatry.* (2004) 28:1109–15. doi: 10.1016/j.pnpbp.2004.05.049
107. Singh SM, Basu D, Kohli A, Prabhakar S. Auditory P300 event-related potentials and neurocognitive functions in opioid dependent men and their brothers. *Am J Addict.* (2009) 18:198–205. doi: 10.1080/10550490902786975
108. Su B, Wang S, Sumich A, Li S, Yang L, Cai Y, et al. Reduction in N2 amplitude in response to deviant drug-related stimuli during a two-choice oddball task in long-term heroin abstainers. *Psychopharmacology.* (2017) 234:3195–205. doi: 10.1007/s00213-017-4707-5
109. Yang L, Xu Q, Li S, Zhao X, Ma L, Zheng Y, et al. The effects of methadone maintenance treatment on heroin addicts with response inhibition function impairments: evidence from event-related potentials. *J Food Drug Analy.* (2015) 23:260–6. doi: 10.1016/j.jfda.2014.06.002
110. Yang B, Yang S, Zhao L, Yin L, Liu X, An S. Event-related potentials in a Go/Nogo task of abnormal response inhibition in heroin addicts. *Sci China Series C Life Sci.* (2009) 52:780–8. doi: 10.1007/s11427-009-0106-4
111. Schupp HT, Junghöfer M, Weike AI, Hamm AO. The selective processing of briefly presented affective pictures: an ERP analysis. *Psychophysiology.* (2004) 41:441–9. doi: 10.1111/j.1469-8986.2004.00174.x
112. Nieuwenhuis S, Yeung N, Van Den Wildenberg W, Ridderinkhof KR. Electrophysiological correlates of anterior cingulate function in a go/no-go task: effects of response conflict and trial type frequency. *Cognit Affect Behav Neurosci.* (2003) 3:17–26. doi: 10.3758/CABN.3.1.17
113. Van Veen V, Carter CS. The anterior cingulate as a conflict monitor: fMRI and ERP studies. *Physiol Behav.* (2002) 77:477–82. doi: 10.1016/S0031-9384(02)00930-7
114. Morie KP, Garavan H, Bell RP, De Sanctis P, Krakowski MI, Foxe JJ. Intact inhibitory control processes in abstinent drug abusers (II): a high-density electrical mapping study in former cocaine and heroin addicts. *Neuropharmacology.* (2014) 82:151–60. doi: 10.1016/j.neuropharm.2013.02.023
115. Zhao Q, Li H, Hu B, Li Y, Gillebert CR, Mantini D, et al. Neural correlates of drug-related attentional bias in heroin dependence. *Front Hum Neurosci.* (2018) 11:646. doi: 10.3389/fnhum.2017.00646
116. Lubman DI, Allen NB, Peters LA, Deakin JFW. Electrophysiological evidence that drug cues have greater salience than other affective stimuli in opiate addiction. *J Psychopharmacol.* (2008) 22:836–42. doi: 10.1177/0269881107083846
117. Diedrich O, Naumann E, Maier S, Becker G, Bartussek D. A frontal positive slow wave in the ERP associated with emotional slides. *J Psychophysiol.* (1997) 1:71–84.
118. Schupp HT, Cuthbert BN, Bradley MM, Cacioppo JT, Ito T, Lang PJ. Affective picture processing: the late positive potential is modulated by motivational relevance. *Psychophysiology.* (2000) 37:257–61. doi: 10.1111/1469-8986.3720257
119. Olvet DM, Hajcak G. The error-related negativity (ERN) and psychopathology: Toward an endophenotype. *Clin Psychol Rev.* (2008) 28:1343–54. doi: 10.1016/j.cpr.2008.07.003
120. Shen Y, Cao X, Tan T, Shan C, Wang Y, Pan J, et al. 10-Hz repetitive transcranial magnetic stimulation of the left dorsolateral prefrontal cortex reduces heroin cue craving in long-term addicts. *Biol Psychiatry.* (2016) 80:e13–4. doi: 10.1016/j.biopsych.2016.02.006
121. Zhou H, Xu J, Jiang J. Deep brain stimulation of nucleus accumbens on heroin-seeking behaviors: a case report. *Biol Psychiatry.* (2011) 69:e41–2. doi: 10.1016/j.biopsych.2011.02.012
122. Zhang C, Huang Y, Zheng F, Zeljic K, Pan J, Sun B. Death from opioid overdose after deep brain stimulation: a case report. *Biol Psychiatry.* (2018) 83:e9–e10. doi: 10.1016/j.biopsych.2017.07.018
123. Chen L, Li N, Ge S, Lozano AM, Lee DJ, Yang C, et al. Long-term results after deep brain stimulation of nucleus accumbens and the anterior limb of the internal capsule for preventing heroin relapse: an open-label pilot study. *Brain Stimul.* (2019) 12:175–83. doi: 10.1016/j.brs.2018.09.006
124. Kuhn J, Möller M, Treppmann JF, Bartsch C, Lenartz D, Gründler TO, et al. Deep brain stimulation of the nucleus accumbens and its usefulness in severe opioid addiction. *Mol Psychiatry.* (2014) 19:145–6. doi: 10.1038/mp.2012.196
125. Peisker CB, Schüller T, Peters J, Wagner BJ, Schilbach L, Müller UJ, et al. Nucleus accumbens deep brain stimulation in patients with substance use disorders and delay discounting. *Brain Sci.* (2018) 8:21. doi: 10.3390/brainsci8020021
126. Lubman DI, Yücel M, Kettle JW, Scaffidi A, MacKenzie T, Simmons JG, et al. Responsiveness to drug cues and natural rewards in opiate addiction: associations with later heroin use. *Arch Gen Psychiatry.* (2009) 66:205–12. doi: 10.1001/archgenpsychiatry.2008.522
127. Fink BC, Steele VR, Maurer MJ, Fede SJ, Calhoun VD, Kiehl KA. Brain potentials predict substance abuse treatment completion in a prison sample. *Brain Behav.* (2016) 6:e00501. doi: 10.1002/brb3.501
128. Steele VR, Fink BC, Maurer JM, Arbabshirani MR, Wilber CH, Jaffe AJ, et al. Brain potentials measured during a Go/NoGo task predict completion of substance abuse treatment. *Biol Psychiatry.* (2014) 76:75–83. doi: 10.1016/j.biopsych.2013.09.030
129. Li Q, Li W, Wang H, Wang Y, Zhang Y, Zhu J, et al. Predicting subsequent relapse by drug-related cue-induced brain activation in heroin addiction:

an event-related functional magnetic resonance imaging study. *Addict Biol.* (2015) 20:968–78. doi: 10.1111/adb.12182

130. Li Q, Liu J, Wang W, Wang Y, Li W, Chen J, et al. Disrupted coupling of large-scale networks is associated with relapse behaviour in heroin-dependent men. *J Psychiatry Neurosci.* (2018) 43:48–57. doi: 10.1503/jpn.170011
131. Steele VR, Maurer JM, Arbabshirani MR, Claus ED, Fink BC, Rao V, et al. Machine learning of functional magnetic resonance imaging network connectivity predicts substance abuse treatment completion. *Biol Psychiatry Cognit Neurosci Neuroimag.* (2018) 3:141–9. doi: 10.1016/j.bpsc.2017.07.003
132. Langleben DD, Ruparel K, Elman I, Loughead JW, Busch EL, Cornish J, et al. Extended-release naltrexone modulates brain response to drug cues in abstinent heroin-dependent patients. *Addict Biol.* (2014) 19:262–71. doi: 10.1111/j.1369-1600.2012.00462.x
133. Shi Z, Wang AL, Jagannathan K, Fairchild VP, O'Brien CP, Childress AR, et al. Effects of extended-release naltrexone on the brain response to drug-related stimuli in patients with opioid use disorder. *J Psychiatry Neurosci.* (2018) 43:254–61. doi: 10.1503/jpn.170036
134. Wang AL, Lowen SB, Elman I, Shi Z, Fairchild VP, Bouril A, et al. Sustained opioid antagonism modulates striatal sensitivity to baby schema in opioid use disorder. *J Subst Abuse Treat.* (2018) 85:70–7. doi: 10.1016/j.jsat.2017.10.007
135. Ye JJ, Li W, Zhang DS, Li Q, Zhu J, Chen JJ, et al. Longitudinal behavioral and fMRI-based assessment of inhibitory control in heroin addicts on methadone maintenance treatment. *Exp Ther Med.* (2018) 16:3202–10. doi: 10.3892/etm.2018.6571
136. Fahmy R, Wasfi M, Mamdouh R, Moussa K, Wahba A, Wittemann M, et al. Mindfulness-based interventions modulate structural network strength in patients with opioid dependence. *Addict Behav.* (2018) 82:50–6. doi: 10.1016/j.addbeh.2018.02.013
137. Marsh JC, Park K, Lin YA, Bersamira C. Gender differences in trends for heroin use and nonmedical prescription opioid use, 2007–2014. *J Subst Abuse Treat.* (2018) 87:79–85. doi: 10.1016/j.jsat.2018.01.001
138. Zakiniaeiz Y, Potenza MN. Gender-related differences in addiction: a review of human studies. *Curr Opin Behav Sci.* (2018) 23:171–5. doi: 10.1016/j.cobeha.2018.08.004
139. Motlagh F, Ibrahim F, Menke JM, Rashid R, Seghatoleslam T, Habil H. Neuroelectrophysiological approaches in heroin addiction research: a review of literatures. *J Neurosci Res.* (2016) 94:297–309. doi: 10.1002/jnr.23703
140. Sinha R. Chronic stress, drug use, and vulnerability to addiction. *Ann N Y Acad Sci.* (2008) 1141:105–30. doi: 10.1196/annals.1441.030
141. Gray MA, Critchley HD. Interoceptive basis to craving. *Neuron.* (2007) 54:183–6. doi: 10.1016/j.neuron.2007.03.024
142. Paulus MP, Stewart JL. Interoception and drug addiction. *Neuropharmacology.* (2014) 76:342–50. doi: 10.1016/j.neuropharm.2013.07.002
143. Paulus MP, Tapert SF, Schulteis G. The role of interoception and alliesthesia in addiction. *Pharmacol Biochem Behav.* (2009) 94:1–7. doi: 10.1016/j.pbb.2009.08.005
144. Verdejo-Garcia A, Clark L, Dunn BD. The role of interoception in addiction: a critical review. *Neurosci Biobehav Rev.* (2012) 36:1857–69. doi: 10.1016/j.neubiorev.2012.05.007
145. Sönmez MB, Kahyaci Kiliç E, Ateş Çöl I, Görgülü Y, Köse Çinar R. Decreased interoceptive awareness in patients with substance use disorders. *J Subst Use.* (2017) 22:60–5. doi: 10.3109/14659891.2016.1143048
146. Garland EL, Bryan CJ, Kreighbaum L, Nakamura Y, Howard MO, Froeliger B. Prescription opioid misusing chronic pain patients exhibit dysregulated context-dependent associations: Investigating associative learning in addiction with the cue-primed reactivity task. *Drug Alcohol Depend.* (2018) 187:13–21. doi: 10.1016/j.drugalcdep.2018.02.014
147. Stewart JL, Parnass JM, May AC, Davenport PW, Paulus MP. Altered frontocingulate activation during aversive interoceptive processing in young adults transitioning to problem stimulant use. *Front Syst Neurosci.* (2013) 7:89. doi: 10.3389/fnsys.2013.00089
148. Stewart JL, May AC, Poppa T, Davenport PW, Tapert SF, Paulus MP. You are the danger: attenuated INS response in methamphetamine users during aversive interoceptive decision-making. *Drug Alcohol Depend.* (2014) 142:110–9. doi: 10.1016/j.drugalcdep.2014.06.003
149. Stewart JL, Juavinett AL, May AC, Davenport PW, Paulus MP. Do you feel alright? attenuated neural processing of aversive interoceptive stimuli in current stimulant users. *Psychophysiology.* (2015) 52:249–62. doi: 10.1111/psyp.12303
150. Fullana MA, Harrison BJ, Soriano-Mas C, Vervliet B, Cardoner N, Àvila-Parcet A, et al. Neural signatures of human fear conditioning: an updated and extended meta-analysis of fMRI studies. *Mol Psychiatry.* (2016) 21:500–8. doi: 10.1038/mp.2015.88
151. Alvarez RP, Biggs A, Chen G, Pine DS, Grillon C. Contextual fear conditioning in humans: cortical-hippocampal and amygdala contributions. *J Neurosci.* (2008) 28:6211–9. doi: 10.1523/JNEUROSCI.1246-08.2008
152. Harnett NG, Shumen JR, Wagle PA, Wood KH, Wheelock MD, Baños JH, et al. Neural mechanisms of human temporal fear conditioning. *Neurobiol Learn Mem.* (2016) 136:97–104. doi: 10.1016/j.nlm.2016.09.019
153. LaBar KS, Gatenby JC, Gore JC, LeDoux JE, Phelps EA. Human amygdala activation during conditioned fear acquisition and extinction: A mixed-trial fMRI study. *Neuron.* (1998) 20:937–45. doi: 10.1016/S0896-6273(00)80475-4
154. Lindner K, Neubert J, Pfannmöller J, Lotze M, Hamm AO, Wendt J. Fear-potentiated startle processing in humans: parallel fMRI and orbicularis EMG assessment during cue conditioning and extinction. *Int J Psychophysiol.* (2015) 98:535–45. doi: 10.1016/j.ijpsycho.2015.02.025
155. Knight DC, Smith CN, Cheng DT, Stein EA, Helmstetter FJ. Amygdala and hippocampal activity during acquisition and extinction of human fear conditioning. *Cognit Affect Behav Neurosci.* (2004) 4:317–25. doi: 10.3758/CABN.4.3.317
156. Phelps EA, O'Connor KJ, Gatenby JC, Gore JC, Grillon C, Davis M. Activation of the left amygdala to a cognitive representation of fear. *Nat Neurosci.* (2001) 4:437–41. doi: 10.1038/86110
157. Baczkowski BM, Johnstone T, Walter H, Erk S, Veer IM. Sliding-window analysis tracks fluctuations in amygdala functional connectivity associated with physiological arousal and vigilance during fear conditioning. *Neuroimage.* (2017) 153:168–78. doi: 10.1016/j.neuroimage.2017.03.022
158. Critchley HD, Mathias CJ, Dolan RJ. Fear conditioning in humans: the influence of awareness and autonomic arousal on functional neuroanatomy. *Neuron.* (2002) 33:653–63. doi: 10.1016/S0896-6273(02)00588-3
159. Fullana MA, Albajes-Eizagirre A, Soriano-Mas C, Vervliet B, Cardoner N, Benet O, et al. Fear extinction in the human brain: a meta-analysis of fMRI studies in healthy participants. *Neurosci Biobehav Rev.* (2018) 88:16–25. doi: 10.1016/j.neubiorev.2018.03.002
160. Barad M, Gean PW, Lutz B. The role of the amygdala in the extinction of conditioned fear. *Biol Psychiatry.* (2006) 60:322–8. doi: 10.1016/j.biopsych.2006.05.029
161. Phelps EA, Delgado MR, Nearing KI, LeDoux JE. Extinction learning in humans: role of the amygdala and vmPFC. *Neuron.* (2004) 43:897–905. doi: 10.1016/j.neuron.2004.08.042
162. Hajcak G, Nieuwenhuis S. Reappraisal modulates the electrocortical response to unpleasant pictures. *Cognit Affect Behav Neurosci.* (2006) 6:291–7. doi: 10.3758/CABN.6.4.291

2

The Effect of High-Frequency Repetitive Transcranial Magnetic Stimulation on Emotion Processing, Reappraisal and Craving in Alcohol use Disorder Patients and Healthy Controls: A Functional Magnetic Resonance Imaging Study

Jochem M. Jansen[1,2], Odile A. van den Heuvel[3,4], Ysbrand D. van der Werf[4], Stella J. de Wit[3,4], Dick J. Veltman[3,4], Wim van den Brink[1] and Anna E. Goudriaan[1,5]*

[1] Department of Psychiatry, Amsterdam Institute for Addiction Research, Amsterdam UMC, University of Amsterdam, Amsterdam, Netherlands, [2] Institute for Criminal Law and Criminology, Faculty of Law, Leiden University, Leiden, Netherlands, [3] Department of Psychiatry, Amsterdam UMC, Vrije Universiteit Amsterdam, Amsterdam, Netherlands, [4] Department of Anatomy and Neurosciences, Amsterdam Neuroscience, Amsterdam UMC, Vrije Universiteit Amsterdam, Amsterdam, Netherlands, [5] Department of Research and Quality of Care, Arkin, Amsterdam, Netherlands

****Correspondence:***
Jochem Milan Jansen
j.m.jansen@law.leidenuniv.nl
jochemjansen89@gmail.com

Impaired cognitive–motivational functioning is present in many psychiatric disorders, including alcohol use disorder (AUD). Emotion regulation is a key intermediate factor, relating to the (cognitive) regulation of emotional and motivational states, such as in regulation of craving or negative emotions that may lead to relapse in alcohol use. These cognitive–motivational functions, including emotion regulation, are a target in cognitive behavioral therapy and may possibly be improved by neurostimulation techniques. The present between-subjects, single-blind study assesses the effects of sham-controlled high-frequency neuronavigated repetitive transcranial magnetic stimulation (10 Hz) of the right dorsolateral prefrontal cortex (dlPFC) on several aspects relevant for emotion regulation (emotion processing and reappraisal abilities) and related brain activity, as well as self-reported craving in a sample of alcohol use disorder patients (AUD; n = 39) and healthy controls (HC; n = 36). During the emotion reappraisal task, participants were instructed to either attend or reappraise their emotions related to the negative, positive, neutral, and alcohol-related images, after which they rated their experienced emotions. We found that repetitive transcranial magnetic stimulation (rTMS) reduces self-reported experienced emotions in response to positive and negative images in AUD patients, whereas experienced emotions were increased in response to neutral and positive images in HCs. In the functional magnetic resonance imaging (fMRI) analyses, we found that rTMS reduces right dlPFC activity during appraisal of affective images relative to sham stimulation only in AUD patients. We could not confirm our hypotheses regarding the effect of rTMS craving levels, or on reappraisal related brain function, since no significant effects of rTMS on craving or reappraisal related brain function were found. These findings imply that rTMS can reduce the emotional impact of images as reflected in blood oxygenation level-dependent

(BOLD) response, especially in AUD patients. Future studies should replicate and expand the current study, for instance, by assessing the effect of multiple stimulation sessions on both explicit and implicit emotion regulation paradigms and craving, and assess the effect of rTMS within subgroups with specific addiction-relevant image preferences.

Clinical Trial Registration: www.ClinicalTrials.gov, identifier NCT02557815.

Keywords: alcohol use disorder, emotion reappraisal, craving, functional magnetic resonance imaging, emotion processing, repetetitive transcranial magnetic stimulation

INTRODUCTION

Harmful alcohol consumption ranks among the top five worldwide contributors of disease, disability, and death (1–3), and alcohol use disorder (AUD) is a common mental health disorder with a 12-month prevalence of 2–3% in the United States (4, 5) and 4% in Europe (6).

AUD is often described as a dual process disorder with reduced cognitive control and alterations in the brain reward system (7–9). Alterations in the reward circuitry include hypersensitivity to addiction relevant cues, in combination with hyposensitivity to natural rewards. This reward deficiency may lead to a disbalance in the reward system favoring addiction-relevant stimuli (10, 11). Brain alterations related to cognitive control include impaired (response) inhibition and emotion regulation (12), resulting in diminished ability to effectively control the emotional impact of certain thoughts or stimuli (13, 14). These changes in the reward circuitry and diminished control over emotions increase alcohol craving and relapse in remitted patients (15–17).

Emotion regulation can be described as the process of moderating the emotional impact of a thought or stimulus and may be achieved through various strategies ranging from relatively automatic and implicit (i.e., extinction) to explicit and cognitively controlled (reappraisal) (18). A recent review indicates that impaired emotion regulation is present in AUD based on various studies employing implicit (e.g., non-effortful) emotion regulation tasks such as emotion reactivity, implicit reappraisal, or behavioral control tasks (12). Impairments in reappraisal are supposed to be related to the development, persistence, and severity of substance dependence (19). Difficulties in coping with negative affect is one of the most prominent clinical factors in substance dependence (20), and the induction of negative affect may increase the urge to drink (16, 21), but studies on more controlled and explicit emotion regulation in substance use disordered patients are scarce. Explicit emotion reappraisal has been linked to several prefrontal brain areas: the dorsolateral prefrontal cortex (dlPFC) (for maintaining attentional and manipulating relevant information), ventrolateral prefrontal cortex (vlPFC) (for selecting the goal-appropriate interpretation), and dorsal anterior cingulate cortex (dACC) and dorsomedial prefrontal cortex (dmPFC) (both for conflict monitoring of the intended versus the actual behavioral outcomes) (18).

In our previous study within this special issue, we showed that *explicit* emotion regulation (reappraisal) abilities and related brain functioning were similar in alcohol use disorder (AUD) patients and healthy controls (HCs), but that in AUD patients compared to HCs, reduced brain activity during implicit emotion processing was present (Jansen et al., submitted). Based on these findings and the current literature, it seems that AUD patients are not impaired in explicit emotion regulation when actively instructed to apply these strategies, but that they do show reduced brain activity while watching emotional stimuli. A reduced response to non-addiction-relevant emotional cues in AUD patients may be related to a reduced salience of these non-addiction-related emotional stimuli.

Motivational interviewing and cognitive behavioral therapies are effective treatments for substance use disorders, including AUDs (22). Research suggests not only that psychological interventions should precede pharmacological treatment, but also that both types of treatment are effective (23, 24). After an initially successful period of abstinence, an estimated 50% of patients relapse into alcohol use within the first year (25–28). Similar results have been obtained for the pharmacotherapy of AUDs (25). These high relapse rates indicate that research into new treatment possibilities is warranted.

Noninvasive neurostimulation of the prefrontal cortex, using techniques such as repetitive transcranial magnetic stimulation (rTMS), may offer a new alternative intervention method for substance use disorder patients (29, 30). rTMS and other forms of neuromodulation can reduce acute craving in patients with a substance use disorder (31), especially when stimulating the (right) dlPFC (29) and improve cognitive functions such as attention, memory, and executive functioning in patients with substance use disorders (32, 33). In recent years, increased attention has been directed toward improving emotion processing and emotion reappraisal with prefrontal rTMS, often directed toward the dlPFC, which is central in explicitly controlled emotion regulation strategies, including reappraisal (18). These studies vary in their methodology and reveal contradictory results with high-frequency *right* dlPFC rTMS being associated with an increase in attentional bias toward negative stimuli (34), whereas high-frequency *left* dlPFC stimulation decreased the amygdala response to negative stimuli (35). Additionally, a recent review concludes that rTMS influences cognitive control and the attentional and affective aspects of emotion regulation and that rTMS should be investigated for substance use disordered patients (33, 36).

The five rTMS studies that are discussed by Choi et al. (36) use varying methodological approaches regarding stimulation location (right and/or left dlPFC, cerebellum), stimulation frequency (high and low frequency), and study outcome (autonomic reactions, attention, mood, and affective processing). De Raedt et al. (37) and Vanderhasselt et al. (34) investigated the effects of sham-controlled high-frequency rTMS of the dlPFC on attentional aspects of emotion regulation, and both conclude that right dlPFC rTMS increased attention toward—or decreased disengagement of—negative stimuli. One study employing sham-controlled high- and low-frequency stimulation of the right dlPFC shows that low-frequency (but not high-frequency) stimulation increased heart rate deceleration in response to negative and neutral, relative to positive, pictures (38). Another study employing low-frequency stimulation of the right dlPFC shows increased responses to fearful faces compared to neutral faces in the right temporal junction (39). Finally, Schutter and van Honk (40) showed that sham-controlled low-frequency stimulation of the cerebellum increased negative mood after an emotion regulation task. Additionally, more recent findings are mixed: high-frequency right dlPFC rTMS stimulation was found not to influence heart rate reactivity to positive or negative images (38) or emotion recognition performance (41). Notzon et al. (42), on the other hand, found high-frequency rTMS of the right DLPFC, compared to low-frequency rTMS, to improve emotion discrimination, leading the authors to conclude that high-frequency rTMS leads to better cognitive control over aversive stimuli. Despite the variety in applied study methods, these studies indicate that rTMS may influence emotion processing and reappraisal in healthy subjects. Other studies suggest that the effect of rTMS may be different in persons with a psychiatric disorder (32), and in a recent study, we have shown that high-frequency *left* dlPFC stimulation may reduce self-reported affect related to negative images in obsessive–compulsive disorder patients and that it reduces dorsomedial prefrontal cortex (PFC) activity relative to sham stimulation, independent of task conditions (43). This study is one of the few studies to investigate the effect of rTMS on both emotion processing and reappraisal at a behavioral and neural level. There are currently no rTMS studies on emotion processing and reappraisal in AUD patients, while these processes are highly relevant for the treatment of this disorder. Cognitive behavioral therapies, for example, often include some form of emotion regulation training (44, 45).

The current study is the first to investigate the effect of high-frequency rTMS on emotion processing and reappraisal in AUD patients and HCs at a behavioral and neural level. Based on previous studies (29), we hypothesize that high-frequency rTMS of the right dlPFC ameliorates reappraisal and the recruitment of the reappraisal-related brain network in both AUD patients and HCs, but this improvement is expected to be greater in the AUD group compared to the HC group [see Ref. (32)]. We expect that high-frequency stimulation will influence (increase or decrease) emotion processing at a behavioral and neural level. Finally, we expect that in AUD patients, high-frequency rTMS decreases reappraisal task-induced craving.

METHODS

This study is part of a larger study, with two fMRI sessions, focusing on differences in emotion regulation performance and related brain activity between AUD patients and HCs during the first (baseline) session and the effect of rTMS on craving, emotion regulation, and related brain activity during the second (rTMS stimulation) session. For a description of the main task effects (e.g., experimental manipulation during the first session), as well as the between-participant group differences at baseline (ADP vs. HC), please see our previous manuscript within this special issue (Jansen et al., submitted). The current manuscript describes the effects of rTMS on emotion processing, reappraisal, craving, and related brain activity.

Participants

A total of 39 AUD patients (26 males) and 36 HCs (20 males) were included in this between-subjects study and were matched on (mean) age, sex, and education. AUD patients were sober for at least 3 weeks and were recruited from addiction treatment centers in the larger city area of Amsterdam, the Netherlands. Sobriety was confirmed with a urine test in the research lab on the test days. None of the participants used psychoactive medication, cannabis, opioids, or stimulants. HCs were recruited through Internet and social media advertisements. All participants were screened for MRI suitability. All subjects were screened (and if positive excluded) for the presence or a history of psychiatric disorders, including substance abuse or dependence, using the Composite International Diagnostic Interview (CIDI) (46). The study was approved by the local Medical Ethical Commission of the Academic Medical Center of the University of Amsterdam and participants signed the informed consent form, consistent with the Declaration of Helsinki, before participating in the study. Participants were remunerated for their participation.

Questionnaires

In addition to the CIDI interview, the Alcohol Use Disorder Identification Test (AUDIT) (47), Beck's Depression Inventory (BDI) (48), Beck's Anxiety Inventory (BAI) (49), the Toronto Alexithymia Scale-20 (TAS-20) (50), and the Emotion Regulation Questionnaire (ERQ) (51) were administered to assess alcohol problem severity, depression severity, anxiety severity, alexithymia, and emotion regulation, respectively. Finally, craving was assessed with the Alcohol Urge Questionnaire (AUQ) (52) before and after the performance of the emotion reappraisal task in both sessions.

Emotion Reappraisal Task

Two matched versions of the task were programmed in E-Prime 2.0 and presented in a counterbalanced order in two different sessions during fMRI scanning. Each session, participants viewed nine negative, nine positive, nine neutral, and nine alcohol-related images on a screen using a mirror attached to the head coil. The negative, positive, and neutral images used in this task were selected from the International Affective Picture Set (IAPS) (53). Negative images had a low valence (≤4.0) and high arousal (≥6.0), neutral images had a mildly positive valence ($4.5 < x < 7.0$) and low arousal ($2.0 < x < 4.2$), and positive images had high valence (≥7.0) and high arousal (≥5.0), based on the original IAPS scores. The alcohol-related images were selected from Vollstädt-Klein et al. (54) and supplemented by alcohol-related images of popular Dutch alcoholic beverages. All alcohol-related images were separately validated in an independent sample of both HCs and AUD patients ($n = 17$) for valence (mildly positive: $3.0 < x < 6.0$) and arousal (low: $2.0 < x < 4.0$).

The images were paired with one of two different instructions: "attend" and "reappraise." In the attend instruction, participants were told to view and identify themselves with the situation in the image (e.g., "how would you feel in this situation"). In the reappraise condition, participants were told to reappraise their emotions related to these images in such a way that the emotional significance was reduced (e.g., "imagine a less negative outcome or interpretation"). Images were presented in 12 blocks of three images of the same emotion type (negative, positive, neutral, and alcohol) with the same instruction (attend and reappraise) and presented in a pseudo-randomized order.

After each image, for both instructions (attend and reappraise), a visual analogue scale (VAS) was presented. Participants had to rate their emotional state ("How do you feel?") by moving a bar to the right or left by pressing a button box multiple times. A moving bar was set in the middle of a line (representing a neutral value of 50) and the range of emotions on this line was indicated by previously validated self-assessment manikins depicting valence (55). Indicated values ranged from 0 (negative, extreme left of the line) to 100 (positive, extreme right of the line). Prior to scanning, the assessment was explained and practiced outside the scanner using example stimuli (not used in the experiments) for approximately 5 min (for more information, see **S1**). The reappraisal task itself took approximately 25 min.

Repetitive Transcranial Magnetic Stimulation

In the stimulation session, participants received either (single-blind) neuro-navigated (Visor2, ANT) sham or active right dlPFC rTMS using a MagStim Rapid2 Air-film coil with a 70-mm diameter (MagStim Co., UK) immediately before entering the MRI. The active rTMS consisted of sixty 5-s trains of 10 Hz at 110% motor threshold (31). These parameters are within the international safety limits for use of rTMS (56). The stimulation location was defined for each individual separately as the most significant peak voxel in the right dlPFC activated during the reappraisal task in the baseline session for the [reappraise minus attend] contrast, as defined by the BrainMap database (57). Sham stimulation was performed using identical parameters, but the rTMS coil was tilted 90° relative to the skull (58).

Analysis

Behavioral Analysis

Data were prepared for analysis by winsorizing extreme values for experienced emotion (mean VAS per condition and session) and craving (AUQ pre- and post-scores), by replacing values below the 5th and above the 95th percentile with the 5th or 95th percentile, respectively, and by confirming that experienced emotion was normally distributed.

In order to assess effects of stimulation (rTMS/sham), image type (positive/neutral/negative/alcohol), instruction (attend/reappraise), and participant group (AUD/HC) on experienced emotion, a four-way general linear model (GLM) Univariate ANOVA was performed, including experienced emotion after rTMS (condition-specific mean VAS) as the dependent variable, and instruction, image type, participant group, and stimulation as fixed factors. Condition-specific experienced emotion during the first session (before rTMS) was incorporated as a covariate. Significant interactions were followed up by Bonferroni-corrected simple effects analyses.

The AUQ was administered before (pre) and after (post) the reappraisal task during each session. Due to the many mistakes that were made in the second and seventh AUQ question—which are reverse coded and were misinterpreted—these were excluded from the analysis. Pre- and post-scores on both sessions were positively skewed and therefore a $\log(x + 1)$ transformation was applied. A GLM Univariate ANOVA was performed including AUQ scores as the dependent variable, time (pre/post) as the within-subjects factor, and both stimulation (rTMS/sham) and participant group (AUD/HC) as the between-group factor.

Functional Magnetic Resonance Imaging

Data Acquisition

MRI scanning was performed on a Philips Achieva 3T scanner at the Spinoza Imaging Centre, Amsterdam, the Netherlands. Functional MRI [echo time (TE) = 27.63 ms; repetition time (TR) = 2,000 ms; field of view (FOV) = 240 × 240 mm, 37 3-mm slices, 0.3-mm slice gap; 80 × 80 matrix; flip angle = 76.1°] was performed to acquire blood oxygenation level-dependent (BOLD) signals using single-shot multi-echo (59) T2*-weighted echo planar imaging (EPI). These T2-weighted flow-compensated eight spin-echo anatomical images were oriented axially along the anterior commissure to the posterior commissure (AC–PC) line. During the baseline session, a T1-weighted 3D data set was obtained for anatomical reference; TR = 8.196 ms, TE = 3.73 ms, field of view (FOV) = 140 × 188 × 220 mm, 240 × 187 matrix, flip angle = 8°, slice thickness = 1 mm, number of slices = 220.

Pre-Processing and First-Level Analysis

Pre-processing was performed with SPM8 (Wellcome Trust Centre for Neuroimaging, London, United Kingdom) in MATLAB (version 2012b) and included realignment to the first image, slice timing correction to the middle (18th) slice, coregistration of the anatomical T1 of the subject to the mean functional scan, and warping of this coregistered T1 to standard space. Next, the volumes were normalized to the Montreal Neurological Institute (MNI) template and smoothed with a 7-mm Gaussian kernel in order to increase signal-to-noise ratio. To account for low-frequency drifts, a high-pass filter (128 Hz) was applied. Three subjects (2 AUD, 1 HC) were removed due to low quality of the fMRI data (e.g., scanner artifacts).

In the first-level model, regressors of no interest were instruction and VAS scoring. Instruction was modeled with boxcars of 3 s, whereas VAS scoring was modeled with a boxcar for the true duration of the scoring process since this was self-paced. The eight regressors of interest included the onsets of the negative, positive, neutral, and alcohol-related images in either attending or reappraising condition, which were modeled as boxcars (duration, 5 s) and convolved with a hemodynamic response function, in the first-level, single-subject, fixed-effects analysis. First-level contrasts for reappraisal [reappraise > attend] were computed per emotion condition (negative, positive, alcohol, and neutral). For emotion processing, separate contrasts were created for attending emotional images (alcohol, positive, or negative) versus neutral images [attend emotion (positive, negative, alcohol) > attend neutral].

Functional Magnetic Resonance Imaging Data Analysis

In order to assess the effects of rTMS on emotion processing and emotion reappraisal, separate second-level fMRI analyses were performed.

For the attend condition (emotion processing), a 3 × 2 × 2 ANOVA was conducted in SPM12, including the [attend emotion > attend neutral] contrast per image type (alcohol, positive, and negative), in order to assess the interaction between image type (alcohol, positive, and negative), group (AUD and HC), and stimulation (rTMS and sham). Additionally, two-way interactions (group by stimulation, image type by stimulation, and group by emotion type) were assessed.

For the reappraise condition, a 4 × 2 × 2 ANOVA was conducted in SPM12, including the [reappraise > attend] contrasts per image type, in order to assess the interaction between image type (alcohol, neutral, positive, and negative), group (AUD and HC), and stimulation (rTMS and sham). Additionally, two-way interactions (group by stimulation, image type by stimulation, and group by image type) were assessed. All results are reported at a whole brain $p < 0.05$ family wise error (FWE)-corrected threshold.

RESULTS

Demographics

AUD patients and HCs were successfully matched on age, gender, and years of education. However, AUD patients reported significantly higher levels of smoking, depression (BDI), anxiety (BAI), and alexithymia (TAS-20). Analyses were not corrected for these differences, because depression, anxiety, and alexithymia levels are well known to be elevated in AUD (60–62) and are related to emotion processing and reappraisal, and thus correction for these factors could results in false-negative findings. Remarkably, there were no group differences in the ERQ scores (**Table 1**). Furthermore, there were no significant differences on any of the questionnaires between participants receiving active rTMS or sham rTMS.

Repetitive Transcranial Magnetic Stimulation Effects

Emotion Processing and Reappraisal

The four-way repeated-measures ANOVA with experienced emotion (mean VAS per condition after rTMS) as the dependent variable, image type (negative, positive, neutral, and alcohol), instruction (attend and reappraise) as within-subject factors, and participant group (AUD and HC) and stimulation (rTMS and sham) as between-subject factors—while correcting for baseline experienced emotion (mean VAS per condition) before rTMS—did not reveal a significant four-way interaction [$F(3,559) = .11$, $p = 0.95$, $d < 0.01$]. There was, however, a significant three-way interaction between image type, participant group, and stimulation [$F(3,559) = 7.18$, $p < 0.001$, $d = 0.39$].

To interpret the significant three-way interaction, we conducted separate GLM Univariate ANOVAs per image type (negative, positive, neutral, and alcohol related), including experienced emotion (mean VAS per condition after rTMS) as the dependent variable, and participant group (AUD and HC) as well as stimulation (rTMS and sham) as between-subject factors—while correcting for baseline experienced emotion (mean VAS per condition) before rTMS. The results of these analyses reveal significant interactions between participant group and stimulation for negative [$F(1,143) = 4.86$, $p = 0.03$, $d = 0.37$], positive [$F(1,143) = 18.38$, $p < 0.001$, $d = 0.11$], and neutral images [$F(1,143) = 6.48$, $p = 0.01$, $d = 0.04$], but not for

TABLE 1 | Sample characteristics.

	Mean AUD (sd) *n* = 39	Mean HC (sd) *n* = 36	Significance
Age	41.64 (8.63)	43.75 (10.90)	$t(1,73) = .93$, $p = 0.35$
Years of education	15.31 (3.05)	15.53 (2.85)	$t(1,71) = .49$, $p = 0.62$
Gender	M = 26	M = 20	$\chi^2(1,73) = .97$, $p = 0.32$
AUDIT	22.11 (10.51)	4.23 (2.52)	$t(1,70) = 9.80$, $p < 0.001$
Current smoker	Yes *n* = 29/35 (82.9%)	Yes *n* = 10/32 (31.3%)	$\chi^2(1,67) = 18.30$, $p < 0.001$
TAS-20 total	51.43 (10.83)	42.97 (8.88)	$t(1,65) = 3.48$, $p = 0.001$
TAS-20 DIDF	31.83 (8.16)	24.82 (7.40)	$t(1,66) = 3.71$, $p < 0.001$
TAS-20 EOT	11.97 (3.30)	11.27 (2.78)	$t(1,69) = .98$, $p = 0.33$
ERQ total	37.81 (7.95)	36.58 (8.42)	$t(1,73) = .90$, $p = 0.37$
ERQ Reappraisal	20.22 (5.87)	19.00 (7.53)	$t(1,71) = .76$, $p = 0.45$
ERQ Suppression	17.72 (5.01)	17.58 (5.08)	$t(1,71) = .01$, $p = 0.99$
Beck Depression Inventory	10.84 (9.58)	4.33 (6.36)	$t(1,72) = 3.41$, $p = 0.001$
Beck Anxiety Inventory	30.40 (8.73)	24.25 (4.67)	$t(1,74) = 3.75$, $p < 0.001$

AUD, alcohol use disorder; HC, healthy controls; SD, standard deviation; AUDIT, Alcohol Use Disorders Identification Test; TAS, Toronto Alexithymia Scale; DIDF, difficulties identifying and describing feelings; EOT, externally oriented thinking; ERQ, emotion regulation questionnaire. ERQ Reappraisal and Suppression are subscales of the ERQ.
This table shows the results for the analyses of the sample characteristics. Values are denoted as mean (standard deviation). Total number of participants per comparison may vary due to a small number of missing values.

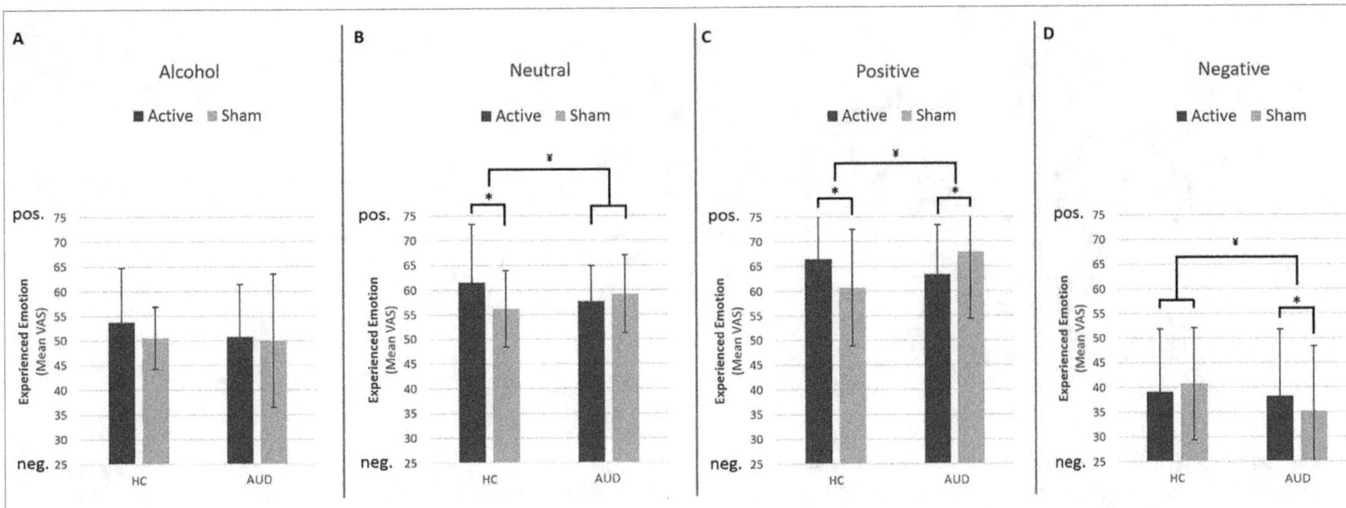

FIGURE 1 | Effect of repetitive transcranial magnetic stimulation (rTMS) on experienced emotion. This figure shows the differential effects of rTMS and sham stimulation on experienced emotion in reaction to alcohol **(A)**, neutral **(B)**, positive **(C)**, and negative **(D)** images. Note that a value of 50 represents "neutral" experienced emotion. Bars represent estimated marginal means, which are corrected for experienced emotion before rTMS. Error bars are standard deviations from the mean. ¥ = significant two-way interaction (group by stimulation), * = significant main effect of stimulation within participant group, pos. = positive, neg. = negative.

alcohol-related images [$F(1,143) = .12$, $p = 0.73$, $d = 0.06$] (see **Figure 1**).

Simple effects analyses show that rTMS dampens experienced emotions in response to positive, neutral, and negative images in AUD patients, whereas in HCs, rTMS intensifies experienced emotions in response to positive and neutral images. For example, experienced emotion in reaction to positive images is more positive after rTMS [mean (m) = 66.50, standard deviation (sd) = 14.66] compared to sham (m = 60.66, sd = 11.82) stimulation in HCs [$F(1,69) = 7.37$, $p = 0.008$, $d = 0.65$], whereas in AUD patients [$F(1,73) = 7.07$, $p = 0.01$, $d = 0.62$], experienced emotion to these images is less positive (e.g., more neutral) after rTMS (m = 63.39, sd = 9.99) compared to sham stimulation (m = 67.87, sd = 13.46). The simple effects analyses for neutral and negative images reveal that rTMS (m = 61.52, sd = 11.77) significantly increases positive experienced emotions to neutral images relative to sham stimulation (m = 56.18, sd = 7.72) in HCs [$F(1,69) = 5.98$, $p = 0.02$, $d = 0.59$], but not in AUD patients [$F(1,73) = 1.00$, $p = 0.32$, $d = 0.24$]. Finally, rTMS (m = 38.26, sd = 13.52) dampens negative emotions in response to negative images in AUD patients relative to sham stimulation [m = 35.18, sd = 13.13; $F(1,73) = 7.07$, $p = 0.01$, $d = 0.62$], but does not affect experienced emotion in HCs [$F(1,69) = .06$, $p = 0.81$, $d = 0.06$].

Craving

The results from the GLM univariate ANOVA with craving levels as the dependent variable, time (pre and post) as within-subjects factor, participant group (AUD and HC), and stimulation (rTMS and sham) as between-subjects factors did *not* reveal a three-way interaction [$F(1,132) = 1.70$, $p = 0.20$, $d = 0.23$]. There was, however, a significant two-way interaction between group and stimulation [$F(1,132) = 4.64$, $p = 0.03$, $d = 0.38$], but not between group and time [$F(1,132) = .36$, $p = 0.55$, $d = 0.11$] or between time and stimulation [$F(1,132) = .90$, $p = 0.34$, $d = 0.17$]. These results indicate that stimulation (rTMS and sham) did not differentially affect the change in craving over time (pre and post) for AUD patients and/or HCs, and therefore do not support our hypothesis that rTMS would reduce craving levels relative to sham stimulation (see **Figure 2**).

Functional Magnetic Resonance Imaging Results

Emotion Processing

Results from the 3 × 2 × 2 ANOVA, including the [attend emotion > attend neutral] contrast per image type, did not reveal a three-way interaction between image type (alcohol, positive, and negative), group (AUD and HC), and stimulation (rTMS and sham). The results do show a significant two-way interaction between group and stimulation within the right dlPFC (see **Figure 3** and **Supplementary Information**), originating from a decrease in dlPFC brain activity after rTMS relative to sham stimulation in the AUD group. The other two-way interactions (emotion by stimulation and group by image type) did not reveal any significant effects.

Emotion Reappraisal

Results from the 4 × 2 × 2 ANOVA, including the [regulate > attend] contrast per emotion, did not reveal a three-way interaction between image type (alcohol, neutral, positive, and negative), group (AUD and HC), and stimulation (rTMS and sham). Although none of the two-way interactions reached significance, there was a trend-significant interaction between image type (alcohol, neutral, positive, and negative) and stimulation (rTMS and sham; $p < 0.1$, FWE corrected). Follow-up analyses revealed that this two-way interaction originated from a difference in the effect of rTMS on brain activity between the reappraisal of positive and negative images in the bilateral superior frontal gyrus for both AUD patients and HCs. rTMS stimulation decreased superior frontal gyrus

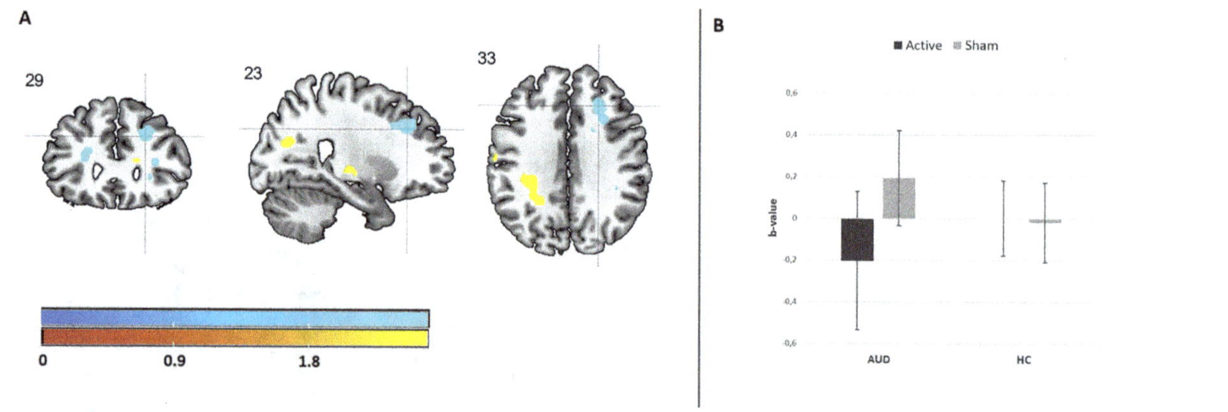

FIGURE 2 | This figure shows the trend-significant interaction between emotion (alcohol, neutral, positive, negative) and stimulation (rTMS, sham) within the superior frontal gyrus. **(A)** This panel shows the location for the interaction in the bilateral superior frontal gyrus. For illustrative purposes, these results are depicted at a $p < 0.001$ uncorrected threshold **(B)**. This panel shows the interaction within the peak voxel in the right superior frontal gyrus, based on the extracted beta weights.

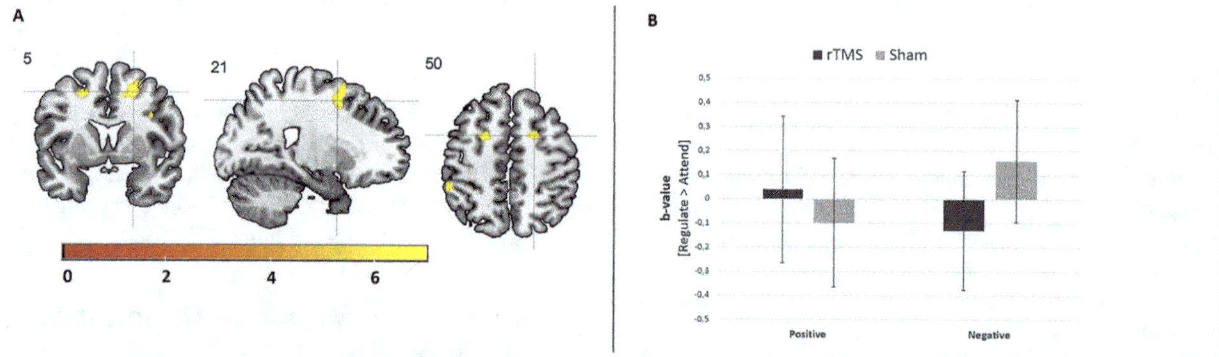

FIGURE 3 | The effect of rTMS on brain activity during emotion processing. **(A)** Cool coloring represents brain activity in the dorsolateral prefrontal cortex (dlPFC), which has decreased due to rTMS relative to sham stimulation in AUD patients. Hot coloring indicates brain activity in the supramarginal gyrus, which has increased due to rTMS stimulation relative to sham stimulation in AUD patients. For illustrative purposes, these results are depicted at a $p < 0.001$ uncorrected threshold. **(B)** This bar chart shows the effect of rTMS and sham stimulation on right dlPFC activity in AUD patients and HCs.

activity in response to negative images relative to sham stimulation, whereas rTMS increased activity in this area in response to positive images (see **Figure 4** and **Supplementary Information**).

DISCUSSION

The purpose of this study was to investigate the effect of sham-controlled high-frequency right dlPFC rTMS on emotion processing, reappraisal ability, and related brain functioning in alcohol use disorder patients (AUD patients) and healthy controls (HCs). We hypothesized that stimulation of the right dlPFC would improve emotion processing and reappraisal—especially in AUD patients—and alter the recruitment of the reappraisal-related brain network. In line with our hypotheses, we found that rTMS reduces self-reported experienced emotions in response to positive and negative images in AUD patients, whereas experienced emotions were increased in response to neutral and positive images in HCs. Instruction (attend or reappraise) did not influence these results. In the fMRI analyses, we found that rTMS reduces right dlPFC activity during appraisal of affective images relative to sham stimulation only in AUD patients. Our results do not support our hypothesis regarding the effect of rTMS on reappraisal-related brain function, since no significant effects of rTMS on reappraisal-related brain function were found. On a lower significance level, however, rTMS—compared to sham stimulation—*decreased* activity during reappraisal of negative images and *increased* activity in the bilateral superior frontal gyrus during reappraisal of positive images in both AUD patients and HCs. rTMS did not influence the change in craving levels compared to sham stimulation.

At a behavioral level, rTMS stimulation reduced the impact of affective (neutral, positive, and negative) images in AUD patients, but increased the impact of positive and neutral images in HCs. No effect of rTMS was found for alcohol-related images in either group, which is not in line with our hypotheses. AUD is characterized by reduced salience of natural stimuli relative to addiction-relevant cues (11), but alcohol consumption has also

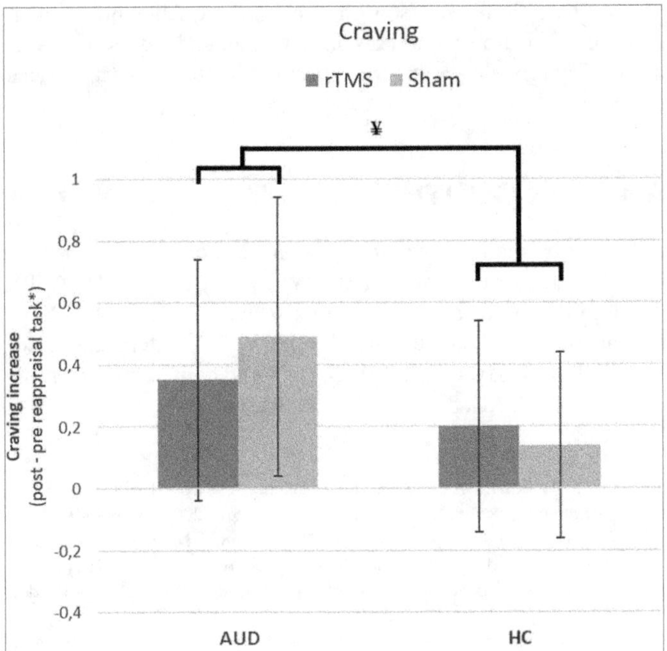

FIGURE 4 | The effect of rTMS and sham stimulation on craving per group. This figure depicts the significant interaction between stimulation (rTMS, sham) and group [alcohol use disorder (AUD), healthy controls (HC)]. * Note that the values are log(x + 1) transformed. ¥ = significant two-way interaction.

been suggested as a self-medication strategy to reduce—relapse-related—stress and negative emotions (63, 64). Therefore, reducing the impact of emotional images in AUD patients through rTMS may be related to reduced emotional impact of affective stimuli, which could possibly reduce stress, craving, and subsequent relapse. This explanation is supported by previous studies, which show positive effects of rTMS on craving reduction (31), cognitive functioning (32, 33), and depressive symptoms (65).

Our results furthermore suggest that rTMS stimulation affects emotion processing and reappraisal in HCs and AUD patients differently, since rTMS reduced emotional experience in AUD patients and reduced right dlPFC activity during emotion processing, whereas experienced emotion was increased in HCs and no effect was found on related brain activity. Although, to our knowledge, there are no other studies on the effect of rTMS on emotion processing and reappraisal in AUD patients, these results are in line with a review that suggests that rTMS effects may differ between healthy and patient populations (32).

These results correspond with previous studies in HCs that reveal that rTMS influences emotion processing (34, 35) and reappraisal (35, 42) in HCs. rTMS increased attentional bias toward negative stimuli in a study in HCs (34) and lead to faster emotion discrimination in HCs (42), which is in line with the strengthened response to (negative) images in HCs after rTMS in our study. Together, these studies imply that high-frequency right dlPFC rTMS impacts emotion processing in HCs, but the neural mechanisms through which these effects occur may partly depend on the paradigm used, which differ between these studies, and are thus in need of further study.

These results are not in line with a recently published multilevel framework on explicit and implicit emotion regulation (18), since the dlPFC is associated with explicitly controlled emotion regulation whereas no effect of dlPFC stimulation on reappraisal was found within this study. The effects on emotion processing reported here may have been caused by (subthreshold) activity changes beyond the site of stimulation that have previously been reported in rTMS studies (66), although none of these effects were found in the fMRI analyses. It is possible that other stimulation targets will render different results; the dmPFC and insula have, for example, been suggested as alternative targets for rTMS stimulation treatment in substance use disorder (67).

Although expected, we did not find any effect of rTMS on experienced emotion, or related brain activity in response to alcohol-related images. This may be explained by the variation in image content, individual preferences for certain alcohol-related contexts, or specific beverage preferences. The images used in the emotion reappraisal task consisted of different variations of alcoholic beverages (beer, wine, and liquor) and alcohol-related contexts (e.g., bar and supermarket). Alcohol-related images may elicit different (e.g., positive and/or negative emotional) responses in AUD patients specifically, due to the psychological burden of having an AUD, and it is possible that these individual differences thus did not result in consistent emotional and brain responses in the AUD group. Increasing the sample size or selecting a subsample of, e.g., beer- or wine-preferring AUD patients, in order to analyze subgroups with specific preferences could clarify these results in future studies.

Finally, in our previous study within this special issue (68), we show that the emotion reappraisal task increases craving levels in both AUD patients and HCs, and that AUD patients have higher overall craving levels. In the current study, we show not only that rTMS affects craving levels differently in AUD patients and HCs but also that the time by stimulation interaction was not significant. These results do not support our hypothesis that rTMS reduces craving levels compared to sham stimulation and are not in line with our meta-analysis on this topic (31), but suggest an accidental preexisting difference in craving levels between the stimulation groups. Furthermore, AUD patients were not eligible for participation when actively using psychoactive medication, including anti-craving medication, due to possible confounding effects on the fMRI data. However, inclusion of non-medicated AUD patients may have resulted in a selection bias. Possibly, these nonmedicated patients are (compared to medicated patient samples) less prone to craving and less susceptible to induction of craving by the emotion reappraisal task. Also, recent reviews (29, 30) suggest that neurostimulation techniques may be more effective in reducing craving for substance use disorder patients when applying more (and longer) stimulation sessions. Finally, although the current study included a larger sample compared to previous neurostimulation and fMRI studies on emotion processing and reappraisal, the sample is still modest, requiring larger effect sizes (or more neurostimulation sessions) to obtain significant results. Future studies should therefore apply more stimulation sessions in a larger AUD sample in order to establish if the rTMS effects reported in this paper are clinically relevant.

Conclusion and Future Directions

This study is the first study that indicates differential effects of sham and high-frequency right dlPFC rTMS on emotion processing, reappraisal ability, and related brain functions in AUD patients and HCs. Subjective experienced emotion during the emotion reappraisal task was reduced after right dlPFC rTMS in AUD patients, but increased the subjective experience in HCs. This possibly indicates an rTMS-related impact on emotion processing of emotional (but not alcohol-related) images in AUD patients. rTMS stimulation changed brain activity in various emotion reappraisal relevant brain areas but did not reduce craving levels in AUD patients. Future studies should replicate and expand the current study, for instance, by assessing the effect of multiple stimulation sessions on both explicit and implicit emotion regulation paradigms and craving, and assess the effect of rTMS within subgroups with specific addiction-relevant image preferences.

AUTHOR CONTRIBUTIONS

All authors made a significant contribution to this article, including acquiring funding (AG, WB), study design (AG, WB), development of the emotion reappraisal task (SW, OH, DV, YD), data acquisition (JJ), data analysis (JJ, DV, SW), interpretation of results (JJ, AG, SW, OH, YD, WB, DV), and contributions to this manuscript (JJ, AG, SW, OH, YD, WB, DV).

REFERENCES

1. Lim SS, Vos T, Flaxman AD, Danaei G, Shibuya K, Adair-Rohani H, et al. A comparative risk assessment of burden of disease and injury attributable to 67 risk factors and risk factor clusters in 21 regions, 1990–2010: a systematic analysis for the Global Burden of Disease Study 2010. *Lancet* (2013) 380(9859):2224–60. doi: 10.1016/S0140-6736(12)61766-8
2. Whiteford HA, Ferrari AJ, Degenhardt L, Feigin V, Vos T. Global burden of disease attributable to mental and substance use disorders: findings from the Global Burden of Disease Study 2010. *Lancet* (2013) 382(9904):1575–86. doi: 10.1016/S0140-6736(13)61611-6
3. World Health Organization. *The global status report on alcohol and health 2011*. Geneva (2011).
4. Compton WM, Thomas YF, Stinson FS, Grant BF. Prevalence, correlates, disability, and comorbidity of DSM-IV drug abuse and dependence in the United States: results from the national epidemiologic survey on alcohol and related conditions. *Arch Gen Psychiatry* (2007) 64(5):566–76. doi: 10.1001/archpsyc.64.5.566
5. Kessler RC, Chiu WT, Demler O, Walters EE. Prevalence, severity, and comorbidity of 12-month DSM-IV disorders in the National Comorbidity Survey replication. *Arch Gen Psychiatry* (2005) 62(6):617–27. doi: 10.1001/archpsyc.62.6.617
6. Wittchen HU, Jacobi F, Rehm J, Gustavsson A, Svensson M, Jonsson B, et al. The size and burden of mental disorders and other disorders of the brain in Europe 2010. *Eur Neuropsychopharmacol* (2011) 21(9):655–79. doi: 10.1016/j.euroneuro.2011.07.018
7. Feil J, Sheppard D, Fitzgerald PB, Yucel M, Lubman DI, Bradshaw JL. Addiction, compulsive drug seeking, and the role of frontostriatal mechanisms in regulating inhibitory control. *Neurosci Biobehav Rev* (2010) 35(2):248–75. doi: 10.1016/j.neubiorev.2010.03.001
8. Hester R, Lubman DI, Yücel M. The role of executive control in human drug addiction. In *Behavioral neuroscience of drug addiction*. Berlin, Heidelberg: Springer (2010). pp. 301–18.
9. Verdejo-García A, Bechara A, Recknor EC, Perez-Garcia M. Executive dysfunction in substance dependent individuals during drug use and abstinence: an examination of the behavioral, cognitive and emotional correlates of addiction. *J Int Neuropsychol Soc* (2006) 12(3):405–15. doi: 10.1017/S1355617706060486
10. Leyton M, Vezina P. Striatal ups and downs: their roles in vulnerability to addictions in humans. *Neurosci Biobehav Rev* (2013) 37(9 pt a):1999–2014. doi: 10.1016/j.neubiorev.2013.01.018
11. Verdejo-Garcia APGM, Pérez-García M, Bechara A. Emotion, decision-making and substance dependence: a somatic-marker model of addiction. *Curr Neuropharmacology* (2006) 4(1):17–31. doi: 10.2174/157015906775203057
12. Wilcox CE, Pommy JM, Adinoff B. Neural circuitry of impaired emotion regulation in substance use disorders. *Am J Psychiatry* (2016) 173(3):344–61. doi: 10.1176/appi.ajp.2015.15060710
13. Ochsner KN, Gross JJ. The cognitive control of emotion. *Trends Cogn Sci* (2005) 9(5):242–9. doi: 10.1016/j.tics.2005.03.010
14. Sher KJ, Grekin ER. Alcohol and affect regulation. In: Gross JJ, editor. *Handbook of emotion regulation*. New York, NY: Guilford Press (2007). p. 560–80.
15. Kim SM, Han DH, Min KJ, Kim BN, Cheong JH. Brain activation in response to craving-and aversion-inducing cues related to alcohol in patients with alcohol dependence. *Drug Alcohol Depend* (2014) 141:124–31. doi: 10.1016/j.drugalcdep.2014.05.017
16. Sinha R, Fox HC, Hong KA, Bergquist K, Bhagwagar Z, Siedlarz KM. Enhanced negative emotion and alcohol craving, and altered physiological responses following stress and cue exposure in alcohol dependent individuals. *Neuropsychopharmacology* (2008) 34(5):1198–208. doi: 10.1038/npp.2008.78
17. Sinha R, Garcia M, Paliwal P, Kreek MJ, Rounsaville BJ. Stress-induced cocaine craving and hypothalamic–pituitary–adrenal responses are predictive of cocaine relapse outcomes. *Arch Gen Psychiatry* (2006) 63(3):324–31. doi: 10.1001/archpsyc.63.3.324
18. Braunstein LM, Gross JJ, Ochsner KN. Explicit and implicit emotion regulation: a multi-level framework. *Soc Cogn Affect Neurosci* (2017) 12(10):1545–57. doi: 10.1093/scan/nsx096
19. Simons JS, Carey KB, Wills TA. Alcohol abuse and dependence symptoms: a multidimensional model of common and specific etiolog. *Psychol Addict Behav* (2009) 23(3):415. doi: 10.1037/a0016003
20. Baker TB, Piper ME, McCarthy DE, Majeskie MR, Fiore MC. Addiction motivation reformulated: an affective processing model of negative reinforcement. *Psychol Rev* (2004) 111(1):33. doi: 10.1037/0033-295X.111.1.33
21. Birch CD, Stewart SH, Wall AM, McKee SA, Eisnor SJ, Theakston JA. Mood-induced increases in alcohol expectancy strength in internally motivated drinkers. *Psychol Addict Behav* (2004) 18(3):231. doi: 10.1037/0893-164X.18.3.231
22. Magill M, Ray LA. Cognitive-behavioral treatment with adult alcohol and illicit drug users: a meta-analysis of randomized controlled trials. *J Stud Alcohol Drugs* (2009) 70(4):516–27. doi: 10.15288/jsad.2009.70.516
23. Martin GW, Rehm J. The effectiveness of psychosocial modalities in the treatment of alcohol problems in adults: a review of the evidence. *Can J Psychiatry* (2012) 57(6):350–8. doi: 10.1177/070674371205700604
24. Reus VI, Fochtmann LJ, Bukstein O, Eyler AE, Hilty DM, Horvitz-Lennon M, et al. The American Psychiatric Association practice guideline for the pharmacological treatment of patients with alcohol use disorder. *Am J Psychiatry* (2017) 175(1):86–90. doi: 10.1176/appi.ajp.2017.1750101
25. Jonas DE, Amick HR, Feltner C, Bobashev G, Thomas K, Wines R, et al. Pharmacotherapy for adults with alcohol use disorders in outpatient settings: a systematic review and meta-analysis. *JAMA* (2014) 311(18):1889–900. doi: 10.1001/jama.2014.3628
26. Merkx MJ, Schippers GM, Koeter MW, Vuijk PJ, Poch M, Kronemeijer H, et al. WM. Predictive validity of treatment allocation guidelines on drinking outcome in alcohol-dependent patients. *Addict Behav* (2013) 38(3):1691–98. doi: 10.1016/j.addbeh.2012.09.011
27. Moos RH, Moos BS. Rates and predictors of relapse after natural and treated remission from alcohol use disorders. *Addiction* (2006) 101(2):212–22. doi: 10.1111/j.1360-0443.2006.01310.x

28. Schippers GM, Broekman TG. The course of alcohol dependence; the course of alcohol dependence. *The State of the Art*. Den Haag: ZonMw. (2006).
29. Coles AS, Kozak K, George TP. A review of brain stimulation methods to treat substance use disorders. *Am J Addict* (2018) 27(2):71–91. doi: 10.1111/ajad.12674
30. Salling MC, Martinez D. Brain stimulation in addiction *Neuropsychopharmacology* (2016) 41(12):2798. doi: 10.1038/npp.2016.80
31. Jansen JM, Daams JG, Koeter MW, Veltman DJ, van den Brink W, Goudriaan AE. Effects of non-invasive neurostimulation on craving: a meta-analysis. *Neurosci Biobehav Rev* (2013) 37(10):2472–80. doi: 10.1016/j.neubiorev.2013.07.009
32. Guse B, Falkai P, Wobrock T. Cognitive effects of high-frequency repetitive transcranial magnetic stimulation: a systematic review. *J Neural Transm* (2010) 117(1):105–22. doi: 10.1007/s00702-009-0333-7
33. Schluter R, Daams J, van Holst RJ, Goudriaan AE. Effects of noninvasive neuromodulation on executive and other cognitive functions in addictive disorders: a systematic review. *Front Neurosci* (2018) 12:642. doi: 10.3389/fnins.2018.00642
34. Vanderhasselt MA, Baeken C, Hendricks M, De Raedt R. The effects of high frequency rTMS on negative attentional bias are influenced by baseline state anxiety. *Neuropsychologia* (2011) 49(7):1824–30. doi: 10.1016/j.neuropsychologia.2011.03.006
35. Möbius M, Lacomblé L, Meyer T, Schutter DJ, Gielkens T, Becker ES, et al. Repetitive transcranial magnetic stimulation modulates the impact of a negative mood induction. *Soc Cogn Affect Neurosci* (2017) 12(4):526–33. doi: 10.1093/scan/nsw180
36. Choi KM, Scott DT, Lim SL. The modulating effects of brain stimulation on emotion regulation and decision-making. *Neuropsychiatr Electrophysiol* (2016) 2(1):4. doi: 10.1186/s40810-016-0018-z
37. De Raedt R, Leyman L, Baeken C, Van Schuerbeek P, Luypaert R, Vanderhasselt MA, et al. Neurocognitive effects of HF-rTMS over the dorsolateral prefrontal cortex on the attentional processing of emotional information in healthy women: an event-related fMRI study. *Biol Psychol* (2010) 85(3):487–95. doi: 10.1016/j.biopsycho.2010.09.015
38. Berger C, Domes G, Balschat J, Thome J, Höppner J. Effects of prefrontal rTMS on autonomic reactions to affective pictures. *J Neural Transm* (2017) 124(1):139–52. doi: 10.1007/s00702-015-1491-4
39. Zwanzger P, Steinberg CR, AM, Bröckelmann AKD, Zavorotnyy M, Junghöfer M. Inhibitory repetitive transcranial magnetic stimulation (rTMS) of the dorsolateral prefrontal cortex modulates early affective processing. *Neuroimage* (2014) 101:193–203. doi: 10.1016/j.neuroimage.2014.07.003
40. Schutter DJ, van Honk J. The cerebellum in emotion regulation: a repetitive transcranial magnetic stimulation study. *Cerebellum* (2009) 8(1):28–34. doi: 10.1007/s12311-008-0056-6
41. Moulier V, Gaudeau-Bosma C, Isaac C, Allard AC, Bouaziz N, Sidhoumi D, et al. Effect of repetitive transcranial magnetic stimulation on mood in healthy subjects. *Socioaffect Neurosci Psychol* (2016) 6(1):29672. doi: 10.3402/snp.v6.29672
42. Notzon S, Steinberg C, Zwanzger P, Junghöfer M. Modulating emotion perception: opposing effects of inhibitory and excitatory prefrontal cortex stimulation. *Biol Psychiatry* (2018) 3(4):329–36. doi: 10.1016/j.bpsc.2017.12.007
43. De Wit SJ, van der Werf YD, Mataix-Cols D, Trujillo JP, van Oppen P, Veltman DJ, et al. Emotion regulation before and after transcranial magnetic stimulation in obsessive compulsive disorder. *Psychol Med* (2015) 45(15):3059–73. doi: 10.1017/S0033291715001026
44. Axelrod SR, Perepletchikova F, Holtzman K, Sinha R. Emotion regulation and substance use frequency in women with substance dependence and borderline personality disorder receiving dialectical behavior therapy. *Am J Drug Alcohol Abuse* (2011) 37(1):37–42. doi: 10.3109/00952990.2010.535582
45. Berking M, Wupperman P, Reichardt A, Pejic T, Dippel A, Znoj H. Emotion-regulation skills as a treatment target in psychotherapy. *Behav Res Ther* (2008) 46(11):1230–7. doi: 10.1016/j.brat.2008.08.005
46. World Health Organisation. *Composite international diagnostic interview.* Geneva. (1990).
47. Babor TF, Higgins-Biddle JC, Saunders JB, Monteiro MG. The alcohol use disorders identification test. In: *Department of mental health and substance dependence (Ed)., Guidelines for use in primary care.* World Health Organisation (2001).
48. Beck AT, Steer RA, Carbin MG. Psychometric properties of the beck depression inventory: twenty-five years of evaluation. *Clin Psychol Rev* (1988) 8(1):77–100. doi: 10.1016/0272-7358(88)90050-5
49. Beck AT, Epstein N, Brown G, Steer RA. An inventory for measuring clinical anxiety: psychometric properties. *J Consult Clin Psychol* (1988) 56(6):893. doi: 10.1037/0022-006X.56.6.893
50. Kooiman CG, Spinhoven P, Trijsburg RW. The assessment of alexithymia: a critical review of the literature and a psychometric study of the Toronto Alexithymia Scale-20. *J Psychosom Res* (2002) 53(6):1083–90. doi: 10.1016/S0022-3999(02)00348-3
51. Gross JJ, John OP. Individual differences in two emotion regulation processes: implications for affect, relationships, and well-being. *J Pers Soc Psychol* (2003) 85(2):348.
52. Bohn MJ, Krahn DD, Staehler BA. Development and initial validation of a measure of drinking urges in abstinent alcoholics. *Alcohol Clin Exp Res* (1995) 19(3):600–6. doi: 10.1111/j.1530-0277.1995.tb01554.x
53. Lang S, Bradley MM, Cuthbert BN. International Affective Picture System (IAPS): technical manual and affective ratings. In: *Center for research in Psychophysiology*. Gainesville: University of Florida (1999).
54. Vollstädt-Klein S, Loeber S, Kirsch M, Bach P, Richter A, Bühler M, et al. Effects of cue-exposure treatment on neural cue reactivity in alcohol dependence: a randomized trial. *Biol Psychiatry* (2011) 69(11):1060–6. doi: 10.1016/j.biopsych.2010.12.016
55. Bradley MM, Lang PJ. Measuring emotion: the self-assessment manikin and the semantic differential. *J Behav Ther Exp Psychiatry* (1994) 25(1):49–59. doi: 10.1016/0005-7916(94)90063-9
56. Rossi S, Hallett M, Rossini PM, Pascual-Leone A, The Safety of TMS Consensus Group. Safety, ethical considerations, and application guidelines for the use of transcranial magnetic stimulation in clinical practice and research. *Clin Neurophysiol* (2009) 120:2008–39. doi: 10.1016/j.clinph.2009.08.016
57. Fox PT, Lancaster JL. Neuroscience on the Net. *Science* (1994) 266(5187):994–6. doi: 10.1126/science.7973682
58. Berlim MT, Broadbent HJ, Van den Eynde F. Blinding integrity in randomized sham-controlled trials of repetitive transcranial magnetic stimulation for major depression: a systematic review and meta-analysis. *Int J Neuropsychopharmacol* (2013) 16(5):1173–81. doi: 10.1017/S1461145712001691
59. Choi JS, Kim MJ, Kim JH, Choi JY, Chung YE, Park MS, et al. Comparison of multi-echo and single-echo gradient-recalled echo sequences for SPIO-enhanced liver MRI at 3 T. *Clin Radiol* (2010) 65(11):916–23. doi: 10.1016/j.crad.2010.07.003
60. Boschloo L, Vogelzangs N, Smit JH, van den Brink W, Veltman DJ, Beekman AT, et al. Comorbidity and risk indicators for alcohol use disorders among persons with anxiety and/or depressive disorders: findings from the Netherlands Study of Depression and Anxiety (NESDA). *J Affect Disord* (2011) 131(1):233–42. doi: 10.1016/j.jad.2010.12.014
61. Cruise KE, Becerra R. Alexithymia and problematic alcohol use: a critical update. *Addict Behav* (2017) 77:232–46. doi: 10.1016/j.addbeh.2017.09.025
62. Stevens J. *Applied multivariate statistics for the social sciences*. 3rd ed. Routledge (1996). p. 323.
63. Fox HC, Bergquist KL, Hong KI, Sinha R. Stress-induced and alcohol cue-induced craving in recently abstinent alcohol-dependent individuals. *Alcohol Clin Exp Res* (2007) 31(3):395–403. doi: 10.1111/j.1530-0277.2006.00320.x
64. Sinha R. How does stress lead to risk of alcohol relapse? *Alcohol Res* (2011) 34(4):432–40.
65. Gaynes BN, Lloyd SW, Lux L, Gartlehner G, Hansen RA, Brode S, et al. Repetitive transcranial magnetic stimulation for treatment-resistant depression: a systematic review and meta-analysis. *Psychol Med* (2014) 44(2):225–39. doi: 10.4088/JCP.13r08815
66. Baeken C, De Raedt R, Van Schuerbeek P, Vanderhasselt MA, De Mey J, Bossuyt A, et al. Right prefrontal HF-rTMS attenuates right amygdala processing of negatively valenced emotional stimuli in healthy females. *Behav Brain Res* (2010) 214(2):450–5. doi: 10.1016/j.bbr.2010.06.029
67. Luigjes J, Segrave R, de Joode N, Figee M, Denys D. Efficacy of invasive and non-invasive brain modulation interventions for addiction. *Neuropsychol Rev* (2018) 1–23. doi: 10.1007/s11065-018-9393-5

3

Network Alterations in Comorbid Chronic Pain and Opioid Addiction: An Exploratory Approach

Rachel F. Smallwood[1†], *Larry R. Price*[2], *Jenna L. Campbell*[3], *Amy S. Garrett*[4], *Sebastian W. Atalla*[5], *Todd B. Monroe*[5], *Semra A. Aytur*[6], *Jennifer S. Potter*[4] and *Donald A. Robin*[3,7*†]

[1] National Institute of Neurological Disorders and Stroke, National Institutes of Health, Bethesda, MD, United States, [2] Methodology, Measurement and Statistical Analysis, Texas State University, San Marcos, TX, United States, [3] Department of Communication Sciences and Disorders, University of New Hampshire, Durham, NH, United States, [4] Department of Psychiatry, University of Texas Health Science Center San Antonio, San Antonio, TX, United States, [5] College of Nursing, The Ohio State University, Columbus, OH, United States, [6] Department of Health Management and Policy, University of New Hampshire, Durham, NH, United States, [7] Interdisciplinary Program in Neuroscience and Behavior, University of New Hampshire, Durham, NH, United States

***Correspondence:**
Donald A. Robin
don.robin@unh.edu

[†] All data were collected and analyzed while RS and DR were at the Research Imaging Institute, University of Texas Health Science Center San Antonio, San Antonio, TX, United States

The comorbidity of chronic pain and opioid addiction is a serious problem that has been growing with the practice of prescribing opioids for chronic pain. Neuroimaging research has shown that chronic pain and opioid dependence both affect brain structure and function, but this is the first study to evaluate the neurophysiological alterations in patients with comorbid chronic pain and addiction. Eighteen participants with chronic low back pain and opioid addiction were compared with eighteen age- and sex-matched healthy individuals in a pain-induction fMRI task. Unified structural equation modeling (SEM) with Lagrange multiplier (LM) testing yielded a network model of pain processing for patient and control groups based on 19 *a priori* defined regions. Tests of differences between groups on specific regression parameters were determined on a path-by-path basis using *z*-tests corrected for the number of comparisons. Patients with the chronic pain and addiction comorbidity had increased connection strengths; many of these connections were interhemispheric and spanned regions involved in sensory, affective, and cognitive processes. The affected regions included those that are commonly altered in chronic pain or addiction alone, indicating that this comorbidity manifests with neurological symptoms of both disorders. Understanding the neural mechanisms involved in the comorbidity is crucial to finding a comprehensive treatment, rather than treating the symptoms individually.

Keywords: chronic low back pain, opioid addiction, fMRI, pain induction, unified structural equation modeling, vector autoregressive modeling, automated search strategy

INTRODUCTION

There is a high prevalence of comorbid chronic pain and opioid addiction, presenting a serious healthcare challenge that has become an epidemic in the United States (Rosenblum et al., 2003; Clark et al., 2008; Barry et al., 2013; Salsitz, 2016). Independently, chronic pain and opioid addiction are difficult to treat, and the comorbidity only increases the difficulty with diagnosis and treatment of the disorders. Patients with a substance use disorder (SUD) and co-occurring physical pain have increased cravings (Tsui et al., 2016) and are more likely to misuse opioids than SUD patients without pain (Potter et al., 2008; Dennis et al., 2015). Impulsive tendencies in chronic pain patients indicate a high risk of illicit opioid use (Vest et al., 2016). As well, opioid use is anticorrelated with pain acceptance and lower pain acceptance rates were associated with higher opioid use rates, but pain intensity had no relationship with opioid use (Lin et al., 2015). Chronic pain is positively associated with substance use disorder severity, psychiatric disorders, psychological distress, medical comorbidities, general physical health problems, medical care utilization, and poorer psychosocial function (Jamison et al., 2000; Rosenblum et al., 2003; Potter et al., 2004; Trafton et al., 2004; Arnow et al., 2006; Tunks et al., 2008; Dominick et al., 2012; Burke et al., 2015; Howe et al., 2015). These comorbid factors are associated with relapse into substance use (Potter et al., 2010) and poor treatment outcomes.

The above challenges are compounded by the fact that opioids are often prescribed as treatment for chronic pain conditions. The effect sizes for opioid treatments are negligible, the associated risks, especially for those of dependency, are high (Ballantyne and LaForge, 2007; Noble et al., 2010). Additionally, chronic opioid use can result in opioid-induced hyperalgesia, increasing pain sensitivity (Lee et al., 2011; Stoicea et al., 2015). Thus, there is a great need for further research addressing the comorbidity of chronic pain (Noble et al., 2010; Chou et al., 2015; Dowell et al., 2016; Volkow and McLellan, 2016). The Centers for Disease Control and Prevention recently released a report providing a set of guidelines for clinicians on prescribing opioids for chronic pain, and the first guideline states that non-pharmacologic and non-opioid pharmacologic treatments should be considered before opioids. If opioids are prescribed, it should be at the lowest effective dose for the shortest duration, and non-pharamcologic therapies, such as mindfulness-based or behavioral therapy approaches, and follow-up monitoring should be used in conjunction (Dowell et al., 2016).

In regard to the brain, pain sensation is not only a peripheral physical phenomenon. Acute pain sensation induces widespread activation spanning regions including the anterior cingulate cortex (ACC), insula, somatosensory cortices, thalamus, basal ganglia, and prefrontal cortices (Tracey, 2005; Chen et al., 2008; May, 2008; Schweinhardt and Bushnell, 2010; Davis and Moayedi, 2013; Schmidt-Wilcke, 2015; Jensen et al., 2016; Morton et al., 2016). Chronic pain disorders often manifest altered processing in and interactions between many of those regions during pain tasks and at rest (Apkarian et al., 2001; Gracely et al., 2002; Moisset and Bouhassira, 2007; Napadow et al., 2010; Baliki et al., 2011; Cifre et al., 2012; Davis and Moayedi, 2013; Schmidt-Wilcke, 2015; Jensen et al., 2016; Martucci and Mackey, 2016; Morton et al., 2016), and chronic pain patients exhibit activation in pain-related structures at lower stimulation levels than healthy controls (Gracely et al., 2002; Giesecke et al., 2004). A recent meta-analysis showed healthy individuals have increased activation likelihood due to painful stimulation in the ACC, insula, and thalamus than chronic pain (Jensen et al., 2016). In addition, gray matter volume and cortical thickness are also decreased in many of the same regions, primarily the ACC, thalamus, basal ganglia, insula, and dorsolateral prefrontal cortex (DLPFC) (Apkarian et al., 2001; May, 2008, 2011; Schmidt-Wilcke, 2008; Davis and Moayedi, 2013; Ivo et al., 2013; Smallwood et al., 2013; Alshuft et al., 2016; Yang et al., 2017). In individuals with CLBP, 1 month of oral morphine consumption resulted in gray matter increases and decreases in pain and reward-related structures (Lin et al., 2016).

Opioid dependence and addiction also affect brain structure and function. Differences in regional dynamics in drug-cue task fMRI have been observed in the ACC, insula, prefrontal cortices, caudate, thalamus, putamen, hippocampus, and amygdala (Langleben et al., 2008; Yang et al., 2009; Wang et al., 2010, 2011, 2014; Lou et al., 2012; Li et al., 2013; Schmidt et al., 2014, 2015b). These regions and the nucleus accumbens exhibit altered functional connectivity at rest in opioid-dependent subjects and heroin addicts (Ma et al., 2010, 2015; Upadhyay et al., 2010; Schmidt et al., 2015a; Zhang et al., 2015). Structurally, opioid-dependent subjects have significantly less gray matter volume bilaterally in the amygdala and nucleus accumbens (Upadhyay et al., 2010; Seifert et al., 2015; Lin et al., 2016) and in frontal and temporal areas (Qiu et al., 2014; Lin et al., 2016; Wollman et al., 2016) and increased gray matter volume in the cingulate (Lin et al., 2016). Administration of oral morphine to healthy subjects undergoing pain stimulation caused the pain-related activations to have smaller spatial extent (Hansen et al., 2015).

Treatment for these disorders must be driven by principles of neural plasticity. Specifically, positive treatment outcomes are linked to targeting neural structures that support a given function. This is known as the "specificity" principle because it has been shown that neural plasticity must specifically target those brain regions or networks that have changed from their normal state (Kleim and Jones, 2008; Cramer et al., 2011). Hence, extensive knowledge of both healthy and abnormal brain structures involved in pain processing and reward circuitry is necessary. While knowledge of the neural substrates of chronic pain or opioid addiction alone is substantial, there are no data on the comorbid disorders, hampering treatment development. It is likely that pain and SUD comorbidity causes complex and unique effects on neural organization. We hypothesize that the comorbidity will result in similar changes but with larger magnitudes than in either of the two disorders alone, and that these synergistic effects will extend to unique brain regions.

Complex functions are supported by a connected network of brain regions, and understanding the function of each region of the network and network connectivity properties is important in determining the underlying neural substrates of disorders. The comorbidity of pain and SUD along with other usual symptoms (e.g., depression, anxiety, and sleep disturbances) makes the typical approach to imaging analysis (e.g., group analysis of conditional contrasts) difficult to use since each impairment contributes distinct neurophysiological response patterns. Hence, this study uses a connectivity approach to understanding this comorbid disorder. Because this clinical population has not been investigated with neuroimaging until now, in this experiment we used an exploratory approach to connectivity analysis that is ideal given the vast possibilities for regional changes. This approach allows for a large number of regions to be entered into the analyses. Further, exploratory connectivity analyses allow for study of neural networks without the bias of preconceived hypotheses and can drive more detailed analyses that focus on the specific neural systems implicated in a disorder.

In this study, the first aim was to identify an optimal network of brain regions and study their connectivity based on coherence of regional activities for patient and healthy control groups. Given that the brain data on the individual comorbid conditions are not available, we argue that we are justified in using a healthy control group in this first study. Much is known about the neuroscience of chronic pain and addiction independently, however, the comorbid patient population is yet unstudied. To accomplish this, we used a unified structural equation modeling (SEM) approach (Kim et al., 2007) that provides a framework for estimating contemporaneous and temporal or lagged relationships through a multivariate vector autoregressive model in conjunction with an automated Lagrange multiplier (LM) model testing strategy (Gates et al., 2010). Our second aim was to determine if statistical differences in magnitude existed between groups based on regional alterations. The network structure identified in aim one was evaluated to determine if statistical differences existed between patient and control groups for each path specific to the magnitude and sign of the regression weights.

TABLE 1 | Participant demographics and assessment results.

	HC	CPOA matched
Subjects (N)	18	18
Gender	10 males, 8 females	10 males, 8 females
Age (years)	39.5 ± 12.4	39.2 ± 12.8
Acceptance and action questionnaire II (AAQ-II)	62.0 ± 9.0*	39.2 ± 9.0
Mindfulness Attention Awareness Scale (MAAS)	4.8 ± 0.9*	3.6 ± 0.9
Visual analog scale (VAS), opioid craving	0.0 ± 0.0	2.4 ± 2.6
Visual analog scale (VAS), interference	0.0 ± 0.0*	3.7 ± 2.0
Visual analog scale (VAS), intensity	0.0 ± 0.0*	3.8 ± 2.1
Roland Morris Disability Questionnaire (RMDQ, %)	–	53.0 ± 24.5

*Averages and standard deviations listed; HC, healthy controls; *healthy controls significantly different from matched patients, $p \leq 0.001$.*

MATERIALS AND METHODS

Eighteen (39.2 ± 12.8 years; 10 males) opioid-addicted individuals with chronic low back pain were recruited from methadone clinics in San Antonio, TX. Eighteen healthy (39.5 ± 12.4 years) individuals were recruited as sex and age (within ±3 years) matches to the patients. Patients met the requirements for current DSM-IV opioid dependence, were currently enrolled in opioid replacement therapy (i.e., methadone maintenance or buprenorphine therapy) for more than 30 days, and had been experiencing chronic low back pain for at least 12 months at a level of 5 or greater on a 0 to 10 rating scale. Control participants had no drug use within the past 30 days, had no drug dependence within the past year, rated their pain-related functional interference as less than 2 on a scale from 0 to 10, and considered themselves healthy. This study was carried out in accordance with the recommendations of the University of Texas Health Science Center San Antonio's Internal Review Board with written informed consent from all subjects. All subjects gave written informed consent in accordance with the Declaration of Helsinki.

Participants completed a battery of paper questionnaires to assess pain and addiction severity, including the Acceptance and Action Questionnaire II (AAQ-II; Bond et al., 2011), the Mindfulness Attention Awareness Scale (MAAS; Brown and Ryan, 2003), the Roland Morris Disability Questionnaire (RMDQ; Roland and Morris, 1983), and the visual analog scale for opioid craving, interference, and intensity (VAS; McMillan and Gilmore-Thomas, 1996). All demographic and assessment data have been included in **Table 1**. While outside of the scanner, participants also underwent a threshold test to determine their individualized pain stimulation levels. Pain stimuli were delivered via pressure to the right thumbnail with a pneumatic device.

Patients underwent a 16-min pain induction fMRI task containing 8 triplets of 5-s painful pressure blocks (pressure the subjects rated as 40/100 on a pain scale) and 8 triplets of 5-s innocuous pressure blocks (pressure that was not rated as painful), each followed by rest periods. An anatomical scan for registration was also collected. Data were collected using a 3T Siemens TIM Trio scanner (fMRI TR/TE/tip angle/slices/voxel size = 2500 ms/30 ms/90°/36/1.72 × 1.72 × 3 mm; aMRI TR/TE/TI/flip angle/voxel size = 2200 ms/2.8 ms/766 ms/13°/1 × 1 × 1 mm). The pain task fMRI data were pre-processed and analyzed using SPM8. To begin, motion parameters were observed across the entire time series of the scan. If a subject had a large spike in motion (≥1 mm/TR), the ArtRepair toolbox was used to interpolate signal from the preceding and following volumes. Then either the raw data (if no motion correction was needed) or the artifact-repaired data were realigned and resliced, coregistered to the anatomical image, transformed into MNI standard space using the transformation derived from the segmented anatomical image, and then smoothed with an 8 mm FWHM kernel. The functional time series for each volume of interest (VOI) was extracted, normalized, and adjusted for motion. Each VOI was centered on the coordinate specified in **Table 2** and was spherical with a 6 mm radius. The 19 regions subjected to analyses are included in **Table 2**. The effective sample size was $N = 1153$ in the control group (pain condition) and $N = 1153$ in the patient group (pain condition). The effective sample size was $N = 6912$ for the control group under all experimental conditions (pain + innocuous + rest) and $N = 6903$ for the patient group under all experimental conditions.

ANALYTIC STRATEGY

In functional connectivity studies, the goal includes modeling the temporal effect of neural activation in one region in relation

TABLE 2 | Volumes of interest included in model 2.

Region	X	Y	Z	Abbreviation
Left insula	−40	6	2	lIns
Right insula	41	15	1	rIns
Dorsal anterior cingulate cortex	3	36	22	dACC
Left amygdala	−23	−3	−17	lAmyg
Right amygdala	23	−4	−16	rAmyg
Left dorsolateral prefrontal cortex	−31	43	22	lDLPFC
Right dorsolateral prefrontal cortex	41	39	24	rDLPFC
Left putamen	−25	0	5	lPut
Right putamen	25	7	2	rPut
Left caudate	−12	4	13	lCaud
Right caudate	15	9	14	rCaud
Left thalamus	−13	−11	16	lThal
Right thalamus	9	−11	7	rThal
Left primary somatosensory cortex	−57	−24	23	lS1
Right primary somatosensory cortex	58	−24	21	rS1
Left precuneus	−18	−57	34	lPrecun
Right precuneus	19	−57	35	rPrecun
Left nucleus accumbens	−9	6	−4	lNAcc
Right nucleus accumbens	9	6	−4	rNAcc

Center coordinates in MNI space of 6 mm radius spheres provided.

to another region. However, each observation (single fMRI volume) is partly a function of the previous within-subject observation due to the multiple volumes collected for each subject. The interdependence among the observations within subjects is manifested in the within-subject residual error of regression for one observation at time t (contemporaneous component) correlating with the previous measurement at time t-1 (temporal component). The autoregressive effect is typically positive thereby biasing the standard errors of regression estimates downward, yielding F-statistics with inflated statistical significance (Bingenheimer and Raudenbush, 2004). Kim et al. (2007) provided a unified SEM approach that allows for estimation of contemporaneous relations (e.g., at time t) among ROIs controlling for sequential dependencies present in fMRI data structures. The unified SEM approach also provides a framework for estimating vector autoregressive parameters (i.e., lagged relationships – time t-1) after controlling for contemporaneous effects. For example, interest may lie in the effect of region X at time t-1 on region Y at time t (current time). This autoregressive analytic approach is then expanded throughout the multivariate regression (network) model to estimate the path loadings throughout the network (Kim et al., 2007; Price, 2012).

Thus, the unified SEM approach advances current techniques by providing a flexible, dynamic approach for simultaneously estimating contemporaneous and lagged relationships between ROIs. Although Granger Causality Modeling can be used to estimate lagged relationships, biased estimates may result from failing to consider contemporaneous relations (Gates et al., 2010). Dynamic causal modeling (DCM) is another approach that can be used to study event-related data. However, DCM is limited to modeling contemporaneous change, whereas the unified SEM is appropriate for simultaneously modeling contemporaneous and lagged effects. Additionally, DCM is used for confirmatory analysis, while the unified SEM approach is appropriate for either confirmatory or exploratory analysis. Because it is entirely data-driven, the unified SEM offers a substantial degree of flexibility when compared to alternative approaches (Gates et al., 2010, 2011; Guàrdia-Olmos et al., 2018).

Identifying the Network Structure

Prior to analyses, we conducted data screening to evaluate the time series properties of the data. Data screening included evaluating (a) the stationarity or non-stationarity of the time series, (b) the time period between observations to determine the lag structure (e.g., lag-1, lag-2, or lag-3) and (c) the autocorrelation and partial autocorrelation functions. Results of the data screening (i.e., autocorrelation and partial autocorrelation plots of residuals) revealed a stationary, white noise process with a lag-1, the time series best representing the series (Box et al., 2015).

The present study was exploratory given the lack of previous research on the comorbidity of chronic pain and opioid addiction. Therefore, although the regions of interest were selected *a priori*, no network model of functional connectivity between those regions was posited *a priori*. Consequently, we employed a search strategy involving LM testing with forward selection starting with a null model (no regression paths among regions) then sequentially added additional parameters one step at a time (Chou and Bentler, 1990; Gates et al., 2010). This process continued until the first non-significant path loading was observed. This search algorithm was conducted using Linear Structural Relations (LISREL), version 9.2 (Jöreskog and Sörbom, 2015). **Table 3** provides the fit statistics for the final model for the patient and control groups. **Supplementary Tables S1, S2** show all the connections present in the optimal models in all subjects for all conditions and the pain condition, respectively. To compare connections between groups, a Z-test was employed on the Fisher's Z for each connection for each group.

RESULTS

Almost every connection in the model was significantly different between groups because there was such a large sample size;

TABLE 3 | Summary fit statistics pain condition, all conditions.

	Control	Patients	Controls	Patients
X^2	2520.64	4594.89	11341.75	23431.75
df	590	590	590	590
p	<0.001	<0.001	<0.001	<0.001
CFI	0.93	0.90	0.92	0.92
RMSEA	0.05	0.07	0.05	0.07
Stability Index	0.46	0.51	0.53	0.53

X^2-test of overall model fit; df, degrees of freedom; p, probability level; CF, comparative fit index; RMSEA, root mean square error of approximation; Stability Index is a measure of system stability in a non-recursive structural equation model (Fox, 1980; Bentler and Freeman, 1983). Pain condition, left; all conditions, right.

therefore, an effect size (Cohen's q; Cohen, 1988) was calculated to distinguish the most relevant and meaningful differences. The results and discussion will focus on the connections that were significantly different between patients and controls with at least a moderate effect size ($q \geq 0.3$). The between group differences for all connections (regardless of effect size) can be seen in **Supplementary Tables S1, S2**. All of the significantly different connection strengths with large or moderate effect sizes were greater in patients than in control subjects. Although there were some connection strengths that were greater in controls than patients, as indicated by a negative z-score, effect sizes for these comparisons were small ($q \leq 0.21$ for all conditions, $q \leq 0.19$ for pain condition only).

For the time series with all conditions included, the connections that differed significantly with large or moderate effect sizes were the connection between the right thalamus and dACC (effect size q = 0.58, lag q = 0.70), the right S1 and left caudate (q = 0.59, lag q = 0.58), the right insula and left NAcc (q = 0.57, lag q = 0.34), the right amygdala to left amygdala (q = 0.53, lag q = 0.57), the right insula and right caudate (lag q = 0.40), the right insula to left caudate (q = 0.38), the right caudate and left caudate (q = 0.37), and the right insula and left insula (q = 0.31). See **Figures 1, 2**.

During the pain conditions, there were only connection strength differences with moderate effect sizes. These connections were between the right S1 and left caudate (q = 0.34, lag q = 0.43), the right insula and right caudate (lag q = 0.41), the right caudate and left caudate (q = 0.38), the right insula and left NAcc (q = 0.35), right insula and left caudate (q = 0.34), right S1 and right thalamus (lag q = 0.34), right thalamus and dACC (lag q = 0.33), and the right caudate and right precuneus (lag q = 0.32). See **Figures 3, 4**.

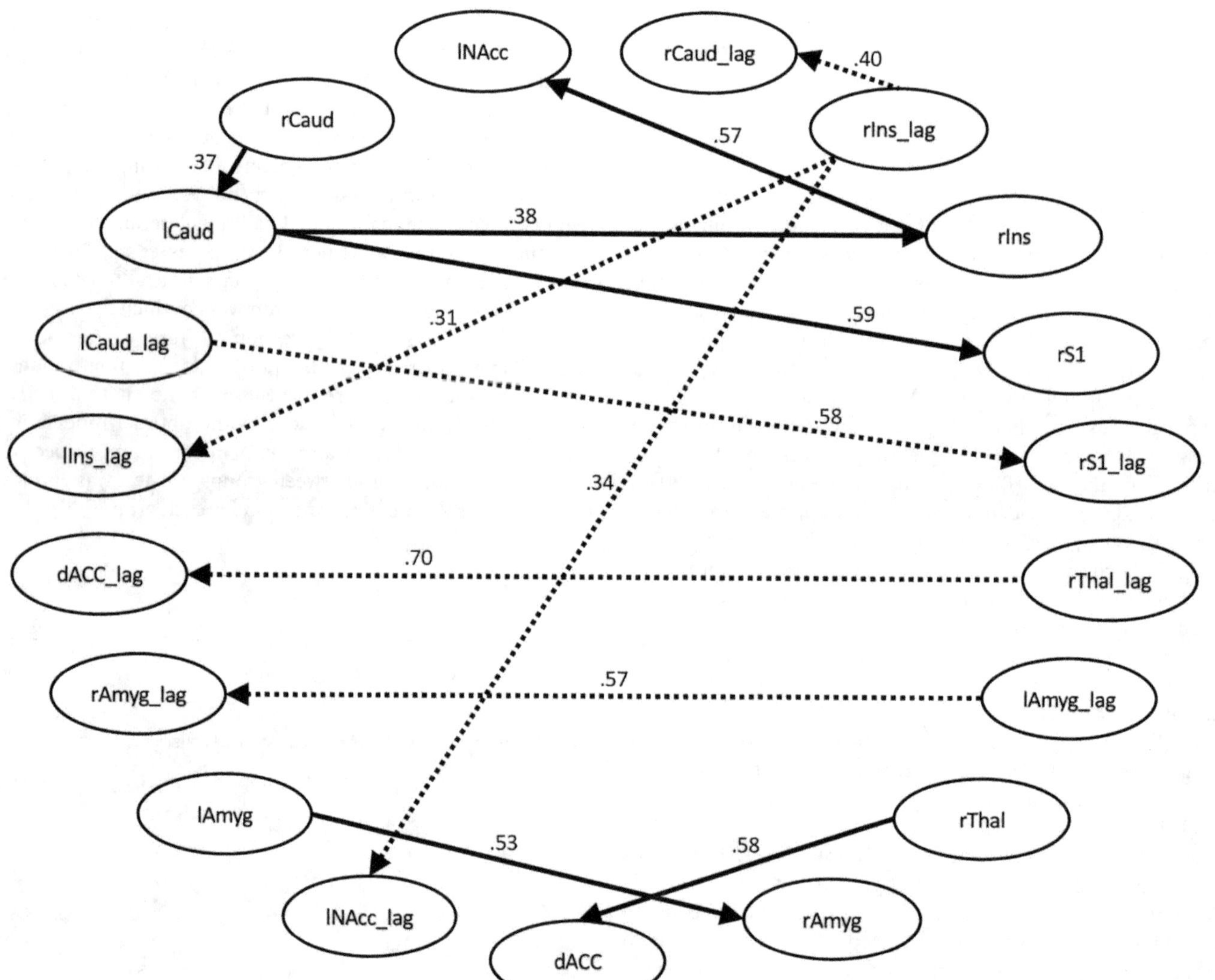

FIGURE 1 | Structural equation modeling network model – all. Patient and Control Groups, All Conditions. Numbers on paths are effect sizes representing the difference between Controls and Patients under all conditions.

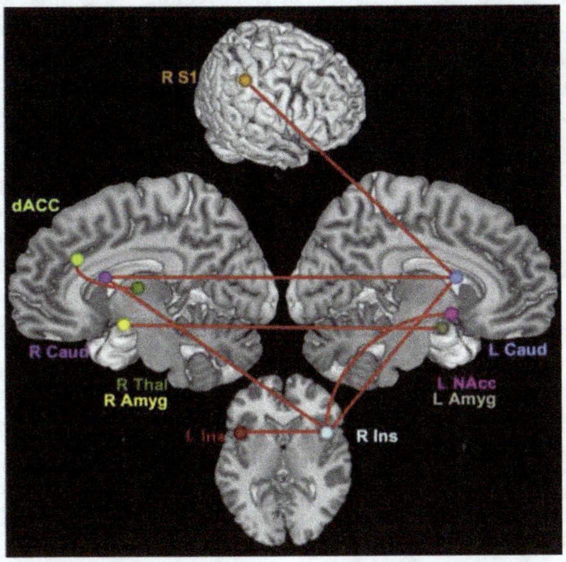

FIGURE 2 | Brain network regions – all. Connections that differed significantly between groups with a moderate or large effect size for all conditions.

DISCUSSION

This study is to our knowledge the first to characterize the neural networks underlying comorbid chronic pain and opioid addiction. Our results indicate that the network changes occurring in patients with this comorbidity reflect a combination of the changes observed in chronic pain and addiction alone. Because of the novelty of the population we used an exploratory analysis to determine the network model via SEM using an automated search algorithm that implements LM testing. Group differences were quantified based on this network model. Hence, the critical analysis from these data is the quantification of coupling properties between model regions. Specifically, higher connection values denote stronger connection strengths, with the inference being two regions with similar temporal activity fluctuations are working in concert during the processing of stimuli. The connections that varied between groups, demonstrating a medium or greater effect size ($|q| \geq 0.3$), reflected *higher connection strengths* in patients compared with controls (positive q). This indicates an increase in coherence of activity between seed regions during painful stimulation in opioid- addicted patients with CLBP compared to healthy subjects.

Previous studies in chronic pain have also reported altered connectivity in patients at rest, showing differences in the default mode network (DMN) (Baliki et al., 2008, 2014; Napadow et al., 2010; Bolwerk et al., 2013; Otti et al., 2013; Kucyi et al., 2014; Hemington et al., 2016; Mansour et al., 2016; Letzen and Robinson, 2017; Yang et al., 2017), executive attention network (Napadow et al., 2010), salience network (Otti et al., 2013; Hemington et al., 2016), in the insula, ACC, and basal ganglia (Malinen et al., 2010; Cifre et al., 2012; Schwedt et al., 2013;

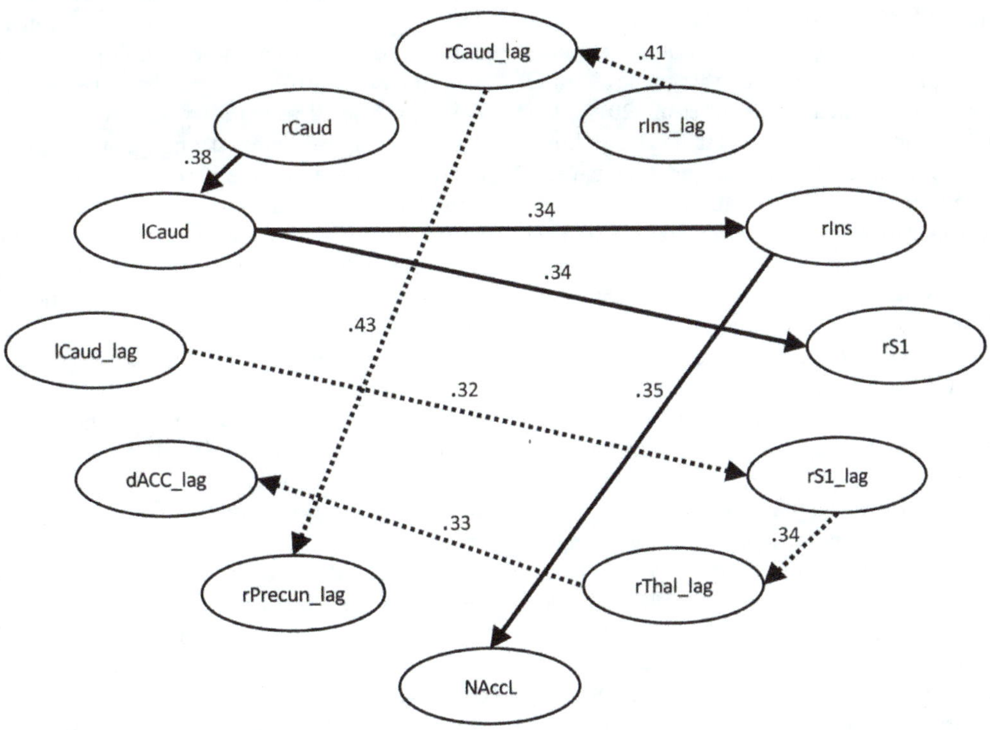

FIGURE 3 | Structural equation modeling network model – pain. Patient and Control Groups, Pain Condition. Numbers on paths are effect sizes representing the difference between Controls and Patients under pain condition only.

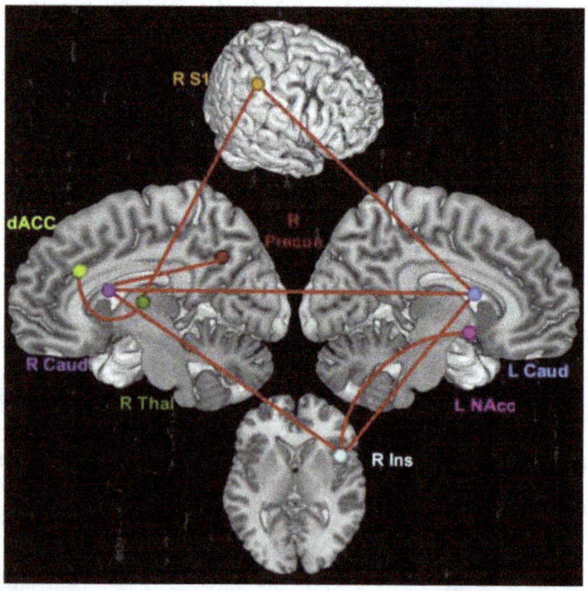

FIGURE 4 | Brain network regions – pain. Connections that differed significantly between groups with a moderate effect size for the pain condition.

Yang et al., 2017), during spontaneous back pain (Hashmi et al., 2013), and during painful stimulation (Baliki et al., 2010; Jensen et al., 2013). Similar connectivity alterations have been observed in opioid-dependent and -addicted populations, with the alterations occurring in amygdala, insula, NAcc, prefrontal cortex (Ma et al., 2010; Upadhyay et al., 2010; Zhang et al., 2011; Schmidt et al., 2014, 2015b), orbitofrontal cortex, caudate, parahippocampus, lingual gyrus, precuneus, middle temporal gyrus (Chang et al., 2016), putamen, posterior cingulate (Schmidt et al., 2015a), and anterior cingulate (Zhang et al., 2015). Our results, coupled with existing literature, indicate both conditions likely contribute to connectivity alterations and that patients' neurophysiological responses to induced pain are characterized by stronger connections between regions than normal controls' responses. This increased synchronicity between regions in patients could reflect an increase in communication with more information being passed between the regions; it could also be indicative of an alteration in a common upstream or regulatory region that is passed to its downstream effectors. Whatever the mechanism, these patterns are consistent with central sensitization (Ng et al., 2017); the neuroplastic changes that occur in chronic pain could lead to regions being more functionally connected than necessary for typical pain processing.

The regions with differing connections are not only regions associated with sensory discrimination of pain (S1, thalamus, insula), but also regions that are involved in the emotional response to pain (insula, caudate, amygdala, dACC) and higher-level regulation and integration of pain signals (caudate, nucleus accumbens, dACC) (Tracey, 2005; Chen et al., 2008; May, 2008; Baliki et al., 2010; Schweinhardt and Bushnell, 2010). If individuals with chronic pain and opioid addiction simply had lower pain thresholds, we would expect to see differences primarily, or even exclusively, in sensorimotor regions. The increased coupling strength of sensory regions with others could partially underlie differences from normal. However, the diverse functional nature of regions with stronger connectivity signifies that this population likely has a heightened multi-dimensional response to pain (i.e., sensory, affective, and cognitive), not just in pain sensation. This is in agreement with a finding that chronification of back pain coincides with a shift of processing from more sensory/acute pain circuits to affective circuits (Hashmi et al., 2013), and CLBP patients appear to have more alterations in regions associated with emotion and cognition than in nociceptive regions (Woolf, 2011). Another interesting trend was many of the significant connections with moderate effect sizes were interhemispheric, indicating that although the painful stimulation was only applied on the right thumb, pain processing in this clinical population seems to be characterized by increased bilateral engagement. This is an intriguing consideration in the context of a recent study of normal pain processing that revealed higher pain stimulus levels resulted in increased interhemispheric DLPFC connectivity (Sevel et al., 2016). Perhaps the constant state of pain in the patients causes these plastic changes in bilateral connections.

Additionally, considering the task used in this study highlights an important trend in the regional connectivity. A pain induction paradigm would assume activation and coordination of thalamus and S1 which primarily encode the sensory aspects of pain. However, another important feature to note in the difference network is that, other than thalamus and S1, all of the regions are altered in both diagnoses independently. The observable differences manifesting in regions that overlap between chronic pain and opioid addiction is consistent with the suggestion of chronic pain and addiction following similar neuroadaptation patterns based on a common neural substrate foundation (Elman and Borsook, 2016). It could be that these are regions where the two disorders work synergistically to cause alterations. This finding provides strong support for the development of treatments that simultaneously treat the two disorders, rather than treating one and/or the other independently. Though there have only been a couple of clinical studies with this approach, they have promising results for patients with comorbid chronic pain and opioid addiction (Ilgen et al., 2016; Smallwood et al., 2016).

The observed increases in connectivity likely are not only related to the actual pain stimulus, but evince aberrant connectivity due to addiction. The NAcc is a central part of reward circuitry (Martin-Soelch et al., 2001) and is altered in opioid-dependent subjects (Ma et al., 2010; Upadhyay et al., 2010). It was also predictive of the effect of pain stimuli on chronic pain in a pain induction study in chronic back pain (Baliki et al., 2010). Its role here suggests its participation could be part of a mechanism underlying the emotional response to pain in the form of a trigger for the substance dependence-related response. This is consistent with the between-group difference in its connection with the insula. The insula has a key role in pain processing, being responsible for both sensory and affective aspects of pain (Tracey, 2005; Chen et al., 2008; Schweinhardt and Bushnell, 2010). In painful stimulation of healthy subjects, it was shown that its connectivity shifted with modulation of attention and emotion (Ploner et al., 2011). The insula is also one of the regions commonly activated in tasks when heroin addicts are shown heroin cues in the scanner (Langleben et al., 2008; Lou et al., 2012). Naqvi and Bechara (2010) proposed a drug cue-induced model of processing that includes a connection between the insula and NAcc. They hypothesized that observing a cue previously associated with partaking of a particular addictive substance would activate a network in which the insula acts as a gate to allow previous experiences of the substance's effects to intensify the urge use, represented by the nucleus accumbens within the reward system. Perhaps in this population painful sensations and their affective sequelae trigger the association of the analgesic effect of opioids, thus increasing the individual's craving for pain relief and the high experienced from the opioids. This highlights a unique challenge to treating addiction and dependence in patients with comorbid chronic pain: if the presence of the pain creates an additional drive for substance use, these individuals could be fighting an even stronger impulse to use. Furthermore, qualitative research suggests that patients with comorbid chronic pain and SUD perceive that healthcare providers are not treating their pain and addiction in an integrated manner (St. Marie, 2014), thereby generating heightened cravings and perpetuating substance misuse.

The caudate is hypothesized to be responsible for regulating the affective response to pain (Borsook et al., 2010), so the connection between S1 and caudate is likely a pathway for transduction from a sensory-only experience to a multi-dimensional experience that includes affective and higher order cognitive/regulatory components. The increased connectivity in patients between the caudate and the precuneus during the pain only condition could be indicative of an increased affective response to pain in patients due to increased pain sensitivity (Goffaux et al., 2014). The amygdala receives nociceptive inputs from the brain, but also encodes a plethora of affective processes (Veinante et al., 2013) and has been linked with craving-relating activation in response to drug cues in opioid-dependent subjects (Murphy et al., 2017). The bilateral amygdala connection differing significantly could imply an increase in the emotional response to pain, but since the difference was observed only in the time series with all conditions (including rest and innocuous pressure) and not during pain induction alone, perhaps it signifies patients having an increased fearful response or negative anticipation of the coming pain compared with controls.

It is important to underline here that since we are not reporting longitudinal or structural MRI data, we cannot conclude on the neural network and morphological changes that may have occurred in the patient group after withdrawing from opioids. All patients had been enrolled in an opioid replacement therapy program for at least 30 days prior to data collection. Fingelkurts et al. (2009) reported that measures of local and remote electroencephalogram (EEG) functional connectivity of opioid-dependent patients treated with methadone for 6 months did not differ significantly from normal values observed in healthy controls. Studies of medication-overuse headache (MOH), which has also been associated with psychiatric comorbidities, report that in some patients gray matter volume changes reverted to normal state after a period of drug withdrawal. Namely, an increase in gray matter in the orbitofrontal cortex and a decrease in periaqueductal gray region of the midbrain were observed and these changes positively correlated with treatment response (Riederer et al., 2013; Lai et al., 2016). To address this issue, future studies should include both longitudinal and voxel-based morphometry (VBM) data.

Our study provides a novel approach to modeling network structure and connectivity patterns, though we address a few limitations here. First, the population of opioid-addicted individuals with chronic pain was very heterogeneous. Ideal exclusion criteria should include a variety of psychiatric disorders. However, this population included participants with a range of comorbid psychiatric conditions such as depression, anxiety, bipolar disorder, and schizophrenia. Nearly every participant self-reported some type of psychiatric condition, often more than one. This is consistent with data reported in a review by Kelly and Daley (2013), stating that 27% of people with SUD have at least one psychiatric disorder and 45% of people with psychiatric conditions actually have two or more disorders (Kessler et al., 2005). These conditions were self-reported, and had they been excluded there would not have been a large enough population to conduct a study with this comorbidity. Second, another constraint that plagues studies of comorbidities is that it is unknown how two (or more) comorbid disorders interact and whether they interact uniformly in all patients. This introduces the potential for more heterogeneity, and these sources of heterogeneity are one of the primary impetuses for using an exploratory approach. Additionally, any differences observed cannot be ascribed to one diagnosis or the other, as we only have the comorbid patient population and a negative control population. Future studies should have positive control groups including subjects with only chronic low back pain and only opioid addiction. However, we feel strongly that although we cannot specifically attribute any of these differences or characteristics to one diagnosis, the other, or the comorbidity, these results still provide essential knowledge about a pragmatic clinical population (Ford and Norrie, 2016) that represents one of our current significant healthcare challenges.

CONCLUSION

The results presented here show that in a network determined via an exploratory SEM analysis, opioid-addicted chronic pain patients had increased connectivity in regions that are affected in both disorders independently. These increases likely indicate altered emotional responses to pain as well as addiction-related neurophysiological reactions, signifying that this comorbidity may act in a synergistic way to exacerbate neural alterations.

This analytic approach represents a novel and interesting way to examine connectivity data. The SEM allowed for defining and refining an optimal network for all subjects. The feature of the SEM that allowed for a large number of regions to be included in the model was invaluable from the exploratory side of the analysis. Because this is a novel population for neuroimaging study, having few restrictions on the number of regions (nodes) of interest included in the model and requiring no *a priori* hypotheses about model structure allowed a broader investigation of the potential relationships and alterations between brain regions in this cohort.

AUTHOR CONTRIBUTIONS

RS conducted all the study aspects, development, implementation, interpretation, and wrote the manuscript. LP developed the connectivity models, assisted in model interpretation, and ran all the statistical tests on model connections and wrote the manuscript. JC, SAA, TM, SWA, and AG contributed to proofreading, provided the input into final document, assisted with writing and interpretation of the data, and contributed pertinent supporting references. JP assisted in study design, interpretation of data, and wrote the manuscript. DR supervised and was invovled in all aspects of study development, implementation, analysis, and interpretation.

ACKNOWLEDGMENTS

The authors thank Harvir Virk and Anneliese New for their contributions in data collection.

REFERENCES

1. Alshuft, H. M., Condon, L. A., Dineen, R. A., and Auer, D. P. (2016). Cerebral cortical thickness in chronic pain due to knee osteoarthritis: the effect of pain duration and pain sensitization. *PLoS One* 11:e0161687. doi: 10.1371/journal. pone.0161687
2. Apkarian, A. V., Thomas, P. S., Krauss, B. R., and Szeverenyi, N. M. (2001). Prefrontal cortical hyperactivity in patients with sympathetically mediated chronic pain. *Neurosci. Lett.* 311, 193–197. doi: 10.1016/s0304-3940(01) 02122-x
3. Arnow, B. A., Hunkeler, E. M., Blasey, C. M., Lee, J., Constantino, M. J., Fireman, B., et al. (2006). Comorbid depression, chronic pain, and disability in primary care. *Psychosom. Med.* 68, 262–268. doi: 10.1097/01. psy.0000204851.15499.fc
4. Baliki, M. N., Baria, A. T., and Apkarian, A. V. (2011). The cortical rhythms of chronic back pain. *J. Neurosci.* 31, 13981–13990. doi: 10.1523/ JNEUROSCI. 1984-11.2011
5. Baliki, M. N., Geha, P. Y., Apkarian, A. V., and Chialvo, D. R. (2008). Beyond feeling: chronic pain hurts the brain, disrupting the default-mode network dynamics. *J. Neurosci.* 28, 1398–1403. doi: 10.1523/ JNEUROSCI.4123-07.2008
6. Baliki, M. N., Geha, P. Y., Fields, H. L., and Apkarian, A. V. (2010). Predicting value of pain and analgesia: nucleus accumbens response to noxious stimuli changes in the presence of chronic pain. *Neuron* 66, 149–160. doi: 10.1016/j. neuron.2010.03.002
7. Baliki, M. N., Mansour, A. R., Baria, A. T., and Apkarian, A. V. (2014). Functional reorganization of the default mode network across chronic pain conditions. *PLoS One* 9:e106133. doi: 10.1371/journal.pone.0106133
8. Ballantyne, J. C., and LaForge, K. S. (2007). Opioid dependence and addiction during opioid treatment of chronic pain. *Pain* 129, 235–255. doi: 10.1016/j.pain. 2007.03.028
9. Barry, D. T., Savant, J. D., Beitel, M., Cutter, C. J., Moore, B. A., Schottenfeld,R. S., et al. (2013). Pain and associated substance use among opioid dependent individuals seeking office-based treatment with buprenorphine-naloxone: a needs assessment study. *Am. J. Addict.* 22, 212–217. doi: 10.1111/j.1521-0391. 2012.00327.x
10. Bentler, P. M., and Freeman, E. H. (1983). Tests for stability in linear structural equation systems. *Psychometrika* 48, 143–145. doi: 10.1007/ bf02314682
11. Bingenheimer, J. B., and Raudenbush, S. W. (2004). Statistical and substantive inferences in public health: issues in the application of multilevel models. *Annu. Rev. Public Health* 25, 53–77. doi: 10.1146/ annurev.publhealth.25.050503. 153925
12. Bolwerk, A., Seifert, F., and Maihofner, C. (2013). Altered resting-state functional connectivity in complex regional pain syndrome. *J. Pain* 14:e8. doi: 10.1016/j. jpain.2013.04.007
13. Bond, F. W., Hayes, S. C., Baer, R. A., Carpenter, K. M., Guenole, N., Orcutt, H. K., et al. (2011). Preliminary psychometric properties of the acceptance and action questionnaire - II: a revised measure of psychological flexibility and experiential avoidance. *Behav. Ther.* 42, 676–688. doi: 10.1016/j.beth.2011.03.007
14. Borsook, D., Upadhyay, J., Chudler, E. H., and Becerra, L. (2010). A key role of the basal ganglia in pain and analgesia–insights gained through human functional imaging. *Mol. Pain* 6, 1–17. doi: 10.1186/1744-8069-6-27
15. Box, G. E., Jenkins, G. M., Reinsel, G. C., and Ljung, G. M. (2015). *Time Series Analysis: Forecasting and Control.* Hoboken, NJ: John Wiley & Sons.
16. Brown, K. W., and Ryan, R. M. (2003). The benefits of being present: mindfulness and its role in psychological well-being. *J. Pers. Soc. Psychol.* 84, 822–848. doi: 10.1037/0022-3514.84.4.822
17. Burke, A. L., Mathias, J. L., and Denson, L. A. (2015). Psychological functioning of people living with chronic pain: a meta-analytic review. *Br. J. Clin. Psychol.* 54, 345–360. doi: 10.1111/bjc.12078
18. Chang, H., Li, W., Li, Q., Chen, J., Zhu, J., Ye, J., et al. (2016). Regional homogeneity changes between heroin relapse and non-relapse patients under methadone maintenance treatment: a resting-state fMRI study. *BMC Neurol.* 16:145. doi: 10.1186/s12883-016-0659-3
19. Chen, F. Y., Tao, W., and Li, Y. J. (2008). Advances in brain imaging of neuropathic pain. *Chin. Med. J.* 121, 653–657. doi: 10.1097/00029330-200804010-00015
20. Chou, C.-P., and Bentler, P. M. (1990). Model modification in covariance structure modeling: acomparison among likelihood ratio. lagrange multiplier, and wald tests. *Multivar. Beh. Res.* 25, 115–136. doi: 10.1207/ s15327906mbr2501_13
21. Chou, R., Turner, J. A., Devine, E. B., Hansen, R. N., Sullivan, S. D., Blazina, I., et al. (2015). The effectiveness and risks of long-term opioid therapy for chronic pain: a systematic review for a national institutes of health pathways to prevention workshop. *Ann. Intern. Med.* 162, 276–286. doi: 10.7326/M14- 2559
22. Cifre, I., Sitges, C., Fraiman, D., Munoz, M. A., Balenzuela, P., Gonzalez-Roldan, A., et al. (2012). Disrupted functional connectivity of the pain network in fibromyalgia. *Psychosom. Med.* 74, 55–62. doi: 10.1097/ PSY.0b013e31824 08f04
23. Clark, M. R., Stoller, K. B., and Brooner, R. K. (2008). Assessment and management of chronic pain in individuals seeking treatment for opioid dependence disorder. *Can. J. Psychiatry* 53, 496–508. doi: 10.1177/070674370805300804

24. Cohen, J. (1988). *Statistical Power Analysis for the Behavioral Sciences*, 2nd Edn. Hillsdale, NJ: Lawrence Erlbaum Associates.
25. Cramer, S. C., Sur, M., Dobkin, B. H., O'Brien, C., Sanger, T. D., Trojanowski, J. Q., et al. (2011). Harnessing neuroplasticity for clinical applications. *Brain* 134, 1591–1609. doi: 10.1093/brain/awr039
26. Davis, K. D., and Moayedi, M. (2013). Central mechanisms of pain revealed through functional and structural MRI. *J. Neuroimmune Pharmacol.* 8, 518– 534. doi: 10.1007/s11481-012-9386-8
27. Dennis, B. B., Bawor, M., Naji, L., Chan, C. K., Varenbut, J., Paul, J., et al. (2015). Impact of chronic pain on treatment prognosis for patients with opioid use disorder: a systematic review and meta-analysis. *Subst. Abuse* 9, 59–80. doi: 10.4137/SART.S30120
28. Dominick, C. H., Blyth, F. M., and Nicholas, M. K. (2012). Unpacking the burden: understanding the relationships between chronic pain and comorbidity in the general population. *Pain* 153, 293–304. doi: 10.1016/j.pain.2011.09.018
29. Dowell, D., Haegerich, T. M., and Chou, R. (2016). CDC guideline for prescribing opioids for chronic pain - United States. *MMWR Recomm. Rep.* 65, 1–49. doi: 10.15585/mmwr.rr6501e1
30. Elman, I., and Borsook, D. (2016). Common brain mechanisms of chronic pain and addiction. *Neuron* 89, 11–36. doi: 10.1016/j.neuron.2015.11.027
31. Fingelkurts, A. A., Fingelkurts, A. A., Kivisaari, R., Autti, T., Borisov, S., Puuskari, V., et al. (2009). Methadone restores local and remote EEG functional connectivity in opioid-dependent patients. *Int. J. Neurosci.* 119, 1469–1493. doi: 10.1080/00207450903007985
32. Ford, I., and Norrie, J. (2016). Pragmatic trials. *N. Engl. J. Med.* 375, 454–463. doi: 10.1056/NEJMra1510059
33. Fox, J. (1980). Effect analysis in structural equation models: extensions and simplified methodsof computation. *Sociol. Methods Res.* 9, 3–28. doi: 10.1177/ 004912418000900101
34. Gates, K. M., Molenaar, P. C., Hillary, F., and Slobounov, S. (2011). Extended unified SEM approach for modeling event-related fMRI data. *Neuroimage* 54, 1151–1158. doi: 10.1016/j.neuroimage.2010.08.051
35. Gates, K. M., Molenaar, P. C., Hillary, F. G., Ram, N., and Rovine, M. J. (2010). Automatic search for fMRI connectivity mapping: an alternative to granger causality testing using formal equivalences among SEM path modeling. VAR, and unified SEM. *Neuroimage* 50, 1118–1125. doi: 10.1016/j.neuroimage.2009. 12.117
36. Giesecke, T., Gracely, R. H., Grant, M. A., Nachemson, A., Petzke, F., Williams, D. A., et al. (2004). Evidence of augmented central pain processing in idiopathic chronic low back pain. *Arthritis Rheum.* 50, 613–623. doi: 10.1002/art.20063
37. Goffaux, P., Girard-Tremblay, L., Marchand, S., Daigle, K., and Whittingstall, K. (2014). Individual differences in pain sensitivity vary as a function of precuneus reactivity. *Brain Topogr.* 27, 366–374. doi: 10.1007/s10548-013-0291-0
38. Gracely, R. H., Petzke, F., Wolf, J. M., and Clauw, D. J. (2002). Functional magnetic resonance imaging evidence of augmented pain processing in fibromyalgia. *Arthritis Rheum.* 46, 1333–1343. doi: 10.1002/art.10225
39. Guàrdia-Olmos, J., Peró-Cebollero, M., and Gudayol-Ferré, E. (2018). Meta- Analysis of the structural equation models' parameters for the estimation of brain connectivity with fMRI. *Front. Behav. Neurosci.* 12:19. doi: 10.3389/fnbeh. 2018.00019
40. Hansen, T. M., Olesen, A. E., Graversen, C., Drewes, A. M., and Frokjaer, J. B. (2015). The effect of oral morphine on pain-related brain activation - an experimental functional magnetic resonance imaging study. *Basic Clin. Pharmacol. Toxicol.* 117, 316–322. doi: 10.1111/bcpt.12415
41. Hashmi, J. A., Baliki, M. N., Huang, L., Baria, A. T., Torbey, S., Hermann, K. M., et al. (2013). Shape shifting pain: chronification of back pain shifts brain representation from nociceptive to emotional circuits. *Brain* 136, 2751–2768. doi: 10.1093/brain/awt211
42. Hemington, K. S., Wu, Q., Kucyi, A., Inman, R. D., and Davis, K. D. (2016). Abnormal cross-network functional connectivity in chronic pain and its association with clinical symptoms. *Brain Struct. Funct.* 221, 4203–4219. doi: 10.1007/s00429-015-1161-1
43. Howe, C. Q., Robinson, J. P., and Sullivan, M. D. (2015). Psychiatric and psychological perspectives on chronic pain. *Phys. Med. Rehabil. Clin. N. Am.* 26, 283–300. doi: 10.1016/j.pmr.2014.12.003
44. Ilgen, M. A., Bohnert, A. S., Chermack, S., Conran, C., Jannausch, M., Trafton, J., et al. (2016). A randomized trial of a pain management intervention for adults receiving substance use disorder treatment. *Addiction* 111, 1385–1393. doi: 10.1111/add.13349
45. Ivo, R., Nicklas, A., Dargel, J., Sobottke, R., Delank, K. S., Eysel, P., et al. (2013). Brain structural and psychometric alterations in chronic low back pain. *Eur. Spine J.* 22, 1958–1964. doi: 10.1007/s00586-013-2692-x
46. Jamison, R. N., Kauffman, J., and Katz, N. P. (2000). Characteristics of methadone maintenance patients with chronic pain. *J. Pain Symptom Manage.* 19, 53–62. doi: 10.1016/s0885-3924(99)00144-x
47. Jensen, K. B., Regenbogen, C., Ohse, M. C., Frasnelli, J., Freiherr, J., and Lundstrom, J. N. (2016). Brain activations during pain: a neuroimaging meta-analysis of patients with pain and healthy controls. *Pain* 157, 1279–1286. doi: 10.1097/j. pain.0000000000000517
48. Jensen, K. B., Srinivasan, P., Spaeth, R., Tan, Y., Kosek, E., Petzke, F., et al. (2013). Overlapping structural and functional brain changes in patients with long-term exposure to fibromyalgia pain. *Arthritis Rheum.* 65, 3293–3303. doi: 10.1002/ art.38170
49. Jöreskog, K. G., and Sörbom, D. (2015). *LISREL. 9*, 20 Edn. Skokie, IL: Scientific Software International, Inc.
50. Kelly, T. M., and Daley, D. C. (2013). Integrated treatment of substance use and psychiatric disorders. *Soc. Work Public Health* 28, 388–406. doi: 10.1080/ 19371918.2013.774673
51. Kessler, R. C., Berglund, P., Demler, O., Jim, R., Merikangas, K. R., and Walters, E. E. (2005). Life time prevalence and age of onset distributions of DSM-IV disorders in the national comorbidity survey replication. *Arch. Gen. Psychiatry* 62, 593–602. doi: 10.1001/archpsyc.62.6.593
52. Kim, J., Zhu, W., Chang, L., Bentler, P. M., and Ernst, T. (2007). Unified structural equation modeling approach for the analysis of multisubject, multivariate functional MRI data. *Hum. Brain Mapp.* 28, 85–93. doi: 10.1002/hbm. 20259
53. Kleim, J. A., and Jones, T. A. (2008). Principles of experience-dependent neural plasticity: implications for rehabilitation after brain damage. *J. Speech Lang. Hear. Res.* 51, S225–S239. doi: 10.1044/1092-4388(2008/018)
54. Kucyi, A., Moayedi, M., Weissman-Fogel, I., Goldberg, M. B., Freeman, B. V., Tenenbaum, H. C., et al. (2014). Enhanced medial prefrontal-default mode network functional connectivity in chronic pain and its association with pain rumination. *J. Neurosci.* 34, 3969–3975. doi: 10.1523/ JNEUROSCI.5055-13. 2014
55. Lai, T. H., Chou, K. H., Fuh, J. L., Lee, P. L., Kung, Y. C., Lin, C. P., et al. (2016). Gray matter changes related to medication overuse in patients with chronic migraine. *Cephalalgia* 36, 1324–1333. doi: 10.1177/0333102416630593
56. Langleben, D. D., Ruparel, K., Elman, I., Busch-Winokur, S., Pratiwadi, R., Loughead, J., et al. (2008). Acute effect of methadone maintenance dose on brain fMRI response to heroin-related cues. *Am. J. Psychiatry* 165, 390–394. doi: 10.1176/appi.ajp.2007.07010070
57. Lee, M., Silverman, S. M., Hansen, H., Patel, V. B., and Manchikanti, L. (2011). A comprehensive review of opioid-induced hyperalgesia. *Pain Phys.* 14, 145–161.

58. Letzen, J. E., and Robinson, M. E. (2017). Negative mood influences default mode network functional connectivity in patients with chronic low back pain: implications for functional neuroimaging biomarkers. *Pain* 158, 48–57. doi: 10.1097/j.pain.0000000000000708
59. Li, Q., Yang, W. C., Wang, Y. R., Huang, Y. F., Li, W., Zhu, J., et al. (2013). Abnormal function of the posterior cingulate cortex in heroin addicted users during resting-state and drug-cue stimulation task. *Chin. Med. J.* 126, 734–739.
60. Lin, J. C., Chu, L. F., Stringer, E. A., Baker, K. S., Sayyid, Z. N., Sun, J., et al. (2016). One month of oral morphine decreases gray matter volume in the right amygdala of individuals with low back pain: confirmation of previously reported magnetic resonance imaging results. *Pain Med.* 17, 1497–1504. doi: 10.1093/pm/pnv047
61. Lin, L. A., Bohnert, A. S., Price, A. M., Jannausch, M., Bonar, E. E., and Ilgen, M. A. (2015). Pain acceptance and opiate use disorders in addiction treatment patients with comorbid pain. *Drug Alcohol Depend.* 157, 136–142. doi: 10.1016/ j.drugalcdep.2015.10.017
62. Lou, M., Wang, E., Shen, Y., and Wang, J. (2012). Cue-elicited craving in heroin addicts at different abstinent time: an fMRI pilot study. *Subst. Use Misuse* 47, 631–639. doi: 10.3109/10826084.2011.646381
63. Ma, N., Liu, Y., Li, N., Wang, C. X., Zhang, H., Jiang, X. F., et al. (2010). Addiction related alteration in resting-state brain connectivity. *Neuroimage* 49, 738–744. doi: 10.1016/j.neuroimage.2009.08.037
64. Ma, X., Qiu, Y., Tian, J., Wang, J., Li, S., Zhan, W., et al. (2015). Aberrant default- mode functional and structural connectivity in heroin-dependent individuals. *PLoS One* 10:e0120861. doi: 10.1371/journal.pone.0120861
65. Malinen, S., Vartiainen, N., Hlushchuk, Y., Koskinen, M., Ramkumar, P., Forss, N., et al. (2010). Aberrant temporal and spatial brain activity during rest in patients with chronic pain. *Proc. Natl. Acad. Sci. U.S.A.* 107, 6493–6497. doi: 10.1073/pnas.1001504107
66. Mansour, A., Baria, A. T., Tetreault, P., Vachon-Presseau, E., Chang, P. C., Huang, L., et al. (2016). Global disruption of degree rank order: a hallmark of chronic pain. *Sci. Rep.* 6, 1–17. doi: 10.1038/srep34853
67. Martin-Soelch, C., Leenders, K. L., Chevalley, A. F., Missimer, J., Kunig, G., Magyar, S., et al. (2001). Reward mechanisms in the brain and their role in dependence: evidence from neurophysiological and neuroimaging studies. *Brain Res. Brain Res. Rev.* 36, 139–149. doi: 10.1016/s0165-0173(01)00089-3
68. Martucci, K. T., and Mackey, S. C. (2016). Imaging pain. *Anesthesiol. Clin.* 34, 255–269. doi: 10.1016/j.anclin.2016.01.001
69. May, A. (2008). Chronic pain may change the structure of the brain. *Pain* 137, 7–15. doi: 10.1016/j.pain.2008.02.034
70. May, A. (2011). Structural brain imaging: a window into chronic pain. *Neuroscientist* 17, 209–220. doi: 10.1177/1073858410396220
71. McMillan, D. E., and Gilmore-Thomas, K. (1996). Stability of opioid craving over time as measured by the visual analog scales. *Drug Alcohol Depend.* 40, 235–239. doi: 10.1016/0376-8716(96)01218-5
72. Moisset, X., and Bouhassira, D. (2007). Brain imaging of neuropathic pain. *Neuroimage* 37, S80–S88. doi: 10.1016/j.neuroimage.2007.03.054
73. Morton, D. L., Sandhu, J. S., and Jones, A. K. (2016). Brain imaging of pain: state of the art. *J. Pain Res.* 9, 613–624. doi: 10.2147/JPR.S60433
74. Murphy, A., Lubman, D. I., McKie, S., Bijral, P. S., Peters, L. A., Faiz, Q., et al. (2017). Time-dependent neuronal changes associated with craving in opioid dependence: an fMRI study. *Addict. Biol.* 23, 1168–1178. doi: 10.1111/adb. 12554
75. Napadow, V., LaCount, L., Park, K., As-Sanie, S., Clauw, D. J., and Harris, R. E. (2010). Intrinsic brain connectivity in fibromyalgia is associated with chronic pain intensity. *Arthritis Rheum.* 62, 2545–2555. doi: 10.1002/ art.27497
76. Naqvi, N. H., and Bechara, A. (2010). The insula and drug addiction: an interoceptive view of pleasure, urges, and decision-making. *Brain Struct. Funct.* 214, 435–450. doi: 10.1007/s00429-010-0268-7
77. Ng, S. K., Urquhart, D. M., Fitzgerald, P. B., Cicuttini, F. M., Hussain, S. M., and Fitzgibbon, B. M. (2017). The relationship between structural and functional brain changes and altered emotion and cognition in chronic low back pain: a systematic review of MRI and fMRI studies. *Clin. J. Pain* 34, 237–261. doi: 10.1097/AJP.0000000000000534
78. Noble, M., Treadwell, J. R., Tregear, S. J., Coates, V. H., Wiffen, P. J., Akafomo, C., et al. (2010). Long-term opioid management for chronic noncancer pain. *Cochrane Database Syst. Rev.* 2010:CD006605. doi: 10.1002/14651858. CD006605.pub2
79. Otti, A., Guendel, H., Henningsen, P., Zimmer, C., Wohlschlaeger, A. M., and Noll-Hussong, M. (2013). Functional network connectivity of pain-related resting state networks in somatoform pain disorder: an exploratory fMRI study. *J. Psychiatry Neurosci.* 38, 57–65. doi: 10.1503/ jpn.110187
80. Ploner, M., Lee, M. C., Wiech, K., Bingel, U., and Tracey, I. (2011). Flexible cerebral connectivity patterns subserve contextual modulations of pain. *Cereb. Cortex* 21, 719–726. doi: 10.1093/cercor/bhq146
81. Potter, J. S., Chakrabarti, A., Domier, C. P., Hillhouse, M. P., Weiss, R. D., and Ling, W. (2010). Pain and continued opioid use in individuals receiving buprenorphine-naloxone for opioid detoxification: secondary analyses from the clinical trials network. *J. Subst. Abuse. Treat.* 38, S80–S86. doi: 10.1016/j.jsat. 2009.12.007
82. Potter, J. S., Hennessy, G., Borrow, J. A., Greenfield, S. F., and Weiss, R. D. (2004). Substance use histories in patients seeking treatment for controlled- release oxycodone dependence. *Drug Alcohol Depend.* 76, 213–215. doi: 10. 1016/j.drugalcdep.2004.05.001
83. Potter, J. S., Prather, K., and Weiss, R. D. (2008). Physical pain and associated clinical characteristics in treatment-seeking patients in four substance use disorder treatment modalities. *Am. J. Addict.* 392, 121–125. doi: 10.1080/ 10550490701862902
84. Price, L. R. (2012). Small sample properties of bayesian multivariate autoregressive time seriesmodels. *Struct. Equ. Modeling Multidiscipl. J.* 19, 51–64. doi: 10.1080/ 10705511.2012.634712
85. Qiu, Y. W., Lv, X. F., Jiang, G. H., Su, H. H., Yu, T., Tian, J. Z., et al. (2014). Reduced ventral medial prefrontal cortex (vmPFC) volume and impaired vmPFC-default mode network integration in codeine-containing cough syrups users. *Drug Alcohol Depend.* 134, 314–321. doi: 10.1016/j. drugalcdep.2013.10.023
86. Riederer, F., Gantenbein, A. R., Marti, M., Luechinger, R., Kollias, S., and Sándor, P. S. (2013). Decrease of gray matter volume in the midbrain is associated with treatment response in medication-overuse headache: possible influence of orbitofrontal cortex. *J. Neurosci.* 33, 15343–15349. doi: 10.1523/JNEUROSCI. 3804-12.2013
87. Roland, M. O., and Morris, R. W. (1983). A study of the natural history of back pain. Part 1: development of a reliable and sensitive measure of disability in low back pain. *Spine* 8, 141–144.
88. Rosenblum, A., Joseph, H., Fong, C., Kipnis, S., Cleland, C., and Portenoy, R. K. (2003). Prevalence and characteristics of chronic pain among chemically dependent patients in methadone maintenance and residential treatment facilities. *JAMA* 289, 2370–2378.
89. Salsitz, E. A. (2016). Chronic pain, chronic opioid addiction: a complex nexus. *J. Med. Toxicol.* 12, 54–57. doi: 10.1007/s13181-015-0521-9
90. Schmidt, A., Borgwardt, S., Gerber, H., Wiesbeck, G. A., Schmid, O., Riecher- Rossler, A., et al. (2014). Acute effects of heroin on negative emotional processing: relation of amygdala activity and stress-related responses. *Biol. Psychiatry* 76, 289–296. doi: 10.1016/j. biopsych.2013.10.019

91. Schmidt, A., Denier, N., Magon, S., Radue, E. W., Huber, C. G., Riecher-Rossler, A., et al. (2015a). Increased functional connectivity in the resting-state basal ganglia network after acute heroin substitution. *Transl. Psychiatry* 5:e533. doi: 10.1038/tp.2015.28
92. Schmidt, A., Walter, M., Gerber, H., Seifritz, E., Brenneisen, R., Wiesbeck, G. A., et al. (2015b). Normalizing effect of heroin maintenance treatment on stress- induced brain connectivity. *Brain* 138, 217–228. doi: 10.1093/brain/awu326
93. Schmidt-Wilcke, T. (2008). Variations in brain volume and regional morphology associated with chronic pain. *Curr. Rheumatol. Rep.* 10, 467–474. doi: 10.1007/ s11926-008-0077-7
94. Schmidt-Wilcke, T. (2015). Neuroimaging of chronic pain. *Best Pract. Res. Clin. Rheumatol.* 29, 29–41. doi: 10.1016/j.berh.2015.04.030
95. Schwedt, T. J., Schlaggar, B. L., Mar, S., Nolan, T., Coalson, R. S., Nardos, B., et al. (2013). Atypical resting-state functional connectivity of affective pain regions in chronic migraine. *Headache* 53, 737–751. doi: 10.1111/head.12081
96. Schweinhardt, P., and Bushnell, M. C. (2010). Pain imaging in health and disease– how far have we come? *J. Clin. Invest.* 120, 3788–3797. doi: 10.1172/JCI43498
97. Seifert, C. L., Magon, S., Sprenger, T., Lang, U. E., Huber, C. G., Denier, N., et al. (2015). Reduced volume of the nucleus accumbens in heroin addiction. *Eur. Arch. Psychiatry Clin. Neurosci.* 265, 637–645. doi: 10.1007/s00406-014-0564-y
98. Sevel, L. S., Letzen, J. E., Staud, R., and Robinson, M. E. (2016). Interhemispheric dorsolateral prefrontal cortex connectivity is associated with individual differences in pain sensitivity in healthy controls. *Brain Connect.* 6, 357–364. doi: 10.1089/brain.2015.0405
99. Smallwood, R. F., Laird, A. R., Ramage, A. E., Parkinson, A. L., Lewis, J., Clauw, D. J., et al. (2013). Structural brain anomalies and chronic pain: a quantitative meta-analysis of gray matter volume. *J. Pain* 14, 663–675. doi: 10.1016/j.jpain. 2013.03.001
100. Smallwood, R. F., Potter, J. S., and Robin, D. A. (2016). Neurophysiological mechanisms inacceptance and commitment therapy in opioid-addicted patients with chronic pain. *Psychiatry Res.* 250, 12–14. doi: 10.1016/j.pscychresns.2016.03.001
101. St Marie, B. (2014). Health care experiences when pain and substance use disorder coexist: just because i'm an addict doesn't mean i don't have pain. *Pain Med.* 15, 2075–2086. doi: 10.1111/pme.12493
102. Stoicea, N., Russell, D., Weidner, G., Durda, M., Joseph, N. C., Yu, J., et al. (2015). Opioid-induced hyperalgesia in chronic pain patients and the mitigating effects of gabapentin. *Front. Pharmacol.* 6:104. doi: 10.3389/fphar.2015.00104
103. Tracey, I. (2005). Nociceptive processing in the human brain. *Curr. Opin. Neurobiol.* 15, 478–487. doi: 10.1016/j.conb.2005.06.010
104. Trafton, J. A., Oliva, E. M., Horst, D. A., Minkel, J. D., and Humphreys, K. (2004). Treatment needs associated with pain in substance use disorder patients: implications for concurrent treatment. *Drug Alcohol Depend.* 73, 23–31. doi: 10.1016/j.drugalcdep.2003.08.007
105. Tsui, J. I., Lira, M. C., Cheng, D. M., Winter, M. R., Alford, D. P., Liebschutz, J. M., et al. (2016). Chronic 387 pain, craving, and illicit opioid use among patients receiving opioid agonist therapy. *Drug Alcohol Depend.* 166, 26–31. doi: 10.1016/j.drugalcdep.2016.06.024
106. Tunks, E. R., Crook, J., and Weir, R. (2008). Epidemiology of chronic pain with psychological comorbidity: prevalence, risk, course, and prognosis. *Can. J. Psychiatry* 53, 224–234. doi: 10.1177/070674370805300403
107. Upadhyay, J., Maleki, N., Potter, J., Elman, I., Rudrauf, D., Knudsen, J., et al. (2010). Alterations in brain structure and functional connectivity in prescription opioid-dependent patients. *Brain* 133, 2098–2114. doi: 10.1093/brain/ awq138
108. Veinante, P., Yalcin, I., and Barrot, M. (2013). The amygdala between sensation and affect: a role in pain. *J. Mol. Psychiatry* 1, 1–14. doi: 10.1186/2049-9256-1-9
109. Vest, N., Reynolds, C. J., and Tragesser, S. L. (2016). Impulsivity and risk for prescription opioid misuse in a chronic pain patient sample. *Addict. Behav.* 60, 184–190. doi: 10.1016/j.addbeh.2016.04.015
110. Volkow, N. D., and McLellan, A. T. (2016). Opioid abuse in chronic pain–misconceptions and mitigation strategies. *N. Engl. J. Med.* 374, 1253–1263. doi: 10.1056/NEJMra1507771
111. Wang, D. J., Rao, H., Korczykowski, M., Wintering, N., Pluta, J., Khalsa, D. S., et al. (2011). Cerebral blood flow changes associated with different meditation practices and perceived depth of meditation. *Psychiatry Res.* 191, 60–67. doi: 10.1016/j.pscychresns.2010.09.011
112. Wang, Y., Wang, H., Li, W., Zhu, J., Gold, M. S., Zhang, D., et al. (2014). Reduced responses to heroin-cue-induced craving in the dorsal striatum: effects of long- term methadone maintenance treatment. *Neurosci. Lett.* 581, 120–124. doi: 10.1016/j.neulet.2014.08.026
113. Wang, Z. X., Zhang, J. X., Wu, Q. L., Liu, N., Hu, X. P., Chan, R. C., et al. (2010). Alterations in the processing of non-drug-related affective stimuli in abstinent heroin addicts. *Neuroimage* 49, 971–976. doi: 10.1016/j.neuroimage.2009. 08.020
114. Wollman, S. C., Alhassoon, O. M., Hall, M. G., Stern, M. J., Connors, E. J., Kimmel, C. L., et al. (2016). Gray matter abnormalities in opioid-dependent patients: a neuroimaging meta-analysis. *Am. J. Drug Alcohol Abuse* 43, 505–517. doi: 10.1080/00952990.2016.1245312
115. Woolf, C. J. (2011). Central sensitization: implications for the diagnosis and treatment of pain. *Pain* 152, S2–S15. doi: 10.1016/j.pain.2010.09.030
116. Yang, Q., Wang, Z., Yang, L., Xu, Y., and Chen, L. M. (2017). Cortical thickness and functionalconnectivity abnormality in chronic headache and low back pain patients. *Hum. Brain Mapp.* 38, 1815–1832. doi: 10.1002/hbm.23484
117. Yang, Z., Xie, J., Shao, Y. C., Xie, C. M., Fu, L. P., Li, D. J., et al. (2009). Dynamic neural responses to cue-reactivity paradigms in heroin-dependent users: an fMRI study. *Hum. Brain Mapp.* 30, 766–775. doi: 10.1002/hbm.20542
118. Zhang, Y., Gong, J., Xie, C., Ye, E. M., Jin, X., Song, H., et al. (2015). Alterations in brain connectivity in three sub-regions of the anterior cingulate cortex in heroin-dependent individuals: evidence from resting state fMRI. *Neuroscience* 284, 998–1010. doi: 10.1016/j.neuroscience.2014.11.007
119. Zhang, Y., Tian, J., Yuan, K., Liu, P., Zhuo, L., Qin, W., et al. (2011). Distinct resting-state brain activities in heroin-dependent individuals. *Brain Res.* 1402, 46–53. doi: 10.1016/j.brainres.2011.05.054

4

Oxytocin-Induced Changes in Intrinsic Network Connectivity in Cocaine use Disorder: Modulation by Gender, Childhood Trauma and Years of use

Jane E. Joseph[1], Brandon K. Vaughan[1], Christopher C. Camp[1], Nathaniel L. Baker[2], Brian J. Sherman[3], Megan Moran-Santa Maria[3], Aimee McRae-Clark[3,4] and Kathleen T. Brady[3,4]*

[1] Department of Neuroscience, Medical University of South Carolina, Charleston, SC, United States, [2] Department of Public Health Sciences, Medical University of South Carolina, Charleston, SC, United States, [3] Department of Psychiatry and Behavioral Sciences, Medical University of South Carolina, Charleston, SC, United States, [4] Ralph H. Johnson VA Medical Center, Charleston, SC, United States

***Correspondence:**
Jane E. Joseph
josep@musc.edu

Cocaine use disorder (CUD) is a major public health concern with devastating social, economic, and mental health implications. A better understanding of the underlying neurobiology and phenotypic variations in individuals with CUD is necessary for the development of effective and targeted treatments. In this study, 39 women and 54 men with CUD completed a 6-min resting-state functional magnetic resonance imaging scan after intranasal oxytocin (OXY) or placebo administration. Graph-theory network analysis was used to quantify functional connectivity changes caused by OXY in striatum, anterior cingulate cortex (ACC), insula, and amygdala nodes of interest. OXY increased connectivity in the right ACC and left amygdala in males, whereas OXY increased connectivity in the right ACC and right accumbens in females. Machine learning was then used to associate treatment response (placebo minus OXY) in nodes of interest with years of cocaine use and severity of childhood trauma separately for males and females. Childhood trauma and years of cocaine use were associated with OXY-induced changes in ACC connectivity for both men and women, but connectivity changes in the amygdala were associated with years of cocaine use in men and connectivity changes in the right insula were associated with years of cocaine use in women. These findings suggest that salience network nodes (ACC and insula) are potential OXY treatment targets in CUD, with the amygdala as a treatment target for men and the accumbens as a treatment target for women.

Keywords: connectome, graph-theory, resting state, gender differences, functional connectivity

INTRODUCTION

Gender differences in addictive and affective disorders are well established (1, 2). Both gonadal and stress hormones can modulate brain function, leading to different levels of susceptibility to neuropsychiatric disorders and treatment response. Biomedical research focused on understanding hormonal modulation and gender differences in brain function may be advanced by including neuroimaging markers of functional brain organization. One such marker is resting-state functional brain connectivity (RSFC), which uses functional magnetic resonance imaging (fMRI) to image the brain while an individual is alert and awake but not engaged in any particular cognitive task; that is, when the brain is at "rest." This continuous resting-state fMRI (rsfMRI) paradigm can reveal brain regions that are temporally synchronized with other brain regions to characterize brain regions that seem to activate (or deactivate) in unison, revealing additional phenotypes that are not captured with current behavioral assessments or neurobiological markers. Therefore, the addition of rsfMRI as a tool in understanding psychiatric illness and gender-specific susceptibility to different disorders may ultimately lead to better treatments and outcomes.

rsfMRI has been widely used in addictions research, including studies in cocaine use disorder (CUD) (3, 4). Differences in RSFC between CUD and control subjects have been reported in numerous circuits, but there is no clear consensus that any particular circuit or resting-state network can be considered a reliable phenotype for CUD. Nevertheless, RSFC has been associated with important clinical variables, such as measures of cocaine use (5–7), impulsivity, inattention, or cognitive control (5, 6, 8–10) and risk for relapse (10–16). For example, years of cocaine use (which will be the primary cocaine use variable in the present study) have been associated with reduced RSFC in the ventromedial prefrontal, hypothalamic, insula, and anterior cingulate cortex (ACC) regions (7, 14). Although not all studies have shown an association between compromised RSFC and years of use (5), the collective findings point to RSFC as a promising imaging biomarker for relapse risk or other behaviors implicated in the addiction process (17).

However, two important variables that are known to modulate addiction neurocircuitry—gender and trauma exposure—have been less studied in rsfMRI studies of CUD. Sex differences were examined in only one RSFC study (7) and revealed greater connectivity between the medial hypothalamus and a critical node of the default mode network, the precuneus, in female cocaine users compared to males. A recent study has also examined modulation of RSFC by history of childhood trauma in CUD (18). The CUD group reported that some childhood trauma showed greater amygdala RSFC with several striatal regions, the insula, medial temporal regions, and the brain stem. These studies are an important step toward understanding individual differences in RSFC, but more studies are needed to characterize RSFC phenotypes that may lead to the development of individualized treatment approaches.

One potential treatment being explored for substance use disorders (SUD) is the neuropeptide oxytocin (OXY). Childhood trauma (19, 20) and chronic substance use (21) can both lead to neuroadaptations in the OXY system. In addition, some studies have shown that exogenous OXY may reverse drug-induced neuroadaptations [see Ref. (21), for review] or can alter neural response in stress-related circuitry (22–24). However, the effect of exogenous OXY may not be the same in men and women because of gender differences in neuropsychiatric sequelae of childhood trauma and the neurobiology of OXY (25, 26).

Few studies, however, have examined gender differences in RSFC changes caused by acute OXY administration, and no studies have examined these changes in individuals with CUD. Seeley and colleagues (27) reviewed 11 studies that examined changes in RSFC caused by acute intranasal OXY administration in healthy controls and individuals with anxiety disorders (posttraumatic stress disorder, generalized social anxiety disorder) or autism spectrum disorder. Most of these studies focused on connectivity of the amygdala with medial prefrontal or cingulate regions. Although findings are mixed as to whether OXY increases or decreases amygdala connectivity, individual differences like gender and psychopathology modulate this connectivity. Whole-brain analyses of RSFC have indicated that acute administration of OXY also increases connectivity in brain regions other than the amygdala, including the striatum, insula, and cingulated (28, 29). In addition, enhanced connectivity under OXY may depend on gender and trauma history, as well as the specific amygdala (24) or striatal nuclei (30) targeted in a given study.

Prior research has demonstrated that females with SUD associate relapse with interpersonal stress and negative affect (31, 32), whereas males with CUD show a more robust reward circuitry response to cocaine cues than females (33, 34). Potenza et al. (35) reported that corticostriatal-limbic hyperactivity was associated primarily with drug cues in men and stress cues in women. These findings suggest that stress circuitry may play a more important role in intrinsic functional brain organization in women with CUD, whereas reward circuitry may play a more prominent role in men with CUD.

To gain a better understanding of gender differences in neural response to OXY in CUD, the present study used RSFC to examine changes in stress- and addiction-related neurocircuitry in response to an acute dose of intranasal OXY in men and women with CUD. More specifically, the goal of this study was to understand the association between graph-theory-based network properties that reflect OXY treatment response and two individual subject variables of interest for SUD: childhood trauma and years of cocaine use. Predictive modeling was used to establish network profiles of OXY response associated with childhood trauma and years of cocaine use in men and women with CUD. The focus was on network connectivity of regions implicated in both substance use and childhood trauma, that is, the striatum, amygdala, insula, and ACC.

Given prior findings, the predictions of this study were that a) childhood trauma was expected to be more strongly associated with OXY connectivity changes in the amygdala because of its involvement in stress reactivity and trauma history (36, 37) and modulation of amygdala RSFC in posttraumatic stress disorder (PTSD) (24) and recent trauma exposure (38); b) years of cocaine use was expected to be more strongly associated with OXY connectivity changes in the striatum because of neuroadaptations of striatal circuitry in addiction (39); c) the major nodes of the salience network (insula, cingulate) were expected to be associated with both childhood trauma and years of cocaine use because of the role of this network in SUD (17) and psychiatric disorders more broadly (40); d) OXY response in network regions associated with childhood trauma and years of cocaine use was expected to be different in men and women. Prior findings suggest that stress circuitry (e.g., amygdala) will exert a stronger network influence in females and reward circuitry (e.g., striatum) will exert a stronger network influence in males.

MATERIALS AND METHODS

Participants

Participants took part in a large study investigating the effect of OXY on subjective and neuroendocrine responses to stressors. The current crossover analysis included only data from the rsfMRI component of the study. A total of 93 non-treatment-seeking CUD individuals who responded to local media advertisements over a 54-month period completed the fMRI scanning procedures. Written informed consent was obtained before study assessments were administered. All procedures were conducted in accordance with Good Clinical Practice Guidelines and the Declaration of Helsinki and received institutional review board (IRB) approval. General exclusion criteria included 1) pregnancy, nursing, or plan to become pregnant during the course of the study; 2) women who had a complete hysterectomy, were postmenopausal, or receiving hormone replacement or hormonal contraceptive therapy; 3) history of or current significant hematological, endocrine, cardiovascular, pulmonary, renal, gastrointestinal, or neurological diseases; 4) history of or current psychotic, panic, eating, or bipolar affective disorders; 5) current major depressive disorder and PTSD; 6) history of or current medical conditions that might affect hypothalamic pituitary axis (HPA)axis activity; 7) synthetic glucocorticoid or exogenous steroid therapy within 1 month of testing; 8) psychotropic medications (with the exception of selective serotonin reuptake inhibitors), opiates or opiate antagonists, benzodiazepines, antipsychotics, beta-blockers, and other medications that might interfere with HPA axis activity or physiologic measurements; 9) acute illness or fever; 10) *Diagnostic and Statistical Manual of Mental Disorders-IV* (DSM-IV) criteria for substance dependence except alcohol, nicotine, or marijuana within the past 60 days; 11) unwillingness or inability to maintain abstinence from cocaine and other drugs of abuse (except nicotine) for 3 days prior to the cue–reactivity sessions; or 12) MRI contraindications.

Assessment

Participants meeting prescreening criteria were evaluated for study eligibility with the Mini-International Neuropsychiatric Interview (MINI) (41). The substance use module of the Structured Clinical Interview for DSM-IV (SCID-IV) was used to assess current and lifetime SUD (42). Substance use in the 90 days before the study was assessed using the Time-Line Follow-Back (43). The Childhood Trauma Questionnaire (CTQ) (44) was used to assess the extent to which individuals experienced five domains of childhood abuse and neglect (sexual abuse, physical abuse, emotional abuse, emotional neglect, and physical neglect). Participants answered each of 25 questions using a 5-point Likert scale ranging from 1 (never true) to 5 (very often true). A medical history and physical examination were completed to assess for medical exclusions. Participants meeting inclusion criteria and no exclusion criteria were scheduled to complete the study procedures and instructed to not use cocaine or other drugs of abuse for a minimum of 3 days before the test sessions.

Study Procedures

Participants completed one 6-min resting-state fMRI session on each of two consecutive days (a cocaine cue reactivity task was also completed on each day, but those results are not reported here). On day 1 of testing, participants arrived at the Medical University of South Carolina's (MUSC) Addiction Sciences Division research clinic at 10:00 a.m. Upon arrival, urine pregnancy tests were administered. Smokers were provided with a nicotine patch. Self-reports, urine drug screens (Roche Diagnostics, Indianapolis, Indiana), and breathalyzer tests (AlcoSensor III, Intoximeters, Inc., St. Louis, Missouri) were used to assess abstinence. If the pregnancy and drug tests were negative [with the exception of Tetrahydrocannabinol (THC)], study procedures continued. At 11:30 a.m., subjective ratings were obtained. A modified version of the Within Session Rating Scale was used to assess subjective ratings of craving, anxiety, and stress (45). This 1–10 visual analogue scale is anchored with the adjectival modifiers ("not at all," "mildly," "moderately," and "extremely"). The Cocaine Craving Questionnaire (CCQ)-Brief was used to assess cocaine craving. The State-Trait Anxiety Inventory (STAI) was used to assess anxiety symptoms (46). Participants were then provided a standardized lunch.

At 1:20 p.m., participants were administered 40 IU of OXY nasal spray or matching placebo (PBO). This dose was selected based on previous studies using similar doses of OXY (47–49) as well as our own previous work (50, 51). Timing of administration was also based on previous studies showing central activity of OXY 40 min after intranasal administration (50, 52). Intranasal OXY and matching PBO were compounded by the MUSC Investigational Drug Service. To achieve balance in sample size with respect to treatment order across genders, a block randomized design with randomly varying block sizes was used. Half of the participants were randomized to OXY on day 1 and half to PBO.

Subjective measures were repeated at 1:55 p.m. Scanning procedures commenced at 2:00 p.m. The 6-min rsfMRI session instructed participants to fixate a centrally presented crosshair but otherwise had no specific instructions other than to remain awake and alert and minimize head movement.

fMRI data images were acquired on a Siemens Trio 3.0 Tesla scanner with a 12-channel head coil (Siemens Medical, Erlangen, Germany) at MUSC for the majority of subjects (36 females, 53 males). Data from four of the subjects (one male) were collected on a Siemens PRISMA FIT 3.0 Tesla scanner with a 32-channel head coil, also at MUSC. During initial scanner tuning, localizing, and structural scanning, participants were shown relaxation images (i.e., 20 scenic pictures, each displayed for 30 s, and repeated if necessary). A high-resolution T1-weighted MPRAGE anatomical scan (TR = 2.25 s, TE = 4.2 ms, flip angle = 9°, 176 sagittal slices, field of view = 256 mm, 256 × 256 matrix, thickness = 1.0 mm) covering the entire brain and positioned using a sagittal scout image was acquired for coregistration and normalization of functional images. T2*-weighted gradient echo EPI images were acquired with the following parameters (parameters were identical for the TRIO and PRISMA): TR = 2,000 ms, TE = 27 ms, flip angle = 76°, 36 axial slices (field of view = 237 mm × 237 mm, thickness = 3.7 mm voxels, in interleaved order). A gradient field map image was collected to match the spatial parameters of the EPI images.

After completion of the first scan, participants returned the next day and completed identical procedures with the opposite treatment condition. At the end of the second scan day, participants were debriefed and compensated.

Data Analysis

Demographics and Subject Characteristics

Baseline demographic and subject characteristics as well as prescan subjective ratings were compared across genders using independent-samples *t*-tests for continuous variables and chi-square tests across categorical characteristics. Data are reported as means and standard deviations for continuous variables and proportions for categorical variables.

An independent-samples *t*-test (unequal variances assumed because of unbalanced sample sizes) compared PBO minus OXY difference score for TRIO versus PRISMA scanner data in each of the 20 nodes of interest for clustering coefficient (CC) or eigenvector centrality (EC). Significance was determined using the false discovery rate (FDR) controlled at a 5% level (53, 54). Similarly, an independent-samples *t*-test (assuming unequal variances) examined whether PBO minus OXY difference score was different for smokers versus nonsmokers in each of the 20 nodes of interest for CC or EC.

Although several measures were taken to minimize the contributions of head motion to the fMRI time series, there are more stringent approaches to control for the influence of head motion on fMRI time series (55) than used here. To address whether any residual head motion was correlated with graph-theory measures of connectivity, we examined Spearman-rank correlations between head motion and any of the 20 nodes × 2 graph-theory measures (EC and CC) × 2 genders × 2 treatment conditions (OXY or PBO) using FDR correction.

Finally, an exploratory analysis examined whether any of the five subjective rating measures collected before scanning on each visit (craving, anxiety, stress, STAI, CCQ) was correlated with graph theory measures. Spearman rank correlations were conducted for each of the five subjective measures × 20 nodes × 2 graph-theory measures (CC and EC) × 2 genders × 2 treatment conditions (OXY or PBO) using FDR correction.

fMRI Preprocessing

FMRIB's FSL package[1] was used unless otherwise noted. Images in each participant's time series on each day were corrected for geometric distortion and head motion. Slice timing correction and spatial filtering (FWHM = 7.5 mm) were applied to each time series, which was then submitted to multiple regression using FSL to remove effects of global signal and head motion. Regressors included global signal [extracted from gray matter, white matter and cerebrospinal fluid (CSF) masks, which were created using FSL's FAST tissue segmentation tool], and six head motion parameters. The residual image from this regression step was then band-pass filtered (0.009 to 0.08 Hz) using AFNI (56). The spatially normalized image was then parcellated using a 294 region atlas—the 264 regions from Power et al. (57) with 30 additional subcortical regions (amygdala, hippocampus, striatum). Each region of interest (ROI) was represented by a 10-mm-diameter sphere. The BOLD signal time series was extracted in each of the 294 ROIs using FSL's "feat query" function.

Connectome Measures

Before computing the 294 × 294 functional connectivity matrix, corrupt time points were identified with fractional displacement values using the "fsl_motion_outliers" command. For each corrupt time point, the preceding time point and two successive time points were removed from the time series for each subject and visit (57) using the RSFC Net toolbox[2] implemented using the R software package (58). The mean percent scrubbed time points averaged over both visits was not significantly different between males ($M = 0.13$, $SD = 0.06$) and females ($M = 0.12$, $SD = 0.06$) according to an independent-samples *t*-test, $t(91) = 0.56$, $p = 0.58$.

The connectivity matrix was a weighted, signed adjacency matrix representing a fully connected undirected graph. Each matrix element reflected the partial correlation between two discreters fMRI time series while controlling for all other time series. We applied a shrinkage factor as to create a well-conditioned covariance matrix (59–61)[3]. The mixing parameter is largely an optimal weight as a function of N to combine the observed covariance and a target matrix, such as a diagonal (i.e., no covariance/correlation between regions).

The RSFC Net toolbox was used to compute two graph-theory measures: EC and CC. EC is a spectral, self-referential measure of centrality (62, 63). A node with a high EC is connected to other nodes with a high eigenvector score. EC considers connections to influential nodes to be more important than connections to marginal nodes. Hence, EC reflects the *global influence* of a node on the network.

$$C_{Eig[i]} = \left| \frac{1}{\lambda'} \sum_{j=1}^{N} M_{i,j} x_j \right|$$

The eigenvector centrality of the ith node, $C_{Eig[i]}$, is defined as the absolute value of the ith number in the eigenvector belonging to the principal eigenvalue of the matrix M, which is denoted λ'.

CC is a local measure of segregation representing the fraction of a node's neighbors that are also neighbors of each other; these patterns effectively form triangles around the node (64–66).

[1] www.fmrib.ox.ac.uk/fsl

[2] https://doi.org/10.5281/zenodo.1403924

[3] http://strimmerlab.org/software/corpcor

We used the CC formula for weighted and signed connectivity matrices provided by (66):

$$CC_i = \frac{\sum_{i,j} w_{s(j,i)} w_{(i,q)} w_{s(j,q)}}{\sum_{i \neq j} \left| w_{s(j,i)} w_{s(i,q)} \right|}$$

CC reflects the degree of *local influence* in a network. In this formula, the triangle is denoted by the direct connection of the ith and j^{th} nodes and an indirect connection through a qth node; $s(i,j,q)$. The numerator is the sum of the products of the signed edge weights between the pairs $s(i,j)$, $s(i,q)$, and $s(j,q)$ divided by the sum of the absolute value of the product of the edge weights for pairs $s(j,i)$ and $s(i,q)$. The denominator represents the maximum magnitude of the value the numerator can obtain.

EC and CC measures were chosen because they reflect different aspects of network organization. Network measures were always calculated using all 294 nodes. Visualization of nodes used BrainNet Viewer (67).

Twenty nodes were used as ROIs in subsequent analyses (**Table 1**): five insula regions, five ACC regions, six amygdala regions, and four striatal regions. ROIs were selected based on being strongly implicated in addiction (3, 17) and trauma (68–71). Of the eight ACC regions available in the Power atlas, two that fell on the midline were eliminated and five of the remaining six that sampled different aspects of the rostral to dorsal gradient were chosen. Of the seven insula regions available in the Power atlas (only two in the left hemisphere), five were chosen that sampled anterior, mid, and posterior aspects of the insula, primarily in the right hemisphere as there were more of those in the Power atlas. All six amygdala, two accumbens, and two caudate regions were selected. Importantly, the network measures reflected the connectivity of a given node with all other nodes in the whole brain network, not just the connectivity among the 20 nodes of interest.

TABLE 1 | Twenty regions of interest used as predictors.

Region name	MNI coordinate		
	x	y	z
Right dorsal ACC	10	−2	45
Right posterior insula	36	−9	14
Right mid insula	37	1	−4
Left ACC	−5	18	34
Left rostral ACC	−11	45	8
Right rostral ACC	12	36	20
Left anterior insula	−35	20	0
Right anterior insula	36	22	3
Right anterior ventral insula	34	16	−8
Right ACC	10	22	27
Left dorsal amygdala	−22	−4	−12
Right dorsal amygdala	22	−4	−12
Left medial amygdala	−14	−4	−20
Right medial amygdala	14	−4	−20
Left ventrolateral amygdala	−28	−4	−22
Right ventrolateral amygdala	28	−4	−22
Left caudate	−13	7	10
Right caudate	14	8	11
Left nucleus accumbens	−10	12	−7
Right nucleus accumbens	10	10	−8

ACC, anterior cingulate cortex; MNI, Montreal Neurological Institute.

Generalized Linear Model Analysis (Analysis 1)

The purpose of this analysis was to isolate regions that showed effects of OXY treatment and establish that changes in connectivity caused by OXY were modified by gender, childhood trauma (CTQ), and years of cocaine use (YRSUSE).

Generalized linear mixed effects models were developed to assess Analysis 1 (IBM SPSS tatistics; Version 24.0; IBM Corp., Armonk, NY). Models were developed to specifically assess the effects of treatment (OXY, PBO) and node (20 ROIs described above) as repeated effects, with gender, head motion, CTQ, and YRSUSE as additional variables. All models further adjust for study-specific design variables, specifically study visit and treatment order. To assess the hypothesis that gender, CTQ, and YRSUSE may modify the relationship between OXY and node response, model interactions were included in subsequent analysis. Both main effects and interactions were considered significant if $p \leq 0.05$. Separate generalized linear models were conducted with CC and EC as outcome variables. This step was conducted before model selection (Analysis 2) to investigate and establish important interactions among variables of interest. Analysis 2 will then examine such interactions in more depth using model selection.

Automatic Linear Modeling (Analysis 2)

The purpose of this analysis was to conduct model selection to select the best set of brain regions and network properties associated with differing levels of childhood trauma and years of cocaine use. Eight different models were examined based on the combination of two different outcome variables (CTQ, YRSUSE), two genders (male, female), and two different network measures (CC, EC). For each of the eight models, model selection was conducted over 10 replications.

Model selection used Automatic Linear Modeling (ALM; IBM SPSS Statistics). ALM is a linear modeling approach in which a set of variables (i.e., network properties in each of the 20 ROIs) predicts an outcome (i.e., CTQ or YRSUSE). The treatment effect was expressed as a difference score in either CC or EC in the PBO condition minus the OXY condition in each of the 20 ROIs. A positive difference score reflected a *reduction* in connectivity because of treatment with OXY, whereas a negative difference score reflected *increased* connectivity because of OXY. ALM automatically trims outliers and transforms variables, if needed. ALM divides the full sample of subjects into a training set (70% of the data) and a test set (30% of the data; called the overfit prevention set in IBM SPSS Statistics). The modeling process used 10 replicated data sets, and training and test sets are randomly selected from each. Replicates were a random sample with replacement.

In ALM, if the number of predictor variables is 20 or fewer, a large subset of possible models is examined using "best subsets" (72). This approach determines the best subset of predictor variables using the average squared error (ASE) of the test set. The model with the lowest ASE is chosen by ALM as the best model. ALM yields a measure of model accuracy, which is 100 times the adjusted R^2 of the final model, Akaike's Information Criterion (AIC), as well as the importance and weight (coefficient) of each predictor.

Predictor importance is a relative measure of how important each variable was in the prediction. IBM SPSS Statistics uses the leave-one-out method to compute importance based on the residual sum of squares by removing one predictor at a time from the final full model. The importance values all sum to 1.

To determine whether EC or CC yielded a better model for predicting CTQ or YRSUSE for males and females separately, the average accuracy across the 10 replications were compared qualitatively, and the number of significant models ($p \leq 0.05$) across the 10 replications was considered. The network measure that yielded the highest average accuracy and more significant replications for a given gender and outcome variable combination was considered the better model. To determine the final set of predictors, the cumulative importance of predictors across the 10 replications was calculated. Predictors with cumulative importance >1 were considered for interpretation. Finally, to address potential collinearity among the predictors in the final models, the predictors with cumulative importance >1 were entered into a simultaneous linear regression, and variance inflation factors (VIFs) were determined for each model covariate; if a VIF exists greater than 4.0 (73), multicollinearity will be mitigated by choosing the collinear variable that produces the greatest model fit when included.

TABLE 2 | Demographics and subject characteristics.

Characteristic	Sex		p value
	Female	Male	
	(*n* = 39)	(*n* = 54)	
Demographics			
Age in years (SD)	40.0 (8.5)	44.5 (9.8)	0.024
Cigarette Smoker % (*n*)	84.6 (33)	75.9 (41)	0.305[a]
Cigarettes per day (SD)	11.5 (6.9)	10.8 (6.9)	0.715
Caucasian % (*n*)	30.1 (12)	22.2 (12)	0.352[a]
Cocaine use characteristics			
Age at first use (SD)	22.1 (5.8)	21.1 (6.3)	0.427
Total years use (SD)	14.1 (7.7)	18.3 (8.2)	0.014
Age at dependence onset[b] (SD)	29.2 (8.1)	29.5 (8.7)	0.849
Using days per month (SD)	17.5 (8.1)	17.0 (7.4)	0.753
Baseline trauma			
CTQ total score[c] (SD)	51.2 (21.4)	43.8 (14.3)	0.079
Prescan subjective ratings—Visit 1			
Craving (SD)	2.3 (2.7)	2.7 (2.5)	0.563
Anxiety (SD)	2.4 (2.4)	2.3 (2.2)	0.857
Stress (SD)	1.5 (2.3)	2.2 (2.4)	0.167
STAI (SD)	32.2 (9.7)	35.2 (12.1)	0.210
CCQ (SD)	5.5 (1.3)	5.5 (1.1)	0.981
Prescan subjective ratings—Visit 2			
Craving (SD)	2.2 (2.5)	2.5 (2.5)	0.534
Anxiety (SD)	2.0 (2.4)	2.1 (2.5)	0.726
Stress (SD)	1.5 (2.4)	1.7 (2.2)	0.747
STAI (SD)	32.4 (12.0)	34.4 (12.0)	0.430
CCQ (SD)	5.7 (1.3)	5.6 (1.2)	0.677

SD, standard deviation; STAI, State-Trait Anxiety Inventory; CCQ, Cocaine Craving Questionnaire.
[a]p value calculated using chi-square test.
[b]Based on responses from 37 females and 53 males.
[c]Based on responses from 36 females and 49 males.

RESULTS

Demographics and Subject Characteristics

Males were older than females and reported more years of cocaine use (**Table 2**). However, males and females were not different on any of the other demographic, cocaine use characteristics, or subjective measures. There were no significant differences between TRIO and PRISMA scanner data in any of the 20 nodes of interest for either CC or EC. There were also no significant differences between smokers and nonsmokers in any of the 20 nodes of interest for either CC or EC. Therefore, scanner type and smoking status were not included as variables in subsequent analyses.

Head motion was not correlated with CC or EC in any of the 20 nodes or treatment conditions. Although none met the threshold for significance, head motion was included in the two primary analyses below as a precaution given that only six head motion parameters were used as nuisance variables in preprocessing.

Finally, the exploratory correlation analysis between subjective ratings and graph theory measures yielded one significant correlation: males in the PBO condition who reported higher stress before scanning also showed higher EC in the left dorsal amygdala, *rho* = 0.53, $p = 0.000046$.

Analysis 1: Establish whether graph-theory measures reflecting treatment response are associated with childhood trauma and years of cocaine use and whether gender moderates these associations.

The generalized linear model with CC as the outcome variable and node, treatment, gender, head motion, CTQ, and YRSUSE as predictors yielded several significant effects and interactions (**Supplement 1**). CC varied by node ($p = 0.0001$), CTQ ($p = 0.009$), and head motion ($p = 0.0001$). The node effect was further modified by treatment (Node × Treatment interaction, $p < 0.0001$), and significant three-way interactions indicated that the treatment effect in different nodes was further modified by gender (Node × Treatment × Gender, $p = 0.0001$), CTQ (Node × Treatment × CTQ, $p = 0.0001$), and YRSUSE (Node × Treatment × YRSUSE, $p = 0.0001$). **Figure 1A** illustrates the Node × Treatment × Gender interaction for CC. OXY increased CC for males in the right ACC and left dorsal amygdala, whereas OXY increased CC for females in the right accumbens.

The generalized linear model with EC as the outcome variable and node, treatment, gender, head motion, CTQ, and YRSUSE as predictors yielded a main effect of node ($p = 0.0001$) and higher-order interactions with node (**Supplement 1**). The node effect was further modified by treatment and gender (Node × Treatment × Gender, $p = 0.0001$), treatment and CTQ (Node × Treatment × CTQ, $p = 0.0001$), and treatment and YRSUSE (Node × Treatment × YRSUSE, $p = 0.0001$). **Figure 1B**

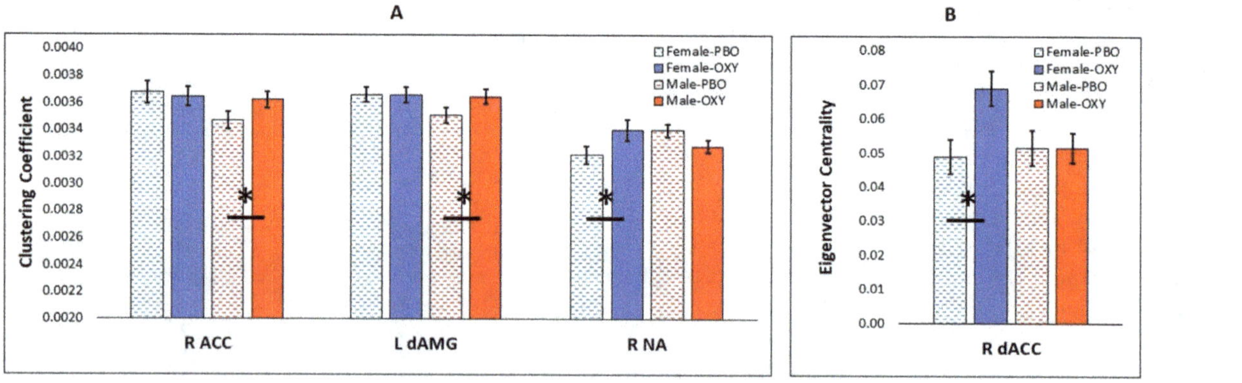

FIGURE 1 | Significant effect of oxytocin (OXY) treatment (solid bars) versus placebo (PBO) (shaded bars) in CUD females (blue) and males (red). **(A)** Effect of OXY on clustering coefficient in three nodes of interest: right anterior cingulate cortex (R ACC), left dorsal amygdala (L dAMG), and right nucleus accumbens (R NA). **(B)** Effect of OXY on eigenvector centrality in one node: right dorsal ACC (R dACC). Error bars are standard error of the mean. Horizontal bars with asterisk indicate a significant difference of OXY versus PBO at $p < 0.05$.

illustrates the Node × Treatment × Gender interaction for EC. OXY increased EC for females in the right dorsal ACC.

These analyses modeled the spatial correlation among the 20 nodes and isolated treatment effects in some of the nodes. For both EC and CC, these treatment effects were modified by gender, CTQ, and YRSUSE. The goal of the next analysis was to use model selection and machine learning to establish the network profiles associated with OXY-related changes in connectivity measures and CTQ or YRSUSE. Because gender modified these effects in Analysis 1, these analyses are conducted separately in males and females.

Analysis 2: Conduct model selection to select the best set of brain regions and network properties associated with childhood trauma and years of cocaine use.

Table 3 summarizes the performance of the 10 replications for each of the 8 models.

Network Profile for CTQ in Males

In males, neither the CC nor the EC model was associated with CTQ reliably across replications. Only one replication was significant for CC, and no replications were significant for EC.

TABLE 3 | Model accuracy (adjusted R^2, top row) and p value (bottom row) for each replication for each model of interest.

			Replication										
Outcome Variable	**Gender**	**Graph-theory Measure**	**1**	**2**	**3**	**4**	**5**	**6**	**7**	**8**	**9**	**10**	**Mean**
CTQ	Male	CC	12%	7%	14%	1%	9%	7%	2%	19%	11%	13%	9%*
			0.11	0.26	0.09	0.40	0.10	0.22	0.36	0.03	0.09	0.07	
	Male	EC	0%	0%	1%	0%	0%	0%	3%	2%	3%	0%	1%
			0.68	0.60	0.42	0.58	0.42	0.79	0.29	0.38	0.31	0.60	
	Female	CC	15%	13%	15%	15%	9%	0%	11%	6%	6%	3%	9%
			0.06	0.17	0.11	0.11	0.17	0.52	0.20	0.23	0.34	0.36	
	Female	EC	28%	29%	39%	37%	23%	35%	31%	24%	21%	7%	27%*
			0.04	0.02	0.01	0.01	0.03	0.01	0.01	0.03	0.03	0.29	
YRSUSE	Male	CC	17%	5%	6%	2%	7%	15%	2%	0%	21%	4%	8%
			0.05	0.18	0.26	0.36	0.17	0.11	0.34	0.64	0.03	0.29	
	Male	EC	18%	23%	19%	10%	15%	17%	27%	3%	1%	22%	16%*
			0.03	0.01	0.01	0.07	0.06	0.03	0.01	0.34	0.30	0.02	
	Female	CC	6%	24%	11%	30%	24%	25%	14%	28%	21%	21%	20%*
			0.23	0.01	0.16	0.01	0.02	0.02	0.10	0.01	0.03	0.05	
	Female	EC	13%	21%	16%	37%	40%	34%	4%	6%	14%	11%	19%
			0.16	0.06	0.06	0.01	0.01	0.02	0.34	0.27	0.09	0.18	

**Indicates best model based on average accuracy and number of significant replications when comparing EC and CC.*
CTQ, Childhood Trauma Questionnaire total score; YRSUSE, years of cocaine se; CC, clustering coefficient; EC, eigenvector centrality.

These results indicate that OXY-related changes in graph-theory measures in the 20 nodes of interest are not associated with individual variations in CTQ scores in males.

Network Profile for CTQ in Females

In females, the best model for CTQ was based on EC. Across 10 replications, this model had an average adjusted R^2 of 0.27. Nine of the 10 replications yielded significant models. The model using CC as the graph-theory metric for CTQ had an average adjusted R^2 of 0.09, and none of the replications was significant.

In the EC model, three predictors had cumulative importance >1 (**Figure 2**). The scatter plots (**Supplement 2**) illustrate that for the right ACC, a higher CTQ was associated with a greater global influence on PBO than OXY, but for the right dorsal ACC and left rostral ACC, a higher CTQ was associated with a greater global influence on OXY than PBO.

Network Profile for YRSUSE in Males

In males, the best model for YRSUSE was based on EC. Across 10 replications, this model had an average adjusted R^2 of 0.16. Six of the 10 replications yielded significant models. In contrast, the model using CC as the graph-theory metric for YRSUSE had an average adjusted R^2 of 0.09 and only two replications were significant.

In the EC model, three predictors had cumulative importance >1 (**Figure 3**). The scatter plots (**Supplement 2**) illustrate that for the right dorsal ACC, higher CTQ was associated with greater global influence on PBO than OXY, but for the left medial amygdala, higher CTQ was associated with a greater global influence on OXY than PBO. Greater head motion was associated with fewer years of cocaine use.

Network Profile for YRSUSE in Females

In females, the best model for YRSUSE was based on CC. Across 10 replications, this model had an average adjusted R^2 of 0.20. Seven of the 10 replications yielded significant models. Although the model using EC as the graph-theory metric for CTQ had an average adjusted R^2 of 0.19, only three of the replications were significant. Although the two models had comparable accuracy, the models using CC as a predictor had more replications that were significant, so it was considered a better model than the EC model.

In the CC model, four predictors had cumulative importance >1 (**Figure 4**). The scatter plots (**Supplement 2**) illustrate that for the right rostral ACC, a higher CTQ was associated with a greater local influence on PBO than OXY, but for the left rostral ACC and right anterior-ventral insula, a higher CTQ was associated with a greater local influence on OXY than PBO. Greater head motion was associated with more years of cocaine use.

For all of the final models, VIFs were less than 2 for all predictors, indicating no collinearity issues, so all variables were retained.

DISCUSSION

The overall goal of this study was to discover how OXY changes functional network organization in men and women with CUD and to isolate network profiles that are associated with severity

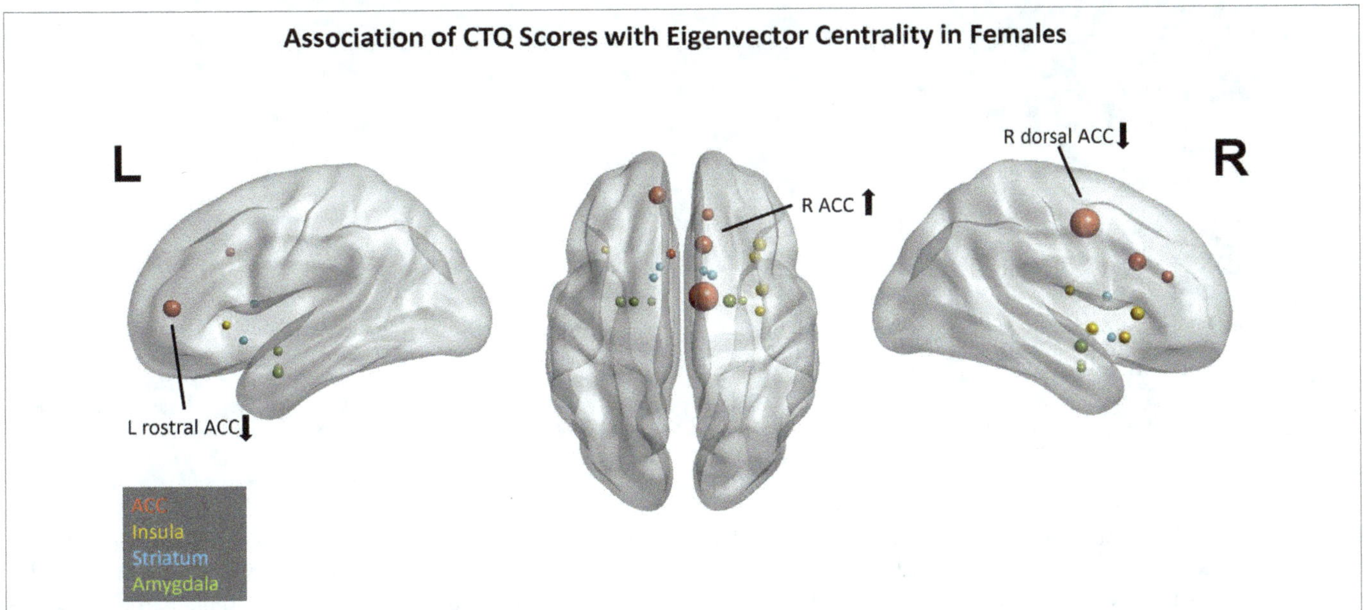

FIGURE 2 | Association of Childhood Trauma Questionnaire (CTQ) scores with eigenvector centrality in females. Network nodes of interest are shown on a template brain in Montreal Neurological Institute (MNI) space, with left lateral (left panel), right lateral (right panel), and axial views (center). Anterior cingulate (ACC) nodes appear in red, insula nodes in yellow, striatum nodes in blue, and amygdala nodes in green. The size of each node reflects its cumulative importance across 10 replications of predictive modeling. Nodes with cumulative importance >1 are labeled anatomically. The arrow next to each label indicates the sign of the regression coefficient for that node. Nodes that failed to appear in any of the 10 replications do not appear in this figure.

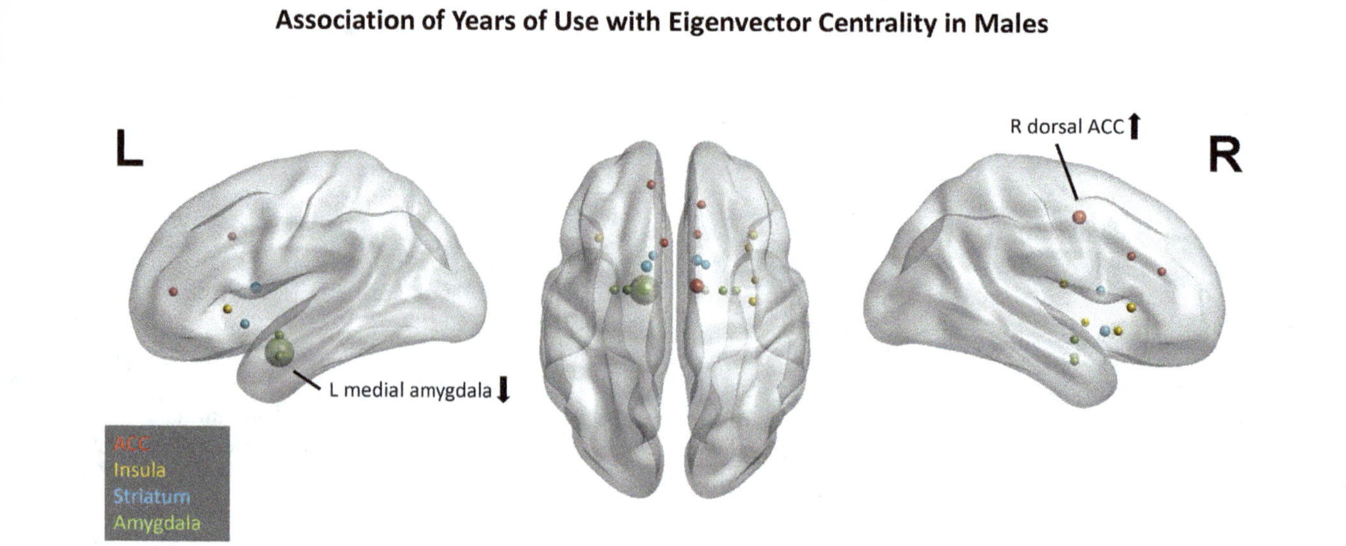

FIGURE 3 | Association of years of cocaine use with eigenvector centrality in males. Network nodes of interest are shown on a template brain in MNI space, with left lateral (left panel), right lateral (right panel), and axial views (center). ACC nodes appear in red, insula nodes in yellow, striatum nodes in blue, and amygdala nodes in green. The size of each node reflects its cumulative importance across 10 replications of predictive modeling. Nodes with cumulative importance >1 are labeled anatomically. The arrow next to each label indicates the sign of the regression coefficient for that node. Nodes that failed to appear in any of the 10 replications do not appear in this figure.

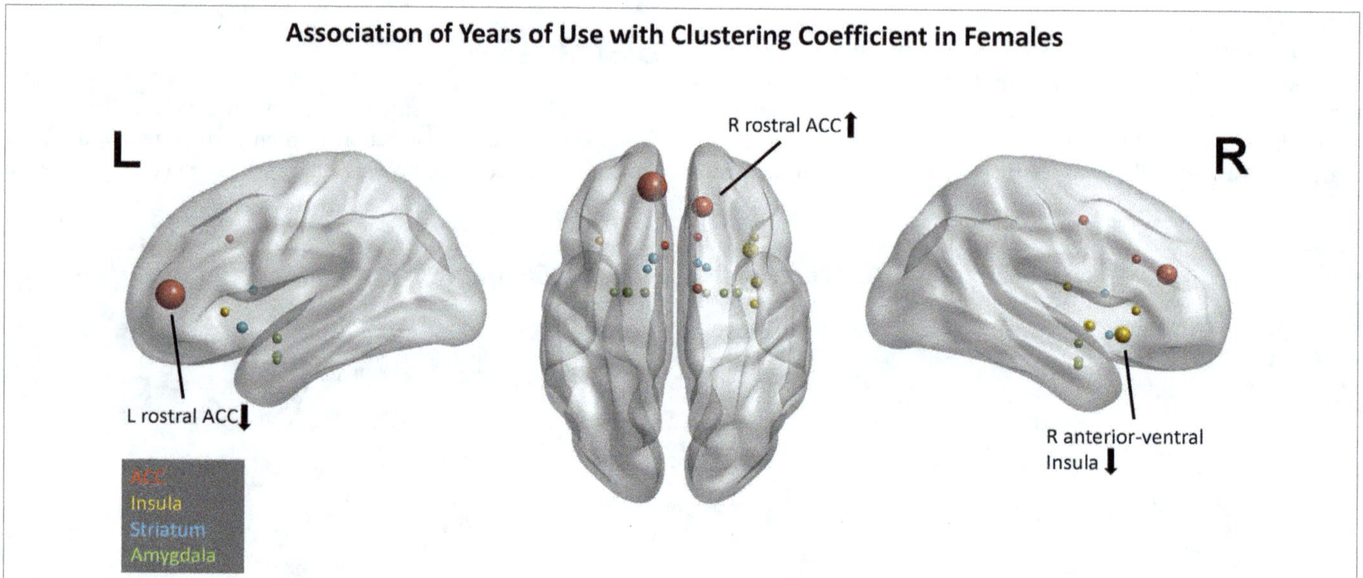

FIGURE 4 | Association of years of cocaine use with clustering coefficient in females. Network nodes of interest are shown on a template brain in MNI space, with left lateral (left panel), right lateral (right panel), and axial views (center). ACC nodes appear in red, insula nodes in yellow, striatum nodes in blue, and amygdala nodes in green. The size of each node reflects its cumulative importance across 10 replications of predictive modeling. Nodes with cumulative importance >1 are labeled anatomically. The arrow next to each label indicates the sign of the regression coefficient for that node. Nodes that failed to appear in any of the 10 replications do not appear in this figure.

of cocaine use and childhood trauma. OXY induced increases in connectivity differently in men and women with CUD. In women, OXY increased local influence of the right accumbens and increased global influence of the right dorsal ACC. In men, OXY increased local influence of the left dorsal amygdala and right ACC.

The first hypothesis that childhood trauma would be associated with OXY-related connectivity changes in the amygdala was not strongly supported. Network profiles associated with individual variations in childhood trauma for females did not include amygdala nodes, and modeling of network profiles in males did not reliably yield significant models. Although the amygdala was not implicated in individual variations in childhood trauma, OXY increased local influence (CC) of the left dorsal amygdala in men. In addition, a higher global influence of this same amygdala region was associated with higher stress ratings in men on PBO. Although the functions of different amygdala nuclei in higher-level human behaviors is still debated, the dorsal (i.e., superficial) amygdala is involved in emotion processing, whereas the other amygdala nuclei play a role in fear, anxiety, and fear conditioning (27). Consequently, the association between dorsal amygdala global influence and stress ratings on PBO (in males) may reflect current emotional state rather than trauma history. In the PBO condition, a higher reported stress in males was associated with stronger global influence and more widespread connectivity of the left dorsal amygdala in males. In other words, the amygdala is exerting a stronger influence on other brain circuitry in the PBO condition, especially for males reporting more stress. Notably, OXY increased *local* influence of the left dorsal amygdala in males, suggesting that OXY shifts the influence of the left dorsal amygdala from global to more local and segregated from other brain circuitry. This shift on OXY may reflect an adaptive process, whereby stress-related amygdala activity is reduced.

The second hypothesis that years of cocaine use would be more strongly associated with OXY connectivity changes in the striatum was also not strongly supported given that none of the striatum nodes in males or females had cumulative importance that exceeded 1. However, OXY increased local influence of the right nucleus accumbens in females, indicating that it was influenced by OXY in females. Bethlehem and colleagues (28) similarly showed that OXY increased connectivity of the striatum with a broad network of brain regions in non-SUD women.

The third hypothesis that the major nodes of the salience network (insula, ACC) were expected to be associated with both childhood trauma and years of cocaine use was largely confirmed. ACC nodes predicted CTQ scores in females, and ACC and insula nodes predicted years of cocaine use in both males and females. The ACC was an important predictor in all models while the insula was an important predictor in one model (prediction of years of use in females). Local influence of the right ACC also increased on OXY in men, and global influence of the right dorsal ACC increased on OXY in women.

The fourth hypothesis was that network profiles associated with childhood trauma and years of cocaine use would be different between men and women. Stress circuitry (e.g., amygdala nodes) was expected to be more influential on network organization in females, whereas reward circuitry (e.g., striatum nodes) was expected to be more influential on network organization in males. Whereas the network profiles were indeed different between males and females, the amygdala was an important predictor of cocaine use in males rather than females (and was modulated by OXY in males), and the striatum was not an important predictor for either males or females, but the right accumbens was modulated by OXY in females.

The finding that amygdala connectivity was modulated by OXY, was associated with stress ratings under PBO, and was a significant component in the network profile for years of cocaine use in males but not females was not predicted. However, preclinical studies have reported that male rodents show greater OXY receptor binding in the amygdala than females, which is also modulated by breeding status in males (74). In addition, maltreated female adolescent rodents show significantly decreased OXY receptor binding in the amygdala compared to female controls (75). Although caution should be taken when translating preclinical findings to human study results, it is possible that the more prominent role for amygdala connectivity in CUD males in the present study is driven by higher OXY receptor binding in males and lower OXY receptor binding in females, particularly in those reporting more severe childhood trauma. This speculation, however, would need to be tested more directly in humans in future studies.

The predominant finding of the present study was that the salience network emerged as a critical component for OXY-induced changes in network profiles for childhood trauma and cocaine use in both males and females. Moreover, the ACC (rather than the insula) was the most prominent component in all models. The ACC is a critical node in the salience network that is functionally coupled to the insula. The ACC serves to influence external behaviors and motoric responses based on input from the insula (76), which processes interoceptive information and internal autonomic states (77). Given that the present study examined intrinsic connectivity (i.e., resting state) in the absence of external environmental input, the most salient information to be processed by subjects likely originated from internal bodily states. This may explain why the salience network was the primary influence on network organization. Had this study used external stimuli that could trigger reward responses, craving, or stress reactivity, the amygdala and striatum may have exerted a stronger influence on network organization.

Another potential explanation for the predominance of ACC nodes in influencing network organization is that the ACC is rich in OXY receptors (25). Because the present analysis focused on change in network connectivity related to OXY administration, those nodes that fall within brain regions with OXY receptors may have dominated network organization compared to regions that have fewer OXY receptors in humans, such as the striatum (25). It should be noted that the amygdala is also rich in OXY receptors, and this brain region emerged as an influential node in network profiles for individual variations in years of cocaine use in males. In addition, the exploratory analysis of subjective stress before scanning showed that higher reported stress was associated with greater global influence (EC) of the left dorsal amygdala in males in the PBO condition. These findings indicate that the amygdala may be an important locus for attenuating stress response in CUD males.

Wilcox and colleagues (17) have suggested that RSFC may be an important biomarker for treatment targets in SUDs. In their review of RSFC studies in SUD, they concluded that reduced connectivity between the salience network and executive control network and reduced connectivity within the executive control network are the most promising treatment targets for SUD. The present study has shown that OXY-related connectivity changes in components of the salience network, ACC, and insula are important for understanding individual variations in childhood trauma severity and cocaine use severity. Consequently, the present findings are consistent with the suggestion that the salience network is a potential treatment target.

It should be noted that associations between OXY-induced connectivity changes and childhood trauma or cocaine use severity were not universally in a single direction. In other words, higher cocaine use and greater childhood trauma were associated with both increases and decreases in connectivity because of OXY relative to PBO. Because this analysis considered a node's relation to all other nodes in the network, it is reasonable that connectivity in one region could increase on OXY, whereas connectivity in another region could decrease. This is particularly true for graph-theory measures like CC and eigenvector centrality, which consider not only the direct connections to a node but also the connections of the connected nodes.

The two graph-theory properties examined here represent different aspects of network organization—local influence (CC) versus global influence (EC) of a node on the whole-brain network. CC has been investigated in prior rsfMRI studies of SUD (78–83), and only one study has examined EC in smokers (83). In the present study, both properties showed utility in characterizing network profiles for CTQ and years of cocaine use in CUD, but EC explained more variance across models and replications. The present findings demonstrate that EC is a potentially more useful graph-theory measure to consider when characterizing network profiles associated with individual differences in CUD. However, CC was more sensitive to changes in RSFC because of OXY.

Limitations

One potential limitation of the present study is that we did not examine executive control network connectivity directly but focused instead on the influence of salience network, amygdala, and striatum nodes on intrinsic network organization. This could be viewed as a missed opportunity given a recent review suggesting that executive control network connectivity is a promising treatment target for SUD (17). However, the reason to limit the number of network nodes in the analysis was to avoid overfitting with automatic linear modeling. Nevertheless, the graph-theory measures used in this study reflect the connectivity of a given node with the entire brain, including frontal regions, thereby allowing for more specific hypotheses involving frontal cortex connectivity to be tested in future investigations.

The present analysis took several approaches to minimize contributions of head motion to graph-theory measures of connectivity (i.e., elimination of data sets with excessive head motion, temporal censoring, inclusion of six rigid-body head motion parameters as nuisance variables), and none of the graph-theory measures in individual nodes of interest was correlated with head motion. Therefore, the effects of head motion did not contaminate the measures of connectivity. Nevertheless, there are many other approaches to head-motion nuisance regression that are more stringent than the approach used in the present study [e.g., Ref. (55)], which could be considered a limitation. In addition, head motion emerged as a significant predictor of years of cocaine use in the final models that resulted from ALM. These findings indicate that head motion was associated with the outcome variable years of cocaine use. However, this association was different in males and females. For males, more years of cocaine use was associated with reduced head motion, but for females, more years of cocaine use was associated with increased head motion. The reason for this gender-specific divergence is not immediately apparent, but the present findings suggest that the extent of head motion is linked to individual variations in cocaine use and should probably be included in analyses even when head motion effects on connectivity are minimized.

Another potential limitation is that several substance use characteristics were not considered in the analyses but could be additional influences on changes in connectivity because of OXY. For example, positive THC tests and length of abstinence period before scanning could all affect resting-state connectivity and change in connectivity because of OXY. Future studies with larger samples should examine the influence of these substance use variables on OXY treatment response in CUD.

CONCLUSION

In conclusion, this study adds to the evidence suggesting that RSFC may be an important biomarker in identifying treatment targets in SUDs. Salience network regions, especially the ACC, emerged as primary loci for OXY-induced changes in connectivity in both men and women with CUD, whereas the amygdala was an additional important locus for OXY response in males with CUD. These brain regions may serve as potential target areas for future OXY-based treatments. In addition, the present findings suggest that treatment strategies for CUD need to consider gender differences in OXY response.

AUTHOR CONTRIBUTIONS

NB, KB, JJ, AM-C, and MM-S contributed to the design and conduct of the study. NB and JJ supervised and conducted the data analysis with contributions from KB, CC, AM-C, and BV. NB, KB, JJ, AM-C, and BS were involved in the interpretation of the data. JJ wrote the first draft of the manuscript. NB, KB, AM-C, BS, and BV helped write sections of and edited the manuscript.

REFERENCES

1. Seedat S, Scott KM, Angermeyer MC, Berglund P, Bromet EJ, Brugha TS, et al. Cross-national associations between gender and mental disorders in the World Health Organization World Mental Health Surveys. *Arch Gen Psychiatry* (2009) 66:785–95. doi: 10.1001/archgenpsychiatry.2009.36
2. Becker JB, Perry AN, Westenbroek C. Sex differences in the neural mechanisms mediating addiction: a new synthesis and hypothesis. *Biol Sex Differ* (2012) 3:14. doi: 10.1186/2042-6410-3-14
3. Sutherland MT, Mchugh MJ, Pariyadath V, Stein EA. Resting state functional connectivity in addiction: lessons learned and a road ahead. *Neuroimage* (2012) 62:2281–95. doi: 10.1016/j.neuroimage.2012.01.117
4. Lu H, Stein EA. Resting state functional connectivity: its physiological basis and application in neuropharmacology. *Neuropharmacology* (2014) 84:79–89. doi: 10.1016/j.neuropharm.2013.08.023
5. Hu Y, Salmeron BJ, Gu H, Stein EA, Yang Y. Impaired functional connectivity within and between frontostriatal circuits and its association with compulsive drug use and trait impulsivity in cocaine addiction. *JAMA Psychiatry* (2015) 72:584–92. doi: 10.1001/jamapsychiatry.2015.1
6. Contreras-Rodriguez O, Albein-Urios N, Vilar-Lopez R, Perales JC, Martinez-Gonzalez JM, Fernandez-Serrano MJ, et al. Increased corticolimbic

connectivity in cocaine dependence versus pathological gambling is associated with drug severity and emotion-related impulsivity. *Addict Biol* (2016) 21:709–18. doi: 10.1111/adb.12242

7. Zhang S, Wang W, Zhornitsky S, Li CR. Resting state functional connectivity of the lateral and medial hypothalamus in cocaine dependence: an exploratory study. *Front Psychiatry* (2018) 9:344. doi: 10.3389/fpsyt.2018.00344
8. Kelly C, Zuo XN, Gotimer K, Cox CL, Lynch L, Brock D, et al. Reduced interhemispheric resting state functional connectivity in cocaine addiction. *Biol Psychiatry* (2011) 69:684–92. doi: 10.1016/j.biopsych.2010.11.022
9. Mchugh MJ, Demers CH, Braud J, Briggs R, Adinoff B, Stein EA. Striatal-insula circuits in cocaine addiction: implications for impulsivity and relapse risk. *Am J Drug Alcohol Abuse* (2013) 39:424–32. doi: 10.3109/00952990.2013.847446
10. Berlingeri M, Losasso D, Girolo A, Cozzolino E, Masullo T, Scotto M, et al. Resting state brain connectivity patterns before eventual relapse into cocaine abuse. *Behav Brain Res* (2017) 327:121–32. doi: 10.1016/j.bbr.2017.01.002
11. Mchugh MJ, Demers CH, Salmeron BJ, Devous MD, Sr., Stein EA, Adinoff B. Cortico-amygdala coupling as a marker of early relapse risk in cocaine-addicted individuals. *Front Psychiatry* (2014) 5:16. doi: 10.3389/fpsyt.2014.00016
12. Adinoff B, Gu H, Merrick C, Mchugh M, Jeon-Slaughter H, Lu H, et al. Basal hippocampal activity and its functional connectivity predicts cocaine relapse. *Biol Psychiatry* (2015) 78:496–504. doi: 10.1016/j.biopsych.2014.12.027
13. Contreras-Rodriguez O, Albein-Urios N, Perales JC, Martinez-Gonzalez JM, Vilar-Lopez R, Fernandez-Serrano MJ, et al. Cocaine-specific neuroplasticity in the ventral striatum network is linked to delay discounting and drug relapse. *Addiction* (2015) 110:1953–62. doi: 10.1111/add.13076
14. Geng X, Hu Y, Gu H, Salmeron BJ, Adinoff B, Stein EA, et al. Salience and default mode network dysregulation in chronic cocaine users predict treatment outcome. *Brain* (2017) 140:1513–24. doi: 10.1093/brain/awx036
15. Mccarthy JM, Zuo CS, Shepherd JM, Dias N, Lukas SE, Janes AC. Reduced interhemispheric executive control network coupling in men during early cocaine abstinence: a pilot study. *Drug Alcohol Depend* (2017) 181:1–4. doi: 10.1016/j.drugalcdep.2017.09.009
16. Mchugh MJ, Gu H, Yang Y, Adinoff B, Stein EA. Executive control network connectivity strength protects against relapse to cocaine use. *Addict Biol* (2017) 22:1790–801. doi: 10.1111/adb.12448
17. Wilcox CE, Abbott CC, Calhoun VD. Alterations in resting-state functional connectivity in substance use disorders and treatment implications. *Prog Neuropsychopharmacol Biol Psychiatry* (2019) 91:79–93. doi: 10.1016/j.pnpbp.2018.06.011
18. Gawrysiak MJ, Jagannathan K, Regier P, Suh JJ, Kampman K, Vickery T, et al. Unseen scars: cocaine patients with prior trauma evidence heightened resting state functional connectivity (RSFC) between the amygdala and limbic-striatal regions. *Drug Alcohol Depend* (2017) 180:363–70. doi: 10.1016/j.drugalcdep.2017.08.035
19. Wismer Fries AB, Ziegler TE, Kurian JR, Jacoris S, Pollak SD. Early experience in humans is associated with changes in neuropeptides critical for regulating social behavior. *Proc Natl Acad Sci U S A* (2005) 102:17237–40. doi: 10.1073/pnas.0504767102
20. Heim C, Bradley B, Mletzko TC, Deveau TC, Musselman DL, Nemeroff CB, et al. Effect of childhood trauma on adult depression and neuroendocrine function: sex-specific moderation by CRH receptor 1 gene. *Front Behav Neurosci* (2009) 3:41. doi: 10.3389/neuro.08.041.2009
21. Lee MR, Rohn MC, Tanda G, Leggio L. Targeting the oxytocin system to treat addictive disorders: rationale and progress to date. *CNS Drugs* (2016) 30:109–23. doi: 10.1007/s40263-016-0313-z
22. Kirsch P, Esslinger C, Chen Q, Mier D, Lis S, Siddhanti S, et al. Oxytocin modulates neural circuitry for social cognition and fear in humans. *J Neurosci* (2005) 25:11489–93. doi: 10.1523/JNEUROSCI.3984-05.2005
23. Labuschagne I, Phan KL, Wood A, Angstadt M, Chua P, Heinrichs M, et al. Oxytocin attenuates amygdala reactivity to fear in generalized social anxiety disorder. *Neuropsychopharmacology* (2010) 35:2403–13. doi: 10.1038/npp.2010.123
24. Koch SB, Van Zuiden M, Nawijn L, Frijling JL, Veltman DJ, Olff M. Intranasal oxytocin normalizes amygdala functional connectivity in posttraumatic stress disorder. *Neuropsychopharmacology* (2016) 41:2041–51. doi: 10.1038/npp.2016.1
25. Boccia ML, Petrusz P, Suzuki K, Marson L, Pedersen CA. Immunohistochemical localization of oxytocin receptors in human brain. *Neuroscience* (2013) 253:155–64. doi: 10.1016/j.neuroscience.2013.08.048
26. Dumais KM, Bredewold R, Mayer TE, Veenema AH. Sex differences in oxytocin receptor binding in forebrain regions: correlations with social interest in brain region- and sex- specific ways. *Horm Behav* (2013) 64:693–701. doi: 10.1016/j.yhbeh.2013.08.012
27. Seeley SH, Chou YH, O'connor MF. Intranasal oxytocin and OXTR genotype effects on resting state functional connectivity: a systematic review. *Neurosci Biobehav Rev* (2018) 95:17–32. doi: 10.1016/j.neubiorev.2018.09.011
28. Bethlehem RAI, Lombardo MV, Lai MC, Auyeung B, Crockford SK, Deakin J, et al. Intranasal oxytocin enhances intrinsic corticostriatal functional connectivity in women. *Transl Psychiatry* (2017) 7:e1099. doi: 10.1038/tp.2017.72
29. Brodmann K, Gruber O, Goya-Maldonado R. Intranasal oxytocin selectively modulates large-scale brain networks in humans. *Brain Connect* (2017) 7:454–63. doi: 10.1089/brain.2017.0528
30. Zhao Z, Ma X, Geng Y, Zhao W, Zhou F, Wang J, et al. Oxytocin differentially modulates specific dorsal and ventral striatal functional connections with frontal and cerebellar regions. *Neuroimage* (2019) 184:781–9. doi: 10.1016/j.neuroimage.2018.09.067
31. Connors GJ, Maisto SA, Zywiak WH. Male and female alcoholics' attributions regarding the onset and termination of relapses and the maintenance of abstinence. *J Subst Abuse* (1998) 10:27–42. doi: 10.1016/S0899-3289(99)80138-2
32. Terry-Mcelrath YM, O'malley PM, Johnston LD. Reasons for drug use among American Youth by consumption level, gender, and race/ethnicity: 1976-2005. *J Drug Issues* (2009) 39:677–714. doi: 10.1177/002204260903900310
33. Kilts CD, Schweitzer JB, Quinn CK, Gross RE, Faber TL, Muhammad F, et al. Neural activity related to drug craving in cocaine addiction. *Arch Gen Psychiatry* (2001) 58:334–41. doi: 10.1001/archpsyc.58.4.334
34. Kilts CD, Gross RE, Ely TD, Drexler KP. The neural correlates of cue-induced craving in cocaine-dependent women. *Am J Psychiatry* (2004) 161:233–41. doi: 10.1176/appi.ajp.161.2.233
35. Potenza MN, Hong KI, Lacadie CM, Fulbright RK, Tuit KL, Sinha R. Neural correlates of stress-induced and cue-induced drug craving: influences of sex and cocaine dependence. *Am J Psychiatry* (2012) 169:406–14. doi: 10.1176/appi.ajp.2011.11020289
36. Teicher MH, Andersen SL, Polcari A, Anderson CM, Navalta CP. Developmental neurobiology of childhood stress and trauma. *Psychiatr Clin North Am* (2002) 25:397–426., vii-viii. doi: 10.1016/S0193-953X(01)00003-X
37. Stevens JS, Van Rooij SJH, Jovanovic T. Developmental contributors to trauma response: the importance of sensitive periods, early environment, and sex differences. *Curr Top Behav Neurosci* (2018) 38:1–22. doi: 10.1007/7854_2016_38
38. Frijling JL, Van Zuiden M, Koch SB, Nawijn L, Veltman DJ, Olff M. Intranasal oxytocin affects amygdala functional connectivity after trauma script-driven imagery in distressed recently trauma-exposed individuals. *Neuropsychopharmacology* (2016) 41:1286–96. doi: 10.1038/npp.2015.278
39. Koob GF, Volkow ND. Neurocircuitry of addiction. *Neuropsychopharmacology* (2010) 35:217–38. doi: 10.1038/npp.2009.110
40. Peters SK, Dunlop K, Downar J. Cortico-striatal-thalamic loop circuits of the salience network: a central pathway in psychiatric disease and treatment. *Front Syst Neurosci* (2016) 10:104. doi: 10.3389/fnsys.2016.00104
41. Sheehan DV, Lecrubier Y, Sheehan KH, Amorim P, Janavs J, Weiller E, et al. The Mini-International Neuropsychiatric Interview (M.I.N.I).: the development and validation of a structured diagnostic psychiatric interview for DSM-IV and ICD-10. *J Clin Psychiatry* (1998) 59 Suppl 20:22–33. ;quiz 34-57.
42. First MB, Spitzer RL, Gibbon M, Williams JB (2002). "Structured clinical interview for DSM-IV-TR axis I disorders, research version, patient edition". SCID-I/P).
43. Sobell LC, Sobell MB. Timeline follow-back: A technique for assessing self-reported alcohol consumption. In: Litten RZ, Allen JP, editors. *Measuring alcohol consumption: Psychosocial and biomedical methods*. Humana Press (1992). p. 41–72. doi: 10.1007/978-1-4612-0357-5_3
44. Bernstein DP, Fink L. *Childhood Trauma Questionnaire: A retrospective self-report manual*. San Antonio, TX: The Psychological Corporation (1998).

45. Childress AR, Mclellan AT, O'brien CP. Conditioned responses in a methadone population: a comparison of laboratory, clinic, and natural settings. *J Subst Abuse Treat* (1986) 3:173–9. doi: 10.1016/0740-5472(86)90018-8
46. Spielberger CD, Gorsuch RL, Lushene R, Vagg PR, Jacobs GA. *Manual for the State-Trait Anxiety Inventory*. Palo Alto, CA: Consulting Psychologists Press (1983).
47. Heinrichs M, Baumgartner T, Kirschbaum C, Ehlert U. Social support and oxytocin interact to suppress cortisol and subjective responses to psychosocial stress. *Biol Psychiatry* (2003) 54:1389–98. doi: 10.1016/S0006-3223(03)00465-7
48. Ditzen B, Schaer M, Gabriel B, Bodenmann G, Ehlert U, Heinrichs M. Intranasal oxytocin increases positive communication and reduces cortisol levels during couple conflict. *Biol Psychiatry* (2009) 65:728–31. doi: 10.1016/j.biopsych.2008.10.011
49. Kubzansky LD, Mendes WB, Appleton A, Block J, Adler GK. Protocol for an experimental investigation of the roles of oxytocin and social support in neuroendocrine, cardiovascular, and subjective responses to stress across age and gender. *BMC Public Health* (2009) 9:481. doi: 10.1186/1471-2458-9-481
50. Mcrae-Clark AL, Baker NL, Moran-Santa Maria M, Brady KT. Effect of oxytocin on craving and stress response in marijuana-dependent individuals: a pilot study. *Psychopharmacology* (2013) 228:623–31. doi: 10.1007/s00213-013-3062-4
51. Flanagan JC, Baker NL, Mcrae-Clark AL, Brady KT, Moran-Santa Maria MM. Effects of adverse childhood experiences on the association between intranasal oxytocin and social stress reactivity among individuals with cocaine dependence. *Psychiatry Res* (2015) 229:94–100. doi: 10.1016/j.psychres.2015.07.064
52. Heinrichs M, Von Dawans B, Domes G. Oxytocin, vasopressin, and human social behavior. *Front Neuroendocrinol* (2009) 30:548–57. doi: 10.1016/j.yfrne.2009.05.005
53. Holm S. A simple sequentially rejective multiple test procedure. *Scand J Stat* (1979), 65–70.
54. Benjamini Y, Hochberg Y. Controlling the false discovery rate: a practical and powerful approach to multiple testing. *J R Stat Soc Series B Stat Methodol* (1995) 57:289–300. doi: 10.1111/j.2517-6161.1995.tb02031.x
55. Satterthwaite TD, Elliott MA, Gerraty RT, Ruparel K, Loughead J, Calkins ME, et al. An improved framework for confound regression and filtering for control of motion artifact in the preprocessing of resting-state functional connectivity data. *Neuroimage* (2013) 64:240–56. doi: 10.1016/j.neuroimage.2012.08.052
56. Cox RW. AFNI: software for analysis and visualization of functional magnetic resonance neuroimages. *Comput Biomed Res* (1996) 29:162–73. doi: 10.1006/cbmr.1996.0014
57. Power JD, Barnes KA, Snyder AZ, Schlaggar BL, Petersen SE. Spurious but systematic correlations in functional connectivity MRI networks arise from subject motion. *Neuroimage* (2012) 59:2142–54. doi: 10.1016/j.neuroimage.2011.10.018
58. Rcoreteam (2018). "R: A language and environment for statistical computing". 3.5.1 ed. (Vienna, Austria: R Foundation for Statistical Computing).
59. Ledoit O, Wolf M. Improved estimation of the covariance matrix of stock retruns with an application to portfolio science. *J Empir Financ* (2003) 10:603–21. doi: 10.1016/S0927-5398(03)00007-0
60. Schafer J, Strimmer K. A shrinkage approach to large-scale covariance matrix estimation and implications for functional genomics. *Stat. Appl. Genet. Mol. Biol.* (2005) 4. doi: 10.2202/1544-6115.1175
61. Opgen-Rhein R, Strimmer K. Accurate ranking of differentially expressed genes by a distribution-free shrinkage approach. *Stat Appl Genet Mol Biol* (2007) 6:Article9. doi: 10.2202/1544-6115.1252
62. Lohmann G, Margulies DS, Horstmann A, Pleger B, Lepsien J, Goldhahn D, et al. Eigenvector centrality mapping for analyzing connectivity patterns in fMRI data of the human brain. *PLoS ONE* (2010) 5:e10232. doi: 10.1371/journal.pone.0010232
63. Fornito A, Harrison BJ, Zalesky A, Simons JS. Competitive and cooperative dynamics of large-scale brain functional networks supporting recollection. *Proc Natl Acad Sci U S A* (2012) 109:12788–93. doi: 10.1073/pnas.1204185109
64. Watts DJ, Strogatz SH. Collective dynamics of 'small-world' networks. *Nature* (1998) 393:440–2. doi: 10.1038/30918
65. Rubinov M, Sporns O. Complex network meansures of brain connectivity: uses and interpretations. *Comput Models Brain* (2010) 52:1059–69. doi: 10.1016/j.neuroimage.2009.10.003
66. Costantini G, Perugini M. Generalization of clustering coefficients to signed correlation networks. *PLoS One* (2014) 9:e88669. doi: 10.1371/journal.pone.0088669
67. Xia M, Wang J, He Y. BrainNet Viewer: a network visualization tool for human brain connectomics. *PLoS ONE* (2013) 8:e68910. doi: 10.1371/journal.pone.0068910
68. Arnsten AF. Stress signalling pathways that impair prefrontal cortex structure and function. *Nat Rev Neurosci* (2009) 10:410–22. doi: 10.1038/nrn2648
69. Lupien SJ, Mcewen BS, Gunnar MR, Heim C. Effects of stress throughout the lifespan on the brain, behaviour and cognition. *Nat Rev Neurosci* (2009) 10:434–45. doi: 10.1038/nrn2639
70. Hart H, Rubia K. Neuroimaging of child abuse: a critical review. *Front Hum Neurosci* (2012) 6:52. doi: 10.3389/fnhum.2012.00052
71. Van Harmelen AL, Hauber K, Gunther Moor B, Spinhoven P, Boon AE, Crone EA, et al. Childhood emotional maltreatment severity is associated with dorsal medial prefrontal cortex responsivity to social exclusion in young adults. *PLoS One* (2014) 9:e85107. doi: 10.1371/journal.pone.0085107
72. Schatzoff M, Tsao R, Fienberg S. Efficient computing of all possible regressions. *Technometrics* (1968) 10:769–79. doi: 10.2307/1267458
73. Hair J, Black WC, Babin BJ, Anderson RE. *Multivariate Data Analysis*. Upper Saddle River, NJ: Pearson Education International (2010).
74. Mooney SJ, Coen CW, Holmes MM, Beery AK. Region-specific associations between sex, social status, and oxytocin receptor density in the brains of eusocial rodents. *Neuroscience* (2015) 303:261–9. doi: 10.1016/j.neuroscience.2015.06.043
75. Hill KT, Warren M, Roth TL. The influence of infant-caregiver experiences on amygdala Bdnf, OXTr, and NPY expression in developing and adult male and female rats. *Behav Brain Res* (2014) 272:175–80. doi: 10.1016/j.bbr.2014.07.001
76. Menon V, Uddin LQ. Saliency, switching, attention and control: a network model of insula function. *Brain Struct Funct* (2010) 214:655–67. doi: 10.1007/s00429-010-0262-0
77. Craig AD. Forebrain emotional asymmetry: a neuroanatomical basis? *Trends Cogn Sci* (2005) 9:566–71. doi: 10.1016/j.tics.2005.10.005
78. Breckel TP, Thiel CM, Giessing C. The efficiency of functional brain networks does not differ between smokers and non-smokers. *Psychiatry Res* (2013) 214:349–56. doi: 10.1016/j.pscychresns.2013.07.005
79. Giessing C, Thiel CM, Alexander-Bloch AF, Patel AX, Bullmore ET. Human brain functional network changes associated with enhanced and impaired attentional task performance. *J Neurosci* (2013) 33:5903–14. doi: 10.1523/JNEUROSCI.4854-12.2013
80. Jiang G, Wen X, Qiu Y, Zhang R, Wang J, Li M, et al. Disrupted topological organization in whole-brain functional networks of heroin-dependent individuals: a resting-state FMRI study. *PLoS ONE* (2013) 8:e82715. doi: 10.1371/journal.pone.0082715
81. Lin F, Wu G, Zhu L, Lei H. Altered brain functional networks in heavy smokers. *Addict Biol* (2015) 20:809–19. doi: 10.1111/adb.12155
82. Wang Z, Suh J, Li Z, Li Y, Franklin T, O'brien C, et al. A hyper-connected but less efficient small-world network in the substance-dependent brain. *Drug Alcohol Depend* (2015) 152:102–8. doi: 10.1016/j.drugalcdep.2015.04.015
83. Moran-Santa Maria MM, Vanderweyen DC, Camp CC, Zhu X, Mckee SA, Cosgrove KP, et al. Network analysis of intrinsic functional brain connectivity in male and female adult smokers: a preliminary study. *Nicotine Tob Res* (2018) 20:810–8. doi: 10.1093/ntr/ntx206.

5

Resonance-Paced Breathing Alters Neural Response to Visual Cues: Proof-of-Concept for a Neuroscience-Informed Adjunct to Addiction Treatments

Marsha E. Bates[1,2], Laura M. Lesnewich[2,3], Sarah Grace Uhouse[2,3], Suril Gohel[4] and Jennifer F. Buckman[1,2]*

[1] Cardiac Neuroscience Laboratory, Department of Kinesiology and Health, Rutgers University-New Brunswick, Piscataway, NJ, United States, [2] Center of Alcohol Studies, Rutgers University-New Brunswick, Piscataway, NJ, United States, [3] Cardiac Neuroscience Laboratory, Department of Psychology, Rutgers University-New Brunswick, Piscataway, NJ, United States, [4] Department of Health Informatics, School of Health Professions, Rutgers University-Newark, Newark, NJ, United States

***Correspondence:**
Marsha E. Bates
mebates@smithers.rutgers.edu

Conscious attempts to regulate alcohol and drug use are often undermined by automatic attention and arousal processes that are activated in the context of salient cues. Response to these cues involves body and brain signals that are linked via dynamic feedback loops, yet no studies have targeted the cardiovascular system as a potential conduit to alter automatic neural processes that maintain cue salience. This proof-of-concept study examined within-person changes in neural response to parallel but unique sets of visual alcohol-related cues at two points in time: prior to versus following a brief behavioral intervention. The active intervention was resonance breathing, a rhythmical breathing task paced at 0.1 Hz (6 breaths per minute) that helps normalize neurocardiac feedback. The control intervention was a low-demand cognitive task. Functional magnetic resonance imaging (fMRI) was used to assess changes in brain response to the cues presented before (A1) and after (A2) the intervention in 41 emerging adult men and women with varying drinking behaviors. The resonance breathing group exhibited significantly less activation to A2 cues compared with A1 cues in left inferior and superior lateral occipital cortices, right inferior lateral occipital cortex, bilateral occipital pole, and temporal occipital fusiform cortices. This group also showed significantly greater activation to A2 cues compared with A1 cues in medial prefrontal, anterior and posterior cingulate, and precuneus cortices, paracingulate, and lingual gyri. The control group showed no significant changes. Thus, following resonance breathing, activation in brain regions involved in visual processing of cues was reduced, while activation in brain areas implicated in behavioral control, internally directed cognition, and brain–body integration was increased. These findings provide preliminary evidence that manipulation of the cardiovascular system with resonance breathing alters neural activation in a manner theoretically consistent with a dampening of automatic sensory input and strengthening of higher-level cognitive processing.

Keywords: alcohol, biofeedback, cardiovascular, neural reactivity, functional magnetic resonance imaging, heart rate variability, respiration, resonance breathing

INTRODUCTION

Moment-to-moment changes in internal states (e.g., cognition, emotion, visceral processes, moods) and environments (e.g., cues, persons) influence decisions to use alcohol and other drugs (1). These dynamic, intra-individual change processes derive from the body's ability to collect and relay information to the brain about the environment (afferent neural traffic), as well as from the brain's ability to integrate this information and generate a behavioral response (efferent neural traffic). In other words, behavior is influenced by both body and brain signals that are linked via reflexive and predictive bidirectional feedback (2, 3).

In the case of the cardiovascular system, this feedback loop (**Figure 1**) has been extensively documented in terms of its neurophysiology and functional anatomy in rodent and primate models [e.g., (4, 5)]; parallel functional anatomy emerged in a meta-analysis of human neuroimaging studies (6). The loop maintains signaling between the brain and heart via the vagus and sympathetic nerves, baroreceptors located on the aortic arch, carotid artery, and other vessel walls, and a network of brain regions referred to as the central autonomic network (4). These bodies of literature reveal how the brain elicits cardiovascular signals that promote arousal (e.g., increasing heart rate and blood pressure) that, in turn, prepare the organism for goal-directed behavior to respond to in-the-moment demands. Through this loop, feedback from the heart and vasculature is integrated with other autonomic information and relayed to forebrain structures that mediate cognitive and emotional experience

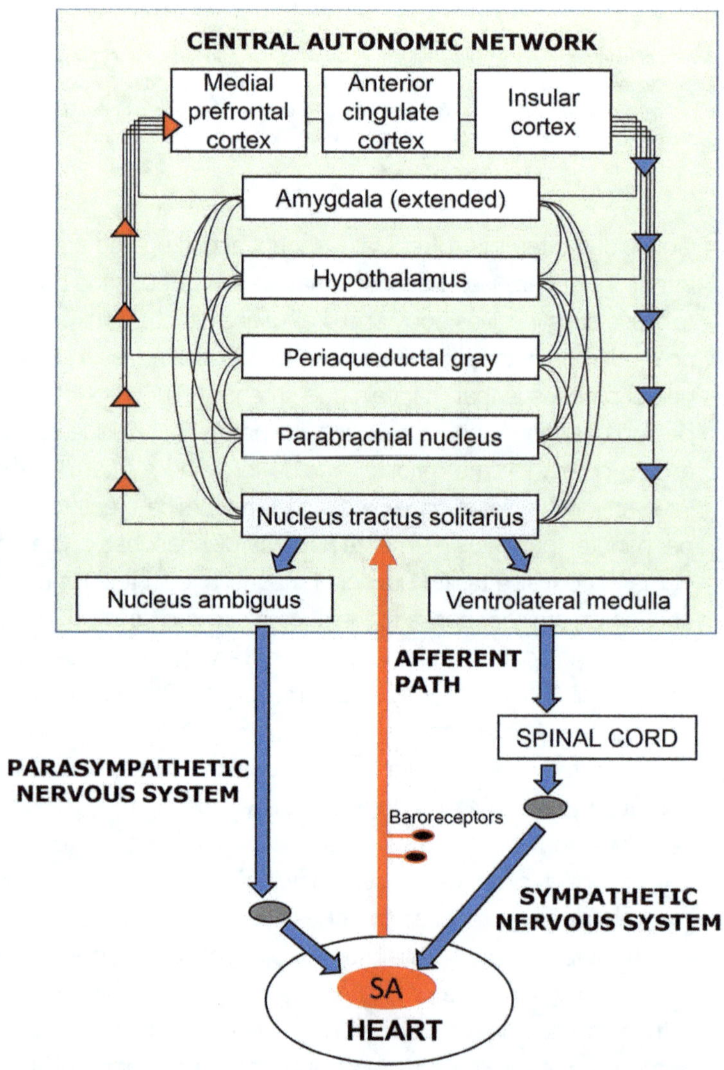

FIGURE 1 | Schematic overview of the neurocardiac feedback loop. Efferent information (blue arrows) emanates from cortical, subcortical, and brain stem structures of the central-autonomic network and flows to the sinoatrial (SA) node of the heart via the sympathetic and parasympathetic branches of the autonomic nervous system. Afferent information (red arrows) from the heart and blood vessels is conveyed back to the brain via baroreceptors located mainly in the walls of the aortic and carotid arteries. Afferent signals enter the brain (shaded in green) via the nucleus tractus solitarius in the brain stem and are integrated with other sensory, cognitive, and affective information as it ascends to cortical regions, including the medial frontal, cingulate, and insular cortices.

(7–9). Consideration of cardiovascular processes as embedded components of affect and cognition implies that these processes contribute to motivated human behavior, including behavioral flexibility toward alcohol and other drugs (10–12). This is important because several non-invasive, low-cost behavioral interventions that help normalize cardiovascular functioning have demonstrated efficacy across various mental and physical health conditions (13–20).

Two compelling qualities of the neurocardiac feedback loop for intervention development are its plasticity and responsivity to relatively simple behavioral interventions. Afferent stream activation of the neurocardiac feedback loop can be accomplished by manipulating peripheral functions, such as respiration and muscle flexion (21–24). Breathing paced at 6 breaths per minute (0.1 Hz) is slower and more rhythmical than typical breathing (12–20 breaths per minute). It creates resonance within the cardiovascular system by synchronizing cardiac oscillations driven by respiratory sinus arrhythmia (i.e., the phenomena of heart rate acceleration with inhalation and deceleration with exhalation) with cardiac oscillations driven by the baroreflex, which links heart rate acceleration/deceleration to corresponding changes in the blood pressure (21, 25). As shown in **Figure 2**, breathing at this frequency lowers systolic blood pressure, increases variability in the time intervals between R-spikes of the electrocardiogram (ECG) (i.e., heart rate variability), generates large oscillations in pulse transit time (i.e., vascular tone variability), and increases the sensitivity of heart rate to changes in blood pressure (i.e., baroreflex gain) (12, 21). A recent meta-analysis found that clinical interventions involving paced breathing at a resonance frequency of the cardiovascular system resulted in large effect size reductions in anxiety and stress (26). Preliminary evidence also suggested paced breathing may reduce craving for appetitive substances (27).

The brain structures of the central autonomic network that participate in cardiovascular signaling overlap considerably with those that process reward, emotion, and habit formation (28), including medial prefrontal, cingulate, and insular cortices, and amygdala. These structures also figure prominently in current translational models of putative addiction neurocircuitry (29–31), with the brain stem serving as the first point of neural integration of afferent autonomic and somatic signals from the body. Psychophysiological evidence suggests that the neurocardiac feedback loop may participate in substance use behaviors through its contribution to attention capture by stimulating cues, affective modulation, and relay of visceral reactivity to the brain [e.g., (32–36)], but little research has extended these findings to the neural structures that comprise the central autonomic network. Nonetheless, converging lines of evidence suggest that ineffective or maladaptive functioning of this feedback loop can set into motion a cascade of biological events that alter one's ability to adaptively modulate affect, arousal, and stress response (2, 37, 38).

Neural cue reactivity studies, wherein brain activation is measured while participants are exposed to salient alcohol- or drug-related cues, have received significant attention in the neuroscience and psychology of addiction literatures (39, 40). Cue reactivity studies typically compare within-person differences in

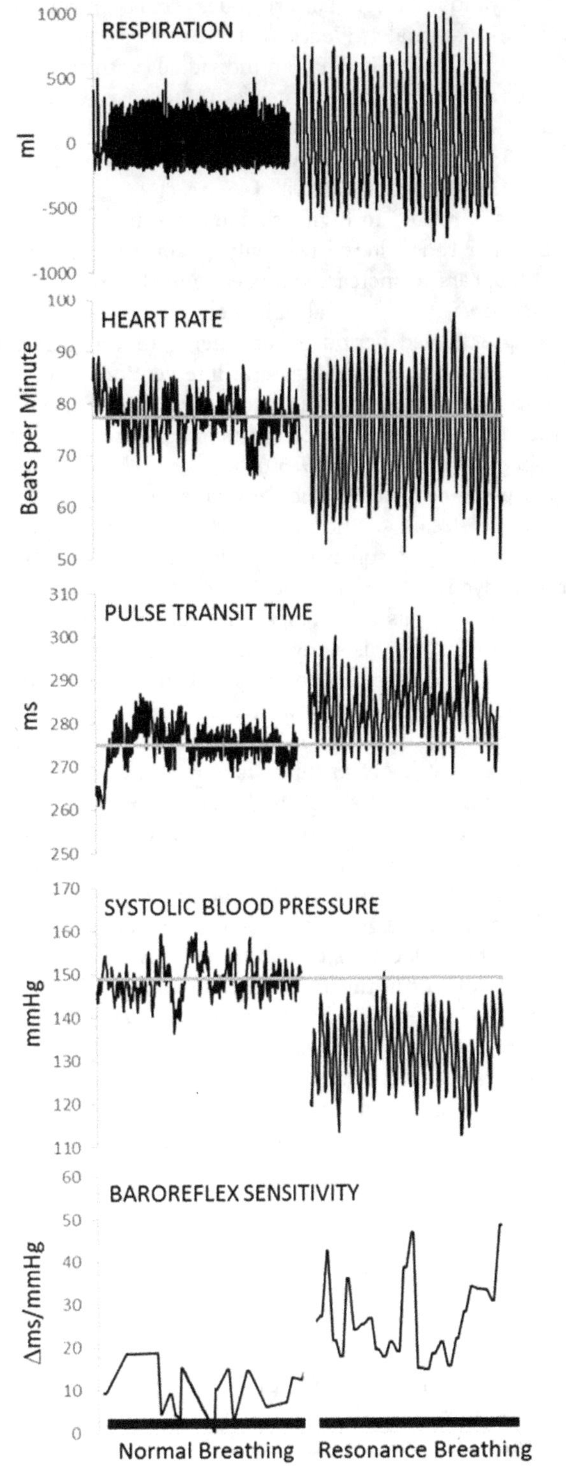

FIGURE 2 | Physiological data from one representative individual collected during a 5-min baseline task (normal breathing) and a 5-min resonance breathing task. Resonance breathing elicited instantaneous changes in respiration, heart rate, pulse transit time (i.e., vascular tone), systolic arterial pressure, and baroreflex sensitivity such that oscillations were magnified and more rhythmic across all measures. In addition, resonance breathing decreased systolic pressure, improved vascular tone, and increased the sensitivity of the neurocardiac feedback loop (i.e., baroreflex). Adapted from (12). Used with permission.

brain activation to alcohol or drug cues versus control cues (40). There is substantial evidence that elevated alcohol and drug cue neural reactivity is found in individuals with substance use disorders (40–42). Increased neural (43) and cardiac (44) cue reactivity also has been associated with increased drug craving (2, 37, 38). Experimental evidence suggests that heightened neural (45) and cardiovascular (46) reactivity to alcohol and drug cues is related to high risk substance use in non-clinical populations. Thus, altered reactivity to affective and appetitive stimuli appears to increase the likelihood that individuals will be susceptible to contextual influences on substance use, even following extended periods of abstinence (47, 48). This raises the question of whether behavioral interventions that enhance the efficiency of neurocardiac signaling might be used to alter neurocardiac activation to contextual challenges that promote substance use and relapse (49, 50).

This proof-of-concept study examined whether stimulating the afferent stream of the neurocardiac feedback loop with a 5-min course of resonance breathing can affect subsequent neural activation to visual alcohol cues. In contrast to cue reactivity paradigms that compare neural activation to alcohol versus control cues, this study examined within-person changes in neural response to alcohol cues at two points in time. We compared neural activation with unique sets of alcohol cues viewed prior to versus following the breathing task. Because this is the first study of its kind, there is no empirical literature to guide predictions about brain activation changes when participants are exposed to visual cues following resonance breathing. Based on the anatomy of the central autonomic network (4, 5) and drug cue salience networks (28, 40), we hypothesized that significant changes in activation may be observed in brainstem, medial prefrontal, cingulate, and insular cortices, as well as in the amygdala. We further allowed for the possibility of spreading activation, wherein structures within the central autonomic network that share additional network circuitry with regions outside the central autonomic network (e.g., the mesocorticolimbic circuit, ventral striatum) may exhibit activation changes as well. Significant changes in neural response were not anticipated in the group that viewed alcohol cues before and after completing a low-demand cognitive task.

METHODS

Participants

Forty-nine men and women, ages 18 to 25 years, were recruited at a large, northeast U.S. university and in the surrounding community through advertisements targeting alcohol drinkers. Initial inclusion criteria for all participants assessed via self-report were fluency in English, right-handedness, near 20/20 vision (corrected), and alcohol consumption at least once per month. Exclusion criteria assessed via self-report included: MRI contraindications (e.g., permanent metal in the body, claustrophobia), abnormal hearing, any serious medical condition (e.g., epilepsy, diabetes), cardiovascular problems (e.g., hypertension, heart murmur), current learning disability or attention difficulties, loss of consciousness for longer than 30 min, and, for women, pregnancy. To reduce heterogeneity related to psychiatric comorbidities and poly-substance use, lifetime diagnosis of a bipolar disorder or psychosis (e.g., schizophrenia, schizoaffective disorder), past year psychiatric/psychological treatment, past year cannabis use exceeding four times per month in the past year, other past year illicit drug use more than twice per month, past or current substance use treatment (including Alcoholics Anonymous/Narcotics Anonymous), and substance use during pregnancy on the part of the biological mother also were exclusionary.

Half of the participants were recruited based on meeting the National Institute on Alcohol Abuse and Alcoholism (NIAAA) "low risk" drinking criteria [i.e., no more than 5 drinks per day for men (4 drinks per day for women), no more than 14 drinks per week for men (7 drinks per week for women)], as well as an additional criterion of not binge drinking more than once in the past 6 months. The other half met DSM-IV-TR criteria (51) for alcohol dependence. This proof-of-concept examination of resonance breathing as a neurally active intervention included all participants with the exception that data from eight participants were excluded due to excessive motion in the scanner. The final sample (n = 41) had a mean age of 21.4 (SD = 1.9) years and was racially and ethnically diverse (27% Asian, 27% black/African American, 29% white, 17% other/multiple race; 11% Latino/a); 46% of the participants identified as female.

Procedures

Potential participants who gave verbal consent completed a telephone screening interview to determine initial eligibility. Eligible participants were asked to abstain from alcohol and drug use (except caffeine and nicotine) for 24 h prior to the experimental session. After screening, they were randomized into the active intervention (i.e., resonance breathing) or the control intervention (i.e., vanilla task), with drinking profiles being approximately equally distributed in both groups.

Upon arrival at the imaging center, participants provided written informed consent, supplied a breath sample to verify zero blood alcohol concentration, and completed a MRI safety screener and self-report questionnaires regarding alcohol use, mood state (Positive and Negative Affect Scale) (52), and stress (Perceived Stress Scale) (53). Basic physiological measures (e.g., temperature, blood pressure, weight) and a urine sample were collected; participants with a positive urine screen for cocaine, methamphetamine, opiates, and/or benzodiazepines (One Step Multi-Drug Screen Test Panel) were excluded. Participants with a positive urine screen for marijuana were asked additional follow-up questions about their drug use, and those with marijuana use exceeding four times per month were excluded. Women were screened for pregnancy using a standard urine dipstick. All participants were trained to use an MRI-compatible response box and to perform their assigned intervention task. Task training lasted approximately 2 min. Participants then were fitted with ECG sensors and a respiration belt and positioned in the scanner.

The overall paradigm (**Figure 3A**) involved four 5-min tasks: 1) viewing a set of nature picture cues, 2) viewing a set

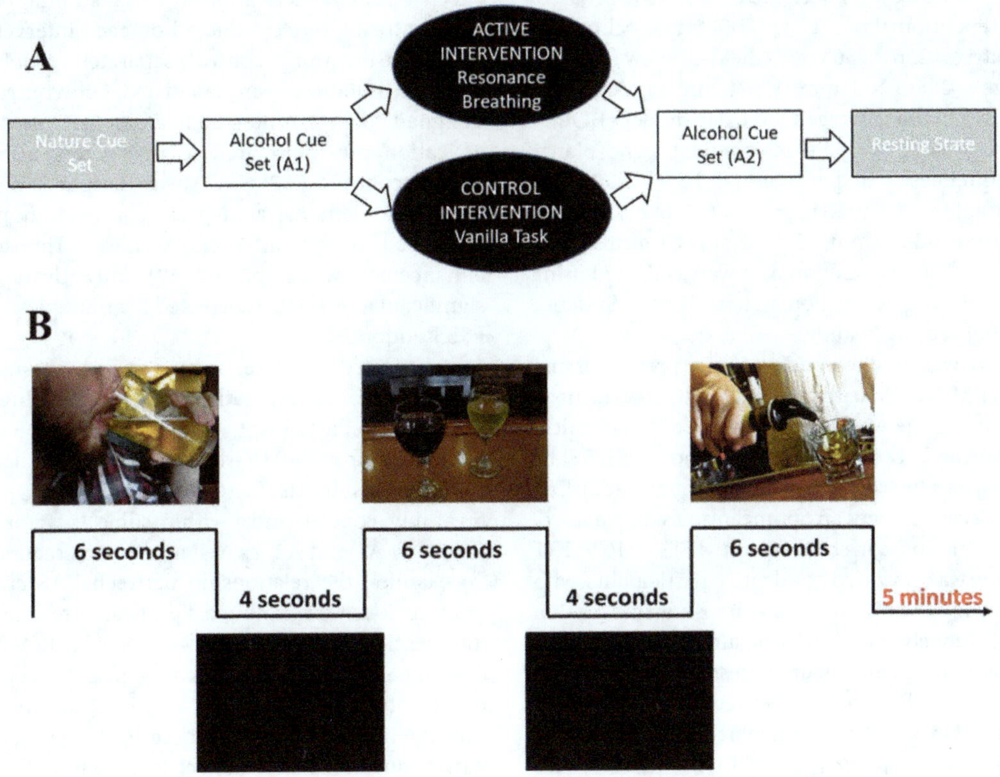

FIGURE 3 | Visual depiction of the study and cue task design. Panel **(A)** shows the complete study design. Participants first viewed a set of nature picture cues (data not shown). Participants then viewed a set of alcohol picture cues (A1), followed by a 5-min intervention task (active condition: resonance breathing; control condition: vanilla task). They then immediately viewed a second, distinct set of alcohol picture cues (A2). The study ended with a 6-min resting state task (data not shown). Panel **(B)** shows representative images from the alcohol cue tasks, both of which involved viewing 30 unique images that were presented for 6 s, with 4-s inter-stimulus intervals.

of alcohol picture cues (A1), 3) performing the intervention task, 4) viewing a second, distinct set of alcohol picture cues (A2); a 6-min resting state task was then performed. After each task, participants responded to the question, "How much are you currently craving alcohol right now?" using a track ball on a visual analogue scale (VAS, 43) anchored from "not at all" (0) to "extremely" (100). Stimulus cues were presented using E-Prime software (Psychology Software Tools Inc.). Images were projected onto a screen positioned at the rear of the scanner bore and viewed through a mirror attached to the head coil. A trigger pulse synchronized the start of each task with the E-Prime software. Total scan time was approximately 45 min.

Data from the two alcohol cue tasks (A1, A2) were analyzed in the present study. Each task included 30 unique images that were presented for 6 s with 4-s inter-stimulus intervals (**Figure 3B**), a design driven by the larger study's broader goal of characterizing the relationship between cardiovascular and neural reactivity. The alcohol cues were drawn from prior studies in our and others' laboratories (34, 54, 55). Each participant's self-reported preferred beverage (i.e., beer, wine, "straight" liquor, or mixed drinks) made up approximately 50% of the images to which they were exposed. Participants were instructed to pay attention to the images and to press a response box button when they saw an image that contained their preferred drink.

Between the A1 and A2 cue sets, participants in the active intervention (resonance breathing) synchronized their breathing with a visual pacer at the rate of 0.1 Hz (i.e., 6 breaths per minute). Compliance to the breathing task was verified via analysis of the respiratory signal. Time series respiratory frequency data were Fourier transformed, and the shape of the spectrum was visually inspected; all participants showed a respiratory peak at 0.1 Hz and spectral characteristics consistent with resonance breathing. Participants in the control intervention group completed a low-demand cognitive "vanilla" task wherein different colored rectangles were presented for 10 s each; they were instructed to silently count the number of blue rectangles (56).

After exiting the scanner, participants were compensated for their time. Those who met the criteria for alcohol dependence were given an informational brochure on alcohol use disorders and treatment options. This study was approved by the university's institutional review board for the protection of human subjects involved in research.

Imaging Parameters and Pre-Processing

Imaging data were collected using a 3T Siemens Trio scanner and 12-channel head coil. Standard localizer, anatomical, scout, and field map scans were collected. High-resolution anatomical images were acquired using a T1-weighted MPRAGE protocol with parameters: repetition time (TR) = 1,900 ms, echo time (TE) = 2.51 ms, matrix = 256 × 256 voxels, field-of-view (FOV) = 256 mm, voxel size = 1 × 1 × 1 mm, 176 1-mm sagittal slices (.5 mm gap). Functional blood oxygen level-dependent (BOLD) data were acquired using single-shot gradient echo-planar imaging (EPI) sequences with parameters: TR = 2,000 ms, TE = 25 ms, flip, angle = 90°, matrix = 64 × 64 voxels, FOV = 192 mm, voxel size = 3 × 3 × 3 mm, 35 contiguous 3-mm sagittal slices (1 mm gap). ECG and respiration data were collected using a MRI-compatible BIOPAC acquisition system (Biopac Systems, Goleta, CA) as part of the larger study.

FSL 5.0.9 software was used to conduct image preprocessing and data analysis (FMIRB's Software Library, https://fsl.fmrib.ox.ac.uk). Non-brain tissue was removed from all anatomical and BOLD images using FSL's Brain Extraction Tool (BET, 57) by estimating each image's center of gravity and manually adjusting BET parameters as necessary until an optimal result was obtained. BOLD data were motion-corrected using FSL's MCFLIRT (58), and the output was reviewed to identify participants with excessive motion during the resting-state scan. Excessive motion was defined conservatively as mean absolute and/or relative displacement greater than .5 mm. A paired t-test was performed to compare mean framewise displacement between the randomized intervention groups. No significant differences were observed in motion between the groups ($p > 0.05$). BOLD images were segmented into gray matter, white matter (WM), and cerebral spinal fluid (CSF) using FSL's FAST (59). Probability maps of CSF and WM were derived, and time-series data for these signals were extracted from each participant. These nuisance parameters (i.e., WM, CSF) along with extended head motion parameters were used as covariates in the linear regression models implemented in FSL to decrease the effects of signals-of-no-interest. BOLD data were registered to standard space with a two-step process using FMRIB's Linear Image Registration Tool (FLIRT) (60). The data were first registered to the T1-weighted anatomical image and then to MNI-152 standard space using 9 degrees-of-freedom and SINC interpolation. All data were visually inspected for gross errors in registration. A high pass temporal filter was set to 50 s, and spatial smoothing was set to a 6-mm full-width at half-maximum Gaussian kernel.

Statistical Analyses

Analyses of the BOLD data from the A1 and A2 cue reactivity tasks were performed using a two-step process. Subject-level effects were calculated using first-level analyses in FSL's FEAT, and group effects were determined using higher-level analyses. In the first-level analysis, each alcohol image event was modeled and convolved with a double-gamma hemodynamic response function (HRF), and the mean task activation for A1 and A2 was calculated for each participant. In the higher-level analysis stage, two sets of analyses were performed using Randomise, the non-parametric permutation-testing tool implemented in FSL (61). First, one-sample t-tests were conducted to characterize neural activation in each intervention group before (A1) and after (A2) the intervention. Next, to examine intervention effects on neural activation to visual stimuli, paired t-tests with two contrasts were conducted on each intervention group (i.e., resonance breathing, control) separately (61). For each contrast, 5,000 permutations were calculated. One contrast (A1 > A2) was designed to determine brain areas that demonstrated greater activation pre- compared to post-intervention task, and the second contrast (A2 > A1) was designed to determine brain areas that demonstrated greater activation post-intervention compared to pre-intervention task. Threshold-free cluster enhancement was employed (62), and activation was considered significant at $p < 0.05$ (corrected for multiple comparisons using FSL Randomise).

A repeated-measures mixed model was used to assess the effect of resonance breathing on VAS craving scores. Craving data for one participant was missing due to equipment failure; thus, data from 40 participants were available for analysis. A between-subjects factor of intervention group (resonance breathing, control) and a within-subjects factor of craving scores following A1 and A2, as well as their interaction, were modeled. To examine the relationship between VAS craving scores and brain regions that exhibited significant pre-intervention to post-intervention changes, regions-of-interest (ROIs) were defined by creating 6-mm spheres around the peak voxel of each significant cluster of activation for the A1 > A2 and A2 > A1 contrasts. Mean activation values of these ROIs were extracted for each participant from the subject-level A1 and A2 cope images. Pearson correlations were then used to test the associations between ROI activation and VAS craving scores at A1 and A2. Point biserial correlations were used to examine the relationship of binary drinking status (low-risk = 0, alcohol dependent = 1) to ROI activation at A2 in the resonance breathing group. These analyses were performed using SAS 9.4 software (SAS Institute, Cary, NC, USA).

RESULTS

Neuroimaging

Both intervention groups exhibited widespread neural activity in response to the visual alcohol cues, including in bilateral posterior parahippocampal gyri, temporal occipital fusiform cortices, lateral occipital cortices (inferior and superior divisions), postcentral gyri, and cerebellum at A1 and A2. The resonance breathing group (n = 22) additionally showed significant activation in bilateral inferior frontal gyri, left insula, left pallidum, left putamen, left amygdala, and left thalamus (A1, A2), and left precentral gyrus (A1). The control group (n = 19) additionally showed significant activation in the right thalamus (A1) and left precentral gyrus (A2). These results are shown in **Figure 4**.

Participants in the resonance breathing group demonstrated greater activation in response to alcohol cues pre-breathing compared with post-breathing (A1>A2) in left inferior and superior lateral occipital cortices and right inferior lateral occipital cortex, as well as bilateral occipital pole and temporal occipital fusiform cortices. They also demonstrated greater activation post-breathing compared with pre-breathing (A2 > A1) in

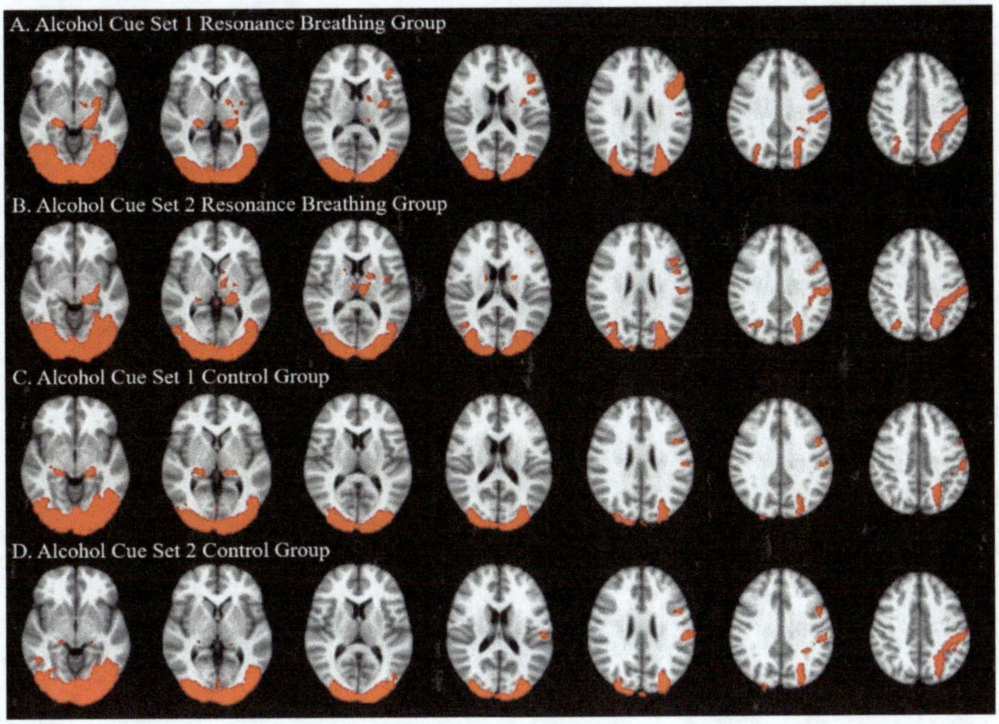

FIGURE 4 | Significant Neural Activation to Visual Alcohol Cue Sets. One-sample *t*-tests were used to identify areas of significant neural activation during alcohol cue set viewing. The neural responses of the active intervention (resonance breathing) group are shown in Panels **(A)** (A1 task, cues viewed prior to the intervention) and **(B)** (A2 task, cues viewed after the intervention). The neural responses of the control intervention (vanilla task) group are shown in Panels **(C)** (A1 task, cues viewed prior to the intervention) and **(D)** (A2 task, cues viewed after the intervention). Axial slices are shown in MNI standard space at z = −6 (first slice) and every fourth subsequent slice. Images are oriented using radiological convention. Areas of significant activation are shown in red.

voxels spanning precuneus cortex, posterior cingulate gyrus, and bilateral lingual gyri, as well as in medial prefrontal cortex (MPFC), paracingulate gyrus, and anterior cingulate cortex (ACC). These results are shown in **Table 1** and **Figure 5**.

The control group analysis yielded no significant activation in either the A1 > A2 or A2 > A1 contrasts, indicating that there were no statistically significant changes in brain activation in response to visual alcohol cues in the group that performed the control task.

Self-Report

Surveys administered prior to the neuroimaging session revealed that the sample as a whole had low-moderate perceived stress (mean ± standard deviation = 17 ± 6), and positive (mean ± standard deviation = 30.7±9.7) and negative (mean ± standard deviation = 13.9 ± 6.2) affect scores that were similar to those reported from the original general adult normative sample (52). There were no differences in affect or stress between the intervention groups nor between the drinking groups (all $p > .05$).

Craving was measured in the scanner after exposure to each cue block. The results of a repeated-measures (A1, A2) mixed model indicated that there was a significant main effect of group on craving, but no main effect of task (i.e., from pre- to post-intervention). Participants randomized to the resonance breathing intervention group reported lower levels

TABLE 1 | Anatomical location at peak voxel coordinates in significant clusters of activation in resonance breathing group.

A1>A2 Contrast					
		MNI Coordinates			
Cluster Size	**Z**	**x**	**y**	**z**	**Peak Voxel Anatomical Location**
2,433	6.80	−30	−96	10	Occipital pole (L)
1,339	6.95	28	−90	4	Occipital pole (R)
10	4.74	28	−38	−24	Temporal fusiform cortex (R)
A2>A1 Contrast					
		MNI Coordinates			
Cluster Size	**Z**	**x**	**y**	**z**	**Peak Voxel Anatomical Location**
2,141	7.81	2	−78	42	Precuneus Cortex
283	5.89	−2	50	0	Paracingulate Gyrus/ Medial Prefrontal Cortex
150	4.74	−16	−50	−2	Lingual Gyrus (L)
16	5.35	6	−24	40	Posterior Cingulate Cortex
15	4.44	2	−22	32	Posterior Cingulate Cortex
2	3.81	0	−56	10	Precuneus Cortex
1	6.87	−2	−6	36	Anterior Cingulate Cortex

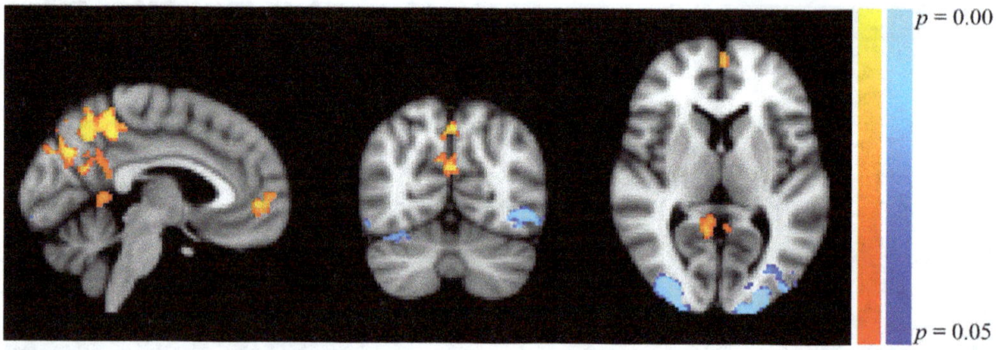

FIGURE 5 | Significant Clusters of Activation in Resonance Breathing Group. Blue-cyan clusters represent regions with greater activation during A1 compared to A2 (A1 > A2), and red-yellow clusters represent regions with greater activation during A2 compared with A1 (A2 > A1). Voxels were thresholded at $p < 0.05$. Image is shown in MNI standard space at x = −4, y = −66, z = 6, and oriented using radiological convention.

of in-the-moment craving compared to those randomized to the control intervention group [$F(76,1) = 5.76$, $p = 0.0188$; least square mean ± standard error of resonance breathing group = 28.1 ± 4.5 and of control group = 43.7 ± 4.7]. The group–task interaction was not statistically significant, suggesting that changes in subjective reports of craving pre- to post-intervention did not significantly differ between the two groups.

No significant correlations were observed at A1 between VAS craving scores and the ten cluster activation scores in the full sample (r range, −0.24 to 0.09, all $p > .05$). In addition, there were no significant correlations at A2 between craving scores and the ten cluster activation scores within either group (resonance breathing group r range, −0.32 to 0.28, all $p >.05$; control group r range, −0.42 to 0.44, all $p > .05$). Lastly, there were no significant correlations at A2 between drinking status (AUD vs. low risk) and the ten-cluster activation scores in the resonance breathing group (r range, −0.27 to 0.28, all $p > .05$).

DISCUSSION

Evidence that visceral afferent signaling influences stimulus processing argues for intervention development aimed at manipulating cardiovascular signals to alter detection and neural processing of affective stimuli (63). The results of the present study provide the first proof-of-concept evidence that a brief behavioral intervention of resonance breathing can significantly alter drinkers' neural activation to visual alcohol cues. The observed changes in brain activity included both decreases and increases in the activation of distinct brain regions.

In the group that performed resonance breathing between the visual cue tasks, but not in the control group, there was reduced activation in occipital regions from the first set of alcohol cues to the second, different set of alcohol cues. This pattern of results suggests that the breathing intervention prompted a subsequent decrease in visual cortex activation when individuals were confronted with alcohol-related visual stimuli. The specificity of these changes to alcohol-related content is unclear as this proof-of-concept study did not include a cue set of non-alcohol–related images presented before and after the intervention. Indeed, visual cortex activation to many types of images, including faces, is modulated by their emotional and social significance (64–66). Multiple lines of evidence also support the involvement of the visual cortex in appetitive cue processing. Several meta-analyses found that drug users consistently showed increased activation in occipital regions in response to drug-related cues compared to controls, even when non-visual drug-related stimuli were presented (41, 67–69). Increased visual cortex activation has been observed in individuals with behavioral addictions, such as pathological gambling, as well (70–72). Thus, although the literature suggests that the role of the visual cortex in alcohol and drug cue reactivity is not specific, decreased activation in the lateral occipital cortices following resonance breathing would be consistent with decreased perception, representation, and recognition of the images (73) and/or may potentially reflect less attention being directed toward the cues by the amygdala (66) or higher cortical areas (74).

In parallel with reduced visual processing of the cues, we observed increased activation in bilateral medial prefrontal, anterior and posterior cingulate, and precuneus cortices during the second alcohol cue task, only in the resonance breathing group. The ACC and MPFC, as regions of the central autonomic network, bi-directionally influence, and are influenced by, afferent cardiovascular signaling. Resonance breathing increases cardiovascular input to the brain via activation of brainstem nuclei that share connectivity with the ACC and MPFC (4) and are thought to give rise to the visceral experience of emotion (75). Functionally, the ACC is a part of the mesocorticolimbic circuit, which is thought to be involved in conflict monitoring and the regulation of cognitive and emotional processing by integrating input and modulating processing in other regions (76, 77). The MPFC is considered to be part of a cognitive control system in the brain that promotes goal-directed behaviors (78) by using incoming information to predict the most adaptive response based on past experience (79).

Hypothetically, increased activation of MPFC and ACC in response to alcohol cues following the breathing intervention would be consistent with heightened internal monitoring of cognitive-emotional state and enhanced cognitive control. At the same time, some studies have identified these regions as sites of heightened reactivity to alcohol and other drug cues (42), and heightened reactivity in these regions has been related to post-treatment drinking and relapse, although the results in this area have not been consistent (80). Thus, it is unclear whether or under what circumstances these and other brain regions accentuate or restrain cue-elicited craving and substance use behaviors. Evidence for individual differences in brain areas most reactive to appetitive cues (42) and inconsistencies in replication add further complication to interpretation. More nuanced examination of intra-individual changes in neural activation across brain areas, and perhaps also across simultaneously operating psychological and physiological systems involved in motivated behavior, are needed.

The posterior cingulate cortex (PCC) and the precuneus showed increased activation to visual alcohol cues following the breathing intervention, but not the control task. Both of these regions are considered core nodes of the default mode network, a functional brain network involved in self-referential thought and mind-wandering (81) that shows preserved connectivity during cognitive load (82). The lingual gyrus, a brain region involved in visual encoding and higher-order analysis of complex visual stimuli (83), also showed increased activation only in the resonance breathing group. This gyrus has been implicated in spontaneous thought and often co-activates with the default mode network (84). Whether increased activation in these regions potentially plays a role in promoting self-regulation in response to alcohol or other affectively valenced cues is unknown, but warrants further investigation. One possibility is that following resonance breathing the brain reverts to its "baseline" resting state (85) for some amount of time despite activation by salient cues, rather than transitioning to a heightened state of arousal.

We did not observe acute changes in self-reported craving levels in the resonance breathing group following the second presentation of alcohol cues (absence of significant cue task by group interaction), nor were craving levels related to brain clusters of activation in response to cues at A1 or A2. Several factors likely contributed to these null findings. Randomization into resonance breathing and control groups in the present study did not result in equivalent mean craving rating scores; the resonance breathing group reported significantly lower craving levels throughout the study. Failures of randomization in small samples are common (86), and future studies may benefit from selecting participants with high levels of self-reported craving and/or matching on craving levels across intervention groups. It may also be that the brief 5-min duration of resonance breathing did not affect conscious self-estimates of craving in the present sample, or that resonance breathing works in a way that affects a different pathway, such as the operation of cue salience (50), rather than consciously experienced craving levels. The present data are limited in not speaking to these alternative speculations.

Implications for Clinical Translation

If replicated and extended, the current findings that a brief, 5-min bout of resonance breathing changed neural activation in brain areas implicated in affective and appetitive stimulus processing could have clinical implications for individuals who show elevated neural reactivity in response to appetitive cues (44). Resonance breathing is the active mechanism of heart rate variability biofeedback, an empirically supported behavioral intervention for disorders with core features of affective and emotional dysregulation (13, 14, 17, 26) including alcohol use disorders (44, 87, 88). Emerging evidence suggests that heart rate variability biofeedback and paced breathing interventions reduce self-reported craving for alcohol and other appetitive stimuli, such as food (27, 89). While standard heart rate variability biofeedback delivery protocols include five to ten 1-h sessions and home practice (90, 91), resonance breathing itself produces immediate physiological effects (see **Figure 2**). This proof-of-concept study was novel in examining whether resonance breathing also elicits immediate neural effects. The findings provide an initial step in validating resonance breathing as an in-the-moment behavioral tool that potentially could be used ad lib in the natural environment to alter neural activation, both before and during contexts of heightened risk for substance use. Accessible smart phone applications are available to self-administer resonance breathing and HRV biofeedback, suggesting promise for a scalable intervention tool if future research is successful in demonstrating that such effects are linked to reduced alcohol and drug use behaviors.

Limitations and Directions for Future Research

As a proof-of-concept study, these findings should be interpreted with caution and used for the generation of future hypotheses regarding the effects of resonance breathing on neural activation to alcohol-related visual stimuli, behavioral correlates of alcohol use such as in-the-moment craving, and actual use behaviors. Importantly, the changes observed in neural activation to the cues following the resonance breathing intervention should not be considered specific to alcohol-cue reactivity, as this study did not include a comparison condition of matched, non-alcohol cues presented before and after the intervention. This study also was limited in not being sufficiently powered to examine sensitively the relation of individual differences in alcohol use behaviors to changes in neural activation following resonance breathing. We note that the cue presentation paradigm of the present study was designed in line with the goal of better understanding afferent cardiovascular input to neural reactivity and thus was not typical of those used in many other fMRI studies of cue reactivity. A recent meta-analysis found that cue paradigm and type did not significantly influence neural response patterns associated with cue reactivity however (28), suggesting the fMRI assessment of neural activation is robust to multiple cue presentation approaches. Future studies should include larger samples to link current and chronic substance use behaviors to cue reactivity, and a design that counterbalances and compares neural response to alcohol-related and non-alcoholic beverage cues. Specificity may be addressed also by comparisons to non-alcohol or drug-related, yet positive or negative affectively valenced, visual cue sets.

Conclusion

In summary, this study presents preliminary evidence that individuals ranging in drinking behaviors from low-risk to alcohol-dependent may be less visually engaged by alcohol cues and initiate greater top-down cognitive processing of cues following resonance breathing. This is consistent with the broader literature on resonance breathing that shows it normalizes neurocardiac feedback and improves autonomic nervous system regulation (25). Moreover, it points to a potential neural foundation for the effects of resonance breathing and adds to the scientific premise for the use of heart rate variability biofeedback as an intervention for brain-based mental and physical health conditions. More highly powered studies are needed to replicate and extend these neural activation results. Critical next steps are to understand how the cardiovascular and neural changes elicited by resonance breathing are linked to changes in the subjective experience of craving and alcohol use behaviors.

AUTHOR CONTRIBUTIONS

MB and JB designed the study. MB and LL wrote the first draft of the article. All authors contributed to writing sections of the manuscript. LL and SU collected all data. LL and SU post-processed the imaging data. LL, SU, and SG performed the data analyses. All authors read and approved the final manuscript.

ACKNOWLEDGMENTS

We acknowledge Dr. Evgeny Vaschillo, an originator of heart rate variability biofeedback and the study of cardiovascular resonance. We also thank the staff and students of the Cardiac Neuroscience Laboratory for their assistance in screening and testing participants.

REFERENCES

1. Shiffman S, Stone AA, Hufford MR. Ecological momentary assessment. *AnnRev Clin Psychol* (2008) 4:1–32. doi: 10.1146/annurev.clinpsy.3.022806.091415
2. Tracey KJ. Reflex control of immunity. *Nat Rev Immunol* (2009) 9:418–28. doi: 10.1038/nri2566
3. Gianaros PJ, Jennings JR. Host in the machine: a neurobiological perspective on psychological stress and cardiovascular disease. *Am Psychol* (2018) 73:1031–44. doi: 10.1037/amp0000232
4. Benarroch EE. The central autonomic network. In: Low PA, editor. *Clinical Autonomic Disorders*. 2nd ed Lippincott-Raven (1997). p. 17–23.
5. Goldstein DS. *The autonomic nervous system in health and disease*. New York: Marcel Dekker, Inc. (2001).
6. Beissner F, Meissner K, Bar KJ, Napadow V. The autonomic brain: an activation likelihood estimation meta-analysis for central processing of autonomic function. *J Neurosci* (2013) 33:10503–11. doi: 10.1523/JNEUROSCI.1103-13.2013
7. Lacey BC, Lacey JI. Some autonomic-central nervous system interrelationships. In: Blank P, editor. *Physiological Correlations of Emotion*. Academic Press (1970). p. 205–27. doi: 10.1016/B978-0-12-102850-3.50016-5
8. Iversen S, Iversen L, Saper CB. The autonomic nervous system and the hypothalamus. In: Kandel ER, Schwartz CE, Jessell TM, editors. *Principle of Neural Science*. McGraw-Hill (2000). p. 960–81.
9. Critchley HD. Neural mechanisms of autonomic, affective, and cognitive integration. *J Compar Neurol* (2005) 493:154–66. doi: 10.1002/cne.20749
10. Bates ME, Buckman JF. Emotional dysregulation in the moment: why some college students may not mature out of hazardous alcohol and drug use. In: White HR, Rabiner DL, editors. *College drinking and drug use*. The Guilford Press (2011). p. 83–101.
11. Bates ME, Buckman JF. Integrating body and brain systems in addiction neuroscience. In: Miller P, editor. *Biological Research on Addiction: Comprehensive Addictive Behaviors and Disorders*. Elsevier (2013). doi: 10.1016/B978-0-12-398335-0.00020-0
12. Buckman JF, Vaschillo EG, Fonoberova M, Mezic I, Bates ME. The translational value of psychophysiology methods and mechanisms: multilevel, dynamic, personalized. *J Stud Alcohol Drugs* (2018) 79:229–38. doi: 10.15288/jsad.2018.79.229
13. Hassett AL, Radvanski DC, Vaschillo E, Vaschillo B, Sigal LH, Karavidas MK, et al. A pilot study of the efficacy of heart rate variability (HRV) biofeedback in patients with fibromyalgia. *Appl Psychophysiol Biofeedback* (2007) 32:1–10. doi: 10.1007/s10484-006-9028-0
14. Karavidas MK, Lehrer PM, Vaschillo E, Vaschillo B, Marin H, Buyske S, et al. Preliminary results of an open label study of heart rate variability biofeedback for the treatment of major depression. *Appl Psychophysiol Biofeedback* (2007) 32:19–30. doi: 10.1007/s10484-006-9029-z
15. Windhorst U. Muscle proprioceptive feedback and spinal networks. *Brain Res Bull* (2007) 73:155–202. doi: 10.1016/j.brainresbull.2007.03.010
16. Reiner R. Integrating a portable biofeedback device into clinical practice for patients with anxiety disorders: results of a pilot study. *Appl Psychophysiol Biofeedback* (2008) 33:55–61. doi: 10.1007/s10484-007-9046-6
17. Siepmann M, Aykac V, Unterdorfer J, Petrowski K, Mueck-Weymann M. A pilot study on the effects of heart rate variability biofeedback in patients with depression and in healthy subjects. *Appl Psychophysiol Biofeedback* (2008) 33:195–201. doi: 10.1007/s10484-008-9064-z
18. Zucker TL, Samuelson KW, Muench F, Greenberg MA, Gevirtz RN. The effects of respiratory sinus arrhythmia biofeedback on heart rate variability and posttraumatic stress disorder symptoms: a pilot study. *Appl Psychophysiol Biofeedback* (2009) 34:135–43. doi: 10.1007/s10484-009-9085-2
19. Sutarto AP, Wahab MN, Zin NM. Resonant breathing biofeedback training for stress reduction among manufacturing operators. *Int J Occup Saf Ergon* (2012) 18:549–61. doi: 10.1080/10803548.2012.11076959
20. Eddie D, Kim C, Bates ME, Lehrer P, Deneke E. A pilot study of brief heart rate variability biofeedback to reduce craving in young adult men receiving inpatient treatment for substance use disorders. *Appl Psychophysiol Biofeedback* (2014) 39:181–92. doi: 10.1007/s10484-014-9251-z
21. Lehrer PM, Vaschillo E, Vaschillo B, Lu SE, Eckberg DL, Edelberg R, et al. Heart rate variability biofeedback increases baroreflex gain and peak expiratory flow. *Psychosomatic Med* (2003) 65:796–805. doi: 10.1097/01.PSY.0000089200.81962.19
22. Vaschillo E, Vaschillo B, Lehrer P. Heartbeat synchronizes with respiratory rhythm only under specific circumstances. *Chest* (2004) 126:1385–6. doi: 10.1016/S0012-3692(15)31329-5
23. Lehrer P, Vaschillo E, Trost Z, France CR. Effects of rhythmical muscle tension at 0.1Hz on cardiovascular resonance and the baroreflex. *Biol Psychol* (2009) 81:24–30. doi: 10.1016/j.biopsycho.2009.01.003
24. Vaschillo EG, Vaschillo B, Pandina RJ, Bates ME. Resonances in the cardiovascular system caused by rhythmical muscle tension. *Psychophysiology* (2010) 48:927–36. doi: 10.1111/j.1469-8986.2010.01156.x
25. Vaschillo EG, Vaschillo B, Buckman JF, Pandina RJ, Bates ME. The investigation and clinical significance of resonance in the heart rate and vascular tone baroreflexes. In: Fred A, Filipe J, Gamboa H, editors. *Biomedical Engineering Systems and Technologies: Communications in Computer and Information Science*. Springer (2011). p. 224–37. doi: 10.1007/978-3-642-18472-7_18

26. Goessl VC, Curtiss JE, Hofmann SG. The effect of heart rate variability biofeedback training on stress and anxiety: a meta-analysis. *Psychol Med* (2017) 47:2578–86. doi: 10.1017/S0033291717001003
27. Alayan N, Eller L, Bates ME, Carmody DP. Current evidence on heart rate variability biofeedback as a complementary anticraving intervention. *J Altern Complement Med* (2018) 24:1039–50. doi: 10.1089/acm.2018.0019
28. Noori HR, Cosa Linan A, Spanagel R. Largely overlapping neuronal substrates of reactivity to drug, gambling, food and sexual cues: a comprehensive meta-analysis. *Eur Neuropsychopharmacol* (2016) 26:1419–30. doi: 10.1016/j.euroneuro.2016.06.013
29. Kelley AE, Berridge KC. The neuroscience of natural rewards: relevance to addictive drugs. *J Neurosci* (2002) 22:3306–11. doi: 10.1523/JNEUROSCI.22-09-03306.2002
30. Naqvi NH, Bechara A. The hidden island of addiction: the insula. *Trends Neurosci* (2009) 32:56–67. doi: 10.1016/j.tins.2008.09.009
31. Koob GF, Volkow ND. Neurocircuitry of addiction. *Neuropsychopharmacology* (2010) 35:217–38. doi: 10.1038/npp.2009.110
32. Sinha R, Fuse T, Aubin LR, O'malley SS. Psychological stress, drug-related cues and cocaine craving. *Psychopharmacology (Berl)* (2000) 152:140–8. doi: 10.1007/s002130000499
33. Thayer JF, Lane RD. A model of neurovisceral integration in emotion regulation and dysregulation. *J Affect Disord* (2000) 61:201–16. doi: 10.1016/S0165-0327(00)00338-4
34. Vaschillo EG, Bates ME, Vaschillo B, Lehrer P, Udo T, Mun EY, et al. Heart rate variability response to alcohol, placebo, and emotional picture cue challenges: effects of 0.1-Hz stimulation. *Psychophysiology* (2008) 45:847–58. doi: 10.1111/j.1469-8986.2008.00673.x
35. Garland EL, Carter K, Ropes K, Howard MO. Thought suppression, impaired regulation of urges, and Addiction-Stroop predict affect-modulated cue-reactivity among alcohol dependent adults. *Biol Psychol* (2012a) 89:87–93. doi: 10.1016/j.biopsycho.2011.09.010
36. Garland EL, Franken IH, Sheetz JJ, Howard MO. Alcohol attentional bias is associated with autonomic indices of stress-primed alcohol cue-reactivity in alcohol-dependent patients. *Exp Clin Psychopharmacol* (2012b) 20:225–35. doi: 10.1037/a0027199
37. Porges SW, Doussard-Roosevelt JA, Maita AK. Vagal tone and the physiological regulation of emotion. *Monogr Soc Res Child Dev* (1994) 59(167–186):250–83. doi: 10.2307/1166144
38. Hugdahl K. Cognitive influences on human autonomic nervous system function. *Curr Opin Neurobiol* (1996) 6:252–8. doi: 10.1016/S0959-4388(96)80080-8
39. Kuhn S, Gallinat J. Common biology of craving across legal and illegal drugs—a quantitative meta-analysis of cue-reactivity brain response. *Eur J Neurosci* (2011) 33:1318–26. doi: 10.1111/j.1460-9568.2010.07590.x
40. Jasinska AJ, Stein EA, Kaiser J, Naumer MJ, Yalachkov Y. Factors modulating neural reactivity to drug cues in addiction: a survey of human neuroimaging studies. *Neurosci Biobehav Rev* (2014) 38:1–16. doi: 10.1016/j.neubiorev.2013.10.013
41. Schacht JP, Anton RF, Myrick H. Functional neuroimaging studies of alcohol cue reactivity: a quantitative meta-analysis and systematic review. *Addict Biol* (2013) 18:121–33. doi: 10.1111/j.1369-1600.2012.00464.x
42. Hanlon CA, Dowdle LT, Gibson NB, Li X, Hamilton S, Canterberry M, et al. Cortical substrates of cue-reactivity in multiple substance dependent populations: transdiagnostic relevance of the medial prefrontal cortex. *Transl Psychiatry* (2018) 8:186. doi: 10.1038/s41398-018-0220-9
43. Myrick H, Anton RF, Li X, Henderson S, Drobes D, Voronin K, et al. Differential brain activity in alcoholics and social drinkers to alcohol cues: relationship to craving. *Neuropsychopharmacology* (2004) 29:393–402. doi: 10.1038/sj.npp.1300295
44. Witteman J, Post H, Tarvainen M, De Bruijn A, Perna Ede S, Ramaekers JG, et al. Cue reactivity and its relation to craving and relapse in alcohol dependence: a combined laboratory and field study. *Psychopharmacology (Berl)* (2015) 232:3685–96. doi: 10.1007/s00213-015-4027-6
45. Dager AD, Anderson BM, Stevens MC, Pulido C, Rosen R, Jiantonio-Kelly RE, et al. Influence of alcohol use and family history of alcoholism on neural response to alcohol cues in college drinkers. *Alcohol Clin Exp Res* (2013) 37 Suppl 1:E161–171. doi: 10.1111/j.1530-0277.2012.01879.x
46. Mun EY, Von Eye A, Bates ME, Vaschillo EG. Finding groups using model-based cluster analysis: heterogeneous emotional self-regulatory processes and heavy alcohol use risk. *Dev Psychol* (2008) 44:481–95. doi: 10.1037/0012-1649.44.2.481
47. Tiffany ST. The role of cognitive factors in reactivity to drug cues. In: Drummond DC, Tiffany ST, editors. *Addictive Behaviour: Cue Exposure Theory and Practice*. Wiley (1995).
48. Robinson TE, Berridge KC. Review. The incentive sensitization theory of addiction: some current issues. *Philos Trans R Soc London— B: Biol Sci* (2008) 363:3137–46. doi: 10.1098/rstb.2008.0093
49. Marlatt GA. Section I. theoretical perspectives on relapse: taxonomy of high-risk situations for alcohol relapse: evolution and development of a cognitive-behavioral model. *Addiction* (1996) 91:S37–49. doi: 10.1111/j.1360-0443.1996.tb02326.x
50. Grusser SM, Wrase J, Klein S, Hermann D, Smolka MN, Ruf M, etal. Cue-induced activation of the striatum and medial prefrontal cortex is associated with subsequent relapse in abstinent alcoholics. *Psychopharmacology* (2004) 175:296–302. doi: 10.1007/s00213-004-1828-4
51. American Psychiatric Association. *Diagnostic and statistical manual of mental disorders*. Washington, DC: American Psychiatric Association (2000).
52. Crawford JR, Henry JD. The Positive and Negative Affect Schedule (PANAS): construct validity, measurement properties and normative data in a large non-clinical sample. *Br J Clin Psychol* (2004) 43:245–65. doi: 10.1348/0144665031752934
53. Cohen S, Karmarck T, Mermelstein R. A global measure of perceived stress. *J Health Soc Behav* (1983) 24:385–96. doi: 10.2307/2136404
54. Tapert SF, Cheung EH, Brown GG, Frank LR, Paulus MP, Schweinsburg AD, et al. Neural response to alcohol stimuli in adolescents with alcohol use disorder. *Arch Gen Psychiatry* (2003) 60:727–35. doi: 10.1001/archpsyc.60.7.727
55. Ray S, Hanson C, Hanson SJ, Bates ME. fMRI BOLD response in high-risk college students (Part 1): during exposure to alcohol, marijuana, polydrug and emotional picture cues. *Alcohol Alcohol* (2010) 45:437–43. doi: 10.1093/alcalc/agq042
56. Jennings JR, Kamarck T, Stewart C, Eddy M, Johnson P. Alternate cardiovascular baseline assessment techniques: vanilla or resting baseline. *Psychophysiology* (1992) 29, 742-50. doi: 10.1111/j.1469-8986.1992.tb02052.x
57. Smith SM. Fast robust automated brain extraction. *Hum Brain Mapp* (2002) 17:143–55. doi: 10.1002/hbm.10062
58. Jenkinson M, Bannister P, Brady M, Smith SA. Improved optimization for the robust and accurate linear registration and motion correction of brain images. *Neuroimage* (2002) 17:825–41. doi: 10.1006/nimg.2002.1132
59. Zhang Y, Brady MS, Smith S. Segmentation of brain MR images through a hidden Markov random field model and the expectation-maximization algorithm. *IEEE Transact Med Imaging* (2001) 20:45–57:S. doi: 10.1109/42.906424
60. Jenkinson M, Smith S. A global optimisation method for robust affine registration of brain images. *Med Image Anal* (2001) 5:143–56. doi: 10.1016/S1361-8415(01)00036-6
61. Winkler AM, Ridgway GR, Webster MA, Smith SM, Nichols TE. Permutation inference for the general linear model. *Neuroimage* (2014) 92:381–97. doi: 10.1016/j.neuroimage.2014.01.060
62. Smith SM, Nichols TE. Threshold-free cluster enhancement: addressing problems of smoothing, threshold dependence and localisation in cluster inference. *Neuroimage* (2009) 44:83–98. doi: 10.1016/j.neuroimage.2008.03.061
63. Critchley HD, Garfinkel SN. Interactions between visceral afferent signaling and stimulus processing. *Front Neurosci* (2015) 9:286. doi: 10.3389/fnins.2015.00286
64. Adolphs R. Neural systems for recognizing emotion. *Curr Opin Neurobiol* (2002) 12:169–77. doi: 10.1016/S0959-4388(02)00301-X
65. Schupp HT, Junghoefer M, Weike AI, Hamm AO. Emotional facilitation of sensory processing in the visual cortex. *Psychol Sci* (2003) 14:7–13. doi: 10.1111/1467-9280.01411
66. Vuilleumier P, Pourtois G. Distributed and interactive brain mechanisms during emotion face perception: evidence from functional neuroimaging. *Neuropsychologia* (2007) 45:174–94. doi: 10.1016/j.neuropsychologia.2006.06.003
67. Chase HW, Eickhoff SB, Laird AR, Hogarth L. The neural basis of drug stimulus processing and craving: an activation likelihood estimation meta-analysis. *Biol Psychiatry* (2011) 70:785–93. doi: 10.1016/j.biopsych.2011.05.025
68. Engelmann JM, Versace F, Robinson JD, Minnix JA, Lam CY, Cui Y, et al. Neural substrates of smoking cue reactivity: a meta-analysis of fMRI studies. *Neuroimage* (2012) 60:252–62. doi: 10.1016/j.neuroimage.2011.12.024

69. Hanlon CA, Dowdle LT, Naselaris T, Canterberry M, Cortese BM. Visual cortex activation to drug cues: a meta-analysis of functional neuroimaging papers in addiction and substance abuse literature. *Drug Alcohol Depend* (2014) 143:206–12. doi: 10.1016/j.drugalcdep.2014.07.028
70. Potenza MN, Steinberg MA, Skudlarski P, Fulbright RK, Lacadie CM, Wilber MK, et al. Gambling urges in pathological gambling: a functional magnetic resonance imaging study. *Arch Gen Psychiatry* (2003) 60:828–36. doi: 10.1001/archpsyc.60.8.828
71. Crockford DN, Goodyear B, Edwards J, Quickfall J, El-Guebaly N. Cue-induced brain activity in pathological gamblers. *Biol Psychiatry* (2005) 58:787–95. doi: 10.1016/j.biopsych.2005.04.037
72. Goudriaan AE, De Ruiter MB, Van Den Brink W, Oosterlaan J, Veltman DJ. Brain activation patterns associated with cue reactivity and craving in abstinent problem gamblers, heavy smokers and healthy controls: an fMRI study. *Addict Biol* (2010) 15:491–503. doi: 10.1111/j.1369-1600.2010.00242.x
73. Grill-Spector K, Kourtzi Z, Kanwisher N. The lateral occipital complex and its role in object recognition. *Vision Res* (2001) 41:1409–22. doi: 10.1016/S0042-6989(01)00073-6
74. Kanwisher N, Wojciulik E. Visual attention: insights from brain imaging. *Nat Rev Neurosci* (2000) 1:91–100. doi: 10.1038/35039043
75. Venkatraman A, Edlow BL, Immordino-Yang MH. The Brainstem in Emotion: A Review. *Front Neuroanat* (2017) 11:15. doi: 10.3389/fnana.2017.00015
76. Bush G, Luu P, Posner MI. Cognitive and emotional influences in anterior cingulate cortex. *Trends Cogn Sci* (2000) 4:215–22. doi: 10.1016/S1364-6613(00)01483-2
77. Botvinick MM, Cohen JD, Carter CS. Conflict monitoring and anterior cingulate cortex: an update. *Trends Cogn Sci* (2004) 8:539–46. doi: 10.1016/j.tics.2004.10.003
78. Ridderinkhof KR, Ullsperger M, Crone EA, Nieuwenhuis S. The role of the medial frontal cortex in cognitive control. *Science* (2004) 306:443–7. doi: 10.1126/science.1100301
79. Euston DR, Gruber AJ, Mcnaughton BL. The role of medial prefrontal cortex in memory and decision making. *Neuron* (2012) 76:1057–70. doi: 10.1016/j.neuron.2012.12.002
80. Courtney KE, Schacht JP, Hutchison K, Roche DJ, Ray LA. Neural substrates of cue reactivity: association with treatment outcomes and relapse. *Addict Biol* (2016) 21:3–22. doi: 10.1111/adb.12314
81. Buckner RL, Andrews-Hanna JR, Schacter DL. The brain's default network: anatomy, function, and relevance to disease. *Ann N Y Acad Sci* (2008) 1124:1–38. doi: 10.1196/annals.1440.011
82. Fransson P, Marrelec G. The precuneus/posterior cingulate cortex plays a pivotal role in the default mode network: evidence from a partial correlation network analysis. *Neuroimage* (2008) 42:1178–84. doi: 10.1016/j.neuroimage.2008.05.059
83. Machielsen WC, Rombouts SA, Barkhof F, Scheltens P, Witter MP. FMRI of visual encoding: reproducibility of activation. *Hum Brain Mapp* (2000) 9:156–64. doi: 10.1002/(SICI)1097-0193(200003)9:3<156::AID-HBM4>3.0.CO;2-Q
84. Fox KC, Spreng RN, Ellamil M, Andrews-Hanna JR, Christoff K. The wandering brain: meta-analysis of functional neuroimaging studies of mind-wandering and related spontaneous thought processes. *Neuroimage* (2015) 111:611–21. doi: 10.1016/j.neuroimage.2015.02.039
85. Gusnard DA, Raichle ME, Raichle ME. Searching for a baseline: functional imaging and the resting human brain. *Nat Rev Neurosci* (2001) 2:685–94. doi: 10.1038/35094500
86. Kang M, Ragan BG, Park JH. Issues in outcomes research: an overview of randomization techniques for clinical trials. *J Athl Train* (2008) 43:215–21. doi: 10.4085/1062-6050-43.2.215
87. Penzlin AI, Siepmann T, Illigens BM, Weidner K, Siepmann M. Heart rate variability biofeedback in patients with alcohol dependence: a randomized controlled study. *Neuropsychiatr Dis Treat* (2015) 11:2619–27. doi: 10.2147/NDT.S84798
88. Penzlin AI, Barlinn K, Illigens BM, Weidner K, Siepmann M, Siepmann T. Effect of short-term heart rate variability biofeedback on long-term abstinence in alcohol dependent patients—a one-year follow-up. *BMC Psychiatry* (2017) 17:325. doi: 10.1186/s12888-017-1480-2
89. Eddie D, Conway FN, Alayan N, Buckman J, Bates ME. Assessing heart rate variability biofeedback as an adjunct to college recovery housing programs. *J Subst Abuse Treat* (2018) 92:70–6. doi: 10.1016/j.jsat.2018.06.014
90. Lehrer PM, Vaschillo E, Vaschillo B. Resonant frequency biofeedback training to increase cardiac variability: rationale and manual for training. *Appl Psychophysiol Biofeedback* (2000) 25:177–91. doi: 10.1023/A:1009554825745
91. Lehrer P, Vaschillo B, Zucker T, Graves J, Katsamanis M, Aviles M, et al. Protocol for Heart Rate Variability Biofeedback Training. *Biofeedback* (2013) 41:98–109 doi: 10.5298/1081-5937-41.3.08.

6

A Roadmap for Integrating Neuroscience into Addiction Treatment: A Consensus of the Neuroscience Interest Group of the International Society of Addiction Medicine

Antonio Verdejo-Garcia[1], Valentina Lorenzetti[2], Victoria Manning[3,4], Hugh Piercy[3,4], Raimondo Bruno[5], Rob Hester[6], David Pennington[7,8], Serenella Tolomeo[9,10], Shalini Arunogiri[3,4], Marsha E. Bates[11], Henrietta Bowden-Jones[12], Salvatore Campanella[13], Stacey B. Daughters[14], Christos Kouimtsidis[15], Dan I. Lubman[3], Dieter J. Meyerhoff[16], Annaketurah Ralph[17], Tara Rezapour[18], Hosna Tavakoli[18,19], Mehran Zare-Bidoky[19,20], Anna Zilverstand[21], Douglas Steele[22], Scott J. Moeller[23], Martin Paulus[24], Alex Baldacchino[8] and Hamed Ekhtiari[24]*

[1] Turner Institute for Brain and Mental Health, Monash University, Melbourne, VIC, Australia, [2] School of Psychology, Faculty of Health Sciences, Australian Catholic University, Canberra, ACT, Australia, [3] Eastern Health Clinical School Turning Point, Eastern Health, Richmond, VIC, Australia, [4] Eastern Health Clinical School, Monash University, Melbourne, VIC, Australia, [5] School of Medicine, University of Tasmania, Hobart, TAS, Australia, [6] School of Psychological Sciences, University of Melbourne, Melbourne, VIC, Australia, [7] San Francisco Veterans Affairs Health Care System (SFVAHCS), San Francisco, CA, United States, [8] Department of Psychiatry, University of California, San Francisco, San Francisco, CA, United States, [9] School of Medicine, University of St Andrews, Medical and Biological Science Building, North Haugh, St Andrews, United Kingdom, [10] Department of Psychology, National University of Singapore, Singapore, Singapore, [11] Department of Kinesiology and Health, Rutgers University, New Brunswick, NJ, United States, [12] Department of Medicine, Faculty of Medicine, Imperial College, London, United Kingdom, [13] Laboratoire de Psychologie Médicale et d'Addictologie, ULB Neuroscience Institute (UNI), CHU Brugmann-Université Libre de Bruxelles (U.L.B.), Brussels, Belgium, [14] Department of Psychology and Neuroscience, University of North Carolina at Chapel Hill, Chapel Hill, NC, United States, [15] Department of Psychiatry, Surrey and Borders Partnership NHS Foundation Trust, Leatherhead, United Kingdom, [16] DVA Medical Center and Department of Radiology and Biomedical Imaging, University of California San Francisco, School of Medicine, San Francisco, CA, United States, [17] School of Psychology, University of Queensland, Brisbane, QLD, Australia, [18] Department of Cognitive Psychology, Institute for Cognitive Sciences Studies, Tehran, Iran, [19] Iranian National Center for Addiction Studies, Tehran University of Medical Sciences, Tehran, Iran, [20] School of Medicine, Shahid-Sadoughi University of Medical Sciences, Yazd, Iran, [21] Department of Psychiatry, University of Minnesota, Minneapolis, MN, United States, [22] Medical School, University of Dundee, Ninewells Hospital, Scotland, United Kingdom, [23] Department of Psychiatry, Renaissance School of Medicine at Stony Brook University, Stony Brook, NY, United States, [24] Laureate Institute for Brain Research, University of Tulsa, Tulsa, OK, United States

***Correspondence:**
Antonio Verdejo-Garcia
antonio.verdejo@monash.edu

Although there is general consensus that altered brain structure and function underpins addictive disorders, clinicians working in addiction treatment rarely incorporate neuroscience-informed approaches into their practice. We recently launched the Neuroscience Interest Group within the International Society of Addiction Medicine (ISAM-NIG) to promote initiatives to bridge this gap. This article summarizes the ISAM-NIG key priorities and strategies to achieve implementation of addiction neuroscience knowledge and tools for the assessment and treatment of substance use disorders. We cover two assessment areas: cognitive assessment and neuroimaging, and two interventional areas: cognitive training/remediation and neuromodulation, where we identify key challenges and proposed solutions. We reason that incorporating cognitive assessment into clinical settings requires the identification of constructs that predict meaningful clinical outcomes. Other requirements are the development of measures that are easily-administered, reliable, and ecologically-valid. Translation of neuroimaging techniques requires the development of diagnostic and prognostic biomarkers and testing the cost-effectiveness of these biomarkers in individualized prediction algorithms for relapse prevention and treatment selection. Integration of cognitive assessments with neuroimaging can provide multilevel targets including neural, cognitive, and behavioral outcomes for neuroscience-informed interventions. Application of neuroscience-informed interventions including cognitive training/remediation and neuromodulation requires clear pathways to design treatments based on multilevel targets, additional evidence from randomized trials and subsequent clinical implementation, including evaluation of cost-effectiveness. We propose to address these challenges by promoting international collaboration between researchers and clinicians, developing harmonized protocols and data management systems, and prioritizing multi-site research that focuses on improving clinical outcomes.

Keywords: neuroscience, addiction medicine, treatment, substance use disorder, fMRI, neuromodulation, neuropsychological assessment, cognitive rehabilitation

INTRODUCTION

The past two decades have seen significant advances in our understanding of the neuroscience of addiction and its implications for practice [reviewed in (1–3)]. However, despite such insights, there is a substantial lag in translating these findings into everyday practice, with few clinicians incorporating neuroscience-informed interventions in their routine practice (4). We recently launched the Neuroscience Interest Group within the International Society of Addiction Medicine (ISAM-NIG) to promote initiatives to bridge this gap between knowledge and practice. This article introduces the ISAM-NIG key priorities and strategies to achieve implementation of addiction neuroscience knowledge and tools in the assessment and treatment of substance use disorders (SUD). We cover four broad areas: (1) cognitive assessment, (2) neuroimaging, (3) cognitive training and remediation, and (4) neuromodulation. Cognitive assessment and neuroimaging provide multilevel biomarkers (neural circuits, cognitive processes, and behaviors) to be targeted with cognitive and neuromodulation interventions. Cognitive training/remediation and neuromodulation provide neuroscience-informed interventions to ameliorate neural, cognitive, and related behavioral alterations and potentially improve clinical outcomes in people with SUD. In the following sections, we review the current knowledge and challenges in each of these areas and provide ISAM-NIG recommendations to link knowledge and practice. Our goal is for researchers and clinicians to work collaboratively to address these challenges and recommendations. Cutting across the four areas, we focus on cognitive and neural systems that predict meaningful clinical outcomes for people with SUD and opportunities for harmonized assessment and intervention protocols.

COGNITIVE ASSESSMENT

Neuropsychological studies consistently demonstrate that many people with SUD exhibit mild to moderately severe cognitive deficits in processing speed, selective, and sustained attention, episodic memory, executive functions (EF: working memory, response inhibition, shifting and higher-order functions such as reasoning, problem-solving, and planning), decision-making and social cognition (5–10). Furthermore, neurobiologically-informed theories and expert consensus have identified additional cognitive changes not typically assessed by traditional neuropsychological measures, namely, negative affectivity and reward-related processes (e.g., reward expectancy, valuation and learning, and habits-compulsivity) (11–13).

Cognitive deficits in SUD have moderate longevity, and although there is abstinence-related recovery (14–16), these deficits may significantly complicate treatment efforts during the first 3 to 6 months after discontinuation of drug use. Thus, one of the most critical implications of cognitive deficits for SUD is their potential negative impact on treatment retention and adherence, in addition to clinical outcomes such as craving, relapse, and quality of life. A systematic review of prospective cognitive studies measuring treatment retention and relapse across different SUD suggested that measures of processing speed and accuracy during attention and reasoning tasks (MicroCog test battery) were the only consistent predictors of treatment retention, whereas tests of decision-making (Iowa and Cambridge Gambling Tasks) were the only consistent predictors of relapse (1). A later review that focused on substance-specific cognitive predictors of relapse found that long-term episodic memory and higher-order EF (including problem-solving, planning, and decision-making) predicted alcohol relapse, whereas attention and higher-order EF predicted stimulant relapse, while only higher-order EF predicted opioid relapse (8). Working memory and response inhibition have also been associated with increased risk of relapse among cannabis and stimulant users (8, 17, 18). Additionally, variation in response inhibition has been shown to predict poorer recovery of quality of life during SUD treatment (19). Therefore, consistent evidence suggests that processing speed, attention, and reasoning are critical targets for current SUD treatments, whereas higher-order EF and decision-making are critical for maintaining abstinence. Response inhibition deficits seem to be specifically associated with relapse prediction in cannabis and stimulant users and also predict quality of life (a key non-drug-related clinical outcome) (20).

Practical Considerations: Characteristics and Needs of the SUD Treatment Workforce

The workforce in the SUD specialist treatment sector is diverse, encompassing medical specialists, allied health professionals, generalist health workers, and peer and volunteer workers (21). For instance, in the Australian context, multiple workforce surveys over the past decade suggest that around half the workforce have attained a tertiary level Bachelor (undergraduate) degree or greater (21–24). Similarly, US and European data has shown that education qualifications in the SUD workforce are lower than in other health services (25). Because the administration and interpretation of many cognitive tests are restricted to individuals with specialist qualifications, this limits their adoption in the sector. In addition, when screening does occur in SUD treatment settings, its primary function is to identify individuals requiring referral to specialist service providers (i.e., neuropsychology, neurology, etc.) for more comprehensive assessment and intervention, rather than to inform individual treatment plans.

Two fields in particular have driven progress in cognitive assessment practice for generalist workers: dementia, with an increasing emphasis on screening in primary care (26, 27), and schizophrenia, where cognitive impairment is an established predictor of functional outcome (28) necessitating the development of a standardized assessment battery specifically for this disorder. In the selection of domain-specific tests for the Measurement and Treatment Research to Improve Cognition in Schizophrenia (MATRICS) standard battery, a particular emphasis was placed on test practicality and tolerability, as well as psychometric quality. Pragmatic issues of administration time, scoring time and complexity, and test difficulty and unpleasantness (such as item repetition) for the client should be considered (28). These domains and issues are particularly relevant for the SUD workforce as well. The dementia screening literature has also emphasized these pragmatic issues, leading to a greater awareness and access to general cognitive screening tools.

Routine Cognitive Assessments in Clinical Practice

To date, the majority of the published literature on routine cognitive screening in SUD contexts has focused on three tests commonly used in dementia screening (29–34): the Mini-Mental State Examination (MMSE) (35), Addenbrooke's Cognitive Examination (ACE) (36), and the Montreal Cognitive Assessment (MoCA) (37). Due to their development for application in dementia contexts, these screening tools placed a heavy emphasis on memory, attention, language and visuospatial functioning (34). Multiple studies have demonstrated superior sensitivity of the MoCA and the ACE scales compared to the MMSE (34, 38). It is possible that this arises from the MoCA and ACE including at least some items assessing EF (letter fluency and trails) which are absent in the MMSE. Indeed, this may demonstrate an important limitation of adopting existing screening tools designed for dementia in the context of SUD treatment. It can be argued that cognitive screening is most beneficial in SUD contexts when focused on SUD-relevant domains, rather than the identification of general cognitive deficits. Therefore, current neuroscience-based frameworks emphasise the importance of assessing EF, incentive salience, and decision-making in SUD (13, 28, 39, 40). As such, there is much to be gained by applying a process similar to the MATRICS effort (28, 39, 40) in the SUD field to identify a 'gold-standard' set of practical and sensitive cognitive tests that can be routinely used in clinical practice.

Cognitive Assessment Approaches in SUD Research

The most commonly used cognitive assessment approach in SUD research has been the "flexible test battery". This approach combines different types of tests to measure selected cognitive domains (e.g., attention, EF). Attention, memory, EF, and decision-making are the most commonly assessed domains, although there is a considerable discrepancy in the tests selected to assess these constructs (41). Even within specific tests, different studies have used several different versions; for example, at least four different versions of the Stroop test have been employed in the SUD literature (1). Another commonly used approach is the "fixed test battery", which involves a comprehensive suite of tests that have been jointly standardized and provide a general profile of cognitive impairment. The Cambridge Automated Neuropsychological Test Battery (CANTAB) (42), the Repeatable Battery for the Assessment of Neuropsychological Status (RBANS) (43), the Neuropsychological Assessment Battery (NAB) – Screening Module (44) and the MicroCog™ (45) are examples of fixed test batteries utilized in SUD research (30, 46–48), although these too have limited assessment of EF. Another limitation of these assessment modules is the lack of construct validity, as they were not originally designed to measure SUD-related cognitive deficits. As a result, they overemphasize assessment of cognitive domains that are relatively irrelevant in the context of SUD and neglect other domains that are pivotal (e.g., decision-making). A common limitation of flexible and fixed batteries is their reliance on face-to-face testing, normally involving a researcher or clinician, and their duration, which is typically around 60-90 min.

To address this gap, a number of semi-automated tests of cognitive performance have been developed, including the Automated Neuropsychological Assessment Metrics (ANAM, developed by the U.S. Department of Defence), Immediate

Post-concussion Assessment and Cognitive Testing battery (ImPACT), and CogState brief battery, have been used more widely, although validation studies to date suggest they may not yet have sufficient psychometric evidence to support clinical use (49–53). Research specifically in addictions has begun to develop and validate cognitive tests that can be delivered in client/participants' homes or *via* smartphone devices (54) (*scienceofbehaviorchange.org*, 2019). Evaluations of the reliability, validity, and feasibility of mobile cognitive assessment in individuals with SUD have been scarce, but promising (55–57).

Cognitive assessment *via* smartphone applications and web-based computing is a rapidly developing field, following many of the procedures and traditions of Ecological Momentary Assessment (EMA) (56). The flexibility and rapidity of assessment offered by mobile applications makes it particularly suited to questions assessing change in cognitive performance over various time scales (within hours to over months). For example, cognitive performance can be assessed in event-based (i.e., participants-initiated assessment entries), time-based and randomly prompted procedures that were not previously feasible, and or valid, in laboratory testing. While the benefits of mobile testing to longitudinal research, particularly large-scale clinical trials, appear obvious (57), the rapidity and frequency of deployment also provide opportunities to test questions of much shorter delays between drug use behavior and cognition. For example, recent studies have examined if daily within-individual variability in cognitive performance, principally response inhibition, was associated with variable likelihood for binge alcohol consumption (58). Similarly, influencing the immediate dynamic relationship between cognition and drug use has also been used for intervention purposes. Web and smartphone platforms have been used to administer cognitive-task based interventions, such as cognitive bias modification (CBM) training (59–61), where cognitive performance is routinely measured as a central element of interventions that span several weeks. The outcomes of these trials show that mobile cognitive-task based interventions are feasible but not efficacious as in a stand-alone context (58, 61). However, the combination of cognitive bias modification (approach bias re-training) and normative feedback significantly reduces weekly alcohol consumption in excessive drinkers (59).

Summary of Evidence and Future Directions

A substantial proportion of people with SUD have cognitive deficits. Alcohol, stimulants and opioid users have overlapping deficits in EF and decision-making. Alcohol users have additional deficits in learning and memory and psychomotor speed. Heavy cannabis users have specific deficits in episodic memory and attention. Cognitive assessments of speed/attention, EF and decision-making are meaningfully associated with addiction treatment outcomes such as treatment retention, relapse and quality of life (1). In addition, there is growing evidence that motivational and affective domains are also implicated in SUD pathophysiology and clinical symptoms (8). For example, both reward expectancy and valuation and negative affect have been proposed to explain SUD chronicity (13). However, to date, there have been no studies linking these "novel domains" with clinical outcomes. Thus, it is important to explore the predictive validity of non-traditional cognitive-motivational and cognitive-affective domains in relation to treatment response. While flexible and fixed test batteries are the most common assessment approaches, data comparability is alarmingly low and future studies should aim to apply harmonized methods (41). Remote monitoring and mobile cognitive assessment remain in a nascent stage for SUD research and clinical care. It is too early to make accurate cost-benefit assessments of different mobile methodologies. Yet, their potential to provide more cost-effective assessment with larger and more representative samples and in greater proximity to drug use behavior justifies continued investment into their development.

Challenges for Implementation Into Practice

One of the main challenges for the cognitive assessment of people with SUD is the disparity of tests applied across sites and studies, and the lack of a common ontology and harmonized assessment approach (13, 62). Furthermore, harmonization efforts must accommodate clinicians' needs, including brevity, simplicity, and automated scoring and interpretation (10). Mobile cognitive testing is a highly promising approach, although its reliability and validity are influenced by a number of key factors. Test compliance, or lack thereof, seems to be problematic. A recent meta-analysis suggested that the compliance rate for EMA (the standard paradigm to administer mobile cognitive testing) with SUD samples was below the recommended rate of 80% (63). Designs including participant-initiated event-based assessments were associated with test compliance issues, whereas duration and frequency of assessment were not. While the latter finding suggests that extensive cognitive assessment may be feasible with mobile methods, caution is advised with regard to the scope and depth of the data that can be obtained with these brief assessments and the validity of data sets collected (64). Remote methods for assessing confounds such as task distraction, malingering, and "cheating" are not well established or validated. As the capability of smartphones, for example, increases, so will the potential to minimize or control for such variables. Face-recognition and fingerprint technology has been proposed for ensuring identity compliance, although this presents ethical issues regarding confidential and de-identified data collection from samples that engage in illicit drug use (65).

ISAM-NIG Recommendations for Cognitive Assessment

As the authors of this ISAM-NIG roadmap, we give the following recommendations for future work:

1. *Selecting theoretically and clinically relevant constructs*: We recommend prioritizing constructs that are theoretically implicated in current neurobiological models of SUD [reviewed in (66)] and meaningfully related to SUD treatment

response and clinical outcomes [e.g., (1, 67, 68)]. These include attention/processing speed, response inhibition, and higher-order EF/decision-making. Episodic and working memory assessments can be particularly indicated in the case of alcohol and cannabis users (8).

2. *Selecting measures with well-established clinical validity in the SUD population*: We recommend using measures with demonstrated predictive and ecological validity (i.e., their scores predict individual variation in meaningful clinical outcomes such as treatment response, craving, drug use/ relapse, and quality of life), in addition to reliability. Unfortunately, few such measures are currently available. The MicroCog test battery and Continuous Performance Test (sustained attention/response inhibition) are highly reliable and excellent predictors of treatment response (1). Delay discounting paradigms and gambling tasks have excellent predictive and ecological validity, but the latter have been criticized for low reliability and construct validity (69). Because the ultimate goal is to incorporate cognitive assessment into clinical practice, we recommend conducting a Delphi consensus study including both cognitive assessment researchers and SUD clinicians to identify a minimum battery of measures with adequate psychometric properties AND clinical significance.
3. *Adopting harmonized cognitive assessment protocols*: We recommend continuing work towards developing a harmonized Cognitive Assessment of Addiction (CAA) battery. This battery should be (1) theoretically grounded in current addiction neuroscience frameworks; (2) brief and easy to administer, to meet the needs and qualifications of the SUD workforce; (3) portable and repeatable, capitalizing when possible on emerging remote monitoring techniques; (4) clinically meaningful in individual-level predictive models, i.e., able to identify risk of cognition-related premature treatment cessation or relapse, cognitive phenotypes relevant for predicting response to different treatment approaches, or changes in cognitive status relevant to treatment progression. The CAA should also address challenges specific to international research collaboration, including culturally-sensitive contents and appropriate translation of instructions.

NEUROIMAGING

The development of functional imaging techniques such as Positron Emission Tomography (PET) and functional Magnetic Resonance Imaging (fMRI), has allowed the high-resolution mapping of the brain in-vivo, in people with SUD. This body of work has provided increasing evidence that SUD is associated with alterations in the anatomy and the functional brain pathways ascribed to reward, learning, and EF. Importantly, emerging evidence suggests that neuroimaging versus subjective measures in SUD may predict with greater precision addiction-relevant cognitive processes (e.g., attentional biases) and treatment outcomes (e.g., abstinence) (70–72).

Neuroimaging Methods and Techniques Applied to SUD

Functional imaging techniques allowed exploration of whether brain dysfunction is implicated in SUD in humans. These create images of brain function by relying on proxies, including metabolic properties of the brain (e.g., oxygen in PET and fMRI, glucose levels in PET) (73). The application of functional imaging has been crucial to reveal the impact of SUD on human brain function in areas ascribed to cognitive processes (e.g., EF, decision-making) and positive and negative emotions (see "Cognitive assessment approaches in SUD research" in the COGNITIVE ASSESSMENT section).

PET studies have also provided early evidence on the neurobiology of SUD (74–77). PET imaging relies on the movement of injected radioactive material to identify whether the metabolic activity of brain regions is related to cognitive functions (73). PET's invasiveness and high financial costs have resulted in a limited number of studies using it, and its low temporal and spatial resolutions (i.e., 20–40 min required for image generation, with a spatial resolution up to 5 mm^3) prevented the identification of subtle brain activity alterations in SUD samples (73).

The development of fMRI provided a way to overcome these limitations. Unlike PET, fMRI is non-invasive, promoting feasibility in unpacking the neural correlates of SUD (73). Specifically, fMRI generates information about brain activity by exploiting the magnetic properties of oxygenated and deoxygenated blood (73). Further, fMRI provides information on the brain's functional activity with higher temporal and spatial resolutions than those of PET, i.e., within seconds and millimeters, respectively (73). These methodological advantages have allowed many studies to map the neural pathways implicated in SUD, while providing information on brain function within a high spatial and temporal resolution. However, a well-described limitation of fMRI analyses is the difficulty to control for multiple tests (i.e., statistical thresholds) and related false positive errors (78). The neuroimaging community has started to implement several strategies to address this limitation (79), but the use of liberal thresholds has probably inflated false positive rates in earlier studies.

Using multi-modal imaging techniques is warranted to further unpack the neural mechanisms of SUD and abstinence. For instance, integrating structural MRI (sMRI) data with Magnetic Resonance Spectroscopy Imaging, an MRI imaging technique that allows investigation of metabolites in the brain, may provide insight into the biochemical changes associated with volumetric alterations in SUD. Further, conducting brief, repeated task-free fMRI studies during treatment/abstinence could provide a better understanding of the impact of clinical changes on intrinsic brain architecture. An advantage of resting-state functional imaging data is the possibility of investigating patterns of brain function without restrictive "forces" on brain function placed by a specific task. Finally, studying SUD with modalities such as Diffusion Tensor Imaging (DTI) may reveal alteration in white matter pathways that connect brain regions that are volumetrically altered. This approach may inform the pathophysiology of volumetric alterations in SUD-relevant brain circuits.

Brain Systems Implicated in Addiction: Insights From Theory

Table 1 overviews key neurobehavioral pathways implicated by prominent neuroscientific theories of addiction and a growing body of work. These include neurobehavioral systems implicated in positive valence, negative valence, interoception, and EF (80–86). Abstinence may recover and mitigate such brain alterations and related cognitive functions, e.g., increase in response inhibition capacity, lower stress and drug reactivity, learning new responses to drugs and related stimuli. This notion is yet to be tested using robust neuroimaging methods that, in conjunction with treatment-relevant clinical and cognitive measures, measure and track the integrity of specific neural pathways during abstinence (see examples in **Table 1**).

The neurobiology of abstinence has been posited to entail two core processes (99). The first is the *restored* integrity of brain function, as drug levels in the central nervous system and bloodstream clear out with abstinence. The second is the *retraining* of neural pathways implicated in cognitive changes that enable abstinence. These include awareness/monitoring of internal

TABLE 1 | Overview of addiction-related neurocognitive constructs and related brain circuits, tasks, and interventions.

	Positive affect, Response (13), (80), (82), (84)	Positive affect, Anticipation (13), (83), (84)	Negative affect (13), (80), (82),	Learning/habit (13), (83), (84)	Cognitive control (13), (82), (83), (84)	Interoception (83), (86)
Brain circuit	Medial OFC, ventral striatum	Medial OFC, sgACC (subgenual)	Amygdala	Lateral OFC, Dorsal striatum (Caudate, putamen), Hippocampus	DLPFC, dACC (dorsal), IFG	Insula, posterior cingulate
fMRI tasks	Monetary incentive delay (reward receipt) (87), probabilistic reward task (88), activity incentive Delay task (98)	Monetary Incentive delay (reward anticipation) (87), cue-reactivity (90), attentional bias (89)	Cue reactivity (90) during withdrawal, negative or stress cue reactivity	Instrumental reward-gain and loss-avoidance task (89)	Stop Signal (91), Go-no go (92), Stroop (93), PASAT-M (97)	heartbeat counting task (94), visceral interoceptive attention task (95)
Cognitive	Reward receipt, response to reward, reward satiation	Motivation, saliency valuation, reward anticipation, drive expectancy, approach/attentional bias	Acute/sustained threat	Stimulus-response conditioned habits, compulsivity, learning reward/loss contingencies	Loss of cognitive control, disinhibition, performance monitoring, action/response selection, low distress tolerance	"Momentary mapping of the body's internal landscape" (96) during craving and withdrawal
Behavior	Experience of reward with drug use, response to substance-free reward	Increased: attention/salience of drugs and related stimuli, reward when anticipating drug use.	Experience of withdrawal, stress, anxiety, anhedonia	Drug use as: repetitive, compulsive drive, conditioned response to seek positive affect & avoid/mitigate negative affect, learnt association with people, situations, places	Drug use even when known as harmful and in response to affective distress	Heightened/lowered awareness to drug-related physical & psychological states; increase distance between cue and behavioral response.
Intervention strategies	Decrease reward value of drug (e.g., methadone or nicotine patches), suppression of mPFC with low frequency rTMS or cTBS; increase reward value of drug-free activities (e.g., behavioral activation, physical activity)	Cognitive bias modification, reappraisal training for drug cues, exposure therapy, motivational interviewing, contingency management	Strategies to address negative affect (e.g., behavioral activation and cognitive reappraisal training), medication that counter stress response, rtfMRI neurofeedback on Insula or sgACC	Strategies that weaken conditioned drug behaviors, memory reconsolidation	Strengthen inhibitory/executive control, inhibitory control training (e.g., Go-No-Go), working memory training, goal management training, stimulating DLPFC with anodal tDCS or high frequency rTMS	Mindfulness-based therapies, physical exercise

Columns reflect key neurocognitive constructs for addiction research. Identified constructs also map onto the three domains of the Addiction Neuroclinical Assessment (ANA) (11) framework: Positive affect (response and anticipation), Negative affect, and Cognitive control map directly onto the three domains of ANA (i.e., Incentive salience, Negative affectivity and Executive function). Learning/habit is part of Incentive salience (reward learning); Interoception is at the interface of the three ANA domains. Rows reflect functional neuroimaging methods (e.g., fMRI tasks), cognitive/behavioral assessments, and examples of neuroscience informed intervention strategies aligned with each of the identified constructs.

ACC, anterior cingulate cortex; cTBS, continuous theta burst stimulation; DLPFC, dorsolateral PFC; IFG, Inferior Frontal Gyrus; mPFC, medial PFC; OFC, orbitofrontal cortex; PFC, prefrontal cortex; rtfMRI, real-time functional MRI; rTMS, repeated transcranial magnetic stimulation; tDCS, transcranial direct current stimulation.

psychological/physiological states (e.g., insula), withdrawal and craving (e.g., amygdala); EF (e.g., dorsal prefrontal regions); monitoring conflict between short-term goals (e.g., pleasure from using drugs, ventral striatum) *versus* long-term goals (e.g., abstinence and improved quality of life; anterior cingulate cortex); motivation to use drugs (e.g., orbitofrontal cortex); and learning new responses to drug-related and other stimuli (e.g., lateral prefrontal and dorsal striatal regions) (99).

Summary of Neuroimaging Evidence in SUD

Most neuroimaging studies to date have mapped dysfunctional neural pathways in SUD. There is a significant lack of work that tracks abstinence-related brain changes over time. This evidence gap prevents neuroimaging studies from informing the identification of treatment targets and clinical practice. It is unclear if abstinence (i) leads to recovery of SUD-related brain dysfunction (i.e., return to pre-drug onset level, or comparable levels to non-drug using controls), (ii) engages additional pathways implicated in abstinence-related cognitive, clinical, and behavioral changes, and (iii) is predicted by specific brain measures assessed pre-treatment. Emerging (but mixed) evidence from standard behavioral (e.g., CBT, Motivational Interview, Contingency Management) and pharmacological treatments that directly affect the central nervous system provides preliminary support for these notions, as reviewed in detail in previous work [see (100–102)]. This section provides an overview of early neuroimaging evidence for brain changes related to abstinence and novel interventions (i.e., cognitive training approaches and mindfulness-based therapies).

Neuroimaging Evidence in Abstinence

Abstinence may "reverse" brain dysfunction and volume loss associated with SUD. Studies have observed increased or normalized volumes in global and prefrontal brain regions related to abstinence in people with alcohol use disorder (103) and cocaine and opiate use disorders (104). PET and DTI studies of alcohol and cocaine users showed recovery of brain dysfunction and white matter integrity following heterogeneous abstinence durations, e.g., from about a month (105, 106), to several months (107, 108) and several years (109, 110). Results from fMRI tasks of response inhibition in abstinent users also showed that reduced brain function typically associated with drug use, was "restored" and increased in prefrontal and cerebellar pathways in former *versus* current cigarette smokers (> 12 month abstinent) (111, 112), and in former cannabis users (> 28 day abstinent) *versus* non-users (113).

Emerging (but mixed) evidence showed that abstinence duration was associated with improved integrity (functional and structure) of cortical and prefrontal pathways (109, 111, 114). Additionally, abstinence related neuroadaptations have been associated with substance use levels [e.g., cocaine dose (115)], and performance was improved during cognitive tasks relevant to addiction [e.g., processing speed, memory, EF-shifting (104, 115)]. Thus, abstinence-related brain changes may in part drive treatment relevant outcomes.

Neuroimaging Predictors of Abstinence

Several neuroimaging studies have examined whether (structural and functional) brain integrity in SUD predicts abstinence, with promising results. Studies of *brain structure* in people with nicotine and alcohol use disorders reported that increased volume and white matter integrity in prefrontal regions, followed by parietal and subcortical areas, most consistently segregated abstainers *versus* relapsers (116–119). Studies have examined *brain function* using fMRI tasks that engage cognitive domains relevant to treatment response (cue reactivity, attentional bias, error-related activity, reward, and emotion processing) (71, 72, 111, 116, 117, 120–124). These studies provided evidence that the function of fronto-striatal regions in particular, followed by other regions (e.g., cingulate, temporal, insular cortices) discriminated responders *versus* non-responders, relapsers *versus* non-relapsers in cigarette smokers and people with methamphetamine, cocaine and alcohol use disorders (71, 72, 111, 116, 117, 120, 121, 123, 124). Also, the activity of fronto-striatal pathways have been shown to predict alcohol dosage at 6 month follow-up (122). Studies that used other functional imaging techniques such as spectroscopy and PET imaging consistently reported that frontal blood flow and metabolites (i.e., in prefrontal, insular, and cerebellar areas) and the density of dopamine receptors (i.e., in the dorsal striatum) predicted treatment outcome in alcohol users (125, 126) and relapse in methamphetamine users (127).

Impact of Cognitive Training Strategies

Novel training strategies that target core cognitive dysfunctions in SUD have shown promise to restore cognitive alterations and help maintain abstinence (128). One example includes cognitive bias modification strategies that reduce attentional biases towards substance related cues [see study in tobacco smokers (129)]. Such strategies may target top-down and bottom-up brain pathways (130) implicated in addiction (131). These include increasing the activity of top-down EF regions that enhance inhibitory control and behavioral monitoring (e.g., dorsal anterior cingulate, lateral orbitofrontal cortex), and decreasing reactivity of bottom-up pathways implicated in reactivity to drug stimuli, and craving (e.g., amygdala).

Early neuroimaging evidence has examined the neuroadaptations that occur pre-to-post-cognitive bias modification training. These findings are revised and discussed in the COGNITIVE TRAINING AND REMEDIATION section below. There is a paucity of neuroimaging research on other cognitive training and remediation approaches, despite promising evidence of neuroplasticity-related changes after cognitive remediation in brain injury (132).

Impact of Mindfulness-Based Interventions

Mindfulness-based interventions are being increasingly used for the treatment of SUD (133). Although mindfulness does not use standard cognitive training/remediation approaches, it has shown to improve SUD-relevant cognitive processes such as attention and EF (134) as well as substance use outcomes (i.e., reduced craving, withdrawal) (135). Mindfulness-based interventions engage two key cognitive processes (i) *focused attention*, which consists of paying attention to a specific stimulus while letting go of distractions (e.g., focus on breathing, while experiencing craving) and (ii) *open monitoring*, which refers to the being aware of internal and external stimuli (e.g., acknowledging the experience of stress, craving, and withdrawal, or environmental triggers) with a non-judgmental attitude and acceptance.

The effectiveness of mindfulness-based interventions has been ascribed to improved function of prefrontal, parietal, and insula regions that are implicated in EF and autonomic regulation (133, 136), and down-regulation of reactivity in striatal/amygdala regions implicated in reward, stress, and habitual substance use (136). Only a handful of neuroimaging studies have examined brain changes that occur with mindfulness-based interventions in SUD. This includes a fMRI study in tobacco smokers that showed a 10-session mindfulness-oriented recovery enhancement (MORE) *versus* placebo intervention, decreased activity of the ventral striatum, and medial prefrontal regions during a craving task and an emotion regulation task (137). Most evidence on mindfulness and SUD consists of behavioral studies that showed robust effects on cognition, substance use, and craving. Given the widespread use of mindfulness-based interventions in clinical settings, we advocate the conduct of active placebo-controlled neuroimaging studies that map the neurobiology of mindfulness in SUD.

Challenges for Implementation Into Practice

Overall, there is a paucity of neuroimaging studies of treatment and abstinence in SUD. The study methods are very heterogeneous which precludes their systematic integration. *First*, there was significant heterogeneity in treatments, with distinct durations and hypothesized neurobehavioral and pharmacological mechanisms of action, and distinct treatment responses across different individuals, SUD and related psychiatric comorbidities. *Second*, control groups varied substantially (e.g., placebo, active control treatment, no control group) and brain changes related to abstinence were compared to different types of controls (e.g., pretreatment baseline in the same group, control group of non-substance users, separate SUD group also assessed post-treatment). *Third*, repeated measures study designs had varying data testing points (e.g., before, during and at varying times post-treatment) that precluded the integration of the study findings and mapping treatment-related, trajectories of brain changes with abstinence/recovery. More systematic evidence is needed to provide sufficient power to measure brain pathways relevant to treatment response and to inform clinically-relevant treatment endpoints. In order to address this gap, the ISAM-NIG Neuroimaging stream recommends the conduct of harmonized, multi-site, neuroimaging studies with systematic testing protocols of relevance for clinical practice. It is hoped that the ISAM-NIG Neuroimaging approach will generate results that can be readily integrated and that increase the power to detect abstinence-related neuroadaptations.

On one hand, the integration of neuroimaging testing into clinical practice can be challenging. MRI scanners are extremely expensive to buy, setup, and run safely, and the acquisition of high-quality brain images requires extensive specialized technical expertise. On the other hand, the availability of MRI scans in many hospitals, universities, and medical institutions, may provide ideal settings to integrate neuroimaging and clinical expertise. MRI scans can be feasible in that they are non-invasive, safe, and can be relatively quick (e.g., anatomical and resting-state brain scans can take <10 min, and some fMRI tasks can last between 10 and 15 min). Outstanding challenges to address remain funding sources, the lack of integration in the theoretical frameworks between basic research, clinical science, and clinical practice. Discipline-specific specialized language and practices can also create barriers. We advocate using team science to develop a harmonized interdisciplinary framework, so that all stakeholders, including clinicians, neuropsychologists, social workers and neuroscientists interact to inform commonly-agreed testing batteries and most profitable directions for future work.

The present review has focused on neuroimaging data mainly acquired through fMRI, allowing for visualization of the brain networks involved in certain conditions (e.g., abstinence vs. relapse). However, it should be noted that the coarse temporal resolution of such techniques (1–2 s) impedes determination of the temporal activation sequence (in the order of the ms), allowing the specific brain activation patterns to be correlated with the various cognitive stages involved in the investigated processes [e.g., (138)]. Other tools, such as cognitive event-related potentials (ERPs) in particular, might be more suitable for this purpose (139). Nowadays, different studies reveal that specific ERP components tagging specific cognitive functions (mainly cue reactivity and inhibition) may be used as neurophysiological biomarkers for addiction treatment outcome prediction (140). Such data may be of great value to clinicians for the identification of cognitive processes that should be rehabilitated on a patient-by-patient basis through cognitive training and/or brain stimulation. However, despite technical facilities (cheap tool easily implementable in each clinical care unit), several decades of research, and clinical relevance, ERPs like other neuroimaging modalities have yet to be implemented in the clinical management of SUD.

ISAM NIG Recommendations for Neuroimaging

We aim to map how advanced multimodal neuroimaging tools—coordinated with relevant clinical and cognitive measures agreed upon with a large multidisciplinary team of experts in the field—can be used to track the neurobiological mechanisms of addiction treatment. As the authors of this ISAM-NIG roadmap, we give the following recommendations for future work:

1. Neuroimaging testing should be *harmonized* with clinical and cognitive tools mapping overlapping systems (see example in **Table 1**).
2. Neuroimaging testing should be *feasible* and rely on short and robust imaging protocols that recruit specific brain pathways implicated in relevant clinical and cognitive features of addiction (e.g., craving, attentional bias, cognitive control).

3. Neuroimaging protocols may also incorporate *neuroimaging measures of brain integrity other than those included in the harmonized protocols when focused on discovery science* (e.g., new fMRI tasks that target novel cognitive constructs, new neuroimaging techniques that test distinct properties of brain integrity). This would mitigate the risks that complete harmonization around existing neuroimaging measures and neurobiological models of addiction would stifle new knowledge. We cannot exclude that current neuroimaging techniques and theories of addiction may not be an accurate/valid representation of brain changes that occur with SUD treatment.
4. Imaging testing batteries should be *amenable to repeated testing* so that changes over time can be tracked (i) *prospectively*, to examine if baseline imaging measures predict follow up outcomes assessed 1+ times at the end of treatment, (ii) *longitudinally*, to track individual trajectories of brain and behavioral change before, during and after treatment, (iii) using rigorous *double-blind randomized controlled studies* to map treatment-specific effects in distinct substance and behavioral addictions.
5. *Multi-site* neuroimaging studies using shared protocols will be necessary to gain sufficient power to track heterogeneity of treatment responses between individuals SUD, to validate the protocols and test their reliability. There are excellent examples of successful international collaborations that are already in place in this area, such as ENIGMA-Addiction (141). We aim to leverage these existing collaboration initiatives to increase neuroimaging methods reliability and validity and studies sample size and representativity, and to expand them by incorporating more clinical researchers and clinicians.
6. As treatments often consist of individual and combined interventions, the distinct and cumulative effects on brain changes should be examined. In addition, investigating moderating roles of age and sex differences on these abstinence-related neuroadaptations is critical. Indeed, younger and older people with SUD may show lower and greater vulnerability to aberrant neurobiology (142). People with different ages and sex may show distinct neuroplastic changes with abstinence and these are largely unknown (99, 143, 144).
7. Brain indices from neuroimaging testing should be *examined in relation to treatment response variables*, whether measured as categories (e.g., responders vs. non-responders, relapsers vs. non-relapsers) or as discrete measures of addiction (severity of addiction symptom scores, number of relapses, duration of abstinence, amount of substance used) and related mental health, cognitive and quality of life outcomes (e.g., stress, mood, socio-occupational functioning).

COGNITIVE TRAINING AND REMEDIATION

Despite recent advances in psychological and pharmacological interventions for SUD, relapse remains the norm. A recent meta-analysis of 21 treatment outcome studies conducted between 2000–2015 found that fewer than 10% of treatment seekers were in remission (i.e., did not meet SUD diagnostic criteria for the past 6 months) in any given year following SUD treatment (145). The past decade has seen a proliferation of cognitive training (CT) intervention trials aimed at remediating or reversing substance-related cognitive deficits (146). However, their implementation into clinical practice is almost non-existent, despite promising results and now having more flexible, precise, engaging and convenient modes of delivery (i.e., computer, web and mobile application-based approaches). Gathering more data in this still-developing area is essential to facilitate translation. Even the most widely tested training interventions, such as cognitive bias modification, need more data to fully appraise their benefit for addiction treatment (147). This section summarizes recent advances in CT, identifies limitations in the evidence base, and highlights priorities and directions for future research to bridge the gap between science and practice. Current CT approaches can be broadly divided into: general cognitive remediation, working memory training (WMT), inhibitory control (or response inhibition) training (ICT), and cognitive bias modification (CBM).

Cognitive Remediation

In SUD, general cognitive remediation approaches such as cognitive enhancement therapy (CET) and cognitive remediation therapy (CRT) aim to reduce substance use (148–150) and craving (151) by targeting EF and self-regulation. Cognitive remediation has been shown to improve cognition in domains of working memory (WM), verbal memory, verbal learning, attention, and processing speed (151–154). Positive outcomes have also been shown to be associated with increased neuroplasticity in emotion regulation-related fronto-limbic networks in individuals with schizophrenia and co-morbid SUD (155). A recent study delivered 12 two-hour group sessions of clinician-guided CRT and computerized CT (Lumosity) (156) over 4 weeks to a sample of female residents completing residential rehabilitation and found significant improvements in EF, response inhibition, self-control, and quality of life relative to treatment as usual (TAU) (157). Similar research has reported comparable improvements in cognitive functioning following CRT (150, 151) and CET (148), and improved cognitive functioning has been associated with reduced substance use at 3- and 6-month follow-ups (148, 150). Importantly, CET and CRT also demonstrate preliminary efficacy for SUD patients with cognitive impairments (e.g., schizophrenia, past head injury) (148, 157). However, their duration, intensity, and high cognitive demand—coupled with a current paucity of large-scale, methodologically rigorous clinical trials—may currently preclude their widespread implementation in clinical settings.

Another manualized therapist-assisted group intervention is Goal Management Training (GMT), which trains EF and sustained attention and emphasizes the transfer of these skills to goal-related tasks and projects in everyday life. When combined with mindfulness meditation, GMT has been found to significantly improve WM, response inhibition and decision-making in alcohol and stimulant outpatients relative to TAU (158) and more recently also in polysubstance users in a therapeutic community (159). A meta-analysis of GMT more broadly concluded that it provides small to moderate improvements in EF which are consistently maintained at 1–6 month follow-ups (160). As such, GMT is likely to be an effective candidate cognitive remediation approach for SUD treatment; however, substantially more research is needed to validate this assertion, particularly regarding the translation of cognitive improvements into improved substance use outcomes.

Working Memory Training (WMT)

The most widely researched EF training intervention, WMT (e.g., Cogmed, PSSCogRehab) (161, 162) requires participants to repeatedly manipulate and recall sequences of shapes and numbers through computerized tasks that become increasingly difficult over time (i.e., they are adaptive to the individual's performance). WMT aims to extend WM capacity, so individuals can better integrate, manipulate, and prioritize important information, with the aim of supporting more adaptive decision-making that leads to reduced substance use (163). Relative to many other approaches, WMT is intensive, typically requiring 19–25 days of training and as such, retention is often poor (164). While WMT has been shown to lead to improvements in near-transfer effects (i.e., improved performance on similar WM tasks), there is limited evidence supporting far-transfer effects of WMT on other measures of EF and importantly, on substance-related outcomes (165). Reduced alcohol consumption 1 month after training was reported following WMT in heavy drinkers (163), but most studies have failed to demonstrate or even measure changes in substance use (165). For example, non-treatment seekers with alcohol use disorder who were trained with Cogmed showed improved verbal memory but no clinically significant reductions in alcohol consumption or problem severity (166). While a study of treatment-seekers improved WM and capacity to plan for the future (i.e., episodic future thinking) on a delay discounting task, there was no measurement of substance use outcomes (167). Similarly, studies of methadone maintenance (168) and cannabis (169) have found no evidence of far-transfer effects (e.g., delay discounting), although Rass et al. (168) showed WMT-related reductions in street drug use among methadone users. Other forms of WMT (e.g., n-back training) have reported similar near-transfer but not substance-use-related findings with methamphetamine patients (170) and a mixed group of substance use patients (alcohol, cannabis, cocaine) (164). As such, the greatest limitation in the WMT literature is the failure to consistently examine substance use outcomes and therefore there is insufficient evidence at this time to support the utility of WMT as an effective adjunctive treatment for SUD.

Inhibitory Control Training (ICT)

Since deficits in inhibitory control are associated with increased drug use (171–174), ICT aims to bolster inhibitory control through the repeated practice of tasks [e.g., go/no-go (GNG), stop-signal task]. Such tasks require individuals to repeatedly inhibit prepotent motor responses to salient stimuli (172). In a seminal study, a beer-GNG task which trained heavily drinking students to inhibit responses to "beer" stimuli resulted in significantly reduced weekly alcohol intake relative to students trained towards "beer" stimuli (175). A recent RCT of 120 heavily drinking students found that a single session of either ICT or approach bias modification (ApBM, described below) led to significant reductions in alcohol consumption relative to matched controls (176). Similarly, Kilwein et al. (177) found that a single session of ICT (GNG) reduced alcohol consumption and alcohol approach tendencies in a small sample (n = 23) of heavily drinking men (177). Despite these promising findings, each of the aforementioned ICT studies used community samples, and it has not yet been established whether these results will generalise to treatment seekers.

Two meta-analyses recently concluded that ICT leads to small but robust reductions in alcohol consumption immediately after training (178, 179). Di Lemma and Field (176) reported reduced alcohol consumption in a bogus taste test after a single session of ICT or cue-avoidance training (approach bias modification). Others have observed reduced alcohol consumption 1 and 2 weeks after ICT (163, 177, 180). These findings highlight the promise of ICT though there remains a paucity of research assessing long-term drinking outcomes outside of laboratory settings. Future studies of ICT with clinical populations should consider testing multi-session approaches akin to WMT. To date, few studies have trialled multi-session ICT: One found it to be ineffective (58) for heavily drinking individuals, while another found that 2 weeks of ICT resulted in modest reductions of alcohol consumption among individuals with AUDs, compared to WMT or a control condition (181).

Cognitive Bias Modification (CBM)

CBM aims to directly interrupt and modify automatic processes in response to appetitive cues. Attentional bias modification (AtBM) aims to modify the preferential allocation of attentional resources to drug cues by repeatedly shifting attention to neutral or positive (non-drug) cues and away from drug-related cues. Despite several null findings (182), significant effects have included the reduction of alcohol consumption in non-treatment seeking heavy or social drinkers (183, 184). Among treatment seekers, five sessions of AtBM have been shown to significantly delay time to relapse (but not relapse rates) relative to controls who received sham training (185). Similarly, six sessions significantly reduced alcohol relapse rates at a one-year follow-up relative to a sham training condition in a sample of treatment seekers with AUD (186). Among methadone maintenance patients, AtBM reduced attentional bias to heroin-related words, temptations to use, and number of lapses relative to TAU (187). However, among individuals with cocaine use disorder, it failed to reduce attentional bias, craving, and cocaine use (188). Likewise, 12 sessions of AtBM vs. sham training during residential treatment for methamphetamine use disorder failed to reduce craving and preferences for methamphetamine images (189). A systematic review of alcohol, nicotine, and opioid AtBM studies concluded that despite numerous negative findings in the literature, eight out of 10 multiple-session studies resulted in reduced addiction symptoms (particularly for alcohol), but without concomitant reductions in attentional bias (190).

Approach bias modification (ApBM), which uses the Approach Avoidance Task, requires an avoidance response to drug cues (pushing a joystick, shrinking image size) and an approach response (pulling a joystick, enlarging image size) to non-drug cues. Several trials have examined alcohol ApBM, with evidence that short-term abstinence is increased by up to 30% with four consecutive training sessions during inpatient withdrawal (32) and by 8%–13% at 12-month follow-up (186, 191, 192). Alcohol ApBM has demonstrated relatively consistent, moderate reductions in drinking behavior when delivered to clinical populations (193), and it was even added to the German guidelines for the treatment of AUD (194).

Early neuroimaging evidence has examined the neuroadaptations that occur pre-to-post-cognitive bias modification training. This work has focused on two samples of abstinent alcoholics undergoing an fMRI cue-reactivity task (alcohol *versus* soft drink stimuli) (61, 195). Participants showed higher baseline reactivity to alcohol cues within the amygdala/nucleus accumbens and the medial prefrontal cortex, respectively (61, 195). The same samples, following a 3-week implicit avoidance task (versus placebo), showed reduced amygdala and medial prefrontal reactivity (61, 195). Notably, these brain changes were associated with reduced craving and approach bias to alcohol stimuli (61, 195) but not abstinence 12 months later. While preliminary, these findings suggest that neuroadaptations associated with cognitive bias modification have clinical relevance and warrant replication in larger SUD samples using robust, active placebo-controlled designs.

To date, only one study has been published that trialled ApBM in an illicit drug-using sample of non-treatment-seeking adults with cannabis use disorder (N = 33). Relative to sham-training, four sessions resulted in blunted cannabis cue-induced craving (196) but not less cannabis use. Overall, evidence suggests that ApBM is associated with reduced approach bias and reduced consumption behaviors for alcohol, smoking, and unhealthy foods (197). Recently, six sessions of ApBM delivered to 1,405 alcohol-dependent patients significantly reduced alcohol relapse rates at a 1-year follow-up relative to a sham-training condition (186). However, as these reductions were also observed following AtBM and a combined AtBM and ApBM condition, the authors concluded that all active CBM training conditions had a small but robust long-term effect on relapse rates.

Finally, a meta-analysis of alcohol and smoking CBM studies (both AtBM and ApBM) showed a small but significant effect on clinical outcomes for alcohol (but not smoking), but a lack of evidence that reduced approach bias led to improved outcomes (198). This assertion was challenged by Wiers et al. (193) who noted that the review conflated proof-of-principle lab-studies and clinical RCTs and different samples (e.g., treatment-seeking alcohol dependent individuals vs non-clinical student populations). Importantly, these populations likely have differences in motivation/awareness for receiving an intervention to reduce alcohol use, which could explain inconsistencies in the reported effectiveness of CBM across populations (193).

Summary of Evidence and Future Directions

Currently CBM, particularly ApBM, appears one of the most promising approaches for individuals seeking treatment for AUDs; however, its effectiveness for other drugs (aside from tobacco) is yet to be established. The most extensively trialled CT approach is WMT, which has shown promising results in alcohol and stimulants users. However, its high cognitive demand, training intensity, and apparent lack of far-transfer effects limit its application to clinical populations. ICT holds much promise for reducing alcohol consumption in heavy drinkers, but requires testing in treatment-seekers. Finally, more intensive group-based approaches such as CRT/CET and GMT may improve EF and quality of life; however, their impact on substance use outcomes remains largely untested. Synergistic approaches now warrant exploration. Indeed, a study that combined WMT and AtBM (199) has shown promising feasibility and improved EF, though substance use outcomes were not assessed. It may also prove fruitful to adopt staggered CT approaches, capitalizing on the brain's capacity to repair itself (neuroplasticity) during withdrawal, early and later abstinence by strengthening cognitive control (e.g., using ICT) and dampening cue-reactivity (e.g., using CBM), prior to engaging in more intensive and cognitively demanding but ecologically valid group training for more extensive remediation (e.g., using GMT).

Challenges for Implementation Into Practice

While there may be logistical challenges to the adoption of CT in clinical practice (e.g., cost, lack of time, training requirements, etc.), the main impediment to implementing CT in clinical practice is the absence of robust evidence for treatment success of any one particular approach. This is largely due to the vast heterogeneity of studies, particularly regarding differences in treatment settings, samples (clinical vs. non-clinical populations), cognitive intervention approaches, number and duration of training sessions, targeted mechanisms, targeted drugs of concern and varying primary outcome measures. Similarly, the absence of brief, ecologically valid, easily-administered measures of cognition precludes the identification of candidates who are most likely to benefit from CT (e.g., individuals with the poorest WM or the strongest attentional bias). As such, the evidence base for CT remains hampered by (1) the marked lack of studies on clinical populations, (2) the counter-intuitive neglect of assessing relevant substance use outcomes, (3) the lack of adequately-powered RCTs, (4) the limitations of research designs, (5) lack of attention to individual-level trajectories of cognitive improvements in relation to substance use and quality of life outcomes (precision medicine approach), and (6) a simple focus on direct relations between cognitive deficits and outcomes without considering person and environmental mediators and moderators of this relation (14). Despite positive signals from proof-of-concept studies and pilot RCTs, they require replication and testing with suitable control conditions in order to demonstrate their applicability in clinical settings. These limitations highlight the need for a harmonization approach that promotes greater standardization in cognitive training protocols and assessment of its effectiveness (i.e., routine assessment of substance use outcomes). Since the software and manuals of some of the most promising interventions (e.g., CBM, GMT) are well-developed and reproducible, we should advance towards optimized shared protocols that can promote international collaborations and multi-site studies. These recommendations will elucidate what works, for whom and under what conditions (i.e., identifying neurocognitive phenotypes). This knowledge will then guide the adoption of CT to improve outcomes for people seeking treatment for SUD.

ISAM-NIG Recommendations for Cognitive Training and Remediation

As the authors of this ISAM-NIG roadmap, we give the following recommendations for future work:

1. *The a priori publishing of research protocols*: To improve the consistency of cognitive training trials we encourage the publishing of research methodologies and protocols. This will permit replication studies to aid the consolidation of a disparate evidence base and help determine the optimal training duration and frequency to be implemented in real world clinical settings.
2. *Adopting consistent training paradigms and tailored, context-relevant stimuli:* A challenge for CBM research is the absence of consensus on optimal sham training conditions (e.g., matched stimuli with different push-pull contingencies) and optimal approach stimuli (e.g., whether to use neutral stimuli or healthier alternatives such as non-alcoholic beverages) (200). In the context of both CBM and ICT, utilizing personalized/tailored stimuli may increase engagement and effectiveness. For avoidance or "no-go" stimuli this might involve only using beverage types/brands that are regularly consumed by an individual, or images of illicit drug use and paraphernalia reflecting their preferred route of administration. Similarly, approach or "go" stimuli could encompass positive motivational images representing an individual's personal goals, values, and aspirations (family, employment, hobbies, etc.), which are drawn on heavily in most psychosocial interventions. Furthermore, co-design with consumers and end-users is a fundamental step to developing interventions that will be implemented successfully in practice.
3. *Ensuring targeted constructs are measured in cognitive training trials:* Future research protocols must adopt pre- and post-intervention measures that will elucidate changes in targeted mechanisms, thereby integrating neuroscience into addiction treatment. Importantly, these protocols should enable moderation and mediation analyses using psychophysiological measures (e.g., EEG, skin-conductance) in order to address issues regarding the notorious lack of reliability of traditional measures (e.g., the implicit association task and the approach avoidance task) (192, 201, 202) and thereby more accurately identify individuals most likely to benefit from adjunctive approaches.
4. *Adopting and standardizing SUD-related outcome measurement*: Future research needs to test cognitive interventions in real-world clinical settings and assess meaningful SUD clinical outcomes (i.e., reduced substance use, reduced cue-craving). Clear evidence of reduced harm and consumption is likely to appeal to both clinicians and individuals under their care, thus driving this improved addiction treatment effort.

NEUROMODULATION

The exponential growth in our understanding of the neural circuits involved in drug addiction over the last 20 years (3, 203–205) has been accompanied by the introduction of non-invasive brain stimulation technologies (NIBS) capable of modulating brain circuits externally (outside of the skull), such as transcranial magnetic stimulation (TMS) and transcranial electrical stimulation (tES). Technical advances in NIBS has increased hopes to find clinical applications for NIBS in addiction medicine (206). New FDA approval of NIBS technologies in depressive and obsessive-compulsive disorders, which have overlapping brain circuits with SUD, has raised these expectations to a higher level. There are other emerging areas of NIBS for addiction medicine, such as focused ultrasound stimulation (FUS) and transcranial nerve stimulation (tNS). Furthermore, other technologies exist that target neural circuits noninvasively that can be classified as "neuromodulation", such as fMRI- or EEG-neurofeedback (NF), whereby individuals can change their own brain activity in real time using a brain-computer interface. However, this section will primarily focus on tES/TMS/NF. We will review potential targets, ideal scenarios, and complexities in the field of neuromodulation for addiction treatment and then conclude with a few recommendations for future research.

Potential Targets for Neuromodulation

Targets in the field of neuromodulation should be defined across multiple levels, from behavior, cognitive process, and neural circuit. The NIMH research domain criteria (RDoC) have provided a research framework for mental health disorders that include these levels of targets for neuroscience-informed interventions including neuromodulation. While this framework was not specifically designed for addiction science, it is still a helpful resource. In RDoC terminologies, three main domains are more frequently considered for addiction medicine: *positive valence*, *negative valence*, and *cognitive systems* with a predominant focus on EF (13, 207). Within the positive valence domain, non-drug and drug-related reward processing (drug craving) are the most favorable multi-level targets for addiction treatment. Within the negative valence domain, acute or chronic withdrawal/negative reinforcement, anhedonia, and negative mood/anxiety comorbidities should be considered. EF with a broad definition has also potential to be targeted in neuromodulation (208). For more details, please see **Table 1**.

Brain Stimulation Studies in SUD

There is a trend of reporting positive results in tDCS and rTMS trials in SUD that is being reflected in systematic reviews and meta-analysis. In a meta-analysis published in 2013 on 17 eligible trials, Jansen, et al., reported that rTMS and tDCS on DLPFC could decrease drug craving (209). A meta-analysis of 10 rTMS studies identified a beneficial effect of high-frequency rTMS on craving associated with nicotine use disorder but not alcohol (210). Another meta-analysis published in 2018 by Song, et al., including 48 tDCS and rTMS studies targeting the DLPFC, reported positive overall effects on reducing drug craving and consumption with larger effect for multi-session interventions compared to single-session interventions (211). A recent meta-analysis with 15 studies using tDCS among nicotine dependents reported positive effect on craving and consumption (212). However, there is a large variation in methodological details (mainly ignored in meta-analyses) that makes it hard to find trials replicating previous findings using same stimulation protocols. Some of these methodological variations are being introduced below with few examples.

Figure 1 depicts the distribution of published tES/TMS studies based on their target areas. Most but not all published tES/TMS studies (90%) have targeted the DLPFC in order to indirectly target other areas within the EF network or other limbic/paralimbic areas through their connections to the DLPFC. As an example, Terraneo et al. showed that applying 15-Hz stimulation to the left DLPFC can reduce self-reported craving [visual analogue scale (VAS)] and cocaine use (urinalysis) among patients with cocaine use disorder randomized to receive active or sham repetitive TMS (rTMS) (213). In another study, Yang et al. showed that electrical stimulation over the DLPFC helps lower cigarette craving in nicotine-dependent individuals (214). Participant smokers underwent 1 session of real and sham transcranial direct current stimulation (tDCS) in a cross-over setting with 30 min duration and 1-mA intensity. There are studies targeting other areas than the DLPFC within the frontal cortex, such as inferior frontal gyrus, ventromedial prefrontal, or middle frontal cortices. As an example, Kearney-Ramos et al. demonstrated that applying continuous theta burst stimulation (cTBS) as a type of TMS to the ventromedial prefrontal cortex could attenuate the cue-related functional connectivity (215). In another study, Ceccanti et al. found out that deep TMS (dTMS) on the medial prefrontal cortex (MPFC) decreased craving and alcohol intake in people with alcohol use disorder. There are also studies targeting motor cortex and temporoparietal areas which have shown that tDCS reduces behavior in tobacco users. To conclude (as shown in **Figure 1**), the distribution of international resources across all these circuit/process/behavior targets provides interesting explorative results to date. Ignoring these methodological variations could result in positive results in meta-analysis reports. However, considering these methodological details would make it hard to introduce a stimulation protocol with enough evidence for clinical use. There is a critical need in the international NIBS research community to focus on one or two main targets to explore any potentially replicable effects that could determine suitable avenues for clinical application.

Application of other areas of NIBS such as FUS, tNS in addiction medicine is limited to a few case reports. Beyond NIBS, invasive brain stimulation technologies like deep brain stimulation (DBS) are only just emerging as approaches in addiction medicine with only a few case reports or pilot trials in the literature. Consequently, the lack of robust evidence for invasive neuromodulation precludes any judgment regarding its clinical utility.

Challenges for Implementation Into Practice

There are 96 original tES/TMS publications in addiction medicine as of May 1, 2019 mainly reporting positive results with one to over 20 sessions of stimulation (**Figure 2**). Large space of methodological parameters to select from, small sample sizes, and lack of replication across different labs make it difficult to draw firm conclusions regarding its effectiveness. Published tES/TMS evidence for addiction treatment has been generated by labs in 14 countries so far (**Figure 3**). To focus these efforts, there is a need for an international roadmap to harmonize the current activities in the field across the world using methodologically rigorous designs. We hope ISAM-NIG along with other international collaborative networks like International Network of tES/TMS

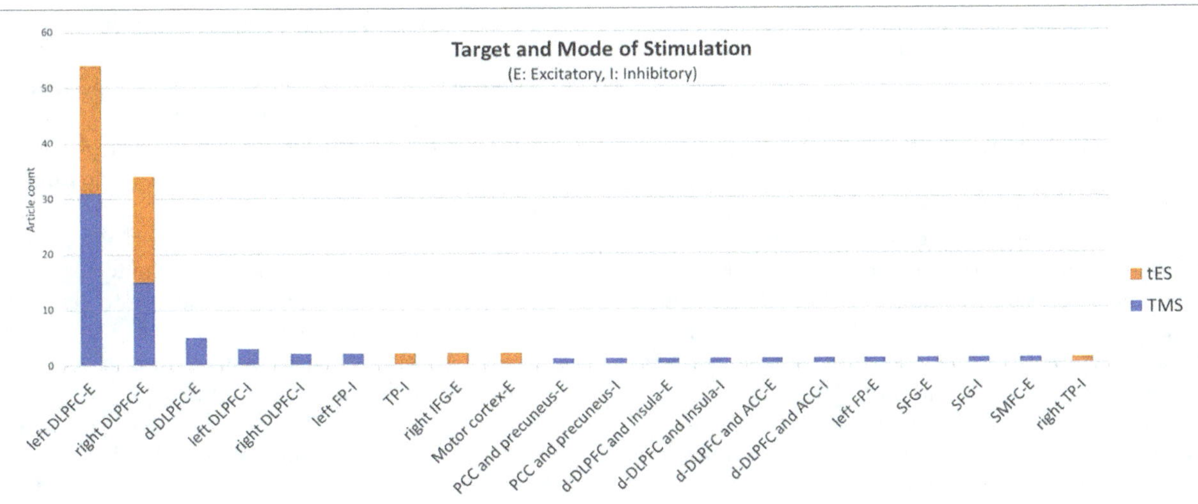

FIGURE 1 | Brain areas targeted with inhibitory (i) and excitatory (e) protocols in 96 tES/TMS studies among people with substance use disorder (as of May 1, 2019) (ACC, anterior cingulate cortex; DLPFC, dorsolateral prefrontal cortex; FP, frontal pole; IFG, inferior frontal gyrus; PCC, posterior cingulate cortex; SFG, superior frontal gyrus; SMFC, superior medial frontal cortex; tES, transcranial electrical stimulation; TMS, transcranial magnetic stimulation; TP, temporoparietal).

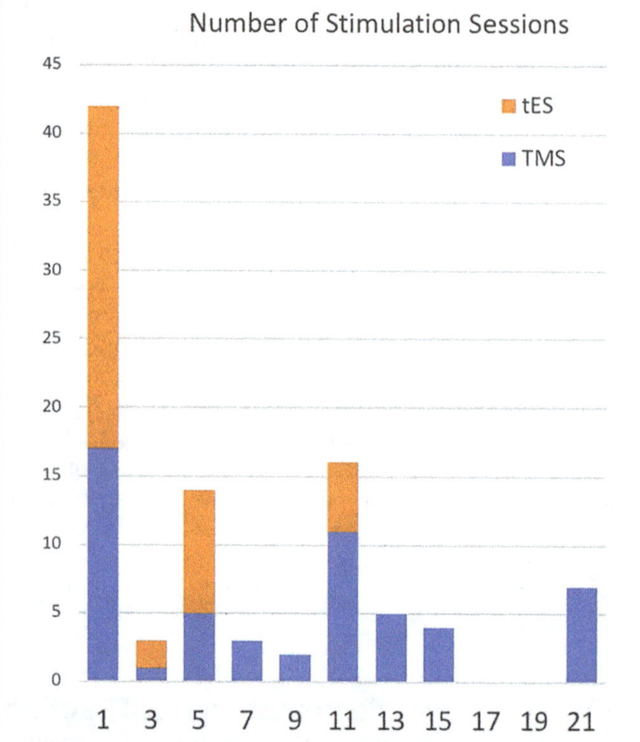

FIGURE 2 | Number of sessions in 96 TMS/tES studies among people with substance use disorder. Around half of the published studies in the field have used just a single session of intervention (as of May 1, 2019). tES, transcranial electrical stimulation; TMS, transcranial magnetic stimulation.

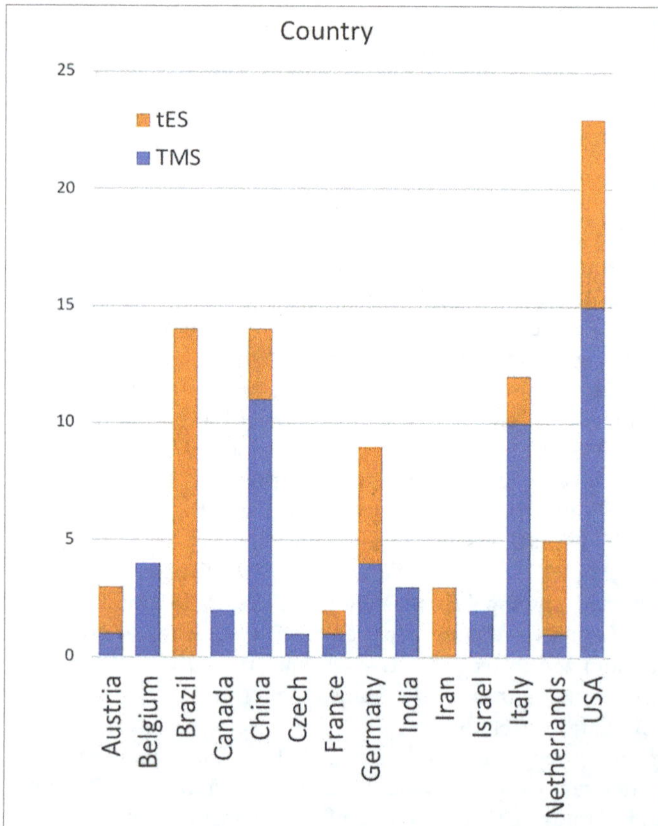

FIGURE 3 | International contribution to the published evidence with tES/TMS in people with substance use disorder. Contribution of 14 different countries (as of May 1, 2019) in the filed confirms the importance of international partnership to improve quality of research in the field. tES, transcranial electrical stimulation; TMS, transcranial magnetic stimulation.

Trials for Addiction Medicine (INTAM) can serve to develop and navigate this roadmap. The ISAM-NIG neuromodulation roadmap should also align with ISAM-NIG roadmaps in other areas like brain imaging, cognitive assessments or cognitive training, and this publication is the first attempt at this initiative. These domains of clinical addiction neuroscience can then work hand-in-hand to create tangible outcomes in daily clinical practice. The challenges for implementing neuromodulation studies into practice are summarized below:

1. *How to move beyond single session interventions:* 44% of the tES/TMS studies have recruited a single session of intervention to investigate potential effects to then move forward to multiple session studies (**Figure 2**). By comparison, most of the medications, we use in daily clinical practice in psychiatry today probably do not show significant effects with a single dose. Even adding a sensitive biomarker like a human brain mapping measure using fMRI will not be sufficient for a "no-go" or "fast-fail" decision. In a recent trial with NIMH fast-fail framework, 8 weeks of medication was being considered as the minimum dosage of intervention (216). Meanwhile, running multi-session trials is costly and decisions between the wide range of available parameters to apply and measure are complex.
2. *How to narrow down key brain targets and relevant SUD-relevant cognitive processes/behaviors:* There is a wide range of potential targets for neuromodulation. There is not a consensus on a framework that specifically defines (i) key neuromodulation targets, (ii) their relevant substance use, cognitive, and clinical outcomes, as different brain pathways are ascribed to heterogeneous neurobehavioral processes (**Table 1**), (iii) measurement instruments of desired outcomes with highest psychometric properties.
3. *How to find the best target population/timing for intervention/contextual treatment:* Timing of neuromodulation intervention [before treatment, before initiating abstinence, during early abstinence (detoxification), after early abstinence (maintenance)] and contextual treatment (pharmacotherapies, psychosocial interventions, cue exposure, cognitive remediation, etc.) in parallel to neuromodulation are important areas for future explorations with specific considerations in different SUDs.
4. *How to optimize the large parameter space within each NIBS technology at the individual level:* There is a new effort to optimize the stimulation parameter for each individual subject based on their subjective responses or objective biomarkers in closed-loop stimulation. Bayesian optimization protocols have introduced an interesting area with initial positive response

with transcranial alternating current (tACS) stimulation (217). Additionally, personalized brain treatment targets can be identified using neurofeedback machine learning approaches that discriminate distinct patterns of brain function within each individual, instead of *a priori* brain regions (or their connectivity) across various individuals (218).

Neurofeedback Studies in SUD

Real-time neurofeedback allows online voluntary regulation of brain activity and has shown promise to enhance ascribed cognitive processes in health and psychopathology (219–221). Participants can monitor their brain function in real time through a brain computer interface (BCI), typically showing a thermometer representing the "temperature" of which increases/decreases in real time, to reflect changes in the level of brain function. Neurofeedback aids participants to voluntarily change brain function online using distinct cognitive strategies (e.g., focus on and away from drug-related stimuli). Neurofeedback has been most consistently tested in ADHD and other psychopathologies, with very early evidence being available in SUD.

Neurofeedback is a promising tool that enables mapping of the causal mechanisms of SUD. As core brain dysfunction is identified within a SUD, neurofeedback can be used as a personalized intervention to enhance and recover underlying dysfunctional neurocognitive pathways. Neurofeedback can source and target brain activity using distinct brain imaging techniques including EEG and fMRI (222).

EEG-based neurofeedback allows individuals to modulate the intensity of brain oscillations at specific frequencies (e.g., alpha, beta, theta, alpha-theta, theta-alpha). These protocols have often been used in conjunction with sensorimotor rhythm training (223) to improve efficacy in SUD. EEG-based neurofeedback studies have targeted brain function in varying SUD groups including alcohol, opioid, and stimulant use disorders [see detailed review here (224)]. This body of work led to mixed evidence of effects (and lack of) on abstinence in the week and months following neurofeedback training, as well as reduced disinhibition, craving, and severity of dependence symptoms. A paucity of studies has shown that these effects were stronger when EEG neurofeedback was used in conjunction with existing standard psychological, pharmacological, and rehabilitation treatments.

Real-time fMRI (rtfMRI)-based neurofeedback has the potential to provide insight in understanding the mechanisms of SUD underpinned by deep brain nuclei [e.g., striatum, amygdala (80)] the activity of which is unlikely to be robustly measured *via* surface EEG. Feedback can be provided on the level of activity of single or multiple *a priori* regions of interest, the strength of the connectivity between multiple regions, and patterns of brain activity identified with machine learning methods (e.g., support vector machine) (218). A handful of studies have used rtfMRI neurofeedback in SUD [for a review, see (12)]. This body of work focused largely on nicotine (225–230) and alcohol use disorders (231, 232).

Most of these studies focused on *a priori* brain regions of interest, most commonly the anterior cingulate cortex, medial prefrontal cortex, and other regions—as well as brain connectivity—were used as source for feedback from single studies (OFC, dorsomedial and dorsolateral prefrontal regions, insula and ventral striatum). Several neurofeedback studies required participants to modulate brain function during craving tasks (e.g., largely cue reactivity tasks that entail watching drug-related pictures). This body of work shows that patients could modulate brain function in the target regions, and provides mixed evidence on the presence and absence (226, 227, 229) of associations between changes in brain activity/connectivity and the severity of drug craving.

In EEG and rtfMRI neurofeedback studies, the significant lack of active placebo controlled and well-powered studies (e.g., comparison with a group with sham feedback) warrants the conduct of more systematic work to determine the efficacy of rEEG and rtfMRI-based neurofeedback.

ISAM NIG Recommendations for Neuromodulation

As discussed above, there is a growing hope that neuromodulation can play a role in the daily practice of addiction medicine. However, the lack of rigorous designs does not provide strong enough evidence to give a green light for clinical use. With frequent negative trials for new pharmacological interventions in addiction medicine, governmental agencies across the world are seriously looking for new hopes for any intervention that can bring positive results in well-powered double-blinded sham/active controlled randomized trials. As the authors of this ISAM-NIG roadmap, we give the following recommendations for future work:

1. Creating international platforms that facilitate consensus on key targets for neuromodulation and outcome measures of efficacy: Addiction neuroscience suffers from the lack of international collaborations based on shared matrix of multilayer targets and outcome measures. We hope that ISAM NIG can bring together a critical mass of expert multidisciplinary scientists across the world to contribute in development of this international consensus.
2. Setting an agreed-upon minimum international standards to produce high quality evidence on the efficacy of neuromodulation in SUD: An overview on the scientific rigor in the published trials on tES/TMS for addiction medicine shows many methodological gaps (233). New potential solutions to address this may include shared protocols across labs internationally with leadership of expert scientists in the field, the development of quality control checklists and Delphi initiatives to reach a consensus on minimum standards.
3. Increase the power of neuromodulation experiments: Over 80% of tES/TMS/NFB studies reported 30 or less subjects in each of their arms. Sample sizes can be boosted using multi-site studies with shared protocols with or without shared funding and replication of previous and ongoing studies and trials across distinct laboratories. Larger samples will be instrumental to (i) increase the power to detect existing effects (or lack of), (ii) increase external validity (while accounting for inter-individual variability), (iii) make predictive modeling for responders and non-responders possible.

4. We also need to have studies with multi-session interventions and long term follow-up to examine the efficacy in tES/TMS/NF over time, particularly if it increases prolonged abstinence.
5. Strategize research efforts to focus available resources to examine the clinical feasibility/efficacy of neuromodulation: Huge parameter space in almost all areas of neuromodulation prevent providing high quality evidence necessary to inform clinical practice. Pharmaceutical companies are one of the main drivers of drug developments. There is no big company in the field of non-invasive neuromodulation and few new ones for TMS are still considered as "small businesses" (less than 250 employees). Efforts that pool sources of research support, e.g., targeted governmental funds and/or "crowd sourcing"-type collective international efforts may support the development and testing of harmonized neuromodulation protocols/target sites for intervention, in order to provide high quality, well-powered evidence.

CONCLUSIONS

We reason that incorporating cognitive assessment into clinical practice in addiction treatment requires identification of constructs that predict meaningful clinical outcomes, streamlining of measures for clinical usability while improving retest reliability and ecological validity, and application of technology for remote monitoring and scalability. Translation of neuroimaging measures to clinically meaningful treatment outcomes requires developing imaging biomarkers that have mechanistic, diagnostic, and prognostic value. It also requires testing the cost-effectiveness of introducing brief, targeted brain scans, and deriving quantitative predictors of successful treatment outcome. Application of cognitive training/remediation and neuromodulation requires additional evidence from randomized trials and clear pathways to implementation. These translation efforts need to address all substance-related disorders. To date, most neuroscience studies have focused on alcohol, nicotine, cannabis, and stimulants, whereas opioids have been underrepresented. The promise of translational neuroscience will only be fulfilled if we can provide novel and effective solutions to pervasive addiction problems, for example, the current opioid crisis. Translation efforts should also factor in the heterogeneity of SUD populations in terms of principal drug of choice, patterns of polysubstance use and psychiatric comorbidities. In this regard, assessment and intervention protocols need to advance towards personalized approaches, by capitalizing on advanced machine learning applications.

Cognitive assessments and neuroimaging methods can elucidate mechanistic multi-level targets (biomarkers) with neural/cognitive/behavioral levels for neuroscience-informed individualized interventions (**Figure 4**). Neuromodulation and cognitive training interventions along with neuropharmacological agents could form multilevel adjunctive interventions based on these targets. The effects of these multilevel interventions in

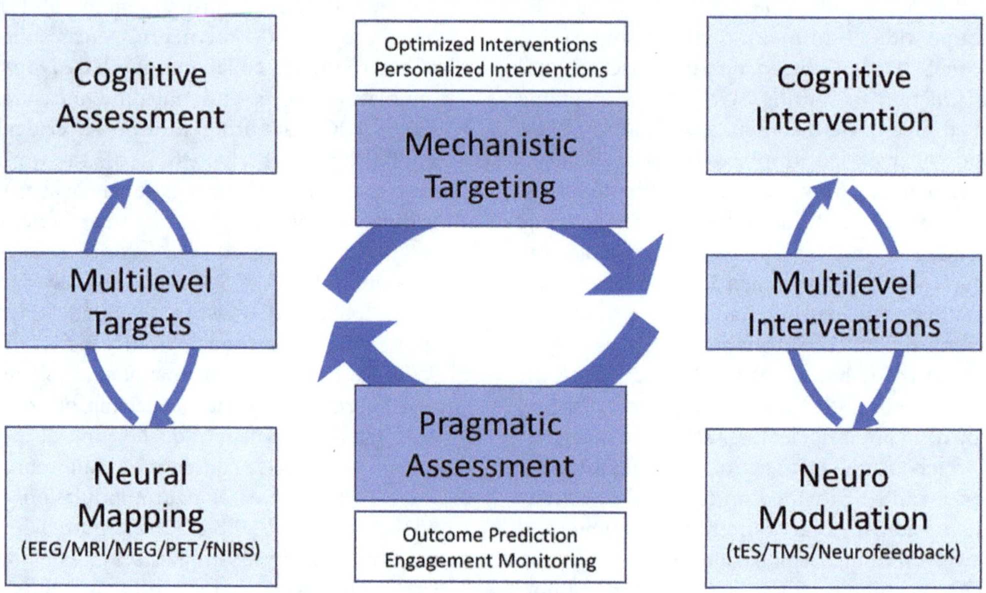

FIGURE 4 | Neuroscience-informed addiction medicine in closed-loops. Cognitive assessments and different neural mapping technologies will introduce mechanistic targets (biomarkers) with neural/cognitive/behavioral levels for a combination of neuromodulation and cognitive interventions. Effects of interventions in successfully modifying these targets (biomarkers) are assessed with cognitive and neural mapping measures. Predictive models for treatment efficacy are optimized with Bayesian algorithms based on the pragmatic multilevel assessments. Interventions can be optimized in closed-loops to engage targets and consider personalized variations toward precision addiction medicine. Psychopharmacological interventions are not included in this roadmap paper; however, they could be delivered alongside and potentially augment cognitive training and neuromodulation.

successfully targeting these mechanisms (biomarkers) should be assessed using cognitive and neural mapping measures. There remain many challenges to implementing neuroscience-informed addiction treatments. We propose to address these challenges by promoting international collaboration between researchers, clinicians, and industry, developing harmonized protocols and data collection/sharing platforms, and prioritizing research that focuses on improving clinical outcomes in SUD.

AUTHOR CONTRIBUTIONS

All authors have contributed in design and preparation of the manuscript. RH, RB, AV-G, VL, VM, DP, and HE created the first draft of assessment, imaging, training, and neuromodulation sections, respectively. AV-G and HE integrated all feedbacks from authors. All authors have agreed on the final manuscript before submission.

REFERENCES

1. Dominguez-Salas S, Diaz-Batanero C, Lozano-Rojas OM, Verdejo-Garcia A. Impact of general cognition and executive function deficits on addiction treatment outcomes: Systematic review and discussion of neurocognitive pathways. *Neurosci Biobehav Rev* (2016) 71:772–801. doi: 10.1016/j.neubiorev.2016.09.030
2. Ekhtiari H, Victor TA, Paulus MP. Aberrant decision-making and drug addiction — how strong is the evidence? *Curr Opin In Behav Sci* (2017) 13:25–33. doi: 10.1016/j.cobeha.2016.09.002
3. Zilverstand A, Huang AS, Alia-Klein N, Goldstein RZ. Neuroimaging impaired response inhibition and salience attribution in human drug addiction: a systematic review. *Neuron* (2018) 98(5):886–903. doi: 10.1016/j.neuron.2018.03.048
4. Passetti F, Verdejo-García A, Checinski K, Robbins TW. Bridging the gap between neurocognitive models and treatment in alcohol, opiates and stimulants addiction. *Front Psychiatry* (2014).
5. Fernandez-Serrano MJ, Perez-Garcia M, Verdejo-Garcia A. What are the specific vs. generalized effects of drugs of abuse on neuropsychological performance? *Neurosci Biobehav Rev* (2011) 35(3):377–406. doi: 10.1016/j.neubiorev.2010.04.008
6. Potvin S, Pelletier J, Grot S, Hebert C, Barr AM, Lecomte T. Cognitive deficits in individuals with methamphetamine use disorder: A meta-analysis. *Addict Behav* (2018) 80:154–60. doi: 10.1016/j.addbeh.2018.01.021
7. Potvin S, Stavro K, Rizkallah E, Pelletier J. Cocaine and cognition: a systematic quantitative review. *J Addict Med* (2014) 8(5):368–76. doi: 10.1097/ADM.0000000000000066
8. Rolland B, D'Hondt F, Montegue S, Brion M, Peyron E, D'Aviau de Ternay J, et al. A patient-tailored evidence-based approach for developing early neuropsychological training programs in addiction settings. *Neuropsychol Rev* (2019) 29(1):103–15. doi: 10.1007/s11065-018-9395-3
9. Stavro K, Pelletier J, Potvin S. Widespread and sustained cognitive deficits in alcoholism: a meta-analysis. *Addict Biol* (2013) 18(2):203–13. doi: 10.1111/j.1369-1600.2011.00418.x
10. Verdejo-Garcia A. Neuroclinical assessment of addiction needs to incorporate decision-making measures and ecological validity. *Biol Psychiatry* (2017) 81(7):e53–4. doi: 10.1016/j.biopsych.2016.07.015
11. Kwako LE, Momenan R, Litten RZ, Koob GF, Goldman D. Addictions neuroclinical assessment: a neuroscience-based framework for addictive disorders. *Biol Psychiatry* (2016) 80(3):179–89. doi: 10.1016/j.biopsych.2015.10.024
12. Luigjes J, Lorenzetti V, de Haan S, Youssef GJ, Murawski C, Sjoerds Z, et al. Defining compulsive behavior. *Neuropsychol Rev* (2019) 29(1):4–13. doi: 10.1007/s11065-019-09404-9
13. Yucel M, Oldenhof E, Ahmed SH, Belin D, Billieux J, Bowden-Jones H, et al. A transdiagnostic dimensional approach towards a neuropsychological assessment for addiction: an international Delphi consensus study. *Addiction* (2019) 114(6):1095–109. doi: 10.1111/add.14424
14. Bates ME, Buckman JF, Nguyen TT. A role for cognitive rehabilitation in increasing the effectiveness of treatment for alcohol use disorders. *Neuropsychol Rev* (2013) 23(1):27–47. doi: 10.1007/s11065-013-9228-3
15. Schmidt P, Haberthur A, Soyka M. Cognitive functioning in formerly opioid-dependent adults after atleast 1 year of abstinence: a naturalistic study. *Eur Addict Res* (2017) 23(6):269–75. doi: 10.1159/000485032
16. Vonmoos M, Hulka LM, Preller KH, Minder F, Baumgartner MR, Quednow BB. Cognitive impairment in cocaine users is drug-induced but partially reversible: evidence from a longitudinal study. *Neuropsychopharmacology* (2014) 39(9):2200–10. doi: 10.1038/npp.2014.71
17. Rubenis AJ, Fitzpatrick RE, Lubman DI, Verdejo-Garcia A. Working memory predicts methamphetamine hair concentration over the course of treatment: moderating effect of impulsivity and implications for dual-systems model. *Addict Biol* (2019) 24(1):145–53. doi: 10.1111/adb.12575
18. Stevens L, Verdejo-Garcia A, Goudriaan AE, Roeyers H, Dom G, Vanderplasschen W. Impulsivity as a vulnerability factor for poor addiction treatment outcomes: a review of neurocognitive findings among individuals with substance use disorders. *J Subst Abuse Treat* (2014) 47(1):58–72. doi: 10.1016/j.jsat.2014.01.008
19. Rubenis AJ, Fitzpatrick RE, Lubman DI, Verdejo-Garcia A. Impulsivity predicts poorer improvement in quality of life during early treatment for people with methamphetamine dependence. *Addiction* (2018) 113(4):668–76. doi: 10.1111/add.14058
20. Tiffany ST, Friedman L, Greenfield SF, Hasin DS, Jackson R. Beyond drug use: a systematic consideration of other outcomes in evaluations of treatments for substance use disorders. *Addiction* (2012) 107(4):709–18. doi: 10.1111/j.1360-0443.2011.03581.x
21. Roche A, Pidd K. *Alcohol & Other Drugs Workforce Development Issues and Imperatives: Setting the Scene*. Adelaide, National Centre for Education and Training on Addiction (NCETA), Flinders University (2010).
22. ACT, A. T. O. D. A. (2016). Strengthening Specialist Alcohol and Other Drug Treatment and Support: Needsand Prioritiesforthe ACT 2016–2017. *A. T. O. D. A. ACT. Canberra, Alcohol Tobacco and Other Drug Association ACT.*
23. Health Q. Mental health alcohol and other drugs workforce development framework. *Queensland State Queensland* (Queensland Health) (2017).
24. Roche A, Kostadinov V, Hodge S, Duralsingham V, McEntee A, Pidd K, et al. *Characteristics and wellbeing of the NSW non-government AOD Workforce.* Adelaide, National Centre for Education and Training on Addiction, Flinders University (2018).
25. Nelson A. *The SAGE Handbook of Drug and Alcohol Studies.* SAGE Publications Ltd.: 55 City Road, London (2016). Retrieved from http://sk.sagepub.com/reference/the-sage-handbook-of-drug-alcohol-studies-v1. doi: 10.4135/9781473921986
26. Boustani M, Peterson B, Hanson L, Harris R, Lohr KN, Force U. S. P. S. T. Screening for dementia in primary care: a summary of the evidence for the U.S. Preventive Services Task Force. *Ann Intern Med* (2003) 138(11):927–37. doi: 10.7326/0003-4819-138-11-200306030-00015
27. Milne A, Culverwell A, Guss R, Tuppen J, Whelton R. Screening for dementia in primary care: a review of the use, efficacy and quality of measures. *Int Psychogeriatr* (2008) 20(5):911–26. doi: 10.1017/S1041610208007394
28. Nuechterlein KH, Green MF, Kern RS, Baade LE, Barch DM, Cohen JD, et al. The MATRICS Consensus Cognitive Battery, part 1: test selection, reliability, and validity. *Am J Psychiatry* (2008) 165(2):203–13. doi: 10.1176/appi.ajp.2007.07010042
29. Alarcon R, Nalpas B, Pelletier S, Perney P. MoCA as a Screening tool of neuropsychological deficits in alcohol-dependent patients. *Alcohol Clin Exp Res* (2015) 39(6):1042–8. doi: 10.1111/acer.12734
30. Copersino ML, Fals-Stewart W, Fitzmaurice G, Schretlen DJ, Sokoloff J, Weiss RD. Rapid cognitive screening of patients with substance use disorders. *Exp Clin Psychopharmacol* (2009) 17(5):337–44. doi: 10.1037/a0017260
31. Copersino ML, Schretlen DJ, Fitzmaurice GM, Lukas SE, Faberman J, Sokoloff J, et al. Effects of cognitive impairment on substance abuse treatment attendance: predictive validation of a brief cognitive screening measure. *Am J Drug Alcohol Abuse* (2012) 38(3):246–50. doi: 10.3109/00952990.2012.670866

32. Manning V, Staiger PK, Hall K, Garfield JB, Flaks G, Leung D, et al. Cognitive bias modification training during inpatient alcohol detoxification reduces early relapse: a randomized controlled trial. *Alcohol Clin Exp Res* (2016) 40(9):2011–9. doi: 10.1111/acer.13163
33. Manning V, Wanigaratne S, Best D, Strathdee G, Schrover I, Gossop M. Screening for cognitive functioning in psychiatric outpatients with schizophrenia, alcohol dependence, and dual diagnosis. *Schizophr Res* (2007) 91(1-3):151–8. doi: 10.1016/j.schres.2006.11.019
34. Ridley N, Batchelor J, Draper B, Demirkol A, Lintzeris N, Withall A. Cognitive screening in substance users: diagnostic accuracies of the mini-mental state examination, addenbrooke's cognitive examination-revised, and montreal cognitive assessment. *J Clin Exp Neuropsychol* (2018) 40(2):107–22. doi: 10.1080/13803395.2017.1316970
35. Folstein MF, Folstein SE, McHugh PR. "Mini-mental state". a practical method for grading the cognitive state of patients for the clinician. *J Psychiatr Res* (1975) 12(3):189–98. doi: 10.1016/0022-3956(75)90026-6
36. Mioshi E, Dawson K, Mitchell J, Arnold R, Hodges JR. The Addenbrooke's Cognitive Examination Revised (ACE-R): a brief cognitive test battery for dementia screening. *Int J Geriatr Psychiatry* (2006) 21(11):1078–85. doi: 10.1002/gps.1610
37. Nasreddine ZS, Phillips NA, Bedirian V, Charbonneau S, Whitehead V, Collin I, et al. The montreal cognitive assessment, MoCA: a brief screening tool for mild cognitive impairment. *J Am Geriatr Soc* (2005) 53(4):695–9. doi: 10.1111/j.1532-5415.2005.53221.x
38. Manning V, Teo HC, Guo S, Wong KE, Li TK. Neurocognitive functioning and treatment outcome following detoxification among asian alcohol-dependent inpatients. *Subst Use Misuse* (2016) 51(2):193–205. doi: 10.3109/10826084.2015.1092985
39. Kern RS, Green MF, Nuechterlein KH, Deng BH. NIMH-MATRICS survey on assessment of neurocognition in schizophrenia. *Schizophr Res* (2004) 72(1):11–9. doi: 10.1016/j.schres.2004.09.004
40. Kern RS, Nuechterlein KH, Green MF, Baade LE, Fenton WS, Gold JM, et al. The MATRICS consensus cognitive battery, part 2: co-norming and standardization. *Am J Psychiatry* (2008) 165(2):214–20. doi: 10.1176/appi.ajp.2007.07010043
41. Conway KP, Vullo GC, Kennedy AP, Finger MS, Agrawal A, Bjork JM, et al. Data compatibility in the addiction sciences: an examination of measure commonality. *Drug Alcohol Depend* (2014) 141:153–8. doi: 10.1016/j.drugalcdep.2014.04.029
42. Robbins TW, James M, Owen AM, Sahakian BJ, Lawrence AD, McInnes L, et al. A study of performance on tests from the CANTAB battery sensitive to frontal lobe dysfunction in a large sample of normal volunteers: implications for theories of executive functioning and cognitive aging. Cambridge Neuropsychological Test Automated Battery. *J Int Neuropsychol Soc* (1998) 4(5):474–90. doi: 10.1017/s1355617798455073
43. Randolph C, Tierney MC, Mohr E, Chase TN. The Repeatable Battery for the Assessment of Neuropsychological Status (RBANS): preliminary clinical validity. *J Clin Exp Neuropsychol* (1998) 20(3):310–9. doi: 10.1076/jcen.20.3.310.823
44. Stern RA, White T. *NAB, Neuropsychological Assessment Battery: Administration, scoring, and interpretation manual.* Psychological Assessment Resources Lutz (FL) (2003).
45. Powell D, Kaplan E, Whitla D, Weinstraub S, Catlin R, Funkenstein H. MicroCog Assessment of cognitive functioning, windows® edition (MicroCog™ for Windows®) San Antonio, TX. *Psychol Corporation* (2004).
46. Cannizzaro DL, Elliott JC, Stohl M, Hasin DS, Aharonovich E. Neuropsychological Assessment Battery-Screening Module (S-NAB): performance in treatment-seeking cocaine users. *Am J Drug Alcohol Abuse* (2014) 40(6):476–83. doi: 10.3109/00952990.2014.916718
47. Latvala A, Castaneda AE, Perala J, Saarni SI, Aalto-Setala T, Lonnqvist J, et al. Cognitive functioning in substance abuse and dependence: a population-based study of young adults. *Addiction* (2009) 104(9):1558–68. doi: 10.1111/j.1360-0443.2009.02656.x
48. Schrimsher GW, Parker JD. Changes in cognitive function during substance use disorder treatment. *J Psychopathol Behav Assess* (2008) 30(2):146–53. doi: 10.1007/s10862-007-9054-0
49. Bauer RM, Iverson GL, Cernich AN, Binder LM, Ruff RM, Naugle RI. Computerized neuropsychological assessment devices: joint position paper of the American Academy of Clinical Neuropsychology and the National Academy of Neuropsychology. *Arch Clin Neuropsychol* (2012) 27(3):362–73. doi: 10.1093/arclin/acs027
50. Cole WR, Arrieux JP, Schwab K, Ivins BJ, Qashu FM, Lewis SC. Test-retest reliability of four computerized neurocognitive assessment tools in an active duty military population. *Arch Clin Neuropsychol* (2013) 28(7):732–42. doi: 10.1093/arclin/act040
51. Fratti S, Bowden SC, Cook MJ. Reliability and validity of the CogState computerized battery in patients with seizure disorders and healthy young adults: comparison with standard neuropsychological tests. *Clin Neuropsychol* (2017) 31(3):569–86. doi: 10.1080/13854046.2016.1256435
52. Nelson LD, LaRoche AA, Pfaller AY, Lerner EB, Hammeke TA, Randolph C, et al. Prospective, head-to-head study of three computerized Neurocognitive Assessment Tools (CNTs): reliability and validity for the assessment of sport-related concussion. *J Int Neuropsychol Soc* (2016) 22(1):24–37. doi: 10.1017/S1355617715001101
53. Resch JE, Schneider MW, Munro Cullum C. The test-retest reliability of three computerized neurocognitive tests used in the assessment of sport concussion. *Int J Psychophysiol* (2018) 132(Pt A):31–8. doi: 10.1016/j.ijpsycho.2017.09.011
54. Enkavi AZ, Eisenberg IW, Bissett PG, Mazza GL, MacKinnon DP, Marsch LA, et al. Large-scale analysis of test-retest reliabilities of self-regulation measures. *Proc Natl Acad Sci U.S.A.* (2019) 116(12):5472–7. doi: 10.1073/pnas.1818430116
55. Bouvard A, Dupuy M, Schweitzer P, Revranche M, Fatseas M, Serre F, et al. Feasibility and validity of mobile cognitive testing in patients with substance use disorders and healthy controls. *Am J Addict* (2018) 27(7):553–6. doi: 10.1111/ajad.12804
56. Moore RC, Swendsen J, Depp CA. Applications for self-administered mobile cognitive assessments in clinical research: a systematic review. *Int J Methods Psychiatr Res* (2017) 26(4):e1562. doi: 10.1002/mpr.1562
57. Sliwinski MJ, Mogle JA, Hyun J, Munoz E, Smyth JM, Lipton RB. Reliability and validity of ambulatory cognitive assessments. *Assessment* (2018) 25(1):14–30. doi: 10.1177/1073191116643164
58. Jones A, McGrath E, Robinson E, Houben K, Nederkoorn C, Field M. A randomized controlled trial of inhibitory control training for the reduction of alcohol consumption in problem drinkers. *J Consult Clin Psychol* (2018) 86(12):991–1004. doi: 10.1037/ccp0000312
59. Crane D, Garnett C, Michie S, West R, Brown J. A smartphone app to reduce excessive alcohol consumption: Identifying the effectiveness of intervention components in a factorial randomised control trial. *Sci Rep* (2018) 8(1):4384. doi: 10.1038/s41598-018-22420-8
60. Jones A, Tiplady B, Houben K, Nederkoorn C, Field M. Do daily fluctuations in inhibitory control predict alcohol consumption? An ecological momentary assessment study. *Psychopharmacol (Berl)* (2018) 235(5):1487–96. doi: 10.1007/s00213-018-4860-5
61. Wiers CE, Ludwig VU, Gladwin TE, Park SQ, Heinz A, Wiers RW, et al. Effects of cognitive bias modification training on neural signatures of alcohol approach tendencies in male alcohol-dependent patients. *Addict Biol* (2015) 20(5):990–9. doi: 10.1111/adb.12221
62. Eisenberg IW, Bissett P, Enkavi AZ, Li J, MacKinnon D, Marsch L, et al. Uncovering mental structure through data-driven ontology discovery. *PsyArXiv* (2018). doi: 10.31234/osf.io/fvqej
63. Jones A, Remmerswaal D, Verveer I, Robinson E, Franken IHA, Wen CKF, et al. Compliance with ecological momentary assessment protocols in substance users: a meta-analysis. *Addiction* (2019) 114(4):609–19. doi: 10.1111/add.14503
64. Bos FM, Schoevers RA, aan het Rot M. Experience sampling and ecological momentary assessment studies in psychopharmacology: a systematic review. *Eur Neuropsychopharmacol* (2015) 25(11):1853–64. doi: 10.1016/j.euroneuro.2015.08.008
65. Ramsey AT, Wetherell JL, Depp C, Dixon D, Lenze E. Feasibility and acceptability of smartphone assessment in older adults with cognitive and emotional difficulties. *J Technol Hum Serv* (2016) 34(2):209–23. doi: 10.1080/15228835.2016.1170649
66. Bickel WK, Mellis AM, Snider SE, Athamneh LN, Stein JS, Pope DA. 21st century neurobehavioral theories of decision making in addiction: review and evaluation. *Pharmacol Biochem Behav* (2018) 164:4–21. doi: 10.1016/j.pbb.2017.09.009
67. Bates ME, Bowden SC, Barry D. Neurocognitive impairment associated with alcohol use disorders: implications for treatment. *Exp Clin Psychopharmacol* (2002) 10(3):193–212. doi: 10.1037//1064-1297.10.3.193

68. Bates ME, Buckman JF, Voelbel GT, Eddie D, Freeman J. The mean and the individual: integrating variable-centered and person-centered analyses of cognitive recovery in patients with substance use disorders. *Front Psychiatry* (2013) 4:177. doi: 10.3389/fpsyt.2013.00177
69. Buelow MT, Suhr JA. Construct validity of the Iowa Gambling Task. *Neuropsychol Rev* (2009) 19(1):102–14. doi: 10.1007/s11065-009-9083-4
70. Field M, Munafò MR, Franken IH. A meta-analytic investigation of the relationship between attentional bias and subjective craving in substance abuse. *J Psychol Bull* (2009) 135(4):589. doi: 10.1037/a0015843
71. Grüsser SM, Wrase J, Klein S, Hermann D, Smolka MN, Ruf M, et al. Cue-induced activation of the striatum and medial prefrontal cortex is associated with subsequent relapse in abstinent alcoholics. *Psychopharmacology* (2004) 175(3):296–302.
72. Kosten T, Scanley B, Tucker K, Oliveto A, Prince C, Sinha R, et al. Cue-induced brain activity changes and relapse in cocaine-dependent patients. *Neuropsychopharmacology* (2006) 31:644–50. doi: 10.1038/sj.npp.1300851
73. Huettel SA, Song AW, McCarthy G. What is fMRI? In: *Functional magnetic research imaging*, 2nd ed., vol. 2. Sinauer: Sunderland, Massachusetts, USA (2009). p. 3–14.
74. Leroy C, Karila L, Martinot JL, Lukasiewicz M, Duchesnay E, Comtat C, et al. Striatal and extrastriatal dopamine transporter in cannabis and tobacco addiction: a high-resolution PET study. *Addict Biol* (2012) 17(6):981–90. doi: 10.1111/j.1369-1600.2011.00356.x
75. Volkow ND, Ding YS, Fowler JS, Wang GJ. Cocaine addiction: hypothesis derived from imaging studies with PET. *J Addict Dis* (1996) 15(4):55–71. doi: 10.1300/J069v15n04_04
76. Williams TM, Davies SJ, Taylor LG, Daglish MR, Hammers A, Brooks DJ, et al. Brain opioid receptor binding in early abstinence from alcohol dependence and relationship to craving: an [11C]diprenorphine PET study. *Eur Neuropsychopharmacol* (2009) 19(10):740–8. doi: 10.1016/j.euroneuro.2009.06.007
77. Yoder KK, Constantinescu CC, Kareken DA, Normandin MD, Cheng TE, O'Connor SJ, et al. Heterogeneous effects of alcohol on dopamine release in the striatum: a pet study. *Alcohol Clin Exp Res* (2007) 31(6):965–73. doi: 10.1111/j.1530-0277.2007.00390.x
78. Yeung AWK. An updated survey on statistical thresholding and sample size of fMRI studies. *Front Hum Neurosci* (2018) 12:16. doi: 10.3389/fnhum.2018.00016 eCollection 2018.
79. Nichols TE, Das S, Eickhoff SB, Evans AC, Glatard T, Hanke M, et al. Best practices in data analysis and sharing in neuroimaging using MRI. *Nat Neurosci* (2017) 20(3):299–303. doi: 10.1038/nn.4500
80. Koob GF, Volkow ND. Neurobiology of addiction: a neurocircuitry analysis. *Lancet Psychiatry* (2016) 3(8):760–73. doi: 10.1016/S2215-0366(16)00104-8
81. Lewis M. Brain change in addiction as learning, not disease. *New Engl J Med* (2018) 379(16):1551–60. doi: 10.1056/NEJMra1602872
82. Morris SE, Cuthbert BN. Research Domain Criteria: cognitive systems, neural circuits, and dimensions of behavior. *Dialogues Clin Neurosci* (2012) 14(1):29–37.
83. Paulus MP, Stewart JL. Interoception and drug addiction. *Neuropharmacology* (2014) 76 Pt B:342–50. doi: 10.1016/j.neuropharm.2013.07.002
84. Volkow ND, Fowler JS, Wang GJ. The addicted human brain viewed in the light of imaging studies: brain circuits and treatment strategies. *Neuropharmacology* (2004) 47 Suppl 1:3–13. doi: 10.1016/j.neuropharm.2004.07.019
85. Yücel M, Oldenhof E, Ahmed SH, Belin D, Billieux J, Bowden-Jones H, et al. A transdiagnostic dimensional approach towards a neuropsychological assessment for addiction: an international Delphi consensus study. (2019). 114(6):1095–1109.
86. Verdejo-Garcia A, Clark L, Dunn BD. The role of interoception in addiction: a critical review. *Neurosci Biobehav Rev* (2012) 36(8):1857–69. doi: 10.1016/j.neubiorev.2012.05.007
87. Oldham S, Murawski C, Fornito A, Youssef G, Yucel M, Lorenzetti V. The anticipation and outcome phases of reward and loss processing: A neuroimaging meta-analysis of the monetary incentive delay task. *Hum Brain Mapp* (2018) 39(8):3398–418. doi: 10.1002/hbm.24184
88. Liu X, Hairston J, Schrier M, Fan J. Common and distinct networks underlying reward valence and processing stages: a meta-analysis of functional neuroimaging studies. *Neurosci Biobehav Rev* (2011) 35(5):1219–36. doi: 10.1016/j.neubiorev.2010.12.012
89. Engelmann JM, Versace F, Robinson JD, Minnix JA, Lam CY, Cui Y, et al. Neural substrates of smoking cue reactivity: a meta-analysis of fMRI studies. *Neuroimage* (2012) 60(1):252–62. doi: 10.1016/j.neuroimage.2011.12.024
90. Schacht JP, Anton RF, Myrick H. Functional neuroimaging studies of alcohol cue reactivity: a quantitative meta-analysis and systematic review. *Addict Biol* (2013) 18(1):121–33. doi: 10.1111/j.1369-1600.2012.00464.x
91. Lipszyc J, Schachar R. Inhibitory control and psychopathology: a meta-analysis of studies using the stop signal task. *J Int Neuropsychol Soc* (2010) 16(6):1064–76. doi: 10.1017/S1355617710000895
92. Simmonds DJ, Pekar JJ, Mostofsky SH. Meta-analysis of Go/No-go tasks demonstrating that fMRI activation associated with response inhibition is task-dependent. *Neuropsychologia* (2008) 46(1):224–32. doi: 10.1016/j.neuropsychologia.2007.07.015
93. Derrfuss J, Brass M, Neumann J, von Cramon DY. Involvement of the inferior frontal junction in cognitive control: meta-analyses of switching and Stroop studies. *Hum Brain Mapp* (2005) 25(1):22–34. doi: 10.1002/hbm.20127
94. Schulz SM. Neural correlates of heart-focused interoception: a functional magnetic resonance imaging meta-analysis. *Philos Trans R Soc Lond B Biol Sci* (2016) 371(1708):20160018. doi: 10.1098/rstb.2016.0018
95. Stewart J, Khalsa S, Kuplicki R, Paulus M. T206. Interoceptive Dysfunction in Stimulant and Opioid Addiction. *Biol Psychiatry* (2019) 85(10):S210. doi: 10.1016/j.biopsych.2019.03.529
96. Paulus MP, Feinstein JS, Khalsa SS. An active inference approach to interoceptive psychopathology. *Annual Review of Clinical Psychology* (2019) 15(1):97–122. doi: 10.1146/annurev-clinpsy-050718-095617
97. Daughters SB, Ross TJ, Bell RP, Yi JY, Ryan J, Stein EA. Distress tolerance among substance users is associated with functional connectivity between prefrontal regions during a distress tolerance task. *Addict Biol* (2017) 22(5):1378–90.
98. Jennifer YY, Dichter GS, Reese ED, Bell RP, Bartuska AD, Stein JR, et al. Neural reward response to substance-free activity images in opiate use disorder patients with depressive symptoms. *Drug Alcohol Dependence* (2019) 198:180–89.
99. Garavan H, Brennan K, Hester R, Whelan R. The neurobiology of successful abstinence. *Curr Opin In Neurobiol* (2013) 23(4):668–74. doi: 10.1016/j.conb.2013.01.029
100. Sofuoglu M. Cognitive enhancement as a pharmacotherapy target for stimulant addiction. *Addict (Abingdon England)* (2010) 105(1):38–48. doi: 10.1111/j.1360-0443.2009.02791.x
101. Sofuoglu M, DeVito EE, Waters AJ, Carroll KM. Cognitive enhancement as a treatment for drug addictions. *Neuropharmacology* (2013) 64(1):452–63. doi: 10.1016/j.neuropharm.2012.06.021
102. Zilverstand A, Parvaz MA, Moeller SJ, Goldstein RZ. Cognitive interventions for addiction medicine: Understanding the underlying neurobiological mechanisms. *Prog Brain Res* (2016) 224:285–304. doi: 10.1016/bs.pbr.2015.07.019
103. Trabert W, Betz T, Niewald M, Huber G. Significant reversibility of alcoholic brain shrinkage within 3 weeks of abstinence. *Acta Psychiatrica Scand* (1995) 92(2):87–90. doi: 10.1111/j.1600-0447.1995.tb09548.x
104. Hanlon CA, Dufault DL, Wesley MJ, Porrino LJ. Elevated gray and white matter densities in cocaine abstainers compared to current users. *Psychopharmacology* (2011) 218(4):681–92.
105. Kril J, Halliday G, Svoboda M, Cartwright H. The cerebral cortex is damaged in chronic alcoholics. *Neuroscience* (1997) 79(4):983–98.
106. Pfefferbaum A, Sullivan E, Mathalon D, Shear P, Rosenbloom M, Lim KJAC, et al. Longitudinal changes in magnetic resonance imaging brain volumes in abstinent and relapsed alcoholics. *Alcohol Clin Exp Res* (1995) 19:(5):1177–91.
107. Roberts AJ, Koob GF. The neurobiology of addiction. *Alcohol Health Res World* (1997) 21(2):101–6.
108. Stephens DN, Duka T. Cognitive and emotional consequences of binge drinking: role of amygdala and prefrontal cortex. *Philos Trans R Soc B: Biol Sci* (2008) 363(1507):3169–79.
109. Bell RP, Foxe JJ, Nierenberg J, Hoptman MJ, Garavan H. Assessing white matter integrity as a function of abstinence duration in former cocaine-dependent individuals. *Drug Alcohol Depend* (2011) 114(2-3):159–68.
110. Gansler DA, Harris GJ, Oscar-Berman M, Streeter C, Lewis RF, Ahmed I, et al. Hypoperfusion of inferior frontal brain regions in abstinent alcoholics: a pilot SPECT study. *J Stud Alcohol* (2000) 61(1):32–7.

111. Connolly CG, Foxe JJ, Nierenberg J, Shpaner M, Garavan H. The neurobiology of cognitive control in successful cocaine abstinence. *Drug Alcohol Depend* (2012) 121(1-2):45–53.
112. Nestor L, McCabe E, Jones J, Clancy L, Garavan H. Differences in "bottom-up" and "top-down" neural activity in current and former cigarette smokers: evidence for neural substrates which may promote nicotine abstinence through increased cognitive control. *Neuroimage* (2011) 56(4):2258–75.
113. Tapert SF, Schweinsburg AD, Drummond SP, Paulus MP, Brown SA, Yang TT, et al. Functional MRI of inhibitory processing in abstinent adolescent marijuana users. *Psychopharmacology* (2007) 194(2):173–83.
114. Gazdzinski S, Durazzo TC, Meyerhoff DJ. Temporal dynamics and determinants of whole brain tissue volume changes during recovery from alcohol dependence. *Drug Alcohol Depend* (2005) 78(3):263–73.
115. Bolla K, Ernst M, Kiehl K, Mouratidis M, Eldreth D, Contoreggi C, et al. Prefrontal cortical dysfunction in abstinent cocaine abusers. *J Neuropsychiatry Clin Neurosci* (2004) 16(4):456–64.
116. Froeliger B, Kozink RV, Rose JE, Behm FM, Salley AN, McClernon FJ. Hippocampal and striatal gray matter volume are associated with a smoking cessation treatment outcome: results of an exploratory voxel-based morphometric analysis. *Psychopharmacology* (2010) 210(4):577–83.
117. Janes AC, Pizzagalli DA, Richardt S, Chuzi S, Pachas G, Culhane MA, et al. Brain reactivity to smoking cues prior to smoking cessation predicts ability to maintain tobacco abstinence. *Biol Psychiatry* (2010) 67(8):722–9.
118. Rando K, Hong K-I, Bhagwagar Z, Li C-SR, Bergquist K, Guarnaccia J, et al. Association of frontal and posterior cortical gray matter volume with time to alcohol relapse: a prospective study. *Am J Psychiatry* (2011) 168(2):183–92.
119. Sorg SF, Taylor MJ, Alhassoon OM, Gongvatana A, Theilmann RJ, Frank LR, et al. Frontal white matter integrity predictors of adult alcohol treatment outcome. *Biol Psychiatry* (2012) 71(3):262–8.
120. Brewer JA, Worhunsky PD, Carroll KM, Rounsaville BJ, Potenza MN. Pretreatment brain activation during stroop task is associated with outcomes in cocaine-dependent patients. *Biol Psychiatry* (2008) 64(11):998–1004.
121. Clark V, Beatty G, Anderson R, Kodituwakku P, Phillips J, Lane T, et al. Reduced fMRI activity predicts relapse in patients recovering from stimulant dependence. *Hum Brain Mapp* (2014) 35(2):414–28.
122. Heinz A, Wrase J, Kahnt T, Beck A, Bromand Z, Grüsser SM, et al. Brain activation elicited by affectively positive stimuli is associated with a lower risk of relapse in detoxified alcoholic subjects. *Alcohol: Clin Exp Res* (2007) 31(7):1138–47.
123. Jia Z, Worhunsky PD, Carroll KM, Rounsaville BJ, Stevens MC, Pearlson GD, et al. An initial study of neural responses to monetary incentives as related to treatment outcome in cocaine dependence. *Biol Psychiatry* (2011) 70: (6):553–60.
124. Paulus M, Tapert S, Schuckit M. Neural activation patterns of methamphetamine-dependent subjects during decision making predict relapse. *Arch Gen Psychiatry* (2005) 62(7):761–8.
125. Durazzo T, Pathak V, Gazdzinski S, Mon A, Meyerhoff D. Metabolite levels in the brain reward pathway discriminate those who remain abstinent from those who resume hazardous alcohol consumption after treatment for alcohol dependence. *J Stud Alcohol Drugs* (2010) 71(2):278–89.
126. Noel X, Sferrazza R, Van der Linden M, Paternot J, Verhas M, Hanak C, et al. Contribution of frontal cerebral blood flow measured by Tc-99m-bicisate spect and executive function deficits to predicting treatment outcome in alcohol-dependent patients. *Alcohol* (2002) 37(4):347–54.
127. Wang GJ, Smith L, Volkow ND, Telang F, Logan J, Tomasi D, et al. Decreased dopamine activity predicts relapse in methamphetamine abusers. *Mol Psychiatry* (2012) 17(9):918.
128. Verdejo-Garcia A. Cognitive training for substance use disorders: Neuroscientific mechanisms. *Neurosci Biobehav Rev* (2016) 68:270–81. doi: 10.1016/j.neubiorev.2016.05.018
129. Field M, Duka T, Tyler E, Schoenmakers T. Attentional bias modification in tobacco smokers. *J Nicotine Tobacco Res* (2009) 11(7):812–22. doi: 10.1093/ntr/ntp067
130. Wiers CE, Wiers RW. Imaging the neural effects of cognitive bias modification training. *Neuroimage* (2017) 151:81–91. doi: 10.1016/j.neuroimage.2016.07.041
131. Volkow ND, Swanson JM, Evins AE, DeLisi LE, Meier MH, Gonzalez R, et al. Effects of cannabis use on human behavior, including cognition, motivation, and psychosis: a review. *JAMA Psychiatry* (2016) 73(3):292–7. doi: 10.1001/jamapsychiatry.2015.3278
132. Chen AJ, Novakovic-Agopian T, Nycum TJ, Song S, Turner GR, Hills NK, et al. Training of goal-directed attention regulation enhances control over neural processing for individuals with brain injury. *Brain* (2011) 134(Pt 5):1541–54. doi: 10.1093/brain/awr067
133. Garland EL, Howard MO. Mindfulness-based treatment of addiction: current state of the field and envisioning the next wave of research. *Addict Sci Clin Pract* (2018) 13(1):14. doi: 10.1186/s13722-018-0115-3
134. Anicha CL, Ode S, Moeller SK, Robinson M. Toward a cognitive view of trait mindfulness: distinct cognitive skills predict its observing and nonreactivity facets. *J Pers* (2012) 80(2):255–85. doi: 10.1111/j.1467-6494.2011.00722.x
135. Li W, Howard MO, Garland EL, McGovern P, Lazar M. Mindfulness treatment for substance misuse: A systematic review and meta-analysis. *J Subst Abuse Treat* (2017) 75:62–96. doi: 10.1016/j.jsat.2017.01.008
136. Brewer JA, Elwafi HM, Davis JH. Craving to Quit: psychological models and neurobiological mechanisms of mindfulness training as treatment for addictions. *Psychol Addict Behav* (2013) 27(2):366–79. doi: 10.1037/a0028490
137. Froeliger B, Mathew AR, McConnell P, Eichberg C, Saladin M, Carpenter M, et al. Restructuring reward mechanisms in nicotine addiction: a pilot fMRI study of mindfulness-oriented recovery enhancement for cigarette smokers. *J Evidence-Based Complementary Altern Med* (2017).
138. Calhoun V, Adali T. (2006). "*Fusion of Multisubject Hemodynamic and Event-Related Potential Data Using Independent Component Analysis*.," in Paper presented at the 2006 IEEE International Conference on Acoustics Speech and Signal Processing Proceedings. (Vol. 5, pp. V-V). IEEE.
139. Picton TW. *Electrophysiology of Mind: Event-Related Brain Potentials and Cognition*. Vol. 33. Rugg MD, Coles MGH, editors. Oxford University Press: Oxford, England (1996) p. 612–3. 1995. *Psychophysiology*. doi: 10.1111/j.1469-8986.1996.tb02439.x
140. Campanella S, Schroder E, Kajosch H, Noel X, Kornreich C. Why cognitive event-related potentials (ERPs) should have a role in the management of alcohol disorders. *Neurosci Biobehav Rev* (2018). 106:234–244 doi: 10.1016/j.neubiorev.2018.06.016
141. Mackey S, Kan KJ, Chaarani B, Alia-Klein N, Batalla A, Brooks S, et al. Genetic imaging consortium for addiction medicine: From neuroimaging to genes. *Prog Brain Res* (2016) 224:203–23. doi: 10.1016/bs.pbr.2015.07.026
142. Gorey C, Kuhns L, Smaragdi E, Kroon E, Cousijn J. Age-related differences in the impact of cannabis use on the brain and cognition: a systematic review. *Eur Arch Psychiatry Clin Neurosci* (2019) 1–22. doi: 10.1007/s00406-019-00981-7
143. Scott JC, Rosen AF, Moore TM, Roalf DR, Satterthwaite TD, Calkins ME, et al. Cannabis use in youth is associated with limited alterations in brain structure. *Neuropsychopharmacology* (2019) 1:1362–69.
144. Scott JC, Wolf DH, Calkins ME, Bach EC, Weidner J, Ruparel K, et al. Cognitive functioning of adolescent and young adult cannabis users in the Philadelphia Neurodevelopmental Cohort. *Psychol Addictive Behav* (2017) 31(4):423.
145. Fleury MJ, Djouini A, Huynh C, Tremblay J, Ferland F, Menard JM, et al. Remission from substance use disorders: A systematic review and meta-analysis. *Drug Alcohol Depend* (2016) 168:293–306. doi: 10.1016/j.drugalcdep.2016.08.625
146. Rezapour T, DeVito EE, Sofuoglu M, Ekhtiari H. Perspectives on neurocognitive rehabilitation as an adjunct treatment for addictive disorders: from cognitive improvement to relapse prevention. *Prog Brain Res* (2016) 224:345–69. doi: 10.1016/bs.pbr.2015.07.022
147. Boffo M, Zerhouni O, Gronau QF, van Beek RJJ, Nikolaou K, Marsman M, et al. Cognitive bias modification for behavior change in alcohol and smoking addiction: bayesian meta-analysis of individual participant data. *Neuropsychol Rev* (2019) 29(1):52–78. doi: 10.1007/s11065-018-9386-4
148. Eack SM, Hogarty SS, Bangalore SS, Keshavan MS, Cornelius JR. Patterns of substance use during cognitive enhancement therapy: an 18-month randomized feasibility study. *J Dual Diagn* (2016) 12(1):74–82. doi: 10.1080/15504263.2016.1145778
149. Eack SM, Hogarty SS, Greenwald DP, Litschge MY, McKnight SA, Bangalore SS, et al. Cognitive Enhancement Therapy in substance misusing schizophrenia: results of an 18-month feasibility trial. *Schizophr Res* (2015) 161(2-3):478–83. doi: 10.1016/j.schres.2014.11.017
150. Rezapour T, Hatami J, Farhoudian A, Sofuoglu M, Noroozi A, Daneshmand R, et al. Cognitive rehabilitation for individuals with opioid use disorder: a

randomized controlled trial. *Neuropsychol Rehabil* (2019) 29(8):1273–89. doi: 10.1080/09602011.2017.1391103

151. Rupp CI, Kemmler G, Kurz M, Hinterhuber H, Fleischhacker WW. Cognitive remediation therapy during treatment for alcohol dependence. *J Stud Alcohol Drugs* (2012) 73(4):625–34. doi: 10.15288/jsad.2012.73.625
152. Bell MD, Laws HB, Petrakis IB. A randomized controlled trial of cognitive remediation and work therapy in the early phase of substance use disorder recovery for older veterans: neurocognitive and substance use outcomes. *Psychiatr Rehabil J* (2017) 40(1):94–102. doi: 10.1037/prj0000211
153. Bell MD, Vissicchio NA, Weinstein AJ. Cognitive training and work therapy for the treatment of verbal learning and memory deficits in veterans with alcohol use disorders. *J Dual Diagn* (2016) 12(1):83–9. doi: 10.1080/15504263.2016.1145779
154. Rezapour T, Wurfel B, Simblett S, Ekhtiari H. Neuropsychological Rehabilitation for Psychiatric Disorders. In: *Neuropsychological Rehabilitation: The International Handbook*, Routledge, New York vol. 136. (2017).
155. Wojtalik JA, Hogarty SS, Cornelius JR, Phillips ML, Keshavan MS, Newhill CE, et al. Cognitive Enhancement therapy improves frontolimbic regulation of emotion in alcohol and/or cannabis misusing schizophrenia: a preliminary study. *Front Psychiatry* (2015) 6:186. doi: 10.3389/fpsyt.2015.00186
156. Labs L. (2019). Lumosity. Retrieved from https://www.lumosity.com/.
157. Marceau EM, Berry J, Lunn J, Kelly PJ, Solowij N. Cognitive remediation improves executive functions, self-regulation and quality of life in residents of a substance use disorder therapeutic community. *Drug Alcohol Depend* (2017) 178:150–8. doi: 10.1016/j.drugalcdep.2017.04.023
158. Alfonso JP, Caracuel A, Delgado-Pastor LC, Verdejo-Garcia A. Combined Goal management training and mindfulness meditation improve executive functions and decision-making performance in abstinent polysubstance abusers. *Drug Alcohol Depend* (2011) 117(1):78–81. doi: 10.1016/j.drugalcdep.2010.12.025
159. Valls-Serrano C, Caracuel A, Verdejo-Garcia A. Goal Management Training and Mindfulness Meditation improve executive functions and transfer to ecological tasks of daily life in polysubstance users enrolled in therapeutic community treatment. *Drug Alcohol Depend* (2016) 165:9–14. doi: 10.1016/j.drugalcdep.2016.04.040
160. Stamenova V, Levine B. Effectiveness of goal management training(R) in improving executive functions: A meta-analysis. *Neuropsychol Rehabil* (2018) 29(10):1569–99. doi: 10.1080/09602011.2018.1438294
161. Cogmed I. (2019). Cogmed. Retrieved from http://www.cogmed.com.au/.
162. Services PS. (2014). PSSCogRehab. Retrieved from http://www.psychological-software.com/psscogrehab.html.
163. Houben K, Nederkoorn C, Wiers RW, Jansen A. Resisting temptation: decreasing alcohol-related affect and drinking behavior by training response inhibition. *Drug Alcohol Depend* (2011) 116(1–3):132–6. doi: 10.1016/j.drugalcdep.2010.12.011
164. Wanmaker S, Leijdesdorff SMJ, Geraerts E, van de Wetering BJM, Renkema PJ, Franken IHA. The efficacy of a working memory training in substance use patients: A randomized double-blind placebo-controlled clinical trial. *J Clin Exp Neuropsychol* (2018) 40(5):473–86. doi: 10.1080/13803395.2017.1372367
165. Lechner WV, Sidhu NK, Kittaneh AA, Anand A. Interventions with potential to target executive function deficits in addiction: current state of the literature. *Curr Opin Psychol* (2019) 30:24–8. doi: 10.1016/j.copsyc.2019.01.017
166. Khemiri L, Brynte C, Stunkel A, Klingberg T, Jayaram-Lindstrom N. Working memory training in alcohol use disorder: a randomized controlled trial. *Alcohol Clin Exp Res* (2019) 43(1):135–46. doi: 10.1111/acer.13910
167. Snider SE, Deshpande HU, Lisinski JM, Koffarnus MN, LaConte SM, Bickel WK. Working memory training improves alcohol users' episodic future thinking: a rate-dependent analysis. *Biol Psychiatry Cognit Neurosci Neuroimaging* (2018) 3(2):160–7. doi: 10.1016/j.bpsc.2017.11.002
168. Rass O, Schacht RL, Buckheit K, Johnson MW, Strain EC, Mintzer MZ. A randomized controlled trial of the effects of working memory training in methadone maintenance patients. *Drug Alcohol Depend* (2015) 156:38–46. doi: 10.1016/j.drugalcdep.2015.08.012
169. Sweeney MM, Rass O, DiClemente C, Schacht RL, Vo HT, Fishman MJ, et al. Working memory training for adolescents with cannabis use disorders: a randomized controlled trial. *J Child Adolesc Subst Abuse* (2018) 27(4):211–26. doi: 10.1080/1067828X.2018.1451793
170. Brooks SJ, Wiemerslage L, Burch KH, Maiorana SA, Cocolas E, Schioth HB, et al. The impact of cognitive training in substance use disorder: the effect of working memory training on impulse control in methamphetamine users. *Psychopharmacol (Berl)* (2017) 234(12):1911–21. doi: 10.1007/s00213-017-4597-6
171. Houben K, Wiers RW. Response inhibition moderates the relationship between implicit associations and drinking behavior. *Alcohol Clin Exp Res* (2009) 33(4):626–33. doi: 10.1111/j.1530-0277.2008.00877.x
172. Luijten M, Machielsen MW, Veltman DJ, Hester R, de Haan L, Franken IH. Systematic review of ERP and fMRI studies investigating inhibitory control and error processing in people with substance dependence and behavioural addictions. *J Psychiatry Neurosci* (2014) 39(3):149–69. doi: 10.1503/jpn.130052
173. Murphy P, Garavan H. Cognitive predictors of problem drinking and AUDIT scores among college students. *Drug Alcohol Depend* (2011) 115(1-2):94–100. doi: 10.1016/j.drugalcdep.2010.10.011
174. Verdejo-Garcia A, Lawrence AJ, Clark L. Impulsivity as a vulnerability marker for substance-use disorders: review of findings from high-risk research, problem gamblers and genetic association studies. *Neurosci Biobehav Rev* (2008) 32(4):777–810. doi: 10.1016/j.neubiorev.2007.11.003
175. Houben K, Wiers RW, Jansen A. Getting a grip on drinking behavior: training working memory to reduce alcohol abuse. *Psychol Sci* (2011) 22(7):968–75. doi: 10.1177/0956797611412392
176. Di Lemma LCG, Field M. Cue avoidance training and inhibitory control training for the reduction of alcohol consumption: a comparison of effectiveness and investigation of their mechanisms of action. *Psychopharmacol (Berl)* (2017) 234(16):2489–98. doi: 10.1007/s00213-017-4639-0
177. Kilwein TM, Bernhardt KA, Stryker ML, Looby A. Decreased alcohol consumption after pairing alcohol-related cues with an inhibitory response. *J Subst Use* (2018) 23(2):154–61. doi: 10.1080/14659891.2017.1378736
178. Allom V, Mullan B, Hagger M. Does inhibitory control training improve health behaviour? A meta-analysis. *Health Psychol Rev* (2016) 10(2):168–86. doi: 10.1080/17437199.2015.1051078
179. Jones A, Di Lemma LC, Robinson E, Christiansen P, Nolan S, Tudur-Smith C, et al. Inhibitory control training for appetitive behaviour change: A meta-analytic investigation of mechanisms of action and moderators of effectiveness. *Appetite* (2016) 97:16–28. doi: 10.1016/j.appet.2015.11.013
180. Houben K, Havermans RC, Nederkoorn C, Jansen A. Beer a no-go: learning to stop responding to alcohol cues reduces alcohol intake *via* reduced affective associations rather than increased response inhibition. *Addiction* (2012) 107(7):1280–7. doi: 10.1111/j.1360-0443.2012.03827.x
181. Strickland JC, Hill JC, Stoops WW, Rush CR. Feasibility, acceptability, and initial efficacy of delivering alcohol use cognitive interventions *via* crowdsourcing. *Alcohol Clin Exp Res* (2019) 43(5):888–99. doi: 10.1111/acer.13987
182. Christiansen P, Schoenmakers TM, Field M. Less than meets the eye: reappraising the clinical relevance of attentional bias in addiction. *Addict Behav* (2015) 44:43–50. doi: 10.1016/j.addbeh.2014.10.005
183. Fadardi JS, Cox WM. Reversing the sequence: reducing alcohol consumption by overcoming alcohol attentional bias. *Drug Alcohol Depend* (2009) 101(3):137–45. doi: 10.1016/j.drugalcdep.2008.11.015
184. McGeary JE, Meadows SP, Amir N, Gibb BE. Computer-delivered, home-based, attentional retraining reduces drinking behavior in heavy drinkers. *Psychol Addict Behav* (2014) 28(2):559–62. doi: 10.1037/a0036086
185. Schoenmakers TM, de Bruin M, Lux IF, Goertz AG, Van Kerkhof DH, Wiers RW. Clinical effectiveness of attentional bias modification training in abstinent alcoholic patients. *Drug Alcohol Depend* (2010) 109(1–3):30–6. doi: 10.1016/j.drugalcdep.2009.11.022
186. Rinck M, Wiers RW, Becker ES, Lindenmeyer J. Relapse prevention in abstinent alcoholics by cognitive bias modification: Clinical effects of combining approach bias modification and attention bias modification. *J Consult Clin Psychol* (2018) 86(12):1005–16. doi: 10.1037/ccp0000321
187. Ziaee SS, Fadardi JS, Cox WM, Yazdi SA. Effects of attention control training on drug abusers' attentional bias and treatment outcome. *J Consult Clin Psychol* (2016) 84(10):861–73. doi: 10.1037/a0040290
188. Mayer AR, Wilcox CE, Dodd AB, Klimaj SD, Dekonenko CJ, Claus ED, et al. The efficacy of attention bias modification therapy in cocaine

use disorders. *Am J Drug Alcohol Abuse* (2016) 42(4):459–68. doi: 10.3109/00952990.2016.1151523

189. Dean AC, Nurmi EL, Moeller SJ, Amir N, Rozenman M, Ghahremani DG, et al. No effect of attentional bias modification training in methamphetamine users receiving residential treatment. *Psychopharmacol (Berl)* (2019) 236(2):709–21. doi: 10.1007/s00213-018-5100-8
190. Heitmann J, Bennik EC, van Hemel-Ruiter ME, de Jong PJ. The effectiveness of attentional bias modification for substance use disorder symptoms in adults: a systematic review. *Syst Rev* (2018) 7(1):160. doi: 10.1186/s13643-018-0822-6
191. Eberl C, Wiers RW, Pawelczack S, Rinck M, Becker ES, Lindenmeyer J. Approach bias modification in alcohol dependence: do clinical effects replicate and for whom does it work best? *Dev Cognit Neurosci* (2013) 4:38–51. doi: 10.1016/j.dcn.2012.11.002
192. Wiers RW, Eberl C, Rinck M, Becker ES, Lindenmeyer J. Retraining automatic action tendencies changes alcoholic patients' approach bias for alcohol and improves treatment outcome. *Psychol Sci* (2011) 22(4):490–7. doi: 10.1177/0956797611400615
193. Wiers RW, Boffo M, Field M. What's in a Trial? on the importance of distinguishing between experimental lab studies and randomized controlled trials: the case of cognitive bias modification and alcohol use disorders. *J Stud Alcohol Drugs* (2018) 79(3):333–43. doi: 10.15288/jsad.2018.79.333
194. Mann K, Hoch E, Batra A, Bonnet U, Gunthner A, Reymann G, et al. Guideline-oriented treatment of alcohol-related disorders. *Nervenarzt* (2016) 87(1):13–25. doi: 10.1007/s00115-015-0022-8
195. Wiers CE, Stelzel C, Gladwin TE, Park SQ, Pawelczack S, Gawron CK, et al. Effects of cognitive bias modification training on neural alcohol cue reactivity in alcohol dependence. *Am J Psychiatry* (2015) 172(4):335–43. doi: 10.1176/appi.ajp.2014.13111495
196. Sherman BJ, Baker NL, Squeglia LM, McRae-Clark AL. Approach bias modification for cannabis use disorder: a proof-of-principle study. *J Subst Abuse Treat* (2018) 87:16–22. doi: 10.1016/j.jsat.2018.01.012
197. Kakoschke N, Kemps E, Tiggemann M. Approach bias modification training and consumption: A review of the literature. *Addict Behav* (2017) 64:21–8. doi: 10.1016/j.addbeh.2016.08.007
198. Cristea IA, Kok RN, Cuijpers P. The effectiveness of cognitive bias modification interventions for substance addictions: a meta-analysis. *PloS One* (2016) 11(9):e0162226. doi: 10.1371/journal.pone.0162226
199. Zhu Y, Jiang H, Su H, Zhong N, Li R, Li X, et al. A newly designed mobile-based computerized cognitive addiction therapy app for the improvement of cognition impairments and risk decision making in methamphetamine use disorder: randomized controlled trial. *JMIR Mhealth Uhealth* (2018) 6(6):e10292. doi: 10.2196/10292
200. Kakoschke N, Kemps E, Tiggemann M. What is the appropriate control condition for approach bias modification? A response to commentary by Becker et al. (2017). *Addict Behav* (2018) 77:295–6. doi: 10.1016/j.addbeh.2017.02.024
201. Lindgren KP, Neighbors C, Teachman BA, Wiers RW, Westgate E, Greenwald AG. I drink therefore I am: validating alcohol-related implicit association tests. *Psychol Addict Behav* (2013) 27(1):1–13. doi: 10.1037/a0027640
202. Peeters M, Wiers RW, Monshouwer K, van de Schoot R, Janssen T, Vollebergh WA. Automatic processes in at-risk adolescents: the role of alcohol-approach tendencies and response inhibition in drinking behavior. *Addiction* (2012) 107(11):1939–46. doi: 10.1111/j.1360-0443.2012.03948.x
203. Ekhtiari H, Faghiri A, Oghabian MA, Paulus MP. Functional neuroimaging for addiction medicine: From mechanisms to practical considerations. *Prog Brain Res* (2016) 224:129–53. doi: 10.1016/bs.pbr.2015.10.001
204. Ekhtiari H, Nasseri P, Yavari F, Mokri A, Monterosso J. Neuroscience of drug craving for addiction medicine: from circuits to therapies. *Prog Brain Res* (2016) 223:115–41. doi: 10.1016/bs.pbr.2015.10.002
205. Ekhtiari H, Paulus M. Preface: Neuroscience for addiction medicine: from prevention to rehabilitation. *Prog Brain Res* (2016) 224:xxv–xxvi. doi: 10.1016/s0079-6123(16)00030-3
206. Parkin BL, Ekhtiari H, Walsh VF. Non-invasive human brain stimulation in cognitive neuroscience: a primer. *Neuron* (2015) 87(5):932–45. doi: 10.1016/j.neuron.2015.07.032
207. Kwako LE, Schwandt ML, Ramchandani VA, Diazgranados N, Koob GF, Volkow ND, et al. Neurofunctional domains derived from deep behavioral phenotyping in alcohol use disorder. *Am J Psychiatry* (2019) 176(9):744–53 doi: 10.1176/appi.ajp.2018.18030357
208. Yavari F, Shahbabaie A, Leite J, Car 12(3):606-618 valho S, Ekhtiari H, Fregni F. Noninvasive brain stimulation for addiction medicine: From monitoring to modulation. *Prog Brain Res* (2016) 224:371–99. doi: 10.1016/bs.pbr.2015.08.007
209. Jansen JM, Daams JG, Koeter MW, Veltman DJ, van den Brink W, Goudriaan AE. Effects of non-invasive neurostimulation on craving: a meta-analysis. *Neurosci Biobehav Rev* (2013) 37(10):2472–80. doi: 10.1016/j.neubiorev.2013.07.009
210. Maiti R, Mishra BR, Hota D. Effect of high-frequency transcranial magnetic stimulation on craving in substance use disorder: a meta-analysis. *J Neuropsychiatry Clin Neurosci* (2016) 29(2):160–71.
211. Song S, Zilverstand A, Gui W, Li HJ, Zhou X. Effects of single-session versus multi-session non-invasive brain stimulation on craving and consumption in individuals with drug addiction, eating disorders or obesity: A meta-analysis. *Brain Stimulation* (2018) 12(3):606–18.
212. Kang N, Kim RK, Kim HJ. Effects of transcranial direct current stimulation on symptoms of nicotine dependence: a systematic review and meta-analysis. *Addictive Behav* (2019) 96:133–9. doi: 10.1016/j.addbeh.2019.05.006
213. Terraneo A, Leggio L, Saladini M, Ermani M, Bonci A, Gallimberti L. Transcranial magnetic stimulation of dorsolateral prefrontal cortex reduces cocaine use: a pilot study. *Eur Neuropsychopharmacol* (2016) 26(1):37–44. doi: 10.1016/j.euroneuro.2015.11.011
214. Yang LZ, Shi B, Li H, Zhang W, Liu Y, Wang H, et al. Electrical stimulation reduces smokers' craving by modulating the coupling between dorsal lateral prefrontal cortex and parahippocampal gyrus. *Soc Cognit Affect Neurosci* (2017) 12(8):1296–302. doi: 10.1093/scan/nsx055
215. Kearney-Ramos TE, Dowdle LT, Lench DH, Mithoefer OJ, Devries WH, George MS, et al. Transdiagnostic effects of ventromedial prefrontal cortex transcranial magnetic stimulation on cue reactivity. *Biol Psychiatry Cognit Neurosci Neuroimaging* (2018) 3(7):599–609. doi: 10.1016/j.bpsc.2018.03.016
216. Krystal AD, Pizzagalli DA, Mathew SJ, Sanacora G, Keefe R, Song A, et al. The first implementation of the NIMH FAST-FAIL approach to psychiatric drug development. *Nat Rev Drug Discovery* (2018) 18(1):82–4. doi: 10.1038/nrd.2018.222
217. Lorenz R, Simmons LE, Monti RP, Arthur JL, Limal S, Laakso I, et al. Assessing tACS-induced phosphene perception using closed-loop Bayesian optimization. *bioRxiv* (2017), 150086. doi: 10.1101/150086
218. Lorenzetti V, Melo B, Basilio R, Suo C, Yucel M, Tierra-Criollo CJ, et al. Emotion regulation using virtual environments and real-time fMRI neurofeedback. *Front Neurol* (2018) 9:390. doi: 10.3389/fneur.2018.00390
219. Gruzelier J. EEG-neurofeedback for optimising performance. III: a review of methodological and theoretical considerations. *Neurosci Biobehav Rev* (2014) 44:159–82.
220. Niv S. Clinical efficacy and potential mechanisms of neurofeedback. *Pers Individ Dif* (2013) 54(6):676–86.
221. Sulzer J, Haller S, Scharnowski F, Weiskopf N, Birbaumer N, Blefari ML, et al. Real-time fMRI neurofeedback: progress and challenges. *Neuroimage* (2013) 76:386–99. doi: 10.1016/j.neuroimage.2013.03.033
222. Carelli L, Solca F, Faini A, Meriggi P, Sangalli D, Cipresso P, et al. Brain-Computer Interface for Clinical Purposes: Cognitive Assessment and Rehabilitation. *BioMed Res Int* (2017), 1695290. doi: 10.1155/2017/1695290
223. Scott WC, Kaiser D, Othmer S, Sideroff S. Effects of an EEG biofeedback protocol on a mixed substance abusing population. *Am J Drug Alcohol Abuse* (2005) 31(3):455–69. doi: 10.1081/ada-200056807
224. Luigjes J, Segrave R, de Joode N, Figee M, Denys D. Efficacy of invasive and non-invasive brain modulation interventions for addiction. *Neuropsychol Rev* (2019) 29(1):116–38. doi: 10.1007/s11065-018-9393-5
225. Canterberry M, Hanlon CA, Hartwell KJ, Li X, Owens M, Lematty T, et al. Sustained reduction of nicotine craving with real-time neurofeedback: exploring the role of severity of dependence. *Nicotine Tobacco Res* (2013) 15(12):2120–4. doi: 10.1093/ntr/ntt122
226. Hanlon CA, Hartwell KJ, Canterberry M, Li X, Owens M, LeMatty T, et al. Reduction of cue-induced craving through realtime neurofeedback in nicotine users: the role of region of interest selection and multiple visits. *Psychiatry Res: Neuroimaging* (2013) 213(1):79–81.

227. Hartwell KJ, Hanlon CA, Li X, Borckardt JJ, Canterberry M, Prisciandaro JJ, et al. Individualized real-time fMRI neurofeedback to attenuate craving in nicotine-dependent smokers. *J Psychiatry Neurosci* (2016) 41(1):48.
228. Hartwell KJ, Prisciandaro JJ, Borckardt J, Li X, George MS, Brady K. Real-time fMRI in the treatment of nicotine dependence: a conceptual review and pilot studies. *J Psychol Addictive Behav* (2013) 27(2):501.
229. Li X, Hartwell KJ, Borckardt J, Prisciandaro JJ, Saladin ME, Morgan PS, et al. Volitional reduction of anterior cingulate cortex activity produces decreased cue craving in smoking cessation: a preliminary real-time fMRI study. *Addict Biol* (2013) 18(4):739–48.
230. Kim D-Y, Yoo S-S, Tegethoff M, Meinlschmidt G, Lee J-H. The inclusion of functional connectivity information into fMRI-based neurofeedback improves its efficacy in the reduction of cigarette cravings. *J Cog Neurosci* (2015) 27(8):1552–72. doi: 10.1162/jocn_a_00802
231. Karch S, Keeser D, Hümmer S, Paolini M, Kirsch V, Karali T, et al. Modulation of craving related brain responses using real-time fMRI in patients with alcohol use disorder. *PloS One* (2015) 10(7):e0133034.
232. Kirsch M, Gruber I, Ruf M, Kiefer F, Kirsch P. Real-time functional magnetic resonance imaging neurofeedback can reduce striatal cue-reactivity to alcohol stimuli. *Addict Biol* (2016) 21(4):982–92.
233. Ekhtiari H, Tavakoli H, Addolorato G, Baeken C, Bonci A, Campanella S, et al. Transcranial electrical and magnetic stimulation (tES and TMS) for addiction medicine: A consensus paper on the present state of the science and the road ahead. *Neurosci Biobehav Rev* (2019) 104:118–40. doi: 10.1016/j.neubiorev.2019.06.007

7

The Endocannabinoid System and Cannabidiol's Promise for the Treatment of Substance use Disorder

Yann Chye[1*]*, Erynn Christensen*[1]*, Nadia Solowij*[2,3] *and Murat Yücel*[1]

[1] *Brain and Mental Health Research Hub, Monash Institute of Cognitive and Clinical Neurosciences, School of Psychological Sciences, Monash University, Melbourne, VIC, Australia,* [2] *School of Psychology and Illawarra Health and Medical Research Institute, University of Wollongong, Wollongong, NSW, Australia,* [3] *The Australian Centre for Cannabinoid Clinical and Research Excellence, New Lambton Heights, NSW, Australia*

Correspondence:
Yann Chye
yannying.chye@monash.edu

Substance use disorder is characterized by repeated use of a substance, leading to clinically significant distress, making it a serious public health concern. The endocannabinoid system plays an important role in common neurobiological processes underlying substance use disorder, in particular by mediating the rewarding and motivational effects of substances and substance-related cues. In turn, a number of cannabinoid drugs (e.g., rimonabant, nabiximols) have been suggested for potential pharmacological treatment for substance dependence. Recently, cannabidiol (CBD), a non-psychoactive phytocannabinoid found in the cannabis plant, has also been proposed as a potentially effective treatment for the management of substance use disorder. Animal and human studies suggest that these cannabinoids have the potential to reduce craving and relapse in abstinent substance users, by impairing reconsolidation of drug-reward memory, salience of drug cues, and inhibiting the reward-facilitating effect of drugs. Such functions likely arise through the targeting of the endocannabinoid and serotonergic systems, although the exact mechanism is yet to be elucidated. This article seeks to review the role of the endocannabinoid system in substance use disorder and the proposed pharmacological action supporting cannabinoid drugs' therapeutic potential in addictions, with a focus on CBD. Subsequently, this article will evaluate the underlying evidence for CBD as a potential treatment for substance use disorder, across a range of substances including nicotine, alcohol, psychostimulants, opioids, and cannabis. While early research supports CBD's promise, further investigation and validation of CBD's efficacy, across preclinical and clinical trials will be necessary.

Keywords: endocannabinoid system, ECS, substance use disorder, treatment efficacy, cannabidiol, CBD, addiction

INTRODUCTION

Substance use disorder (SUD) is a global problem, with over 30 million individuals estimated to have an SUD (1). Within the United States alone, SUD-related expenditure (e.g., treatment and productivity cost) exceeded 23 billion USD per year (2), presenting a worrisome issue. Treatment to date has had minimal success, with a high likelihood of relapse (3). There is also no reliably established pharmacotherapy for SUDs, such as cannabis, and stimulant use disorder; and current pharmacotherapies (e.g., opiate substitution with methadone; naltrexone for alcohol use disorder;

nicotine replacement) have limited efficacy in relapse prevention (4, 5). SUD has been conceptualized as a maladaptive and relapsing cycle of intoxication, binging, withdrawal and craving that results in excessive substance use despite adverse consequences (6). Recent models implicate major brain circuits involved in reward saliency, motivation, and memory/learned associations in maintaining addiction (7). Critically, these circuits may largely be modulated by the endocannabinoid system (ECS), presenting a promising pharmaceutical avenue for treating SUDs.

THE ENDOCANNABINOID SYSTEM

The ECS consists of cannabinoid receptors (e.g., CB1R, CB2R), the endogenous ligands that bind to these cannabinoid receptors [e.g., anandamide and 2-arachidonoylglycerol (2-AG)], and enzymes for their biosynthesis and degradation [e.g., fatty acid amide hydrolase (FAAH) and monoacylglyrecol lipase (MAGL)] (8). Over the past decade, primary interest has focused on CB1Rs, for their purported role across a range of physiological functions, including directing the psychoactive effect of delta9-tetrahydrocannabinol (THC), a phytocannabinoid present in cannabis (8, 9). CB1Rs are one of the most common G-protein-coupled receptors in the central nervous system, preferentially residing on presynaptic neurons across diverse regions including the neocortex, striatum, and hippocampus (10, 11). Their widespread distribution allows them to guide a host of functions ranging from cognition, memory, mood, appetite, and sensory responses (8). Endocannabinoids themselves function as neuromodulators that are released by post-synaptic neurons, and bind to the presynaptic CB1Rs to moderate the release of neurotransmitters, such as gamma-aminobutyric-acid (GABA), glutamate, and dopamine (DA) (10, 12, 13). While the specific CB1R function depends on the cell population and region in which they reside, their role in retrograde signaling permits them to regulate signaling activity across cognitive, emotive, and sensory functions, lending therapeutic capacity (14).

ECS ROLE IN REWARD SIGNALING

Of the functions that the ECS is involved in, of critical interest, is its influence on the brain reward circuitry, particularly in response to substances of abuse. The rewarding effect of substances of abuse is thought to be primarily mediated by the mesolimbic DA pathway, originating from dopaminergic cell bodies in ventral midbrain [ventral tegmental area (VTA)], carrying reward-related information to the ventral striatum [nucleus accumbens (NAc)] (15). The acute reinforcing effect of addictive substances is thought to be due to their direct or indirect activation of DA neurons along this pathway (16). The VTA-NAc pathway as such plays a key function in reward assessment, anticipation, and valuation, making it a critical component underlying substance use and addiction (17).

DA activity is intrinsically tied to cannabinoid activity. CB1Rs are particularly densely located across the striatal regions that mediate reward function (i.e., NAc and VTA) (18), and their regulatory role on the VTA-NAc pathway may be crucial in modulating overall reward tone (19, 20). Rodent studies have demonstrated that THC increases neuronal firing rates in the VTA (21), likely through local disinhibition of DA-ergic neurons, by binding to CB1Rs present on glutamatergic and/or GABAergic neurons (although it is prudent to note that THC's capacity to potentiate DAergic release differs between rodents and humans) (15, 20, 22, 23). Similarly, other substances of abuse (e.g., opioids, cocaine) have also been demonstrated to potentiate dopaminergic activity via the ECS (24, 25). For example, alcohol is found to have a downstream potentiation effect on the ECS in rats (26), such as an increase in endogenous cannabinoid (anandamide and 2-AG) levels (27, 28) and downregulation of CB1R expression (29). Alcohol-induced DAergic release is furthermore dependent on the presence of CB1Rs (30). Nicotine activates DA neurons in the VTA either directly through stimulation of nicotinic cholinergic receptors or indirectly through glutaminergic nerve terminals that are modulated by the ECS (31). Meanwhile opioid receptors are often co-located with CB1Rs in the striatum (32), and may be modulated by and interact with CB1R activity reciprocally (33, 34). Only psychostimulants are suggested to act directly on DAergic axon terminals in the NAc, potentially avoiding upstream endocannabinoid involvement in the VTA (35).

CB1R's role in the motivational and reinforcing effects of rewards has been demonstrated in animal models with CB1R agonists. For example, acute exposure to CB1R agonists (e.g., THC; CP 55,940; WIN 55,212-2; HU 210) augments NAc DA transmission (36), lowers the brain-reward threshold (17), induces conditioned place preference (CPP) (37), and establishes persistent self-administration of substances of abuse, including cannabis and alcohol (17, 38). Meanwhile, CB1R antagonists (e.g., rimonabant) have been shown to attenuate reinforcing effects of these substances, blocking the increase of DA release in the NAc (37, 39). While substances of abuse, such as alcohol, stimulants, nicotine and opioids have differing upstream mechanisms of action (14, 40), the evidence suggest the downstream involvement of the ECS in their reward mechanism.

In summary, the ECS, by direct CB1R activity, modulates and is modulated by mesolimbic DA activity (41). While the action of individual substances may differ, they share a common effect of precipitating DAergic activity from the VTA neurons (42), with this DA-ergic activity mediated by the ECS (14). It is thus thought that the disruption of endocannabinoid signaling may prove effective in treating SUDs (41). Nevertheless, it is necessary to note that this is a simplistic understanding, given the potential involvement of non-DA-ergic neurons in the VTA, and additional neuronal circuits including those involving glutamatergic and opioids, that are yet to be fully elucidated (39, 43).

ECS ROLE IN SUBSTANCE USE DISORDER (SUD)

Besides the ECS role in reward, it is necessary to acknowledge that substance reward and reinforcement are different from substance dependence. Where the former explain initial substance use, and are suggested to be related to increased DA in striatal and limbic (NAc and amygdala) regions (44, 45); the latter reflects further compulsive substance intake, loss of control, and persistent intake despite the substance's adverse effects and tolerance to its pleasurable responses (44, 46, 47).

Several lines of thought suggest SUD to be a learned habit (48, 49) mediated by persistent changes in striatal function (e.g., synaptic plasticity occurring during learning) (50). Substances of abuse are thought to influence long-lasting plastic changes across corticostriatal circuits, through repeated perturbation of DA activity, thus making it difficult for addicts to cease their substance use, and enhancing risk of relapse (48, 50–52). In this role, CB1Rs present across the corticostriatal circuits, such as the PFC and striatum, mediate synaptic transmission, in their capacity as neuromodulators (35, 53). Evidence demonstrates the necessity of cannabinoid signaling on CB1Rs to induce long-lasting synaptic plasticity, such as long-term depression (LTD) of glutamatergic release across the dorsal and ventral striatum (19, 54). Such functional changes, particularly across the striatal structures responsible for the rewarding and motivational effects of substances of abuse, are not only necessary in providing reward salience, but also in establishing compulsive substance use habit (39, 55). The ECS thus represents a necessary contributor toward cellular adaptations in the transition from recreational substance use to a use disorder (50, 56).

A further function of ECS-mediated synaptic plasticity may be to facilitate emotional learning and memory processes, which promote increased emotional response to substance-related cues (57). The limbic system, in particular the amygdala and hippocampus, by supporting the formation of associative memory, promotes positive and negative reinforcement of rewards including those of substances of abuse (58). Indeed, animal models demonstrate memory performance to not only be dependent on emotional processes, but may be modulated by augmentation of ECS signaling (59–62). Phytocannabinoids, such as THC and CBD for example have been found to modulate brain activity level across limbic regions during emotional processing tasks (63, 64). Endocannabinoids may further induce long-term changes in synaptic strength across the hippocampus, mediating associative memory formation (65–67). Literature investigating cannabinoid agonists and antagonists on SUD solidifies the role of the ECS in emotional learning and memory processes. CB1R agonists and antagonists have respectively been demonstrated to facilitate and attenuate memory extinction in various fear and reward conditioning paradigms in animal models [see (57) for review]. Within the context of SUD, cannabinoid modulation of emotional memory may have implications for extinction, consolidation, and reinstatement of substance-related memory (68). These processes are primarily assessed through place conditioning paradigms, such as CPP. CB1R antagonism by rimonabant for example, has been demonstrated to disrupt the reconsolidation and facilitate the extinction of CPP to substances of abuse, such as methamphetamine and cocaine, potentially via disrupting reward-associated memory (69, 70). Nevertheless, evidence on SUD behavior is mixed and potentially dependent on type and dose of cannabinoids (70, 71).

The ECS's role in reward signaling and learning may as such shape addictive behavior in SUD. The following section details evidence of CB1R's involvement in SUD as demonstrated by cannabinoid agonism and antagonism in animal models.

Agonism of CB1R

CB1R agonism (either studied with the synthetic cannabinoid agonist WIN 55-212,2 or contrasted against CB1R knockout mice) has been shown to facilitate alcohol self-administration, CPP, and binge-like behavior in animals (38, 72–74). WIN 55,212-2 has also been found to increase motivation to self-administer nicotine, and facilitate cue-induced reinstatement in rats (75). Similar results are found in the heroin literature, with THC-induced CB1R agonism increasing substance self-administration in rats (76, 77).

Agonist substitution with CB1R agonists may have potential for treatment of cannabis use disorder by reducing withdrawal symptoms and the reinforcing effect of cannabis (78). Dronabinol—a stereoisomer of THC, and Nabilone—a synthetic analog of THC, originally intended for nausea and weight loss (55), have both been shown to have efficacy for cannabis withdrawal (79, 80). However, Dronabinol and Nabilone may not prevent cannabis use or relapse (78). It is likely that while these substances are efficacious in attenuating withdrawal symptoms by acting as a "proxy-substances," they do not directly normalize substance use-related circuits and behavior.

Antagonism of CB1R

CB1R antagonism has originally been assumed to be a promising target for SUD treatment. SR141716, known as rimonabant, an inverse agonist of CB1R, has been extensively investigated in SUD for its antagonist effect on drug seeking and relapse behavior in both animal and human models.

Animal studies have shown rimonabant as effective in reducing self-administration of alcohol (81, 82), nicotine (83, 84), and heroin (85). Antagonism of CB1R by rimonabant, reduces alcohol-induced sensitization and reinstatement of nicotine-seeking in rats (83, 84, 86). When investigating the efficacy of CB1R antagonists on stimulant use however, the literature is mixed. While rimonabant's CB1R antagonism has been shown to block CPP and attenuate cue- and substance-induced relapse to psychostimulants, such as cocaine and methamphetamines (87–89), evidence pertaining to self-administration is inconsistent (90–92).

Human studies have also been conducted investigating the efficacy of rimonabant in cannabis, nicotine, and alcohol use. Cannabis and nicotine use have both shown sensitivity to rimonabant antagonism. Rimonabant attenuated the acute physiological effects of cannabis including subjective level of intoxication (93, 94), and clinical trials demonstrate rimonabant to be effective in increasing smoking cessation (95). However, the efficacy of rimonabant for alcohol cessation has been less promising. In a 12-weeks clinical trial of relapse rate in recently detoxified alcohol-dependant patients, rimonabant only had a modest effect (that did not reach significance) compared to placebo (96). Rimonabant also had no effect on alcohol consumption for non-treatment seeking heavy alcohol drinkers (97).

Despite promising findings of rimonabant against substance use and relapse, it has been found to produce significant negative psychiatric effects including depression, anxiety, and an elevated suicide rate, preventing it from being a viable treatment option (98). Nevertheless, the evidence indicates CB1R antagonism to have robust effects on some SUDs, highlighting a potential target for SUD treatment. One such candidate drug that antagonizes CB1R, and is increasingly being investigated as a therapeutic option for SUD, is cannabidiol (CBD).

CANNABIDIOL (CBD)

CBD is a phytocannabinoid found in cannabis that has recently emerged as a promising treatment for SUDs (99, 100). CBD is non-rewarding, and acts on a number of receptor systems including the opioid (101), serotonergic (102, 103), and cannabinoid (22) systems. Within the cannabinoid system, it is a non-competitive antagonist of CB1R with a low affinity for CB1Rs' primary ligand site (104, 105), instead acting through negative allosteric modulation (105, 106). CBD is found to inhibit endocannabinoid signaling in a dose-dependent manner, likely by binding to CB1Rs' allosteric site and altering the potency of other primary ligands (e.g., endocannabinoids, THC) (106, 107). Its ability to modulate overall ECS tone despite lacking intrinsic efficacy (105) meant that it may decrease CB1R activity without CB1 inverse agonist-related side effects, such as those produced by rimonabant (108, 109). Indeed, CBD has a good safety profile, with generally mild side effects in animal preclinical studies or human studies (110, 111). This, coupled by the limited abuse liability of CBD (112, 113), makes it a good therapeutic candidate. Systemically administered CBD has also been demonstrated to regulate mesolimbic DA activity (114), and potentially attenuate substance-induced dysregulation of the mesolimbic circuitry (115, 116), suggesting its utility against SUDs. Though its efficacy may be dependent on a range of factors including the sequence of administration (i.e., whether CBD is administered in conjunction with, prior to, or post substance-use), and dose ratio (117). A number of papers are urging for the investigation of CBD as a therapeutic option for SUD of multiple substances including stimulants (118), opioids (119, 120), and nicotine use disorder (31). The following section details evidence of CBD treatments for cannabis, alcohol, nicotine, opioid, and stimulants. **Table 1** further lists this evidence by SUD constructs.

Cannabis

Pharmacological approaches to treating cannabis dependence via agonist replacement (i.e., Dronabinol and Nabilone) have limited efficacy (141). CBD itself has been trialed in rats, and found to be effective in ameliorating conditioned place aversion (CPA) produced by THC injection, but did not alter CPP (142). In human case studies, CBD has also been found to reduce self-reported cannabis use to non-use in a dependent male (128), and to reduced cannabis withdrawal in another (135), although the latter case study did find the subject to have relapsed after a 6-months follow up (135). CBD may have potential in reducing euphoria associated with cannabis use, despite not directly reducing cannabis use (124). However, investigative efforts with pure CBD have been limited. Instead most studies have focused on nabiximols—an oromucosal spray containing 2.7 mg of THC and 2.5 mg of CBD—for cannabis dependence (143).

A number of human case studies suggest nabiximols to be efficacious, in combination with behavioral therapy, in reducing cannabis use and withdrawal symptoms (129). However, case study evidence should be taken cautiously. Further case-control studies indicate nabiximols to be effective in reducing withdrawal, but not cannabis use (123, 130, 144). Nor did it improve abstinence rate (123). It was noted that while therapeutics may assist in short-term withdrawal, it is unlikely that ongoing abstinence can be achieved without psychosocial or clinical support (145). Additionally, the THC component of nabiximols causes the drug to have abuse potential and should not be used lightly (146).

Alcohol

In animal studies, CBD was effective in reducing ethanol self-administration, and at high enough concentration (120 mg/kg but not 60 mg/kg) attenuated ethanol relapse (131). Further animal studies show CBD (at 15 mg/kg) to effectively reduce cue and stress induced reinstatement of ethanol administration, up to 138 days post-CBD treatment (140). However, one study found CBD alone to be ineffective in attenuating ethanol sensitization, which is suggested to be the first step in drug-associated plasticity (121). Comparatively, pure THC and a 1:1 ratio of THC:CBD was found to be more efficacious in reducing ethanol sensitization. In a human trial of 10-weeks of daily CBD administration in cannabis users, no changes in alcohol or tobacco use was observed either, although the study sample was not dependent on alcohol (124).

Tobacco

In a placebo controlled study of 24 smokers, those who received a CBD inhaler significantly reduced the number of smoked cigarettes relative to the placebo group, despite no reported difference in craving between groups (125). In another study, oral CBD reduced the salience of cigarette cues, after overnight abstinence in smokers, relative to placebo, but did not reduce craving or withdrawal (126).

Opioids

Initial studies on the efficacy of cannabinoids in alleviating morphine withdrawal and abstinence symptoms occurred 40 years ago, with rodent models suggesting that CBD alone has low efficacy in alleviating signs of abstinence in rats, but CBD in combination with THC (5:1 ratio) did so significantly (136). THC itself was demonstrated to be more effective than CBD in inhibiting morphine abstinence syndrome in mice (137, 138). Nevertheless, more recent studies demonstrate that treatment with CBD blocked the reward-facilitating effect of morphine (132), reduced morphine CPP and CPA, and prevented drug and stress-induced reinstatement of CPP (71, 127). CBD was also found to have some efficacy in heroin studies in rats. While it did not specifically alter maintenance of self-administration, nor did it aid extinction of self-administration, it did attenuate cue-induced (but not drug-primed) self-administration following

TABLE 1 | CBD's efficacy for the treatment of substance use disorders.

Study	Sample	Substance	Treatment*	Outcome*	Effect
SENSITIZATION					
Filev et al. (121)	Mice	Ethanol	CBD (2.5 mg/kg)	Locomotor activity	–
			THC:CBD (2.5:2.5 mg/kg)	Locomotor activity	↓
Gerdeman et al. (54)	Rats	Heroin	THC:CBD (10:10 mg/kg)	Locomotor activity	–
Luján et al. (122)	Mice	Cocaine	CBD (20 mg/kg)	Locomotor activity	–
REWARD FACILITATION					
Trigo et al. (123)	Humans	Cannabis	THC:CBD (27:25 mg/ml) as needed + MET and CBT	Craving—MCQ	–
Solowij et al. (124)	Humans	Cannabis	Daily oral CBD (200 mg)	CEQ euphoria	↓
Morgan et al. (125)	Humans	Nicotine	CBD as needed	Craving—TCQ	–
Hindocha et al. (126)	Humans	Nicotine	CBD (800 mg)	Craving—QSU-B	–
			CBD (800 mg)	Attentional bias—visual probe task	↓
			CBD (800 mg)	Pleasantness rating	↓
Markos et al. (127)	Mice	Morphine	CBD (2.5 mg/kg)	CPP	–
			CBD (5 mg/kg)	CPP	–
			CBD (10 mg/kg)	CPP	↓
			CBD (20 mg/kg)	CPP	–
Luján et al. (122)	Mice	Cocaine	CBD (5 mg/kg)	CPP	–
			CBD (10 mg/kg)	CPP	↓
			CBD (20 mg/kg)	CPP	↓
			CBD (30 mg/kg)	CPP	–
Parker et al. (113)	Rats	Amphetamine	CBD (5 mg/kg)	CPP	–
SELF-ADMINISTRATION					
Shannon et al. (128)	Human: case study	Cannabis	CBD (24-18 mg)	Abstinence	↓
Trigo et al. (129)	Humans: case series	Cannabis	THC:CBD (27:25 mg/ml) as needed + MET and CBT	Self-reported use	↓
Trigo et al. (123)	Humans	Cannabis	THC:CBD (27:25 mg/ml) as needed + MET and CBT	Abstinence	–
Allsop et al. (130)	Humans	Cannabis	THC:CBD (27:25 mg/ml) + psychosocial intervention	Abstinence	–
Solowij et al. (124)	Humans	Cannabis	Daily oral CBD (200 mg)	Self-reported use	–
Viudez-Martínez et al. (131)	Rats	Ethanol	CBD (30 mg/kg)	Self-administration	↓
Morgan et al. (125)	Humans	Nicotine	CBD as needed	Self-reported use	↓
Ren et al. (115)	Rats	Heroin	CBD (5 mg/kg)	Self-administration	–
			CBD (20 mg/kg)	Self-administration	–
Katsidoni et al. (132)	Rats	Morphine	CBD (5 mg/kg)	ICSS threshold	–
		Cocaine	CBD (5 mg/kg)	ICSS threshold	↓
Luján et al. (122)	Mice	Cocaine	CBD (20 mg/kg)	Self-administration	↓
Mahmud et al. (133)	Rats	Cocaine	CBD (5 mg/kg)	Self-administration	–
			CBD (10 mg/kg)	Self-administration	–
Hay et al. (134)	Rats	Methamphetamine	CBD (20 mg/kg)	Self-administration	–
			CBD (40 mg/kg)	Self-administration	–
			CBD (80 mg/kg)	Self-administration	↓
EXTINCTION					
Parker et al. (113)	Rats	Cocaine	CBD (5 mg/kg)	CPP	↓
		Amphetamine	CBD (5 mg/kg)	CPP	↓
WITHDRAWAL					
Crippa et al. (135)	Human: case study	Cannabis	CBD (600 mg)	MWC	↓
Allsop et al. (130)	Humans	Cannabis	THC:CBD (27:25 mg/ml) + psychosocial intervention	CWS	↓
Trigo et al. (123)	Human	Cannabis	THC:CBD (27:25 mg/ml) as needed + MET and CBT	MWC	–

(Continued)

TABLE 1 | Continued

Study	Sample	Substance	Treatment	Outcome	Effect
Hindocha et al. (126)	Humans	Nicotine	CBD (800 mg)	MPSS	–
de Carvalho and Takahashi (71)	Rats	Morphine	CBD (10 mg/kg)	CPP following naltrexone-precipitated withdrawal	↓
Hine et al. (136)	Rats	Morphine	CBD (10 mg/kg)	Abstinence symptoms	–
			THC:CBD (2:10 mg/kg)	Abstinence symptoms	↓
Bhargava (137)	Mice	Morphine	CBD (5 mg/kg)	Naloxone-precipitated withdrawal	↓
			CBD (10 mg/kg)	Naloxone-precipitated withdrawal	↓
			CBD (20 mg/kg)	Naloxone-precipitated withdrawal	↓
Chesher and Jackson (138)	Rats	Morphine	CBD (5 mg/kg)	Naloxone-precipitated withdrawal	–
			CBD (20 mg/kg)	Naloxone-precipitated withdrawal	–
			CBD (80 mg/kg)	Naloxone-precipitated withdrawal	–
REINSTATEMENT					
Drug-primed					
Ren et al. (115)	Rats	Heroin	CBD (5–20 mg/kg)	Self-administration	–
de Carvalho and Takahashi (71)	Rats	Morphine	CBD (10 mg/kg)	CPP	↓
Luján et al. (122)	Mice	Cocaine	CBD (20 mg/kg)	Self-administration	–
Karimi-Haghighi and Haghparast (139)	Rats	Methamphetamine	CBD (10 μg/5 μl)	CPP	↓
Hay et al. (134)	Rats	Methamphetamine	CBD (20 mg/kg)	Self-administration	–
			CBD (40 mg/kg)	Self-administration	–
			CBD (80 mg/kg)	Self-administration	↓
Context-induced					
Viudez-Martínez et al. (131)	Rats	Ethanol	CBD (60 mg/kg)	Self-administration	–
			CBD (120 mg/kg)	Self-administration	↓
Gonzalez-Cuevas et al. (140)	Rats	Alcohol	CBD (15 mg/kg)	Self-administration	↓
		Cocaine	CBD (15 mg/kg)	Self-administration	↓
		Cocaine	CBD (10 mg/kg)	CPP	↓
de Carvalho and Takahashi (71)	Rats	Morphine	CBD (5 mg/kg)	CPP	–
			CBD (10 mg/kg)	CPP	↓
Cue-induced					
Ren et al. (115)	Rats	Heroin	CBD (5–20 mg/kg)	Self-administration	↓
Mahmud et al. (133)	Rats	Cocaine	CBD (5 mg/kg)	Self-administration	–
			CBD (10 mg/kg)	Self-administration	–
Stress-induced					
Gonzalez-Cuevas et al. (140)	Rats	Alcohol	CBD (15 mg/kg)	Self-administration	↓
		Cocaine	CBD (15 mg/kg)	Self-administration	↓

**CBD, cannabidiol; THC, delta-9-tetrahydrocannabinol; MET, motivational enhancement therapy; CBT, cognitive behavioral therapy; MCQ, marijuana craving questionnaire; CEQ, Cannabis Experiences Questionnaire; TCQ, tiffany craving scale; QSU-B, questionnaire of smoking urges–brief; CPP, conditioned place preference; ICSS, intercranial self-stimulation; MWC, marijuana withdrawal checklist; CWS, cannabis withdrawal scale; MPSS, mood and physical symptoms scale craving.*

14 days of abstinence, with CBD's effect lasting up to 2 weeks post-administration (115).

Stimulants

Evidence of CBD efficacy for stimulant use is mixed. Neither CBD, nor a 1:1 ratio of THC:CBD reversed the cocaine sensitization effect (although rimonabant did) (54, 122). Some studies suggest that acute CBD administration does not block the reward-facilitating effect of cocaine (132), reduce cocaine self-administration, or attenuate cue-induced cocaine seeking in rats (133). However, others did find CBD to disrupt acquisition of cocaine self-administration and CPP (122), and impair drug-primed reinstatement of CPP for methamphetamine (139). Further studies on relapse are similarly mixed with one demonstrating CBD's ability to attenuate reconsolidation of CPP (1 week post-CPP acquisition) for cocaine in mice (71), and effectively reduce cue and stress-induced reinstatement of cocaine seeking up to 48 days post-CBD treatment (140), whilst another suggested no effect of CBD on drug-primed reinstatement post-extinction (122). Dose dependency may explain contradictory findings, as Hay et al. (134) demonstrated that 80 mg/kg (and not less) of CBD was needed to significantly reduce motivation to self-administer methamphetamine and reinstatement post-extinction. While evidence for CBD use for stimulant addiction in animals is weak, a longitudinal observational study of 122 participants did find cocaine users who self-report using cannabis to control their cocaine use, to have reduced their cocaine use over a 3 years period (147). Nevertheless, street cannabis generally has low amounts of CBD (148) and findings cannot be extrapolated to CBD's therapeutic efficacy.

The relatively weaker evidence of CBD in disrupting the reward-facilitating effect and self-administration of substances of abuse, despite its comparative efficacy in CPP reinstatement paradigms, may reflect its role in attenuating reward-related memory, without altering the rewarding properties of substances *per se*. Evidence of CBD's role in regulating emotional memory is supported by studies of other conditions, such as anxiety and PTSD-related fear memory [see (47) and (141) for a more extensive review of cannabinoid's role in emotional memory processing across other paradigms]. However, evidence of CBD's role in the consolidation and extinction of substance-related memory in humans is yet limited.

SUMMARY AND FUTURE DIRECTIONS

CBD shows some promise in alleviating negative withdrawal effects and reducing motivation to self-administer or reinstatement of drug use in animals. However, evidence on its efficacy is limited and mixed. CBD alone may not be sufficiently effective in maintaining long-term abstinence without ongoing support and behavioral therapy, as evidenced by its lack of efficacy over treatments, such as cognitive behavioral therapy and motivational enhancement therapy (123, 129). A combination of pharmacotherapy and behavioral therapy may increase treatment potency and adherence (149), and CBD may be better suited as an adjunct treatment to primary behavioral or psychosocial therapy (124).

There is also much that is unknown about how CBD may be targeting and alleviating SUD-related effects. Recent evidence suggests that within the mesolimbic system, CBD also influences the serotonergic system, as an agonist of the serotonin 1A (5-HT_{1A}) receptor (102, 103), which in addition to contributing to reduction in stress and anxiety (150), may be responsible for (i) blunting the reward-facilitating effect of substances of abuse (e.g., morphine in rats) (132); and (ii) modulating the formation of associative emotional memory related to substances of abuse (151). A number of studies have suggested the potential of selective serotonin reuptake inhibitors and other antidepressants in reducing substance (e.g., alcohol and nicotine) use via alleviating mood symptoms (152). CBD's capacity to alleviate stress, anxiety, and depressive symptoms may be mediating its treatment effect on SUDs (124, 153, 154). Indeed, CBD has been found to have therapeutic potential in alleviating affective and cognitive processing disturbances that may be induced by chronic substance (e.g., cannabis) use (63, 64, 155), proving potential utility in moderating the deleterious course of impairment, particularly in adolescent initiates of substance use (156). Additionally, other receptor and enzyme functions targeted by CBD, such as cannabinoid CB2Rs, non-cannabinoid transient receptor potential vanilloid type-1 (TRPV1) and type-2 (TRPV2) receptors, and ECS' catabolic enzymes FAAH and MAGL, should also be investigated for their role in the ECS and SUD (157–161).

In sum, some early research supports CBD's promise as pharmacotherapy against SUD. However, further investigation into CBD's mechanism of action, and validation of its efficacy, across preclinical and clinical trials will be necessary.

AUTHOR CONTRIBUTIONS

YC wrote the core sections of the manuscript with the assistance of EC. NS and MY provided intellectual input and edits.

REFERENCES

1. United Nations Office on Drugs and Crime. *World Drug Report 2017*. United Nations Publication, Sales No. E.17.XI.6 (2017).
2. Institute for Health Metrics and Evaluation. *Global Burden of Disease Data*. Available online at: www.healthdata.org
3. McLellan AT, Lewis DC, O'Brien CP, Kleber HD. Drug dependence, a chronic medical illness. *JAMA* (2000) 284:1689. doi: 10.1001/jama.284.13.1689
4. Pashaei T, Shojaeizadeh D, Rahimi Foroushani A, Ghazitabatabae M, Moeeni M, Rajati F, et al. Effectiveness of relapse prevention cognitive-behavioral model in opioid-dependent patients participating in the methadone maintenance treatment in Iran. *Iran J Public Health* (2013) 42:896–902.
5. Dermody SS, Wardell JD, Stoner SA, Hendershot CS. Predictors of daily adherence to naltrexone for alcohol use disorder treatment during a mobile health intervention. *Ann Behav Med.* (2018) 52:787–97. doi: 10.1093/abm/kax053
6. Goldstein RZ, Volkow ND. Dysfunction of the prefrontal cortex in addiction: neuroimaging findings and clinical implications. *Nat Rev Neurosci.* (2011) 12:652–69. doi: 10.1038/nrn3119
7. Volkow ND, Fowler JS, Wang G-J. The addicted brain: insights from imaging studies. *J Clin Invest.* (2003) 111:1444–51. doi: 10.1172/JCI18533
8. Svíženská I, Dubový P, Šulcová A. Cannabinoid receptors 1 and 2 (CB1 and CB2), their distribution, ligands and functional involvement in nervous system structures–a short review. *Pharmacol Biochem Behav.* (2008) 90:501–11. doi: 10.1016/j.pbb.2008.05.010
9. Gaoni Y, Mechoulam R. Isolation, structure, and partial synthesis of an active constituent of hashish. *J Am Chem Soc.* (1964) 86:1646–7. doi: 10.1021/ja01062a046
10. Di Marzo V, Bifulco M, De Petrocellis L. The endocannabinoid system and its therapeutic exploitation. *Nat Rev Drug Discov.* (2004) 3:771–84. doi: 10.1038/nrd1495
11. Herkenham M, Lynn AB, Little MD, Johnson MR, Melvin LS, de Costa BR, et al. Cannabinoid receptor localization in brain. *Proc Natl Acad Sci USA.* (1990) 87:1932–6. doi: 10.1073/pnas.87.5.1932

12. Terry GE, Liow J, Zoghbi SS, Hirvonen J, Farris AG, Lerner A, et al. Quantitation of cannabinoid CB1 receptors in healthy human brain using positron emission tomography and an inverse agonist radioligand. *Neuroimage* (2009) 48:362–70. doi: 10.1016/j.neuroimage.2009.06.059
13. McAllister SD, Glass M. CB1 and CB2 receptor-mediated signalling: a focus on endocannabinoids. *Prostaglandins Leukot Essent Fat Acids* (2002) 66:161–71. doi: 10.1054/plef.2001.0344
14. Lupica CR, Riegel AC. Endocannabinoid release from midbrain dopamine neurons: a potential substrate for cannabinoid receptor antagonist treatment of addiction. *Neuropharmacology* (2005) 48:1105–16. doi: 10.1016/j.neuropharm.2005.03.016
15. Gardner EL. Addictive potential of cannabinoids: the underlying neurobiology. *Chem Phys Lipids* (2002) 121:267–90. doi: 10.1016/S0009-3084(02)00162-7
16. Volkow ND, Wang G-J, Fowler JS, Logan J, Schlyer D, Hitzemann R, et al. Imaging endogenous dopamine competition with [11C]raclopride in the human brain. *Synapse* (1994) 16:255–62. doi: 10.1002/syn.890160402
17. Gardner EL. Endocannabinoid signaling system and brain reward: emphasis on dopamine. *Pharmacol Biochem Behav.* (2005) 81:263–84. doi: 10.1016/j.pbb.2005.01.032
18. Glass M, Dragunow M, Faull RL. Cannabinoid receptors in the human brain: a detailed anatomical and quantitative autoradiographic study in the fetal, neonatal and adult human brain. *Neuroscience* (1997) 77:299–318. doi: 10.1016/S0306-4522(96)00428-9
19. Robbe D, Kopf M, Remaury A, Bockaert J, Manzoni OJ. Endogenous cannabinoids mediate long-term synaptic depression in the nucleus accumbens. *Proc Natl Acad Sci USA.* (2002) 99:8384–8. doi: 10.1073/pnas.122149199
20. Riegel AC, Lupica CR. Independent presynaptic and postsynaptic mechanisms regulate endocannabinoid signaling at multiple synapses in the ventral tegmental area. *J Neurosci.* (2004) 24:11070–8. doi: 10.1523/JNEUROSCI.3695-04.2004
21. Cheer JF, Marsden CA., Kendall DA., Mason R. Lack of response suppression follows repeated ventral tegmental cannabinoid administration: an *in vitro* electrophysiological study. *Neuroscience* (2000) 99:661–7. doi: 10.1016/S0306-4522(00)00241-4
22. Pertwee RG. The diverse CB1 and CB2 receptor pharmacology of three plant cannabinoids: delta9-tetrahydrocannabinol, cannabidiol and delta9-tetrahydrocannabivarin. *Br J Pharmacol.* (2008) 153:199–215. doi: 10.1038/sj.bjp.0707442
23. Bossong MG, Mehta MA, Berckel BNM Van, Howes OD, S Kahn RS, Stokes PRA. Further human evidence for striatal dopamine release induced by administration of Δ9-tetrahydrocannabinol (THC): selectivity to limbic striatum. *Psychopharmacology (Berl).* (2015) 232:2723–9. doi: 10.1007/s00213-015-3915-0
24. Mascia MS, Obinu MC, Ledent C, Parmentier M, Böhme GA, Imperato A, et al. Lack of morphine-induced dopamine release in the nucleus accumbens of cannabinoid CB1receptor knockout mice. *Eur J Pharmacol.* (1999) 383:99–100.
25. Wang H, Treadway T, Covey DP, Cheer JF, Lupica CR. Cocaine-induced endocannabinoid mobilization in the ventral tegmental area. *Cell Rep.* (2015) 12:1997–2008. doi: 10.1016/j.celrep.2015.08.041
26. Serrano A, Rivera P, Pavon FJ, Decara J, Suárez J, Rodriguez de Fonseca F, et al. Differential effects of single versus repeated alcohol withdrawal on the expression of endocannabinoid system-related genes in the rat amygdala. *Alcohol Clin Exp Res.* (2012) 36:984–94. doi: 10.1111/j.1530-0277.2011.01686.x
27. Basavarajappa BS, Saito M, Cooper TB, Hungund BL. Stimulation of cannabinoid receptor agonist 2-arachidonylglycerol by chronic ethanol and its modulation by specific neuromodulators in cerebellar granule neurons. *Biochim Biophys Acta* (2000) 1535:78–86. doi: 10.1016/S0925-4439(00)00085-5
28. Basavarajappa BS, Saito M, Cooper TB, Hungund BL. Chronic ethanol inhibits the anandamide transport and increases extracellular anandamide levels in cerebellar granule neurons. *Eur J Pharmacol.* (2003) 466:73–83. doi: 10.1016/S0014-2999(03)01557-7
29. Ortiz S, Oliva JM, Pérez-Rial S, Palomo T, Manzanares J. Chronic ethanol consumption regulates cannabinoid CB1 receptor gene expression in selected regions of rat brain. *Alcohol Alcohol.* (2004) 39:88–92. doi: 10.1093/alcalc/agh036
30. Hungund BL, Szakall I, Adam A, Basavarajappa BS, Vadasz C. Cannabinoid CB1 receptor knockout mice exhibit markedly reduced voluntary alcohol consumption and lack alcohol-induced dopamine release in the nucleus accumbens. *J Neurochem.* (2003) 84:698–704. doi: 10.1046/j.1471-4159.2003.01576.x
31. Gamaleddin IH, Trigo JM, Gueye AB, Zvonok A, Makriyannis A, Goldberg SR, et al. Role of the endogenous cannabinoid system in nicotine addiction: novel insights. *Front Psychiatry* (2015) 6:1–12. doi: 10.3389/fpsyt.2015.00041
32. Pickel VM, Chan J, Kash TL, Rodríguez JJ, Mackie K. Compartment-specific localization of cannabinoid 1 (CB1) and μ-opioid receptors in rat nucleus accumbens. *Neuroscience* (2004) 127:101–12. doi: 10.1016/j.neuroscience.2004.05.015
33. Rios C, Gomes I, Devi LA. μ opioid and CB1 cannabinoid receptor interactions: reciprocal inhibition of receptor signaling and neuritogenesis. *Br J Pharmacol.* (2009) 148:387–95. doi: 10.1038/sj.bjp.0706757
34. Corchero J, Fuentes JA, Manzanares J. Chronic treatment with CP-55,940 regulates corticotropin releasing factor and proopiomelanocortin gene expression in the hypothalamus and pituitary gland of the rat. *Life Sci.* (1999) 64:905–11. doi: 10.1016/S0024-3205(99)00016-8
35. Maldonado R, Valverde O, Berrendero F. Involvement of the endocannabinoid system in drug addiction. *Trends Neurosci.* (2006) 29:225–32. doi: 10.1016/j.tins.2006.01.008
36. French ED. Δ9-Tetrahydrocannabinol excites rat VTA dopamine neurons through activation of cannabinoid CB1 but not opioid receptors. *Neurosci Lett.* (1997) 226:159–62. doi: 10.1016/S0304-3940(97)00278-4
37. Braida D, Iosuè S, Pegorini S, Sala M. Δ9-Tetrahydrocannabinol-induced conditioned place preference and intracerebroventricular self-administration in rats. *Eur J Pharmacol.* (2004) 506:63–9. doi: 10.1016/j.ejphar.2004.10.043
38. Linsenbardt DN, Boehm SL. Agonism of the endocannabinoid system modulates binge-like alcohol intake in male C57BL/6J mice: involvement of the posterior ventral tegmental area. *Neuroscience* (2009) 164:424–34. doi: 10.1016/j.neuroscience.2009.08.007
39. Lupica CR, Riegel AC, Hoffman AF. Marijuana and cannabinoid regulation of brain reward circuits. *Br J Pharmacol.* (2004) 143:227–34. doi: 10.1038/sj.bjp.0705931
40. González S, Fernández-Ruiz J, Sparpaglione V, Parolaro D, Ramos JA. Chronic exposure to morphine, cocaine or ethanol in rats produced different effects in brain cannabinoid CB1 receptor binding and mRNA levels. *Drug Alcohol Depend.* (2002) 66:77–84. doi: 10.1016/S0376-8716(01)00186-7
41. Solinas M, Yasar S, Goldberg SR. Endocannabinoid system involvement in brain reward processes related to drug abuse. *Pharmacol Res.* (2007) 56:393–405. doi: 10.1016/j.phrs.2007.09.005
42. Di Chiara G, Imperato A. Drugs abused by humans preferentially increase synaptic dopamine concentration in the mesolimbic system of freely moving rats. *Proc Natl Acad Sci USA.* (1988) 85:5274–8. doi: 10.1073/pnas.85.14.5274
43. Melis M, Pstis M, Perra S, Muntoni AL, Pillolla G, Gessa GL. Endocannabinoids mediate presynaptic inhibition of glutamatergic transmission in rat ventral tegmental area dopamine neurons through activation of CB1 receptors. *J Neurosci.* (2004) 24:53–62. doi: 10.1523/JNEUROSCI.4503-03.2004
44. Volkow ND, Fowler JS. Addiction, a disease of compulsion and drive: involvement of the orbitofrontal cortex. *Cereb Cortex* (2000) 10:318–25. doi: 10.1093/cercor/10.3.318
45. Pontieri FE, Tanda G, Orzi F, Di Chiara G. Effects of nicotine on the nucleus accumbens and similarity to those of addictive drugs. *Nature* (1996) 382:255–7. doi: 10.1038/382255a0
46. Koob GF, Bloom FE. Cellular and molecular mechanisms of drug dependence. *Science* (1988) 242:715–23. doi: 10.1126/science.2903550
47. Fischman MW, Schuster CR, Javaid J, Hatano Y, Davis J. Acute tolerance development to the cardiovascular and subjective effects of cocaine. *J Pharmacol Exp Ther.* (1985) 235:677–82.
48. Hyman SE, Malenka RC. Addiction and the brain: the neurobiology of compulsion and its persistence. *Nat Rev Neurosci.* (2001) 2:695–703. doi: 10.1038/35094560

49. Robinson TE, Berridge KC. The psychology and neurobiology of addiction: an incentive-sensitization view. *Addiction* (2000) 95 Suppl. 2:S91–117. doi: 10.1046/j.1360-0443.95.8s2.19.x
50. Gerdeman GL, Partridge JG, Lupica CR, Lovinger DM. It could be habit forming: drugs of abuse and striatal synaptic plasticity. *Trends Neurosci.* (2003) 26:184–92. doi: 10.1016/S0166-2236(03)00065-1
51. Waelti P, Dickinson A, Schultz W. Dopamine responses comply with basic assumptions of formal learning theory. *Nature* (2001) 412:43–8. doi: 10.1038/35083500
52. Berridge KC, Robinson TE. What is the role of dopamine in reward: hedonic impact, reward learning, or incentive salience? *Brain Res Rev.* (1998) 28:309–69. doi: 10.1016/S0165-0173(98)00019-8
53. De Vries TJ, Schoffelmeer ANM. Cannabinoid CB1 receptors control conditioned drug seeking. *Trends Pharmacol Sci.* (2005) 26:420–6. doi: 10.1016/j.tips.2005.06.002
54. Gerdeman GL, Schechter JB, French ED. Context-specific reversal of cocaine sensitization by the CB1 cannabinoid receptor antagonist rimonabant. *Neuropsychopharmacology* (2008) 33:2747–59. doi: 10.1038/sj.npp.1301648
55. Sloan ME, Gowin JL, Ramchandani VA, Hurd YL, Le Foll B. The endocannabinoid system as a target for addiction treatment: trials and tribulations. *Neuropharmacology* (2017) 124:73–83. doi: 10.1016/j.neuropharm.2017.05.031
56. Hoffman AF, Riegel AC, Lupica CR. Functional localization of cannabinoid receptors and endogenous cannabinoid production in distinct neuron populations of the hippocampus. *Eur J Neurosci.* (2003) 18:524–34. doi: 10.1046/j.1460-9568.2003.02773.x
57. Stern CAJ, Carvalho CR de, Bertoglio LJ, Takahashi RN. Effects of cannabinoid drugs on aversive or rewarding drug-associated memory extinction and reconsolidation. *Neuroscience* (2018) 370:62–80. doi: 10.1016/j.neuroscience.2017.07.018
58. Parsons LH, Hurd YL. Endocannabinoid signalling in reward and addiction. *Nat Rev Neurosci.* (2015) 16:579–94. doi: 10.1038/nrn4004
59. Brancato A, Cavallaro A, Lavanco G, Plescia F, Cannizzaro C. Reward-related limbic memory and stimulation of the cannabinoid system: an upgrade in value attribution? *J Psychopharmacol.* (2018) 32:204–14. doi: 10.1177/0269881117725683
60. Brancato A, Lavanco G, Cavallaro A, Plescia F, Cannizzaro C. The use of the emotional-object recognition as an assay to assess learning and memory associated to an aversive stimulus in rodents. *J Neurosci Methods* (2016) 274:106–15. doi: 10.1016/j.jneumeth.2016.09.010
61. Campolongo P, Ratano P, Manduca A, Scattoni ML, Palmery M, Trezza V, et al. The endocannabinoid transport inhibitor AM404 differentially modulates recognition memory in rats depending on environmental aversiveness. *Front Behav Neurosci.* (2012) 6:1–10. doi: 10.3389/fnbeh.2012.00011
62. Draycott B, Loureiro M, Ahmad T, Tan H, Zunder J, Laviolette SR. Cannabinoid transmission in the prefrontal cortex bi-phasically controls emotional memory formation via functional interactions with the ventral tegmental area. *J Neurosci.* (2014) 34:13096–109. doi: 10.1523/JNEUROSCI.1297-14.2014
63. Fusar-Poli P, Crippa JA, Bhattacharyya S, Bogwardt SJ, Allen P, Martin-Santos R, et al. Distinct effects of D9-tetrahydrocannabinol and cannabidiol on neural activation during emotional processing. *Arch Gen Psychiatry* (2009) 66:95–105. doi: 10.1001/archgenpsychiatry.2008.519
64. Bhattacharyya S, Morrison PD, Fusar-Poli P, Martin-Santos R, Borgwardt S, Winton-Brown T, et al. Opposite effects of Δ-9-tetrahydrocannabinol and cannabidiol on human brain function and psychopathology. *Neuropsychopharmacology* (2010) 35:764–74. doi: 10.1038/npp.2009.184
65. Heifets BD, Castillo PE. Endocannabinoid signaling and long-term synaptic plasticity. *Annu Rev Physiol.* (2009) 71:283–306. doi: 10.1146/annurev.physiol.010908.163149
66. Hyman SE, Malenka RC, Nestler EJ. Neural mechanisms of addiction: the role of reward-related learning and memory. *Annu Rev Neurosci.* (2006) 29:565–98. doi: 10.1146/annurev.neuro.29.051605.113009
67. Chambers RA. Impulsivity, dual diagnosis, and the structure of motivated behavior in addiction. *Behav Brain Sci.* (2008) 31:443–4. doi: 10.1017/S0140525X08004792
68. Lee JLC, Bertoglio LJ, Guimarães FS, Stevenson CW. Cannabidiol regulation of emotion and emotional memory processing: relevance for treating anxiety-related and substance abuse disorders. *Br J Pharmacol.* (2017) 174:3242–56. doi: 10.1111/bph.13724
69. Yu L, Wang X, Zhao M, Liu Y, Li Y, Li F, et al. Effects of cannabinoid CB1 receptor antagonist rimonabant in consolidation and reconsolidation of methamphetamine reward memory in mice. *Psychopharmacology (Berl).* (2009) 204:203–11. doi: 10.1007/s00213-008-1450-y
70. Hu SS, Liu Y, Yu L. Medial prefrontal cannabinoid CB 1 receptors modulate consolidation and extinction of cocaine-associated memory in mice. *Psychopharmacology (Berl).* (2015) 232:1803–15. doi: 10.1007/s00213-014-3812-y
71. de Carvalho CR, Takahashi RN. Cannabidiol disrupts the reconsolidation of contextual drug-associated memories in Wistar rats. *Addict Biol.* (2017) 22:742–51. doi: 10.1111/adb.12366
72. Colombo G, Serra S, Brunetti G, Gomez R, Melis S, Vacca G, et al. Stimulation of voluntary ethanol intake by cannabinoid receptor agonists in ethanol-preferring sP rats. *Psychopharmacology (Berl).* (2002) 159:181–7. doi: 10.1007/s002130100887
73. Thanos PK, Dimitrakakis ES, Rice O, Gifford A, Volkow ND. Ethanol self-administration and ethanol conditioned place preference are reduced in mice lacking cannabinoid CB1 receptors. *Behav Brain Res.* (2005) 164:206–13. doi: 10.1016/j.bbr.2005.06.021
74. Houchi H, Babovic D, Pierrefiche O, Ledent C, Daoust M, Naassila M. CB1 receptor knockout mice display reduced ethanol-induced conditioned place preference and increased striatal dopamine D2 receptors. *Neuropsychopharmacology* (2005) 30:339–49. doi: 10.1038/sj.npp.1300568
75. Gamaleddin I, Wertheim C, Zhu AZX, Coen KM, Vemuri K, Makryannis A, et al. Cannabinoid receptor stimulation increases motivation for nicotine and nicotine seeking. *Addict Biol.* (2012) 17:47–61. doi: 10.1111/j.1369-1600.2011.00314.x
76. Solinas M, Panlilio LV, Goldberg SR. Exposure to Δ-9-tetrahydrocannabinol (THC) increases subsequent heroin taking but not heroin's reinforcing efficacy: a self-administration study in rats. *Neuropsychopharmacology* (2004) 29:1301–11. doi: 10.1038/sj.npp.1300431
77. Solinas M, Panlilio LV, Tanda G, Makriyannis A, Matthews SA, Goldberg SR. Cannabinoid agonists but not inhibitors of endogenous cannabinoid transport or metabolism enhance the reinforcing efficacy of heroin in rats. *Neuropsychopharmacology* (2005) 30:2046–57. doi: 10.1038/sj.npp.1300754
78. Levin FR, Mariani JJ, Brooks DJ, Pavlicova M, Cheng W, Nunes EV. Dronabinol for the treatment of cannabis dependence: A randomized, double-blind, placebo-controlled trial. *Drug Alcohol Depend.* (2011) 116:142–50. doi: 10.1016/j.drugalcdep.2010.12.010
79. Vandrey R, Stitzer ML, Mintzer MZ, Huestis MA, Murray JA, Lee D. The dose effects of short-term dronabinol (oral THC) maintenance in daily cannabis users. *Drug Alcohol Depend.* (2013) 128:64–70. doi: 10.1016/j.drugalcdep.2012.08.001
80. Herrmann ES, Cooper ZD, Bedi G, Ramesh D, Reed SC, Comer SD, et al. Effects of zolpidem alone and in combination with nabilone on cannabis withdrawal and a laboratory model of relapse in cannabis users. *Psychopharmacology (Berl).* (2016) 233:2469–78. doi: 10.1007/s00213-016-4298-6
81. Maccioni P, Colombo G, Carai MA. Blockade of the cannabinoid CB1 receptor and alcohol dependence: preclinical evidence and preliminary clinical data. *CNS Neurol Disord Drug Targets* (2010) 9:55–9. doi: 10.2174/187152710790966623
82. Arnone M, Maruani J, Chaperon F, Thiébot MH, Poncelet M, Soubrié P, et al. Selective inhibition of sucrose and ethanol intake by SR 141716, an antagonist of central cannabinoid (CB1) receptors. *Psychopharmacology (Berl).* (1997) 132:104–6.
83. Diergaarde L, de Vries W, Raasø H, Schoffelmeer ANM, De Vries TJ. Contextual renewal of nicotine seeking in rats and its suppression by the cannabinoid-1 receptor antagonist Rimonabant (SR141716A). *Neuropharmacology* (2008) 55:712–6. doi: 10.1016/j.neuropharm.2008.06.003
84. Cohen C, Perrault G, Griebel G, Soubrié P. Nicotine-associated cues maintain nicotine-seeking behavior in rats several weeks after nicotine withdrawal: reversal by the cannabinoid (CB1) receptor antagonist, rimonabant (SR141716). *Neuropsychopharmacology* (2005) 30:145–55. doi: 10.1038/sj.npp.1300541

85. De Vries TJ, Homberg JR, Binnekade R, Raasø H, Schoffelmeer ANM. Cannabinoid modulation of the reinforcing and motivational properties of heroin and heroin-associated cues in rats. *Psychopharmacology (Berl).* (2003) 168:164–9. doi: 10.1007/s00213-003-1422-1
86. Cohen C, Perrault G, Voltz C, Steinberg R, Soubrié P. SR141716, a central cannabinoid (CB1) receptor antagonist, blocks the motivational and dopamine-releasing effects of nicotine in rats. *Behav Pharmacol.* (2002) 13:451–63. doi: 10.1097/00008877-200209000-00018
87. Braida D, Iosuè S, Pegorini S, Sala M. 3,4 Methylenedioxymethamphetamine-induced conditioned place preference (CPP) is mediated by endocannabinoid system. *Pharmacol Res.* (2005) 51:177–82. doi: 10.1016/j.phrs.2004.07.009
88. Chaperon F, Soubrié P, Puech AJ, Thiébot MH. Involvement of central cannabinoid (CB1) receptors in the establishment of place conditioning in rats. *Psychopharmacology (Berl).* (1998) 135:324–32.
89. De Vries TJ, Shaham Y, Homberg JR, Crombag H, Schuurman K, Dieben J, et al. A cannabinoid mechanism in relapse to cocaine seeking. *Nat Med.* (2001) 7:1151–4. doi: 10.1038/nm1001-1151
90. Cossu G, Ledent C, Fattore L, Imperato A, Böhme GA, Parmentier M, et al. Cannabinoid CB1 receptor knockout mice fail to self-administer morphine but not other drugs of abuse. *Behav Brain Res.* (2001) 118:61–5. doi: 10.1016/S0166-4328(00)00311-9
91. Caillé S, Parsons LH. Cannabinoid modulation of opiate reinforcement through the ventral striatopallidal pathway. *Neuropsychopharmacology* (2006) 31:804–13. doi: 10.1038/sj.npp.1300848
92. Soria G, Mendizábal V, Touriño C, Robledo P, Ledent C, Parmentier M, et al. Lack of CBI cannabinoid receptor impairs cocaine self-administration. *Neuropsychopharmacology* (2005) 30:1670–80. doi: 10.1038/sj.npp.1300707
93. Huestis MA, Boyd SJ, Heishman SJ, Preston KL, Bonnet D, Le Fur G, et al. Single and multiple doses of rimonabant antagonize acute effects of smoked cannabis in male cannabis users. *Psychopharmacology (Berl).* (2007) 194:505–15. doi: 10.1007/s00213-007-0861-5
94. Gorelick DA, Heishman SJ, Preston KL, Nelson RA, Moolchan ET, Huestis MA. The cannabinoid CB1 receptor antagonist rimonabant attenuates the hypotensive effect of smoked marijuana in male smokers. *Am Heart J.* (2006) 151:1–5. doi: 10.1016/j.ahj.2005.11.006
95. Cahill K, Ussher MH. Cannabinoid type 1 receptor antagonists for smoking cessation. *Cochrane Database Syst Rev.* (2011) 2017:1–26. doi: 10.1002/14651858.CD005353.pub4
96. Soyka M, Koller G, Schmidt P, Lesch OM, Leweke M, Fehr C, et al. Cannabinoid receptor 1 blocker rimonabant (SR 141716) for treatment of alcohol dependence: results from a placebo-controlled, double-blind trial. *J Clin Psychopharmacol.* (2008) 28:317–24. doi: 10.1097/JCP.0b013e318172b8bc
97. Cohen RA, Harezlak J, Schifitto G, Hana G, Clark U, Gongvatana A, et al. Effects of nadir CD4 count and duration of human immunodeficiency virus infection on brain volumes in the highly active antiretroviral therapy era. *J Neurovirol.* (2010) 16:25–32. doi: 10.3109/13550280903552420
98. Christensen R, Kristensen PK, Bartels EM, Bliddal H, Astrup A. Efficacy and safety of the weight-loss drug rimonabant: a meta-analysis of randomised trials. *Lancet* (2007) 370:1706–13. doi: 10.1016/S0140-6736(07) 61721-8
99. Pertwee RG. Cannabinoid pharmacology: the first 66 years. *Br J Pharmacol.* (2006) 147:S163–71. doi: 10.1038/sj.bjp.0706406
100. Santos RG dos, Hallak JEC, Zuardi AW, Crippa JA de S. Cannabidiol for the treatment of drug use disorders. In: V. P. Preedy, Editor. *Handbook of Cannabis and Related Pathologies*, London: Elsevier Inc. (2017). p. 939–46.
101. Kathmann M, Flau K, Redmer A, Tränkle C, Schlicker E. Cannabidiol is an allosteric modulator at mu- and delta-opioid receptors. *Arch Pharmacol.* (2006) 372:354–61. doi: 10.1007/s00210-006-0033-x
102. Russo EB, Burnett A, Hall B, Parker KK. Agonistic properties of cannabidiol at 5-HT1a receptors. *Neurochem Res.* (2005) 30:1037–43. doi: 10.1007/s11064-005-6978-1
103. Campos AC, Guimarães FS. Involvement of 5HT1A receptors in the anxiolytic-like effects of cannabidiol injected into the dorsolateral periaqueductal gray of rats. *Psychopharmacology (Berl).* (2008) 199:223–30. doi: 10.1007/s00213-008-1168-x
104. Thomas A, Baillie GL, Phillips AM, Razdan RK, Ross RA, Pertwee RG. Cannabidiol displays unexpectedly high potency as an antagonist of CB1 and CB2 receptor agonists *in vitro*. *Br J Pharmacol.* (2007) 150:613–23. doi: 10.1038/sj.bjp.0707133
105. Laprairie RB, Bagher AM, Kelly MEM, Denovan-Wright EM. Cannabidiol is a negative allosteric modulator of the cannabinoid CB 1 receptor. *Br J Pharmacol.* (2015) 172:4790–805. doi: 10.1111/bph.13250
106. Tham M, Yilmaz O, Alaverdashvili M, Kelly MEM, Denovan-wright EM, Laprairie RB. Allosteric and orthosteric pharmacology of cannabidiol and cannabidiol-dimethylheptyl at the type 1 and type 2 cannabinoid receptors. *Br J Pharmacol.* (2018). doi: 10.1111/bph.14440. [Epub ahead of print].
107. Straiker A, Dvorakova M, Zimmowitch A, Mackie K. Cannabidiol inhibits endocannabinoid signaling in autaptic hippocampal neurons. *Mol Pharmacol.* (2018) 94:743–8. doi: 10.1124/mol.118.111864
108. Bergamaschi MM, Queiroz RHC, Zuardi AW, Crippa JAS. Safety and side effects of cannabidiol, a Cannabis sativa constituent. *Curr Drug Saf.* (2011) 6:237–49. doi: 10.2174/157488611798280924
109. Rohleder C, Müller JK, Lange B, Leweke FM. Cannabidiol as a potential new type of an antipsychotic. A critical review of the evidence. *Front Pharmacol.* (2016) 7:422. doi: 10.3389/fphar.2016.00422
110. Iffland K, Grotenhermen F. An update on safety and side effects of cannabidiol: a review of clinical data and relevant animal studies. *Cannabis Cannabinoid Res.* (2017) 2:139–54. doi: 10.1089/can.2016.0034
111. Taylor L, Gidal B, Blakey G, Tayo B, Morrison G. A phase I, randomized, double-blind, placebo-controlled, single ascending dose, multiple dose, and food effect trial of the safety, tolerability and pharmacokinetics of highly purified cannabidiol in healthy subjects. *CNS Drugs* (2018) 32:1053–67. doi: 10.1007/s40263-018-0578-5
112. Babalonis S, Haney M, Malcolm RJ, Lofwall MR, Votaw VR, Sparenborg S, et al. Oral cannabidiol does not produce a signal for abuse liability in frequent marijuana smokers. *Drug Alcohol Depend.* (2017) 172:9–13. doi: 10.1016/j.drugalcdep.2016.11.030
113. Parker LA, Burton P, Sorge RE, Yakiwchuk C, Mechoulam R. Effect of low doses of Δ9-tetrahydrocannabinol and cannabidiol on the extinction of cocaine-induced and amphetamine-induced conditioned place preference learning in rats. *Psychopharmacology (Berl).* (2004) 175:360–6. doi: 10.1007/s00213-004-1825-7
114. Murillo-Rodríguez E, Palomero-Rivero M, Millán-Aldaco D, Mechoulam R, Drucker-Colín R. Effects on sleep and dopamine levels of microdialysis perfusion of cannabidiol into the lateral hypothalamus of rats. *Life Sci.* (2011) 88:504–11. doi: 10.1016/j.lfs.2011.01.013
115. Ren Y, Whittard J, Higuera-Matas A, Morris CV, Hurd YL. Cannabidiol, a nonpsychotropic component of cannabis, inhibits cue-induced heroin seeking and normalizes discrete mesolimbic neuronal disturbances. *J Neurosci.* (2009) 29:14764–9. doi: 10.1523/JNEUROSCI.4291-09.2009
116. Renard J, Loureiro M, Rosen LG, Zunder J, de Oliveira C, Schmid S, et al. Cannabidiol counteracts amphetamine-induced neuronal and behavioral sensitization of the mesolimbic dopamine pathway through a novel mTOR/p70S6 kinase signaling pathway. *J Neurosci.* (2016) 36:5160–9. doi: 10.1523/JNEUROSCI.3387-15.2016
117. Zuardi AW, Hallak JEC, Crippa JAS. Interaction between cannabidiol (CBD) and Δ9-tetrahydrocannabinol (THC): influence of administration interval and dose ratio between the cannabinoids. *Psychopharmacology (Berl).* (2012) 219:247–9. doi: 10.1007/s00213-011-2495-x
118. Fischer B, Kuganesan S, Gallassi A, Malcher-Lopes R, van den Brink W, Wood E. Addressing the stimulant treatment gap: a call to investigate the therapeutic benefits potential of cannabinoids for crack-cocaine use. *Int J Drug Policy* (2015) 26:1177–82. doi: 10.1016/j.drugpo.2015.09.005
119. Hurd YL, Yoon M, Manini AF, Hernandez S, Olmedo R, Ostman M, et al. Early phase in the development of cannabidiol as a treatment for addiction: opioid relapse takes initial center stage. *Neurotherapeutics* (2015) 12:807–15. doi: 10.1007/s13311-015-0373-7
120. Hurd YL. Cannabidiol: swinging the marijuana pendulum from 'weed' to medication to treat the opioid epidemic. *Trends Neurosci.* (2017) 40:124–7. doi: 10.1016/j.tins.2016.12.006
121. Filev R, Engelke DS, Da Silveira DX, Mello LE, Santos-Junior JG. THC inhibits the expression of ethanol-induced locomotor sensitization in mice. *Alcohol* (2017) 65:31–5. doi: 10.1016/j.alcohol.2017.06.004

122. Luján MÁ, Castro-Zavala A, Alegre-Zurano L, Valverde O. Repeated Cannabidiol treatment reduces cocaine intake and modulates neural proliferation and CB1R expression in the mouse hippocampus. *Neuropharmacology* (2018) 143:163–75. doi: 10.1016/j.neuropharm.2018.09.043
123. Trigo JM, Soliman A, Quilty LC, Fischer B, Selby P, Barnes AJ, et al. Nabiximols combined with motivational enhancement/cognitive behavioral therapy for the treatment of cannabis dependence: a pilot randomized clinical trial. *PLoS ONE* (2018) 13:e0190768. doi: 10.1371/journal.pone.0190768
124. Solowij N, Broyd SJ, Beale C, Prick J-A, Greenwood L, van Hell H, et al. Therapeutic effects of prolonged cannabidiol treatment on psychological symptoms and cognitive function in regular cannabis users: a pragmatic open-label clinical trial. *Cannabis Cannabinoid Res.* (2018) 3:21–34. doi: 10.1089/can.2017.0043
125. Morgan CJA, Das RK, Joye A, Curran HV, Kamboj SK. Cannabidiol reduces cigarette consumption in tobacco smokers: preliminary findings. *Addict Behav.* (2013) 38:2433–6. doi: 10.1016/j.addbeh.2013.03.011
126. Hindocha C, Freeman TP, Grabski M, Stroud JB, Crudgington H, Davies AC, et al. Cannabidiol reverses attentional bias to cigarette cues in a human experimental model of tobacco withdrawal. *Addiction* (2018) 113:1696–705. doi: 10.1111/add.14243
127. Markos JR, Harris HM, Gul W, Elsohly MA, Sufka KJ. Effects of cannabidiol on morphine conditioned place preference in mice. *Planta Med.* (2018) 84:221–4. doi: 10.1055/s-0043-117838
128. Shannon S, Opila-lehman J. Cannabidiol oil for decreasing addictive use of marijuana: a case report. *Integr Med.* (2015) 14:31–5.
129. Trigo JM, Soliman A, Staios G, Quilty L, Fischer B, George TP, et al. Sativex associated with behavioral-relapse prevention strategy as treatment for cannabis dependence: a case series. *J Addict Med.* (2016) 10:274–9. doi: 10.1097/ADM.0000000000000229
130. Allsop DJ, Copeland J, Lintzeris N, Dunlop AJ, Montebello M, Sadler C, et al. Nabiximols as an agonist replacement therapy during cannabis withdrawal: a randomized clinical trial. *JAMA Psychiatry* (2014) 71:281–91. doi: 10.1001/jamapsychiatry.2013.3947
131. Viudez-Martínez A, García-Gutiérrez MS, Navarrón CM, Morales-Calero MI, Navarrete F, Torres-Suárez AI, et al. Cannabidiol reduces ethanol consumption, motivation and relapse in mice. *Addict Biol.* (2018) 23:154–64. doi: 10.1111/adb.12495
132. Katsidoni V, Anagnostou I, Panagis G. Cannabidiol inhibits the reward-facilitating effect of morphine: involvement of 5-HT 1A receptors in the dorsal raphe nucleus. *Addict Biol.* (2013) 18:286–96. doi: 10.1111/j.1369-1600.2012.00483.x
133. Mahmud A, Gallant S, Sedki F, D'Cunha T, Shalev U. Effects of an acute cannabidiol treatment on cocaine self-administration and cue-induced cocaine seeking in male rats. *J Psychopharmacol.* (2017) 31:96–104. doi: 10.1177/0269881116667706
134. Hay GL, Baracz SJ, Everett NA, Roberts J, Costa PA, Arnold JC, et al. Cannabidiol treatment reduces the motivation to self-administer methamphetamine and methamphetamine-primed relapse in rats. *J Psychopharmacol.* (2018) 32:1369–78. doi: 10.1177/0269881118799954
135. Crippa JAS, Hallak JEC, Machado-de-Sousa JP, Queiroz RHC, Bergamaschi M, Chagas MHN, et al. Cannabidiol for the treatment of cannabis withdrawal syndrome: a case report. *J Clin Pharm Ther.* (2013) 38:162–4. doi: 10.1111/jcpt.12018
136. Hine B, Torrelio M, Gershon S. Interactions between cannabidiol and Δ9-THC during abstinence in morphine-dependent rats. *Life Sci.* (1975) 17:851–8. doi: 10.1016/0024-3205(75)90435-X
137. Bhargava HN. Effect of some cannabinoids on naloxone-precipitated abstinence in morphine-dependent mice. *Psychopharmacology (Berl).* (1976) 49:267–70. doi: 10.1007/BF00426828
138. Chesher GB, Jackson DM. The quasi-morphine withdrawal syndrome: effect of cannabinol, cannabidiol and tetrahydrocannabinol. *Pharmacol Biochem Behav.* (1985) 23:13–5. doi: 10.1016/0091-3057(85)90122-4
139. Karimi-Haghighi S, Haghparast A. Cannabidiol inhibits priming-induced reinstatement of methamphetamine in REM sleep deprived rats. *Prog Neuro-Psychopharmacology Biol Psychiatry* (2018) 82:307–13. doi: 10.1016/j.pnpbp.2017.08.022
140. Gonzalez-Cuevas G, Martin-Fardon R, Kerr TM, Stouffer DG, Parsons LH, Hammell DC, et al. Unique treatment potential of cannabidiol for the prevention of relapse to drug use: preclinical proof of principle. *Neuropsychopharmacology* (2018) 43:2036–45. doi: 10.1038/s41386-018-0050-8
141. Budney AJ, Vandrey RG, Stanger C. Pharmacological and psychosocial interventions for cannabis use disorders. *Rev Bras Psiquiatr.* (2010) 32:46–55. doi: 10.1590/S1516-44462010000500008
142. Vann RE, Gamage TF, Warner JA, Marshall EM, Taylor NL, Martin BR, et al. Divergent effects of cannabidiol on the discriminative stimulus and place conditioning effects of Δ9-tetrahydrocannabinol. *Drug Alcohol Depend.* (2008) 94:191–8. doi: 10.1016/j.drugalcdep.2007.11.017
143. Robson P. Abuse potential and psychoactive effects of δ-9-tetrahydrocannabinol and cannabidiol oromucosal spray (Sativex), a new cannabinoid medicine. *Expert Opin Drug Saf.* (2011) 10:675–85. doi: 10.1517/14740338.2011.575778
144. Trigo JM, Lagzdins D, Rehm J, Selby P, Gamaleddin I, Fischer B, et al. Effects of fixed or self-titrated dosages of Sativex on cannabis withdrawal and cravings. *Drug Alcohol Depend.* (2016) 161:298–306. doi: 10.1016/j.drugalcdep.2016.02.020
145. Allsop DJ, Lintzeris N, Copeland J, Dunlop A, McGregor IS. Cannabinoid replacement therapy (CRT): Nabiximols (Sativex) as a novel treatment for cannabis withdrawal. *Clin Pharmacol Ther.* (2015) 97:571–4. doi: 10.1002/cpt.109
146. Schoedel KA, Chen N, Hilliard A, White L, Stott C, Russo E, et al. A randomized, double-blind, placebo-controlled, crossover study to evaluate the subjective abuse potential and cognitive effects of nabiximols oromucosal spray in subjects with a history of recreational cannabis use. *Hum Psychopharmacol Clin Exp.* (2011) 26:224–36. doi: 10.1002/hup.1196
147. Socías ME, Kerr T, Wood E, Dong H, Lake S, Hayashi K, et al. Intentional cannabis use to reduce crack cocaine use in a Canadian setting: a longitudinal analysis. *Addict Behav.* (2017) 72:138–43. doi: 10.1016/j.addbeh.2017.04.006
148. Swift W, Wong A, Li KM, Arnold JC, McGregor IS. Analysis of cannabis seizures in NSW, Australia: cannabis potency and cannabinoid profile. *PLoS ONE* (2013) 8:e0070052. doi: 10.1371/journal.pone.0070052
149. Carroll KM, Onken LS. Behavioral therapies for drug abuse. *Am J Psychiatry* (2005) 162:1452–60. doi: 10.1176/appi.ajp.162.8.1452
150. Fusar-Poli P, Allen P, Bhattacharyya S, Crippa JA, Mechelli A, Borgwardt S, et al. Modulation of effective connectivity during emotional processing by delta-9-tetrahydrocannabinol and cannabidiol. *Int J Neuropsychopharmacol.* (2010) 13:421–32. doi: 10.1017/S1461145709990617
151. Norris C, Loureiro M, Kramar C, Zunder J, Renard J, Rushlow W, et al. Cannabidiol modulates fear memory formation through interactions with serotonergic transmission in the mesolimbic system. *Neuropsychopharmacology* (2016) 41:2839–50. doi: 10.1038/npp.2016.93
152. Torrens M, Fonseca F, Mateu G, Farré M. Efficacy of antidepressants in substance use disorders with and without comorbid depression: a systematic review and meta-analysis. *Drug Alcohol Depend.* (2005) 78:1–22. doi: 10.1016/j.drugalcdep.2004.09.004
153. Zlebnik NE, Cheer JF. Beyond the CB1 receptor: is cannabidiol the answer for disorders of motivation? *Annu Rev Neurosci.* (2016) 39:1–17. doi: 10.1146/annurev-neuro-070815-014038
154. Crippa JA, Guimarães FS, Campos AC, Zuardi AW. Translational Investigation of the therapeutic potential of cannabidiol (CBD): toward a new age. *Front Immunol.* (2018) 9:2009. doi: 10.3389/fimmu.2018.02009
155. Gruber SA, Rogowska J, Yurgelun-Todd DA. Altered affective response in marijuana smokers: an FMRI study. *Drug Alcohol Depend.* (2009) 105:139–53. doi: 10.1016/j.drugalcdep.2009.06.019
156. Trezza V, Campolongo P, Manduca A, Morena M, Palmery M, Vanderschuren LJMJ, et al. Altering endocannabinoid neurotransmission at critical developmental ages: impact on rodent emotionality and cognitive performance. *Front Behav Neurosci.* (2012) 6:2. doi: 10.3389/fnbeh.2012.00002
157. De Petrocellis L, Ligresti A, Moriello AS, Allarà M, Bisogno T, Petrosino S, et al. Effects of cannabinoids and cannabinoid-enriched Cannabis extracts on TRP channels and endocannabinoid metabolic enzymes. *Br J Pharmacol.* (2011) 163:1479–94. doi: 10.1111/j.1476-5381.2010.01166.x

158. Adamczyk P, Miszkiel J, McCreary AC, Filip M, Papp M, Przegalinski E. The effects of cannabinoid CB1, CB2 and vanilloid TRPV1 receptor antagonists on cocaine addictive behavior in rats. *Brain Res.* (2012) 1444:45–54. doi: 10.1016/j.brainres.2012.01.030
159. Trigo JM, Le Foll B. Inhibition of monoacylglycerol lipase (MAGL) enhances cue-induced reinstatement of nicotine-seeking behavior in mice. *Psychopharmacology (Berl).* (2016) 233:1815–22. doi: 10.1007/s00213-015-4117-5
160. Forget B, Guranda M, Gamaleddin I, Goldberg SR, Le Foll B. Attenuation of cue-induced reinstatement of nicotine seeking by URB597 through cannabinoid CB1 receptor in rats. *Psychopharmacology (Berl).* (2016) 233:1823–8. doi: 10.1007/s00213-016-4232-y
161. Balter RE, Cooper ZD, Haney M. Novel pharmacologic approaches to treating cannabis use disorder. *Curr Addict Rep.* (2014) 1:137–43. doi: 10.1007/s40429-014-0011-1

8

Addiction, Anhedonia and Comorbid Mood Disorder: A Narrative Review

*Marianne Destoop[1,2], Manuel Morrens[1,3], Violette Coppens[1,3] and Geert Dom[1,2]**

[1] Collaborative Antwerp Psychiatric Research Institute (CAPRI), Faculty of Medicine and Health Sciences, University of Antwerp, Antwerp, Belgium, [2] Psychiatric Hospital Multiversum, Campus Alexianen, Boechout, Belgium, [3] University Department of Psychiatry, Campus Duffel, Duffel, Belgium

***Correspondence:**
Geert Dom
geert.dom@uantwerpen.be

Background: Recently, anhedonia has been recognized as an important Research Domain Criterion (RDoC) by the National Institute of Mental Health. Anhedonia is proposed to play an essential role in the pathogenies of both addictive and mood disorders, and possibly their co-occurrence with a single individual. However, up to now, comprehensive information about anhedonia concerning its underlying neurobiological circuitries, the neurocognitive correlates, and their role in addiction, mood disorder, and comorbidity remains scarce.

Aim: In this literature review of human studies, we bring together the current state of knowledge with respect to anhedonia in its relationship with disorders in the use of substances (DUS) and the comorbidity with mood disorders.

Method: A PubMed search was conducted using the following search terms: (Anhedonia OR Reward Deficiency) AND ((Drug Dependence OR Abuse) OR Alcohol OR Nicotine OR Addiction OR Gambling OR (Internet Gaming)). Thirty-two articles were included in the review.

Results: Anhedonia is associated with substance use disorders, and their severity is especially prominent in DUS with comorbid depression. Anhedonia may be both a trait and a state dimension in its relation to DUS and tends to impact DUS treatment outcome negatively.

Keywords: anhedonia, disorders in the use of substances, substance abuse, addiction, depression, mood disorder, gambling, internet gaming

INTRODUCTION

Disorders in the use of substances (DUS) as defined by the *Diagnostic and Statistical Manual of Mental Disorder-5 (DSM-5)* are a set of highly prevalent disorders with an enormous negative impact on individuals, their families, and society as a whole (1). From a neuroscientific perspective, DUS can be conceptualized as complex disorders, i.e., multiple symptom clusters and underlying neurobiological circuitries/systems play a role. In its core lay both a hypersensitivity to drug-related stimuli and an impairment in (executive) control over these impulses. On the other hand, and increasingly as the disorder progresses, a "darker" side has been suggested where an increase of brain-stress system, impaired stress tolerance, negative affect, and anhedonia take the upper hand (2).

From a clinical perspective, anhedonia, i.e., a markedly diminished interest or pleasure in activities that are naturally rewarding, is an essential characteristic for many addicted individuals. Anhedonia-like symptoms have been reported in the context of active chronic substance use, (protracted) withdrawal, and during sustained abstinence. Also, anhedonia may, for some individuals, act as a pre-existing vulnerability for substance initiation, regular use, and the subsequent development transition to addiction (3). The symptoms characterizing anhedonia may reflect underlying neurochemical changes, typically associated with the "dark side" of addiction, where negative reinforcement drives continuing substance use and the neurochemical picture is dominated by dysregulation of brain-stress systems (2). These may also include peripheric inflammation processes that have been reported in the context of chronic substance use and associated with depression and anhedonia (4). In line with this are the recent findings indicating that antidepressants, i.e., agomelatine, might affect anhedonia, possibly *via* decreasing C-reactive protein and increasing BDNF serum levels (5–7). Furthermore, anhedonia may have specific clinical importance, i.e., for outcome and treatment response. Indeed, anhedonia increases the likelihood of relapse and is associated with craving (3).

Characteristic of DUS is the high prevalence of comorbidity with other psychiatric disorders. This might be the result of the diagnostic vagueness inherent to the currently used diagnostic categorical systems such as DSM and ICD. Alternatively, common underlying factors may drive different behavioral–phenotypical presentations that when diagnosed "categorical" on a behavioral level results in statistical high levels of comorbidity (8). Disorders of mood (MD) are one of the psychiatric disorders that have been reported to co-occur frequently with DUS are mood disorders (MD). The co-occurrence of MD and DUS has been well established with an estimated two- to fivefold increase in odds of having an MD when the other condition is present (9). With respect to the pathogenesis of psychiatric disorders, anhedonia has been considered as a principal, transdiagnostic characteristic, within the phenotypic concept of different mental disorders, e.g., mood disorders, schizophrenia, and also DUS (10). Recent studies suggest that reward hyposensitivity within unipolar depression will be most strongly associated with a state of anhedonia characterized by motivational versus hedonic deficits (11, 12). From this perspective, it might be hypothesized that anhedonia as an underlying neurobiological construct acts as a driver explaining the high prevalence of the DUS–depression comorbidity. Alternatively, anhedonia might be a symptom within both disorders but of which its origin is based on different pathogenetic pathways, e.g., anhedonia as a result of down-regulation of reward pathways in a response of chronic substance (ab)use.

Anhedonia is by far not the only common construct underlying comorbidities between DUS and other psychiatric disorders. Indeed, using the Research Domain Criterion (RDoC) terminology, deficits in threat-related processes (Negative Valence Systems), executive control (Arousal/Regulatory Systems), and working memory (Cognitive Systems) are observed across many psychiatric disorders in both the "internalizing" spectrum (e.g., depression, anxiety) and the "externalizing" spectrum, i.e., DUS (8, 11). However, up to now, the role of anhedonia in both the pathogenesis of addiction and in the comorbidity with mood disorders has been mainly left understudied. This is an essential caveat since an increasing number of studies indicate that anhedonia, e.g., within the context of depression, is a factor that negatively impacts treatment outcome. Indeed, anhedonia is a predictor of poor longitudinal course of symptoms of major depression, suicidality, and suicidal ideation and poor response on pharmacological treatment (13–16).

Within the scope of this review, we first present ideas on conceptualizing and assessing anhedonia. Next, we review the literature exploring the relationship between anhedonia and substance use disorders. In the discussion, we extend on how these findings match with current concepts on anhedonia and how this, potentially, reflect on treatment and future research.

CONCEPTUALIZATION OF ANHEDONIA

Anhedonia refers to a decreased interest or pleasure in response to stimuli that are either by nature or previously perceived as rewarding. As such, anhedonia is inherently associated with reward processing. Reward processing involves multiple components that can be dissected experimentally in animal models but are likely intermingled in real life-situations: sensory detection of a stimulus, affective hedonic reaction, pleasure itself (liking), motivation to obtain the reward and work for it (wanting or incentive salience), and reward-related learning processes (17).

At least two broad dimensions underlying anhedonia have been identified through animal and human research: 1) reward hyposensitivity and 2) reduced approach motivation. Of importance, both aspects can be dissected regarding their underlying neurobiological pathways and neurochemical hallmarks (11).

Reward hyposensitivity has been suggested to be associated with the functionalities related to the "consummatory" part of reward processing, i.e., often reflected by the term "liking." Pleasure experience is suggested to be mediated by the endogenous opioid and endocannabinoid receptor pathways in different brain areas (18). This component could be called the hedonic dimension of anhedonia, i.e., "hedonic anhedonia."

Approach motivation is viewed as the driver that facilitates approach or goal-directed behavior to obtain rewards. Information encoded by dopaminergic transmission within the mesolimbic system is suggested to play a role in reward motivational value and motivational salience (17). The primary system is proposed to be dopaminergic frontostriatal circuitries. Reducing dopaminergic functioning has an adverse effect on the motivation to pursue and work for rewarding stimuli. This dimension could be called the motivational component of anhedonia, i.e., "motivational anhedonia." Of interest, administration of a dopamine agonist (d-amfetamine) produces an increase in the willingness to work for rewards in animal models (11, 19).

Taken together, growing evidence from self-report, behavioral, and neurophysiological studies suggest that reward hyposensitivity and reduced approach motivation reflect anhedonia (11). From this perspective, two distinct neural circuits underlying motivational (anticipation, wanting; i.e., associated with dopamine signaling within the frontostriatal circuitry) versus hedonic (consumption, liking; i.e., associated with endogenous opioids signaling) reward-related states can be hypothesized (11). For this review, we conceptualize anhedonia to these two basic dimensions (**Figure 1**).

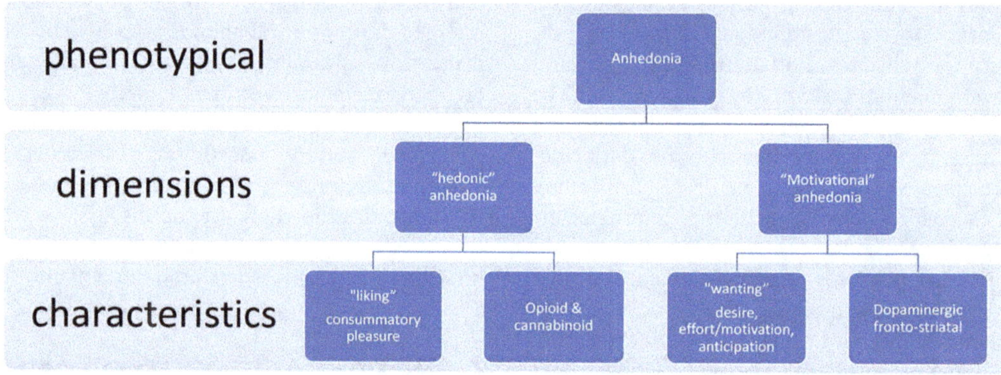

FIGURE 1 | Anhedonia dimensions (11, 18).

REVIEW: AIM AND QUESTIONS

Within the scope of this explorative–narrative review part of this manuscript, we aim to explore the following questions:

- What is the prevalence of anhedonia within human DUS individuals?
- What types of measurement instruments of anhedonia are used in human studies within DUS samples?
- Is there a differentiation according to hedonic versus motivation anhedonia?
- How does anhedonia relate to DUS–depression comorbidity?
- What is the role of anhedonia in DUS course and treatment response?

METHOD

The most recent systematic review on the relation between substance use disorders (SUD) and anhedonia reviewed the literature up to 23 May 2013 (3). So, with this review, we aimed at expanding this body of work by reviewing the literature published after this date, i.e., last 5 years. A search was performed in PubMed using the same search terms as in this latter publication (3). We included pathological gambling and internet gaming in this search because they recently were included in the DUS chapter of the *DSM-5* (and will be in the next ICD11) as addictive disorders.

In order to obtain original studies investigating the link between anhedonia and DUS, a PubMed search (May 2013–November 2018) for English language articles was conducted using the following search terms: (Anhedonia OR Reward Deficiency) AND ((Drug Dependence OR Abuse) OR Alcohol OR Nicotine OR Addiction OR Gambling OR (Internet Gaming)). The papers were filtered for human studies only. An overview of the inclusion process can be found in **Figure 2**. The PubMed search yielded 171 results; abstract screening led to the exclusion of 136 papers, leaving 35 papers. Of these, one full paper could not be retrieved, and two validation studies were excluded, so 32 articles were included in the review.

RESULTS

The majority of studies (n = 13) focused on tobacco smoking compared to alcohol (n = 4), cannabis (n = 4), cocaine (n = 5), benzodiazepines (n = 1), and opioids (n = 4). Behavioral addictions remain poorly studied, i.e., one study on gambling and none on online gaming. See **Table 1** for an overview of all studies.

Types of Measures of Anhedonia Used Within DUS Studies

Self-report measures were, by far, the most used instruments, i.e., all studies included self-report measures. Of these, the Snaith–Hamilton Pleasure Scale (SHAPS) (50) was most frequently used, i.e., in 15 of the 32 studies. Within the depression research, the SHAPS has been validated and remains the gold standard. It measures the consummatory pleasure (51) typically. However, given the recommendation that any scale should be validated in the population of interest prior to use, it needs to be noted that none of the self-report scales found in this review was ever validated within DUS populations. This particularly warrants interpretation of the current results.

Of interest, three studies used ecological momentary assessments (EMAs) during four times a day in a smoking cessation trial (25, 28, 34). It was questioned how much pleasure the participants experienced during the day on three domains (social, recreation, and performance/accomplishment). EMA might be a promising methodology providing data better covering the actual evolution of symptoms than (retrospective) self-report and is increasingly used in both depression and addiction research (52, 53). However, as yet, no validated set of EMA-implementable questions on anhedonia have been developed.

Few studies (n = 4) used behavioral tasks. Guillot et al. used the Picture Rating Task, which is a measure of affective valence related to positive, negative, and smoking cues (27). In this task, participants were instructed to rate the pleasantness of each stimulus by pressing keys corresponding to seven-point Likert scale from −3 (very unpleasant) to 3 (very pleasant). Positive,

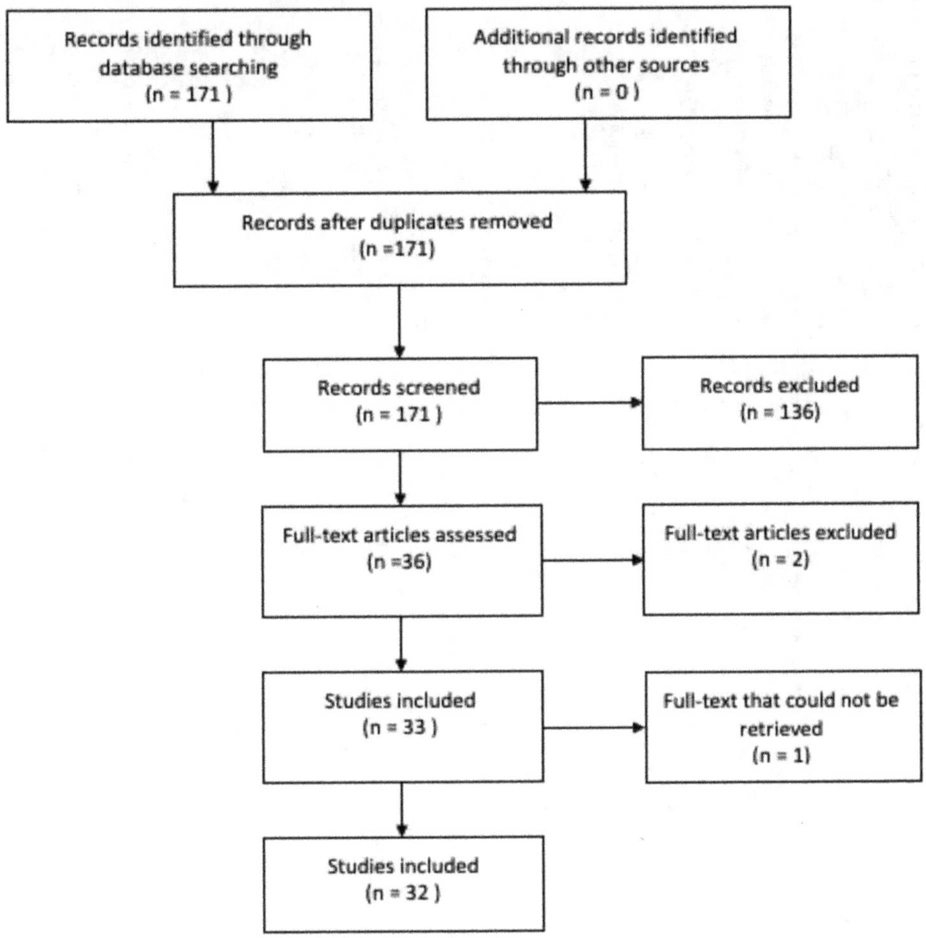

FIGURE 2 | Search strategy for research papers in PubMed.

negative, smoking, and neutral images are shown. In this task, anhedonia has been inversely related to pleasantness ratings of positive or reward-related stimuli.

Liverant et al. (33) used a signal detection task designed to assess modulation of behavior in response to rewards, which was already used in trials with MDD and bipolar disorders (54). In the latter studies, an inverse relationship between response bias and anhedonia was already demonstrated.

Leventhal et al. used a behavioral task measuring the relative reward value of smoking (36). This task yields objective behavioral measures of the relative value of a) initiating smoking versus delaying smoking for money and b) self-administering cigarettes for money when given the opportunity to smoke.

Wardle et al. used a progressive ratio procedure as a behavioral measure of anhedonia (19). Participants can choose two options in which option A results in greater rewards in exchange for greater effort while option C results in less reward but requires less effort. Fewer key presses for A indicates motivational anhedonia. It has to be noted that this type of behavioral measure is not strongly related to the SHAPS (55).

Taken together, the four studies using behavioral tasks all used a different paradigm. It remains unclear as to which aspect/dimension of anhedonia they tap in and how they relate with self-reported anhedonia.

Seven studies used neurobiological, i.e., neurophysiological or imaging, measures of anhedonia. First, an functional magnetic resconance imaging (fMRI) study in young cannabis users implemented a two-card guessing game that assessed response to anticipation and receipt of monetary reward (38). In this paradigm, anhedonia was associated with a pattern of negative Nucleus Accumbens (NAcc)–medial Prefrontal Cortex (mPFC) connectivity.

Parvaz et al. used a gambling task predicting whether they would win or lose money on each trial, while ERP data were required (40). Reward Positivity component (RewP) in response to predicted win trials was extracted from the ERPs. RewP is attributed to the same brain regions that are also implicated in anhedonia (i.e., ventral striatum and mPFC). The results showed that RewP amplitude in response to rewarded trials correlated with anhedonia severity in CUD.

Morie et al. performed two ERP studies in cocaine abusers and healthy controls (41, 42). In Morie et al. (41), a speeded response task with varying probabilities of reward is used. Cocaine users showed blunted response to reward-predictive cues and to feedback about task success or failure. Anhedonia measured by

TABLE 1 | Results from the literature review.

	Author	Sample	Anhedonia measure			Comorbidity	Result
			Self-report	Behavioral task	Neuro-biologic		
Alcohol	(20)	MDD (n = 4,339) MDD+AUD (n = 413)	MINI	/	/	MDD	Anhedonia is associated with alcohol abuse
	(21)	Trauma-exposed US military veterans (n = 913)	PCL-5	/	/	PTSD symptoms	Anhedonia associated with past-year alcohol consequences
	(22)	18- to 25-year Hispanic emerging adults (n = 181)	CES-D	/	/	/	Higher levels of anhedonia were associated with higher alcohol use severity
	(23)	College students (18–22 years) (n = 820)	MASQ-SF	/	fMRI while participants completed a card-guessing task, which elicits ventral striatum reactivity	/	Reduced ventral striatum reactivity to reward is associated with increased risk for anhedonia in individuals exposed to early life stress. Such stress-related anhedonia is associated with problematic alcohol use
Nicotine	(24)	Non-daily cigarette smokers (18–24 years) (n = 518): smoking more than 1/m more than 6m	SHAPS online after 3, 6, and 9 months follow-up	/	/	/	Anhedonia is not predictive for other tobacco products use (OTP), but those with anhedonia used hookah more frequently
	(25	Adults in a smoking cessation clinical trial (n = 1,122), min 10 sig/d min 6 m: placebo (n = 131), bupropion (n = 401), or NRT (n = 590)	Ecological momentary assessments 4 times a day 5 days prior and 10 days after target quit day	/	/	/	Anhedonia is associated with dependence and was suppressed by agonist administration
	(26)	Ninth-grade students (13–15 years) (n = 3299): ever-smokers (n = 343), never-smokers (n = 2,956)	SHAPS	/	/	/	Anhedonia is associated with smoking initiation in the overall sample and higher initiation susceptibility in the subsample never-smokers
	(27)	Non-treatment-seeking smokers (more than 10 sig/d, more than 2 years) (n = 125) attending 2 counterbalanced experimental sessions (abstinent (for 16 h) vs. none abstinent)	SHAPS	Picture Rating Task	/	/	Greater anhedonia associated with less negative affective reactivity to negative pictures
	(28)	Smoking participants in a double-blind cessation clinical trial (n = 1,236): nicotine patch (n = 216), nicotine lozenge (n = 211), bupropion (n = 213), patch + lozenge (n = 228), bupropion + lozenge (n = 221), placebo (n = 147)	Ecological momentary assessments 4 times a day 5 days prior and 10 days after target quit day	/	/	/	High craving anhedonia group reported higher dependence, were less likely to have received combination nicotine replacement, reported lower week 8 abstinence rates and relapsed sooner
	(29)	Smokers (more than 5 sig/d) (n = 1125)	MASQ-S	/	/	/	Urgency is associated with smoking at average or higher levels of anhedonia; it was unrelated to smoking when few anhedonia symptoms were endorsed

(Continued)

TABLE 1 | Continued

Author	Sample	Anhedonia measure			Comorbidity	Result
		Self-report	Behavioral task	Neuro-biologic		
(30)	Adult smokers (n = 525) (more than 10/d) from a cessation clinical trial on 21 mg/day nicotine patch therapy during 8 weeks	SHAPS	/	/	/	70 participants (13%) were anhedonic, men were more anhedonic, anhedonic smokers were more likely to be abstinent
(31)	Ninth-grade students (n = 807): 294 no history of SUD, 166 lifetime history of drug/alcohol use without tobacco, 115 lifetime history of drug/alcohol use with tobacco	SHAPS	/	/	/	Teens with lifetime alcohol/drug use without tobacco had higher anhedonia
(32)	Ninth-grade students (n = 3,310): 2,557 neither conventional nor e-cigarettes, 412 e-cigarettes only, 152 conventional cigarettes only, 189 conventional and e-cigarettes	SHAPS	/	/	/	Anhedonia was higher in e-cigarette only vs. non-users. An ordered effect of dual-use vs. e-cigarette use only vs. non-use was found for anhedonia
(33)	Veterans with MDD or dysthymia (n = 80): 36 depressed smokers and 44 depressed non-smokers	MASQ-S BIS/BAS	Probabilistic reward task that measures reward-learning	/	MDD-dysthymia	Depressed smokers reported higher trait anhedonia and reduced BAS reward responsiveness compared to non-smokers. Depressed smokers demonstrated greater acquisition of reward-based learning
(34)	Adults from smoking cessation clinical trial (n = 1,175) (min 10 sig/d last 6 months): bupropion, nicotine lozenge, nicotine patch + lozenge, bupropion + nicotine lozenge or placebo	Ecological momentary assessments 4 times a day from 5 days prior to 10 days after target quit day	/	/	/	Anhedonia showed an inverted U- pattern of change in response to tobacco cessation and was associated with the severity of withdrawal symptoms and tobacco dependence. Post-quit anhedonia was associated with decreased latency to relapse and with lower 8-week point prevalence abstinence. NRT suppressed the increase in abstinence-related anhedonia
(35)	Adults recruited *via* announcements (n = 275) (more than 10 sig/d): participants attended a baseline visit that involved anhedonia followed by 2 counterbalanced visits after 16 h smoking abstinence and non-abstinent	SHS TEPS CAI	Behavioral smoking task measuring relative reward value of smoking	/	/	Higher anhedonia predicted quicker smoking initiation and more cigarettes purchased, partially mediated by low and high negative mood states. Abstinence amplified the extent to which anhedonia predicted cigarette consumption among those who responded to the abstinence manipulation, but not the entire sample
(36)	Smokers enrolled in a smoking cessation treatment study (n = 1,469) (more than 10 sig/d more than 6 m): bupropion (n = 264), nicotine lozenge (n = 260), nicotine patch (n = 262), bupropion + lozenge (n = 262), placebo (n = 189)	Life time anhedonia *via* CIDI	/	/	depression	Anhedonia predicted cessation outcome

(Continued)

TABLE 1 | Continued

	Author	Sample	Anhedonia measure			Comorbidity	Result
			Self-report	Behavioral task	Neuro-biologic		
Cannabis	(37)	Cannabis users between 15 and 24 years (*n* = 162): 47 early onset, before 16 years; 115 late onset	Online OLIFE	/	/	Schizotypy	Early-onset cannabis use is associated with higher levels of anhedonia in females only
	(32)	Student at the age of 14 (*n* = 3,394) at baseline, 6-, 12-, and 18-month follow-up	SHAPS	/	/	/	Anhedonia is associated with subsequent marijuana use escalation amplified by cannabis-using friends, but baseline marijuana use is not related to the rate of change in anhedonia.
	(38)	20-year-old men (*n* = 158), recruited at the age of 6–17 m	SHAPS	/	fMRI during a 24-trial slow event-related card-guessing game that assesses response to anticipation and receipt of monetary reward		The escalating trajectory group displayed a pattern of negative NAcc–mPFC connectivity that was linked to higher levels of anhedonia
	(39)	MDD subgroup from a national survey (*n* = 2,348): users with CUD vs. users without CUD	*DSM-IV* criteria	/	/	MDD	Level of cannabis use is associated with anhedonia
Stimulants	(19)	Treatment-seeking adults with cocaine dependence: on contingency management (*n* = 85): 40 placebo, 45 levodopa	SHAPS	PR task	/	/	L-dopa did not improve outcomes of CM, nor was the effect moderated by anhedonia; anhedonia may be a modifiable individual difference associated with poorer outcome of CM
	(40)	CUD participants (*n* = 46)	CSSA	/	RewP of ERP	/	RewP is correlated with anhedonia, and anhedonia explained a significant amount of variance in the RewP amplitude
	(41)	Current cocaine abusers (*n* = 23) and participants with no drug history (*n* = 24)	SHAPS	/	ERP after reward receipt	/	Anhedonia is associated with reward motivation, diminished reward feedback, and diminished monitoring
	(42)	Current cocaine abusers, outpatients (*n* = 23) and controls with no drug history (*n* = 27)	SHAPS CPCSAS	/	Go/NoGo task while EEG was recorded. Valenced pictures from the International Affective Picture System	/	Cocaine users performed more poorly than controls on the inhibitory control task. Cocaine users were more anhedonic. Higher levels of anhedonia were associated with more severe substance use. Inhibitor control and anhedonia were correlated only in controls
	(43)	Cocaine-dependent patients, free from cocaine during the last 3 weeks (*n* = 23) and healthy controls (*n* = 38)	Chapman psychosis-proneness scales (with revised physical anhedonia and revised social anhedonia)	/	A paired-stimulus paradigm to elicit three mid-latency auditory evoked responses (MLAER), namely, P50, N100, and P200	Psychosis proneness	Social anhedonia scores accounted for the largest proportion of variance in P200 gating. Poorer P50 gating is related to higher scores on the social anhedonia scale in healthy controls and across mixed samples of cocaine-dependent patients

(Continued)

TABLE 1 | Continued

	Author	Sample	Anhedonia measure			Comorbidity	Result
			Self-report	Behavioral task	Neuro-biologic		
Opioids	(44)	Heroin-dependent participants on opioid maintenance (n = 90): on methadone (n = 55) or on buprenorphine (n = 35); and recently abstinent (up to 12 months) opioid-dependent participants (n = 31); and healthy controls (n = 33)	SHAPS TEPS	/	/	/	Elevation in anhedonia in opioid-dependent participants
	(45)	Patients (mostly inpatients) with opioid dependence (n = 306): 1,000 mg naltrexone implant + oral placebo (n = 102), placebo implant and 50 mg oral naltrexone (n = 102), both placebo (n = 102)	FAS CSPSA	/	/	/	Anhedonia was elevated at baseline and reduced to normal within the first 1–2 months for patients who remained in treatment and did not relapse, no difference between groups
	(46)	Opioid-dependent patients 10–14 days after withdrawal (PODP) (n = 36) and healthy controls (n = 10)	SHAPS	Affect-modulated startle response (AMSR)	Cue reactivity task during which participant's RPFC and VLPFC were monitored with functional near-infrared spectroscopy	/	PODP reported greater anhedonia on self-report, reduced hedonic response to positive stimuli in the AMSR task, reduced bilateral RPFC and left VLPFC activity to food images and reduced left VLPFC to positive social situations compared to controls. Patients with anhedonia showed reduced response to positive social stimuli and food
	(47)	Detoxified heroin-dependent patients recruited from addiction-treatment centers (n = 12) 2 weeks after detoxification starting extended-release naltrexone (XRNT) and healthy subjects (n = 11)	SHAPS	/	[^{123}I]FP-CIT SPECT-scan imaging striatal DAT binding: 1 before and 1 2 weeks after injection with XRNT	/	XRNT does not affect anhedonia, but with a significant reduction of depressive symptoms
Gambling	(48)	Outpatients with Parkinson's disease (n = 154): 34 fulfilled criteria for impulse control disease (ICD), of which 11 met criteria of pathological gambling (PG)	SHAPS	/	/	Parkinson's disease	PG had a higher incidence of anhedonia
Internet gaming		/	/	/	/	/	/
Benzodiazepines	(49)	MDD outpatients of the MDPU database (Mood Disorder Psychopharmacology Unit) (n = 326): 79 benzodiazepine users, 247 nonbenzodiazepine users	MADRS	/	/	MDD	Anhedonia was greater in the benzodiazepine group, and anhedonia was the strongest predictor of regular benzodiazepine use

OLIFE, Oxford-125 Liverpool Inventory of Feeling and Experiences; PCL-5 = PTSD Checklist for DSM-5; SHAPS, Snaith–Hamilton Pleasure Scale; TEPS, Temporal Experience of Pleasure Scale; REI, Rewarding Events Inventory; CES-D, Center Epidemiological Studies Depression Scale; PR task, progressive ratio task; FAS, Ferguson Anhedonia Scale; CSPSA, Chapman Scale of Physical and Social anhedonia; MASQ-S, Mood and Anxiety Symptoms Questionnaire-Short Form (with Anhedonic Depression subscale); CSSA, Cocaine Selective Severity Assessment Scale; RewP, Reward Positivity component; TEPS, Temporal Experience of Pleasure Scale; BIS/BAS, Behavioral Inhibition/Behavioral Activation Scale; CPCSAS, Chapman Physical and Chapman Social Anhedonia Scales; SHS, Subjective Happiness Scale; CAI, Composite Anhedonia Index; MINI, Mini International Neuropsychiatric Interview; CIDI, Composite International Diagnostic Interview; MADRS, Montgomery–Asberg Depression Rating Scale.

the SHAPS was also associated with diminished monitoring and reward feedback in cocaine users. The measures of anhedonia were associated with reward motivation in both cocaine users and healthy controls (41). Morie et al. (42) used a Go/NoGo task in response to valenced pictures. Though this is more a measure for executive functioning, i.e., inhibition and performance monitoring, a correlation was found between inhibitory control and anhedonia, but only in controls.

In a small group of detoxified heroin-dependent patients, striatal dopamine transporter binding was assessed by [^{123}I]FP-CIT single photon emission computed tomography (SPECT) before and 2 weeks after injection with extended-release naltrexone (47). Although depression scores were higher for patients at baseline and depression scores were lower after extended-release naltrexone (XRNT) treatment, no associations could be found for anhedonia.

Finally, a large fMRI study with 820 college students used a ventral striatum reactivity task, a blocked number-guessing paradigm, consisting of three blocks of positive feedback, three blocks of negative feedback, and three control blocks (23). Reduced ventral striatum reactivity to reward is associated with increased risk for anhedonia in individuals exposed to early life stress. This interaction is linked to other depressive symptoms and problematic alcohol use.

In only one study were self-report, behavioral, and neurobiological measures combined (46). Thirty-six opioid-dependent patients and 10 healthy controls filled in the SHAPS and performed the affect-modulated startle response (AMSR), a psychophysiological measure of emotional valence, that was used before to assess hedonic responses to standardized reward-related stimuli. Four categories of stimuli can be derived: positive, negative, neutral, and drug-related. Meanwhile, acoustic startle probes were presented at variable points and the eye-blink component of the startle reflex was recorded by EMG. All participants completed a standard visual cue activity paradigm while being monitored with functional near-infrared spectroscopy (fNIRS). Stimuli consisted of three hedonically positive categories (highly palatable food, positive social interaction, and emotional intimacy) as well as emotionally neutral stimuli. Opioid-dependent patients reported greater anhedonia on self-report, reduced hedonic response to positive stimuli in the AMSR task, and reduced bilateral RPFC and left VLPFC to food imaged and reduced left VLPFC to positive social situations compared to controls.

Taken together, although more studies used a neurobiological measure as compared to behavioral task only, again all of them used a different paradigm, making a comparison of the results difficult. Also, it remains de be defined what dimensions/aspects of anhedonia are captured by these different paradigms, although some studies provide indications for the motivational component (e.g., fronto-striatal connectivity).

Anhedonia Within DUS Populations

Very few studies compared anhedonia between a sample of DUS patients with non-DUS controls. Other studies focused on the relationship between substance abuse and severity-related variables in relation with anhedonia in samples of DUS individuals.

Studies with a healthy control group showed consistently that cocaine abusers, heroin-dependent individuals, and benzodiazepine-dependent individuals were more anhedonic versus controls. Also, higher levels of anhedonia associated with more severe substance use (42, 44, 46, 47, 49).

Studies within DUS samples without control revealed a similar result; i.e., anhedonia was associated with substance use variables. Three studies on alcohol showed a positive association between anhedonia and alcohol use severity and related consequences (20–22). Within cigarette smokers, most studies provide indications of an adverse effect of anhedonia on smoking: initiation, smoking susceptibility, and severity (24, 26, 29, 35). Finally, early onset of cannabis use, subsequent escalation of marijuana use, and level of use have been associated with higher levels of anhedonia (32, 37, 39). One study on gambling showed higher levels of anhedonia in a gambling subsample of Parkinson's disease patients (48). However, this study included only 11 gamblers, warranting careful interpretation.

Taken together, across different substances, indications are consistent that 1) DUS individuals have higher levels of anhedonia than controls and that 2) anhedonia might be related with early onset of substance use and subsequent severity of DUS.

Time Course of Anhedonia: Trait or State?

For nicotine-dependent individuals, there is evidence that anhedonia is both a state and a trait factor. First, in a longitudinal study with 518 young participants, the presence of anhedonia predicted the use of hookah (24). Evidence for anhedonia as a trait can also be found in the study of Leventhal (36), which is already described above (36). The trait anhedonia predicted quicker smoking initiation and more cigarettes purchased, and 16-h smoking abstinence amplified the extent to which anhedonia predicted cigarette consumption. In addition, a recent study showed that 1) anhedonia is associated with smoking initiation and 2) adolescents with higher (vs. lower) anhedonia who have never tried smoking may be more susceptible to smoking initiation perhaps due to stronger pro-smoking intentions or willingness to smoke (26).

Data supporting trait anhedonia for other substances are few. For cannabis, anhedonia has been associated with both early onset of cannabis use and marijuana use escalation in early adolescence (32, 37).

On the other hand, anhedonia can be a part of smoking withdrawal. Cook et al. (34) demonstrated an inverted U-pattern in response to tobacco cessation, which was associated with the severity of withdrawal symptoms and tobacco dependence (34). In the 6-month follow-up study with opioid-dependent patients (mostly inpatients), elevated anhedonia levels at baseline reduced to normal after 1 to 2 months for patients who did not relapse (45). In the study of Garfield et al. (44), elevation of anhedonia was found in opioid-dependent participants compared to healthy controls (44). Among participants on opioid pharmacotherapy (i.e., methadone and buprenorphine), a significant association was found between the frequency of recent illicit opioid use and anhedonia scores, which supports the hypothesis that opioids can cause anhedonia. On the other hand, no association was found between duration of abstinence and anhedonia in the group of abstinent opioid-dependent participants.

Anhedonia and DUS and Depression Comorbidity

Two out of four studies concerning alcohol use disorder (AUD) focused on comorbidity as well. In an major depressive disorder (MDD)-subsample of the Mental Health in the General Population (MHGP), 4,339 subjects met the criteria for MDD (20). In the MDD population, 413 AUD subjects were identified, including 138 subjects with alcohol abuse and 275 with alcohol dependence. Anhedonia was associated with alcohol abuse in the group with MDD and AUD compared to the group without AUD (OR 1.66).

A sample of 916 trauma-exposed US military veterans was drawn from a larger dataset from the National Health and Resilience in Veterans Study (NHRVS, 21). A subsample was chosen that endorsed a "worst" traumatic event on the Traumatic History Screen. In this nonclinical sample, associations between the seven-factor hybrid model of PTSD symptoms and alcohol consumption and consequences were found. Lifetime anhedonia, together with dysphoric arousal and negative affect, was most strongly associated with past-year alcohol consequences.

MDD comorbidity is studied in nicotine papers as well. In an MDD/dysthymia subsample of veterans from a large VA Healthcare System in the Northeast United States, 36 depressed smokers were compared to 44 depressed non-smokers (28). Depressed smokers reported more anhedonia and reduced reward responsiveness. However, on a probabilistic learning task, depressed smokers showed a stronger preference for the more frequently rewarded stimulus, which suggests that depressed smokers demonstrated more robust acquisition of reward-based learning.

Leventhal et al. (36) adjusted the relation between anhedonia and depressed mood with relapse in nicotine for lifetime depressive disorder based on the CIDI. Depressed mood did not predict cessation outcome, while anhedonia did (36).

For cannabis, only one study focused on comorbidity between CUD and MDD. Feingold et al. (39) selected an MDD subgroup from a national survey and concluded that the level of cannabis use was associated with more symptoms at follow-up, notably anhedonia, while remission rates did not differ between MDD with or without CUD (39).

Rizvi et al. (49) demonstrated that anhedonia was more significant in MDD patients using benzodiazepines, with anhedonia being the strongest predictor of regular benzodiazepine use (49).

One fMRI study showed a decreased ventral striatum reactivity to the (monetary) reward associated with an increased risk for anhedonia, especially for those participants who were exposed to early life stress (23). This might suggest that for these individuals specifically, motivational anhedonia is impaired.

Anhedonia and Effect on Treatment of DUS

Most studies showed an adverse effect of anhedonia on treatment effect. In a large randomized, double-blind placebo-controlled smoking cessation trial, four distinct types of quit-day withdrawal were identified: the moderate withdrawal class were the least likely to report high levels of any individual symptom for hunger and anhedonia. The high-craving anhedonia group reported high levels of craving and anhedonia. The affective withdrawal group was scoring high on poor concentration and negative affect. The hunger group reported high quit-day hunger, but low on other indicators. The high-craving anhedonia group reported lower week 8 abstinence and relapsed sooner but were also less likely to have received combination nicotine replacement in this trial (28).

In another smoking cessation treatment study with 1,469 participants, lifetime anhedonia predicted increased odds of relapse after 8 weeks and 6 months (36). Moreover, post-quit anhedonia was associated with decreased latency to relapse and with lower 8-week point prevalence abstinence. Similar findings were demonstrated in the study of Piper using the same design and method (28). They reported lower abstinence after 8 weeks for the high craving anhedonia group.

Wardle et al. (19) demonstrated that anhedonia was associated with poor treatment outcome (i.e., cocaine-negative urines) for cocaine-dependent participants following contingency management. Also, a dopamine-agonist (L-DOPA) did not improve outcomes in this study, nor was the effect of L-DOPA moderated by anhedonia (19).

Only in one study did anhedonia have a positive effect on treatment (30). In the clinical cessation trial on 21-mg nicotine patch a day for 8 weeks, 70 participants were anhedonic based on the SHAPS. The anhedonic smokers were more likely to be abstinent on a nicotine patch.

DISCUSSION

In this exploratory–narrative review, we identified 32 original research papers exploring anhedonia and its relationship with substance use disorders. Results provide indications that 1) anhedonia is associated with substance use problems/disorders and their severity, 2) anhedonia is especially prominent in DUS with comorbid depression and early life stress experiences, 3) anhedonia may be both a trait and a state dimension in its relation to DUS, and 4) anhedonia tends to negatively impact DUS treatment outcome. Finally, most evidence points to motivational anhedonia as the most involved subdimension of anhedonia within its relationship with DUS.

Overall, the findings in this review, focusing on articles over the last 5 years, are in line with the earlier review of Garfield et al. (3). Across the different substances of abuse, findings in this review provide indications that anhedonia—as a broad concept—is associated with DUS and DUS severity. However, these findings need to be looked upon prudently. Indeed, the number of studies using a control group remains very limited. Also, the severity measures used throughout the different studies are very variable, leaving consistent interpretation difficult. Altogether, the number of studies remains very limited especially when compared to the number of studies published on impulse/executive control in SUD. This is remarkable. Indeed, in a recent consensus paper, RDoC Positive Valence System (Reward Valuation, Expectancy, Action Selection, Reward Learning, Habit) was put forward as an essential domain with respect to the pathogenesis of addictive disorders, implicated in vulnerabilities for initiation, continuation, and chronicity of the disorder (8). Anhedonia can be positioned on the bridge of both negative and positive Valence Systems, but associates close to Reward Valuation, Reward Expectancy, and Reward Learning. This theoretical ground and the findings of our review indicate that anhedonia deserves more attention.

Moreover, anhedonia is looked upon as an important "transdiagnostic" concept underlying many different psychiatric disorders, e.g., depression, bipolar disorder, and schizophrenia (11). All these disorders relate, in different ways, to altered reward processing. Finally, anhedonia might have relevance bridging with a growing literature on the role of inflammation in the pathogenesis of psychiatric disorders such as mood disorders or addictive disorders (56). From this perspective, it can be hypothesized that a neurobiological vulnerability to inflammatory stimuli may drive the link between chronic substance use (early life stress) and anhedonia.

A sizable number of (large) studies in this review focused on comorbidity and provided indications that DUS patients with a comorbid mood disorder had higher levels of anhedonia as compared to single diagnosis groups. These findings give some ground for the hypothesis that anhedonia might be a common factor underlying both types of disorder or at least a subtype of each. Subtypes in depression with anhedonia being the prominent feature have recently been suggested. Specifically, an "inflammatory" subtype has been proposed with a neurobiological vulnerability to inflammatory stimuli that drive the link between stress and anhedonic symptoms (56). Of interest, early childhood adversity may be one of the most critical factors modulating this neurobiological vulnerability. It is remarkable that two studies in this review showed a clear association between anhedonia and substance use severity, specifically in a population of individuals exposed to trauma (21, 23). Given the high prevalence of early childhood adversity within individuals with DUS, future studies need to explore whether this subgroup is associated with anhedonia.

Research on anhedonia in other psychiatric disorders, e.g., depression, can also help to provide more insight into how research on anhedonia in SUD needs to be done. As mentioned above, self-reports are the most used instrument, while they are mostly unable to distinguish the different aspects of reward processing and reward learning. In depression literature, however, various aspects of reward in relation to anhedonia could be disentangled based on numerous studies combining behavioral tasks and neurobiological measures, mainly event related potential (ERP) studies. Neuroimaging studies could be useful as well, taking into account the idea that fMRI paradigms are mostly unable to dissect into anticipatory, consummatory, and learning components of reward processing (23). A multimodal approach using the same paradigms in future research projects is recommended.

Data from this review show mixed results as to the trait versus state characteristic of anhedonia within the context of substance use. Some studies give support to the hypothesis that anhedonia might be a trait that underlies a vulnerability for early substance use initiation and early escalation. This is in line with the self-medication theory whereby substances are used to mediate mood disorders or innate reward deficiencies (9). Also, adolescents with high stress and amygdala reactivity are more likely to consume a full standard alcoholic drink, are more likely to experience early intoxication, and are at a heightened risk for the onset of an alcohol use disorder (57). In line with this, anhedonia can be hypothesized as a vulnerability trait for early substance use trajectories and subsequent increase of DUS risk. A hypothesis is also in line with the reward deficiency hypothesis (58). Inversely, different studies in this review indicate that anhedonia is associated with ongoing substance use and withdrawal while improving over time in abstinence. This is in line with earlier studies showing improvement in reward responsiveness during treatment and abstinence (59). These findings are indicative of a state characteristic. However, longitudinal studies remain very scarce, i.e., in this review, only one study followed the course of anhedonia over a 6-month abstinence period showing improvement over time (45). So, any conclusion concerning trait or state is at best preliminary.

Several studies in this review showed a negative influence of anhedonia on DUS course and treatment effect, i.e., shorter posttreatment abstinence and higher relapse rates. This is confirmation of findings presented in the earlier review on this topic showing that anhedonia increases the likelihood of relapse and is associated with craving (3). In the depression research, anhedonia negatively influences disease course. This has also been documented within the context of treating depression (13–16). It can be hypothesized that anhedonia as a transdiagnostic characteristic modulates disease course and outcome.

Within the context of depression treatment, existing psychological and pharmacological treatments have proved to be rather ineffective for treating anhedonia. Some of the more commonly used antidepressants, e.g., fluoxetine, may even worsen anhedonic symptoms (60–62). Of importance, newer treatments such as ketamine are shown to have improvement of anhedonia, even in treatment-resistant depression (63, 64). This is of interest, also from the perspective of indication that ketamine can be used within the context of treatment of DUS (65). Although, at this point, no study has been published exploring the effectiveness of ketamine as a treatment for patients with DUS and depression/anhedonia comorbidity, this is an exciting idea. Of interest in this review is the finding that substitution treatment (i.e., nicotine patch) might be beneficial specifically for smokers scoring high on anhedonia. Powers et al. (30) showed an increased likelihood of short-term abstinence using a 21-mg/day nicotine patch therapy. Cook et al. (34) observed that administering nicotine replacement therapy suppressed abstinence-induced anhedonia and alleviated nicotine withdrawal symptoms during short-term abstinence. Moreover, depressed non-smokers show significant declines in depressive symptoms during nicotine patch treatment, suggesting that NRT (and nicotine patch in particular) may have antidepressant-like effects (66). It has been hypothesized that nicotine exposure ameliorates the hypoactivation in crucial structures of the reward pathway (including caudate, nucleus accumbens, putamen) among depressed smokers, with data showing increased activation after nicotine administration in the dorsal striatum during anticipatory reward responding and in the medial prefrontal cortex associated with sensitivity to reward (67). It has to be noted that the sample of anhedonic participants in the study of Powers et al. (30) was small, and the lack of a placebo condition made it difficult to draw inferences about the impact of nicotine patch therapy on pretreatment anhedonia or depression more generally. Finally, there is preliminary evidence that aripiprazole might promote alcohol abstinence and reduce anhedonia, possibly *via* dopaminergic and serotonergic modulations at the fronto-subcortical circuitries (68). However, this needs future replication.

Taken together, although anhedonia is notably challenging to treat and can negatively impact disease course, these preliminary studies hold promises for developing future—pharmacological—treatments.

Findings in this review need be looked upon critically. Several limitations need to be taken into account. First, the vast majority of studies focus on tobacco smoking. Other substances of abuse remain largely understudied, and regarding behavioral addictions, the information is zero. Next and most importantly, throughout the studies, a variety of anhedonia measures has been used. For none of these measures it is known what exact anhedonia dimension they measure, neither is enough information available on how these measures relate. This makes a comparison between studies impossible and may be responsible for sometimes contradictory findings. Third, different study designs and samples are used, which makes it difficult to draw general conclusions about the temporal and causal relationships between anhedonia and DUS. Finally, ours is an explorative, narrative review highlighting the broad field of the anhedonia–DUS relationship. Future hypothesis-driven studies are needed both on the clinical consequences and on elucidating the exact underlying mechanisms and neurocognitive dimensions.

CONCLUSIONS

Findings from this review provide indications that anhedonia might be of relevance for a better understanding of the pathogenesis of addictive disorders and their comorbidities. Anhedonia might prove to be an unimportant transdiagnostic dimension underlying many disorders in their relationship with different reward processing impairments. Within the National Institute of Mental Health's (NIH) Research Domain Criteria (RDoC), anhedonia is conceptualized as an RDoC Element (behavior) within the following Domains and Constructs: 1) Domain: Negative Valence Systems; 2) Construct: Loss and Construct. However, anhedonia might also be linked to other domains, i.e., Positive Valence Systems (11), so anhedonia might be important in bridging these systems and/or reflect different subgroups/mechanisms.

However, in contrast to the field of impulsivity, the study of anhedonia in the relationship with DUS is only nascent. Reflective of this is not only the relatively small number of studies but also the variability of measures and concepts used in the different studies. There is a great need of consensus in defining the neurocognitive dimensions and best measurement instruments/paradigms to help the field move on more quickly. Within this context, the recent international consensus paper identifying the most critical cognitive domains within neuroscience of addictions is a vital initiative (8). Let us see how and when anhedonia finds a place in this model.

AUTHOR CONTRIBUTIONS

All authors contributed to the manuscript conception design and writing.

REFERENCES

1. Alcohol GBD, Drug Use C. The global burden of disease attributable to alcohol and drug use in 195 countries and territories, 1990–2016: a systematic analysis for the Global Burden of Disease Study 2016. *Lancet Psychiatry* (2018) 5(12):987–1012. doi: 10.1016/S2215-0366(18)30337-7
2. Koob GF. The dark side of addiction: the Horsley Gantt to Joseph Brady connection. *J Nerv Ment Dis* (2017) 205(4):270–2. doi: 10.1097/NMD.0000000000000551
3. Garfield JB, Lubman DI, Yucel M. Anhedonia in substance use disorders: a systematic review of its nature, course and clinical correlates. *Aust N Z J Psychiatry* (2014) 48(1):36–51. doi: 10.1177/0004867413508455
4. de Timary P, Starkel P, Delzenne NM, Leclercq S. A role for the peripheral immune system in the development of alcohol use disorders? *Neuropharmacology* (2017) 122:148–60. doi: 10.1016/j.neuropharm.2017.04.013
5. De Berardis D, Fornaro M, Orsolini L, Iasevoli F, Tomasetti C, de Bartolomeis A, et al. Effect of agomelatine treatment on C-reactive protein levels in patients with major depressive disorder: an exploratory study in "real-world," everyday clinical practice. *CNS Spectr* (2017) 22(4):342–7. doi: 10.1017/S1092852916000572
6. De Berardis D, Fornaro M, Serroni N, Campanella D, Rapini G, Olivieri L, et al. Agomelatine beyond borders: current evidences of its efficacy in disorders other than major depression. *Int J Mol Sci* (2015) 16(1):1111–30. doi: 10.3390/ijms16011111
7. Martinotti G, Pettorruso M, De Berardis D, Varasano PA, Lucidi Pressanti G, De Remigis V, et al. Agomelatine increases BDNF serum levels in depressed patients in correlation with the improvement of depressive symptoms. *Int J Neuropsychopharmacol* (2016) 19(5). doi: 10.1093/ijnp/pyw003
8. Yücel M, Oldenhof E, Ahmed SH, Belin D, Billieux J, Bowden-Jones H, et al. A transdiagnostic dimensional approach towards a neuropsychological assessment for addiction: an international Delphi consensus study. *Addiction* (2019) 114(6):1095–109. doi: 10.1111/add.14424
9. Turner S, Mota N, Bolton J, Sareen J. Self-medication with alcohol or drugs for mood and anxiety disorders: a narrative review of the epidemiological literature. *Depress Anxiety* (2018) 35(9):851–60. doi: 10.1002/da.22771
10. Craske MG, Meuret AE, Ritz T, Treanor M, Dour HJ. Treatment for anhedonia a neuroscience driven approach. *Depress Anxiety* (2016) 33(10):927–38. doi: 10.1002/da.22490
11. Nusslock R, Alloy LB. Reward processing and mood-related symptoms: an RDoC and translational neuroscience perspective. *J Affect Disord* (2017) 216:3–16. doi: 10.1016/j.jad.2017.02.001
12. Treadway MT. The neurobiology of motivational deficits in depression—an update on candidate pathomechanisms. *Curr Top Behav Neurosci* (2016) 27:337–55. doi: 10.1007/7854_2015_400
13. Fawcett J, Scheftner WA, Fogg L, Clark DC, Young MA, Hedeker D, et al. Time-related predictors of suicide in major affective disorder. *Am J Psychiatry* (1990) 147(9):1189–94. doi: 10.1176/ajp.147.9.1189
14. Morris BH, Bylsma LM, Rottenberg J. Does emotion predict the course of major depressive disorder?A review of prospective studies. *Br J Clin Psychol* (2009) 48(Pt 3):255–73. doi: 10.1348/014466508X396549
15. Uher R, Perlis RH, Henigsberg N, Zobel A, Rietschel M, Mors O, et al. Depression symptom dimensions as predictors of antidepressant treatment

outcome: replicable evidence for interest-activity symptoms. *Psychol Med* (2012) 42(5):967–80. doi: 10.1017/S0033291711001905

16. Winer ES, Nadorff MR, Ellis TE, Allen JG, Herrera S, Salem T. Anhedonia predicts suicidal ideation in a large psychiatric inpatient sample. *Psychiatry Res* (2014) 218(1–2):124–8. doi: 10.1016/j.psychres.2014.04.016
17. Scheggi S, De Montis MG, Gambarana C. Making sense of rodent models of anhedonia. *Int J Neuropsychopharmacol* (2018) 21(11):1049–65. doi: 10.1093/ijnp/pyy083
18. Treadway MT, Zald DH. Reconsidering anhedonia in depression: lessons from translational neuroscience. *Neurosci Biobehav Rev* (2011) 35(3):537–55. doi: 10.1016/j.neubiorev.2010.06.006
19. Wardle MC, Vincent JN, Suchting R, Green CE, Lane SD, Schmitz JM. Anhedonia is associated with poorer outcomes in contingency management for cocaine use disorder. *J Subst Abuse Treat* (2017) 72:32–9. doi: 10.1016/j.jsat.2016.08.020
20. Carton L, Pignon B, Baguet A, Benradia I, Roelandt JL, Vaiva G, et al. Influence of comorbid alcohol use disorders on the clinical patterns of major depressive disorder: a general population-based study. *Drug Alcohol Depend* (2018) 187:40–7. doi: 10.1016/j.drugalcdep.2018.02.009
21. Claycomb Erwin M, Charak R, Durham TA, Armour C, Ly C, Southwick SM, et al. The 7-factor hybrid model of DSM-5 PTSD symptoms and alcohol consumption and consequences in a national sample of trauma-exposed veterans. *J Anxiety Disord* (2017) 51:14–21. doi: 10.1016/j.janxdis.2017.08.001
22. Cano MA, de Dios MA, Correa-Fernandez V, Childress S, Abrams JL, Roncancio AM. Depressive symptom domains and alcohol use severity among Hispanic emerging adults: examining moderating effects of gender. *Addict Behav* (2017) 72:72–8. doi: 10.1016/j.addbeh.2017.03.015
23. Corral-Frias NS, Nikolova YS, Michalski LJ, Baranger DA, Hariri AR, Bogdan R. Stress-related anhedonia is associated with ventral striatum reactivity to reward and transdiagnostic psychiatric symptomatology. *Psychol Med* (2015) 45(12):2605–17. doi: 10.1017/S0033291715000525
24. Brikmanis K, Petersen A, Doran N. Do personality traits related to affect regulation predict other tobacco product use among young adult non-daily smokers? *Addict Behav* (2017) 75:79–84. doi: 10.1016/j.addbeh.2017.07.008
25. Cook JW, Lanza ST, Chu W, Baker TB, Piper ME. Anhedonia: its dynamic relations with craving, negative affect, and treatment during a quit smoking attempt. *Nicotine Tob Res* (2017) 19(6):703–9. doi: 10.1093/ntr/ntw247
26. Stone MD, Audrain-McGovern J, Leventhal AM. Association of anhedonia with adolescent smoking susceptibility and initiation. *Nicotine Tob Res* (2017) 19(6):738–42. doi: 10.1093/ntr/ntw177
27. Guillot CR, Halliday TM, Kirkpatrick MG, Pang RD, Leventhal AM. Anhedonia and abstinence as predictors of the subjective pleasantness of positive, negative, and smoking-related pictures. *Nicotine Tob Res* (2017) 19(6):743–9. doi: 10.1093/ntr/ntx036
28. Piper ME, Vasilenko SA, Cook JW, Lanza ST. What a difference a day makes: differences in initial abstinence response during a smoking cessation attempt. *Addiction* (2017) 112(2):330–9. doi: 10.1111/add.13613
29. Roys M, Weed K, Carrigan M, MacKillop J. Associations between nicotine dependence, anhedonia, urgency and smoking motives. *Addict Behav* (2016) 62:145–51. doi: 10.1016/j.addbeh.2016.06.002
30. Powers JM, Carroll AJ, Veluz-Wilkins AK, Blazekovic S, Gariti P, Leone FT, et al. Is the effect of anhedonia on smoking cessation greater for women versus men? *Nicotine Tob Res* (2017) 19(1):119–23. doi: 10.1093/ntr/ntw148
31. Chuang CW, Chan C, Leventhal AM. Adolescent emotional pathology and lifetime history of alcohol or drug use with and without comorbid tabacco use. *J Dual Diagn* (2016) 12:27–35. doi: 10.1080/15504263.2016.1146557
32. Leventhal AM, Cho J, Stone MD, Barrington-Trimis JL, Chou CP, Sussman SY, et al. Associations between anhedonia and marijuana use escalation across mid-adolescence. *Addiction* (2017) 112(12):2182–90. doi: 10.1111/add.13912
33. Liverant GI, Sloan DM, Pizzagalli DA, Harte CB, Kamholz BW, Rosebrock LE, et al. Associations among smoking, anhedonia, and reward learning in depression. *Behav Ther* (2014) 45(5):651–63. doi: 10.1016/j.beth.2014.02.004
34. Cook JW, Piper ME, Leventhal AM, Schlam TR, Fiore MC, Baker TB. Anhedonia as a component of the tobacco withdrawal syndrome. *J Abnorm Psychol* (2015) 124(1):215–25. doi: 10.1037/abn0000016
35. Leventhal AM, Trujillo M, Ameringer KJ, Tidey JW, Sussman S, Kahler CW. Anhedonia and the relative reward value of drug and nondrug reinforcers in cigarette smokers. *J Abnorm Psychol* (2014) 123(2):375–86. doi: 10.1037/a0036384
36. Leventhal AM, Piper ME, Japuntich SJ, Baker TB, Cook JW. Anhedonia, depressed mood, and smoking cessation outcome. *J Consult Clin Psychol* (2014) 82(1):122–9. doi: 10.1037/a0035046
37. Albertella L, Le Pelley ME, Copeland J. Cannabis use in early adolescence is associated with higher negative schizotypy in females. *Eur Psychiatry* (2017) 45:235–41. doi: 10.1016/j.eurpsy.2017.07.009
38. Lichenstein SD, Musselman S, Shaw DS, Sitnick S, Forbes EE. Nucleus accumbens functional connectivity at age 20 is associated with trajectory of adolescent cannabis use and predicts psychosocial functioning in young adulthood. *Addiction* (2017) 112(11):1961–70. doi: 10.1111/add.13882
39. Feingold D, Rehm J, Lev-Ran S. Cannabis use and the course and outcome of major depressive disorder: a population based longitudinal study. *Psychiatry Res* (2017) 251:225–34. doi: 10.1016/j.psychres.2017.02.027
40. Parvaz MA, Gabbay V, Malaker P, Goldstein RZ. Objective and specific tracking of anhedonia *via* event-related potentials in individuals with cocaine use disorders. *Drug Alcohol Depend* (2016) 164:158–65. doi: 10.1016/j.drugalcdep.2016.05.004
41. Morie KP, De Sanctis P, Garavan H, Foxe JJ. Regulating task-monitoring systems in response to variable reward contingencies and outcomes in cocaine addicts. *Psychopharmacology (Berl)* (2016) 233(6):1105–18. doi: 10.1007/s00213-015-4191-8
42. Morie KP, De Sanctis P, Garavan H, Foxe JJ. Executive dysfunction and reward dysregulation: a high-density electrical mapping study in cocaine abusers. *Neuropharmacology* (2014) 85:397–407. doi: 10.1016/j.neuropharm.2014.05.016
43. Gooding DC, Gjini K, Burroughs SA, Boutros NN. The association between psychosis proneness and sensory gating in cocaine-dependent patients and healthy controls. *Psychiatry Res* (2013) 210:1092–100. doi: 10.1016/j.psychres.2013.08.049
44. Garfield JBB, Cotton SM, Allen NB, Cheetham A, Kras M, Yucel M, et al. Evidence that anhedonia is a symptom of opioid dependence associated with recent use. *Drug Alcohol Depend* (2017) 177:29–38. doi: 10.1016/j.drugalcdep.2017.03.012
45. Krupitsky E, Zvartau E, Blokhina E, Verbitskaya E, Wahlgren V, Tsoy-Podosenin M, et al. Anhedonia, depression, anxiety, and craving in opiate dependent patients stabilized on oral naltrexone or an extended release naltrexone implant. *Am J Drug Alcohol Abuse* (2016) 42(5):614–20. doi: 10.1080/00952990.2016.1197231
46. Huhn AS, Meyer RE, Harris JD, Ayaz H, Deneke E, Stankoski DM, et al. Evidence of anhedonia and differential reward processing in prefrontal cortex among post-withdrawal patients with prescription opiate dependence. *Brain Res Bull* (2016) 123:102–9. doi: 10.1016/j.brainresbull.2015.12.004
47. Zaaijer ER, van Dijk L, de Bruin K, Goudriaan AE, Lammers LA, Koeter MW, et al. Effect of extended-release naltrexone on striatal dopamine transporter availability, depression and anhedonia in heroin-dependent patients. *Psychopharmacology (Berl)* (2015) 232(14):2597–607. doi: 10.1007/s00213-015-3891-4
48. Pettorruso M, Martinotti G, Fasano A, Loria G, Di Nicola M, De Risio L, et al. Anhedonia in Parkinson's disease patients with and without pathological gambling: a case–control study. *Psychiatry Res* (2014) 215(2):448–52. doi: 10.1016/j.psychres.2013.12.013
49. Rizvi SJ, Sproule BA, Gallaugher L, McIntyre RS, Kennedy SH. Correlates of benzodiazepine use in major depressive disorder: the effect of anhedonia. *J Affect Disord* (2015) 187:101–5. doi: 10.1016/j.jad.2015.07.040
50. Snaith RP, Hamilton M, Morley S, Humayan A, Hargreaves D, Trigwell P. A scale for the assessment of hedonic tone the Snaith–Hamilton Pleasure Scale. *Br J Psychiatry* (1995) 167(1):99–103. doi: 10.1192/bjp.167.1.99
51. Rizvi SJ, Pizzagalli DA, Sproule BA, Kennedy SH. Assessing anhedonia in depression: potentials and pitfalls. *Neurosci Biobehav Rev* (2016) 65:21–35. doi: 10.1016/j.neubiorev.2016.03.004
52. Andreoni M, Babudieri S, Bruno S, Colombo M, Zignego AL, Di Marco V, et al. Current and future challenges in HCV: insights from an Italian experts panel. *Infection* (2018) 46(2):147–63. doi: 10.1007/s15010-017-1093-1

53. Colombo D, Palacios AG, Alvarez JF, Patane A, Semonella M, Cipresso P, et al. Current state and future directions of technology-based ecological momentary assessments and interventions for major depressive disorder: protocol for a systematic review. *Syst Rev* (2018) 7(1):233. doi: 10.1186/s13643-018-0899-y
54. Pizzagalli DA, Holmes AJ, Dillon DG, Goetz EL, Birk JL, Bogdan R, et al. Reduced caudate and nucleus accumbens response to rewards in unmedicated individuals with major depressive disorder. *Am J Psychiatry* (2009) 166(6):702–10. doi: 10.1176/appi.ajp.2008.08081201
55. Treadway MT, Buckholtz JW, Schwartzman AN, Lambert WE, Zald DH. Worth the 'EEfRT'? The effort expenditure for rewards task as an objective measure of motivation and anhedonia. *PLoS One* (2009) 4(8):e6598. doi: 10.1371/journal.pone.0006598
56. Cooper JA, Arulpragasam AR, Treadway MT. Anhedonia in depression: biological mechanisms and computational models. *Curr Opin Behav Sci* (2018) 22:128–35. doi: 10.1016/j.cobeha.2018.01.024
57. Elsayed NM, Kim MJ, Fields KM, Olvera RL, Hariri AR, Williamson DE. Trajectories of alcohol initiation and use during adolescence: the role of stress and amygdala reactivity. *J Am Acad Child Adolesc Psychiatry* (2018) 57(8):550–60. doi: 10.1016/j.jaac.2018.05.011
58. Blum K, Gondre-Lewis MC, Baron D, Thanos PK, Braverman ER, Neary J, et al. Introducing precision addiction management of reward deficiency syndrome, the construct that underpins all addictive behaviors. *Front Psychiatry* (2018) 9:548. doi: 10.3389/fpsyt.2018.00548
59. Boger KD, Auerbach RP, Pechtel P, Busch AB, Greenfield SF, Pizzagalli DA. Co-occurring depressive and substance use disorders in adolescents: an examination of reward responsiveness during treatment. *J Psychother Integr* (2014) 24(2):109–21. doi: 10.1037/a0036975
60. McCabe C, Mishor Z, Cowen PJ, Harmer CJ. Diminished neural processing of aversive and rewarding stimuli during selective serotonin reuptake inhibitor treatment. *Biol Psychiatry* (2010) 67(5):439–45. doi: 10.1016/j.biopsych.2009.11.001
61. Nierenberg AA, Keefe BR, Leslie VC, Alpert JE, Pava JA, Worthington JJ, et al. Residual symptoms in depressed patients who respond acutely to fluoxetine. *J Clin Psychiatry* (1999) 60(4):221–5. doi: 10.4088/JCP.v60n0403
62. Price J, Cole V, Goodwin GM. Emotional side-effects of selective serotonin reuptake inhibitors: qualitative study. *Br J Psychiatry* (2009) 195(3):211–7. doi: 10.1192/bjp.bp.108.051110
63. Lally N, Nugent AC, Luckenbaugh DA, Ameli R, Roiser JP, Zarate CA. Anti-anhedonic effect of ketamine and its neural correlates in treatment-resistant bipolar depression. *Transl Psychiatry* (2014) 4:e469. doi: 10.1038/tp.2014.105
64. Thomas RK, Baker G, Lind J, Dursun S. Rapid effectiveness of intravenous ketamine for ultraresistant depression in a clinical setting and evidence for baseline anhedonia and bipolarity as clinical predictors of effectiveness. *J Psychopharmacol* (2018) 32(10):1110–7. doi: 10.1177/0269881118793104
65. Jones JL, Mateus CF, Malcolm RJ, Brady KT, Back SE. Efficacy of ketamine in the treatment of substance use disorders: a systematic review. *Front Psychiatry* (2018) 9:277. doi: 10.3389/fpsyt.2018.00277
66. Korhonen T, Kinnunen TH, Garvey AJ. Impact of nicotine replacement therapy on post-cessation mood profile by pre-cessation depressive symptoms. *Tob Induc Dis* (2006) 3:17–33. doi: 10.1186/1617-9625-3-2-17
67. Rose EJ, Ross TJ, Salmeron BJ, Lee M, Shakleya DM, Huestis MA, et al. Acute nicotine differentially impacts anticipatory valence- and magnitude-related striatal activity. *Biol Psychiatry* (2013) 73(3):280–8. doi: 10.1016/j.biopsych.2012.06.034
68. Martinotti G, Orsolini L, Fornaro M, Vecchiotti R, De Berardis D, Iasevoli F, et al. Aripiprazole for relapse prevention and craving in alcohol use disorder: current evidence and future perspectives. *Expert Opin Investig Drugs* (2016) 25(6):719–28. doi: 10.1080/13543784.2016.1175431

9

Neurocognitive Precursors of Substance Misuse Corresponding to Risk, Resistance and Resilience Pathways: Implications for Prevention Science

Emma Jane Rose[1], *Giorgia Picci*[1] *and Diana H. Fishbein*[1,2]*

[1] *Program for Translational Research on Adversity and Neurodevelopment (P-TRAN), The Edna Bennett Pierce Prevention Research Center, The Pennsylvania State University, University Park, PA, USA,* [2] *Department of Human Development and Family Studies, The Pennsylvania State University, University Park, PA, USA*

***Correspondence:**
Diana Hanna Fishbein
dfishbein@psu.edu

Studies of substance misuse prevention generally focus on characteristics that typify risk, with the assumption that the prevalence of the problem will be optimally reduced by identifying, targeting, and reducing or eliminating risk factors. However, this risk-centered approach neglects variations in individual-level and environmental characteristics that portend differential pathways that are distinguishable by timing of substance use initiation (e.g., early versus delayed), the likelihood of use escalation versus eventual desistance, and enduring abstinence, despite exposure to significant risk factors. Considering the various underpinnings of these distinct substance use trajectories is critical to a more nuanced understanding of the effects, potency, and malleability of factors that are known to increase risk *or* confer protection. Here, we discuss three pathways relative to substance use patterns and predictors in the context of adversity, a well-known, highly significant influence on propensity for substance misuse. The first pathway is designated as "high risk" based on early onset of substance use, rapid escalation, and proneness to substance use disorders. Individuals who defy all odds and eventually exhibit adaptive developmental outcomes despite an initial maladaptive reaction to adversity, are referred to as "resilient." However, another categorization that has not been adequately characterized is "resistant." Resistant individuals include those who do not exhibit problematic substance use behaviors (e.g., early onset and escalation) and do not develop substance use disorders or other forms of psychopathology, despite significant exposure to factors that normally increase the propensity for such outcomes (e.g. trauma and/or adversity). In this paper, we apply this conceptualization of risk, resistance, and resilience for substance misuse to a more fine-grained analysis of substance use pathways and their corresponding patterns (e.g., non-use, initiation, escalation, desistance). The significance of the progression of neurocognitive functioning over the course of development is discussed as well as how this knowledge may be translated to make a science-based determination of intervention targets. This more encompassing theoretical model has direct implications for primary prevention and clinical approaches to disrupt risk pathways and to optimize long-term outcomes.

Keywords: neurocognitive, neuroimaging, substance misuse/abuse, risk, resilience, resistance, prevention science

INTRODUCTION

Adolescents who initiate substance use and later develop substance use disorders (SUDs) transition through multiple sequential stages, including experimental or social use, escalation of use, maintenance, abuse, and eventual dependence (1, 2). However, a linear progression along this pathway is not often realized, with individuals showing considerable variability in the likelihood of early, experimental use and significant fluctuations in patterns of usage, escalation, and desistance (3, 4). For example, there are subgroups of users who may never escalate, maintaining nondependent use for decades. While some exhibit intermittent periods of cessation or abstain permanently, others rapidly escalate and go on to develop SUDs. Discriminating between these different user types and delineating which individuals are more likely to follow different pathways is key to identifying critical windows of opportunity for preventing substance misuse.

A potent risk factor influencing the transition from social/experimental use to problematic use and eventual dependence is the experience of traumatic and other chronic or severely stressful events in childhood (5, 6). Indeed, exposure to adversities such as child maltreatment, poverty, and witnessing or experiencing violence have been repeatedly implicated in trajectories leading to SUDs (7–9). The literature is replete with studies documenting the impact of early adversity on neurocognitive development throughout childhood and adolescence and, in turn, how adversity-related deficits or delays in neurocognitive function in youth can increase vulnerability to a myriad of risk behaviors, such as substance misuse (10–12). Integrity of neurocognitive development translates to the ability to self-regulate behavior and emotion via "top-down" cognitive control over affective responses to life's challenges. The development of these processes may be particularly influential in adaptations to adversity. Thus, variations in neurocognitive trajectories are likely more pronounced in populations where adversity prevails, which, in turn, may correspond to a wide range of behavioral pathways and outcomes, from low to high risk (13–15). In other words, adversity can result in diverse outcomes (*multifinality*) depending largely upon the ways in which the nervous system is affected in exposed individuals.

Substance use outcomes in response to adversity, including its impacts on the brain, may manifest in the following general developmental pathways: *risk* (initial and sustained reactions to adversity, resulting in maladaptive outcomes), *delayed risk* (apparent early resistance to adversity but eventual decline toward maladaptive outcomes), *resilience* (initial reaction followed by gradual degradation of response to adversity with eventual restoration of adaptive developmental outcomes), and *resistance* (absence of change in developmental trajectory despite exposure to adversity). Developmental periods that correspond with these patterns may include an initial departure in direction (e.g., risk vs. resistance), the time point at which trajectories may diverge (e.g., resistance vs. delayed risk *or* risk vs. resilience), and the time beyond which specific risk outcomes emerge (e.g., substance abuse). Developing more precision-based interventions will require a clearer delineation of critical time points when influential factors in substance misuse act on emergent neurocognitive systems in a manner that increases the likelihood of following one of these pathways versus another.

As described herein, our *Accumulative Risk Model* (see **Figure 1**) depicts the interactive influence of genetic risk markers and environmental contexts (both detrimental and protective) on intermediate phenotypes, including distinct or interwoven cognitive, affective, and behavioral trajectories and associated neural factors (i.e., variability in brain structure and function) that underpin pathways for outcomes ranging from adaptive to maladaptive. In our model, the dynamic interplay of factors in the developmental context exerts differential impacts on these intermediate phenotypes and their neurobiological substrates in a manner that is contingent upon developmental stage. As such, missing time-dependent opportunities to intervene and redirect development translates to a higher probability of individuals exceeding a liability threshold for high risk behaviors, including substance misuse. In this paper, we review the evidence in support of this integrative framework and its relevance to the ability of evidence-based prevention programming to strengthen these neurodevelopmental processes, thereby attenuating negative effects of risk factors and reinforcing resilience and/or resistance. Such a science-based strategy has potential to redirect developmental pathways away from risky behaviors such as substance abuse.

The content presented in this review was selected via a nonsystematic/narrative review process, whereby we searched standard sources (e.g., PubMed; www.ncbi.nlm.nih.gov) for relevant but broad terms. This included various combinations of the following terms: substance abuse/misuse; SUD(s); development; risk; resilience; genetics; environment; and prevention/intervention. In addition to the articles that resulted from these searches, we engaged in an iterative process by which relevant publications that were cited in specific articles were also included in our review.

The Accumulative Risk Model

Defining Risk: The Accumulative Developmental Context

Risk is commonly thought of as binary and deterministic, as reflected in the tendency to designate individuals as either "at risk" or not, and the assumption that those who are "at risk" are more likely to assume a maladaptive pathway, characterized by

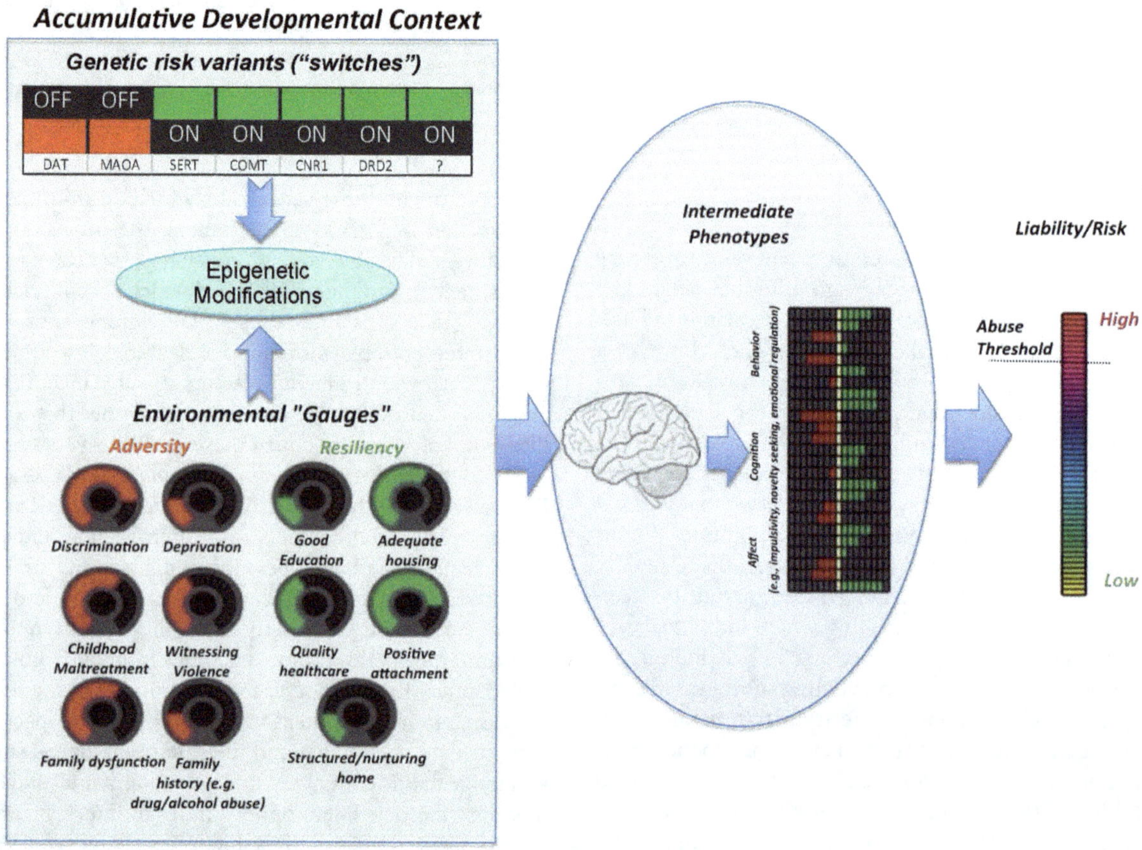

FIGURE 1 | The Accumulative Risk Model. Shown here are the two main categories of factors that constitute the accumulative developmental context, i.e., genetic and environmental factors. The combined effect of the number, type, and severity of these factors confers risk for substance abuse. Genetic variants are considered as switches, which are either "on" or "off." This conceptualization reflects the common binary consideration of genetic risk (i.e., individuals are often considered at risk or not depending on the particular variant of a given gene that they happen to carry). To reflect their more continuous nature, environmental factors are presented as dials, turned up or down depending on the magnitude of the experience. The unique combination of genetic switches and environmental dials drives neurodevelopmental trajectories that underlie particular cognitive, behavioral, and affective intermediate phenotypes, which, in turn, can result in an increased liability threshold, beyond which an individual is considered to be at greater likelihood of developing problematic substance use behaviors and eventual SUD. Importantly, the functional relationship between factors is not linear, and some environmental factors may exacerbate or attenuate the effects of the particular genes via epigenetic modifications.

high-risk behaviors such as substance abuse. However, risk is better conceptualized as a continuous trait—*liability*—with values ranging from low to high. An individual's positioning along the liability continuum is determined by a number of pertinent intermediate phenotypes—such as patterns of behavior, cognition, and affect—modulated by an individual's unique brain structure and function. This neurobiological variability is, itself, a function of a highly complex and individualized range of factors, including those that are potentially malleable, such as environmental and contextual conditions, and those that are not so amenable to change or manipulation, such as genetic factors.

The constellation of factors that confer adaptive or maladaptive neurodevelopmental trajectories can be conceptualized as the "accumulative developmental context." Within this context are factors that either increase (i.e., risk factors) or decrease (i.e., protective factors) liability (**Figure 1**). Importantly, the number and type of risk and protective factors are presumed to be unique between individuals and the interplay between factors determines an individual's level of liability more so than any one factor alone. The influence of each factor, whether risk or protective, is not necessarily linear and some factors may act as moderators of other relevant factors, either amplifying or decreasing their risk or protective potential. Understanding these relationships and how the accumulative developmental context increases liability for SUD or, alternatively, offers protection and fosters resilience or resistance, promises to provide critical information on which to base the development of approaches to prevent SUDs.

Putatively Distinct Developmental Trajectories

Liability for high-risk behaviors or other suboptimal outcomes is commonly considered from the perspective of being either at risk or resilient, with the corresponding assumption being that either trajectory is strongly associated with the prevalence (or sheer number) of risk or protective influences, respectively (16–19). While there is a wealth of experimental evidence to support this characterization, possible developmental pathways arising from any given context includes a range of potential positive and negative trajectories (20, 21) (see **Figure 2a**). Pathways that lead to maladaptive outcomes include the typically considered "risk" pathway; i.e., adverse external conditions and the development of suboptimal intermediate phenotypes, together that increase an individual's likelihood of crossing the liability threshold for high-risk outcomes, such as SUD and other psychopathologies. Typically, risk is described as occurring in close temporal proximity to the factors that promote its expression (e.g., changes in cognitive or behavioral functioning that more or less immediately follow some stressful life event). A related, but not commonly considered, negative trajectory is "delayed risk," which occurs when there is a temporal delay or disconnect between the factors that promote a high-risk trajectory and the observable changes the portend a maladaptive outcome. Though not often distinguished in the literature, determining those aspects of the developmental context that confer risk vs. delayed risk may be helpful in the design of preventive interventions. In particular, such information may lead to programs aimed at individuals who may not immediately appear to be at risk but for whom early evidence-based intervention may be particularly advantageous (i.e., potentially stemming the proliferation of maladaptive phenotypes).

At the positive end of the spectrum are resilience and the related, but theoretically distinct, concept of "resistance." Resilience can be defined as the later expression of adaptive/optimal outcomes despite initially exhibiting negative responses to challenging or threatening circumstances (e.g., adversities and traumas, such as poverty, maltreatment, violence). Resilience-related factors are those that enable an individual to rebound from adversity- or trauma-related dysfunctions or deficits and to achieve their original state or otherwise adaptive outcome(s). In contrast, *resistance* is characterized by the maintenance of the original state despite exposure to stressful events or contexts; i.e., developmental pathways remain unaltered despite significant stress/trauma. A third possible positive trajectory—"recovery"—involves the resumption of function following the development of a maladaptive outcome, such as SUD, and subsequent intervention/treatment (**Figure 2a**). Although possibly driven by the same or similar factors as resistance and resilience (e.g., more optimal levels of neurocognitive functioning or emotional regulation), it is probable that recovery is at least partially distinct in terms of the pathway itself, the factors that promote it, and the timing (i.e., only following intervention). As such, recovery may constitute a third distinct class of positive adaptation. In support of this notion, and in the context of SUD specifically, recovery is highly likely to be distinguishable from resistance and resilience since SUD-related neuroadaptations may not be reversible (23); thus, individuals who recover from SUD do so without regaining a substantial degree of original functioning. Instead, other compensatory mechanisms may facilitate overall functioning in a way that is adaptive and allows individuals with SUD to achieve recovery and avoid relapse (24–26).

PUTATIVE UNDERPINNINGS OF DISTINCT DEVELOPMENTAL TRAJECTORIES

Determining which experimental or social substance users will progress to abuse (i.e., a maladaptive pattern of substance use manifested by recurrent and significant adverse consequences) and dependence (i.e., a chronic relapsing brain disease characterized by compulsive drug seeking despite harmful consequences) is a longstanding question that has compelled researchers and practitioners to better understand, predict, and effectively intervene in maladaptive patterns of substance use. As depicted in the Accumulative Risk Model, the interplay between an individual's genetics and their environmental and contextual experiences during critical periods of development give rise to patterns of neurobiological functioning, stress physiology, personality/temperament, and emerging coping strategies that determine the individual's response to the prevailing social and environmental conditions. The nature of this response contributes to eventual substance use outcomes, including whether an individual will or will not engage in substance use and whether use will progress to abuse and dependence. A critical step in delineating the distinct etiological pathways under consideration here is understanding how relevant person-level characteristics predict or moderate outcomes and interact with environmental influences in unique and complex ways to either promote or preclude substance misuse.

Neurocognitive Pathways to Substance Misuse

As noted above, there are commonalities in the key factors (risk and protective) that give rise to particular types of substance use pathways (i.e., adaptive or maladaptive); distinguishing between those that are more tightly coupled to one specific pathway (i.e., risk, delayed risk, resilience, or resistance) is not possible based on current knowledge and given limitations of the extant research. For example, most studies consider outcomes as either positive/adaptive or negative/maladaptive (e.g., having an SUD or not) at a single time point and lack the longitudinal perspective and temporal specificity needed to distinguish the putative pathways under consideration here. Nonetheless, defining the differential constellations of influences that lead to distinctive pathways toward or away from substance abuse is a paramount task; one holds considerable potential to lead to more personalized interventions with potential for population level impacts. Working backwards within the Accumulative Risk Model, from cognitive and behavioral phenotypes to their more basic substrates, risk and protective factors that cross trajectories are described briefly below. The following subsections consider evidence that implicates neurocognitive factors in the four divergent pathways under consideration here (i.e., risk, delayed risk, resistance, and resilience).

Risk for Substance Misuse

Genetic Vulnerabilities

There have been many genetic risk studies for SUDs that have delineated gene variants that appear to be associated with specific types of abuse (e.g., alcohol/alcohol dehydrogenase genes;

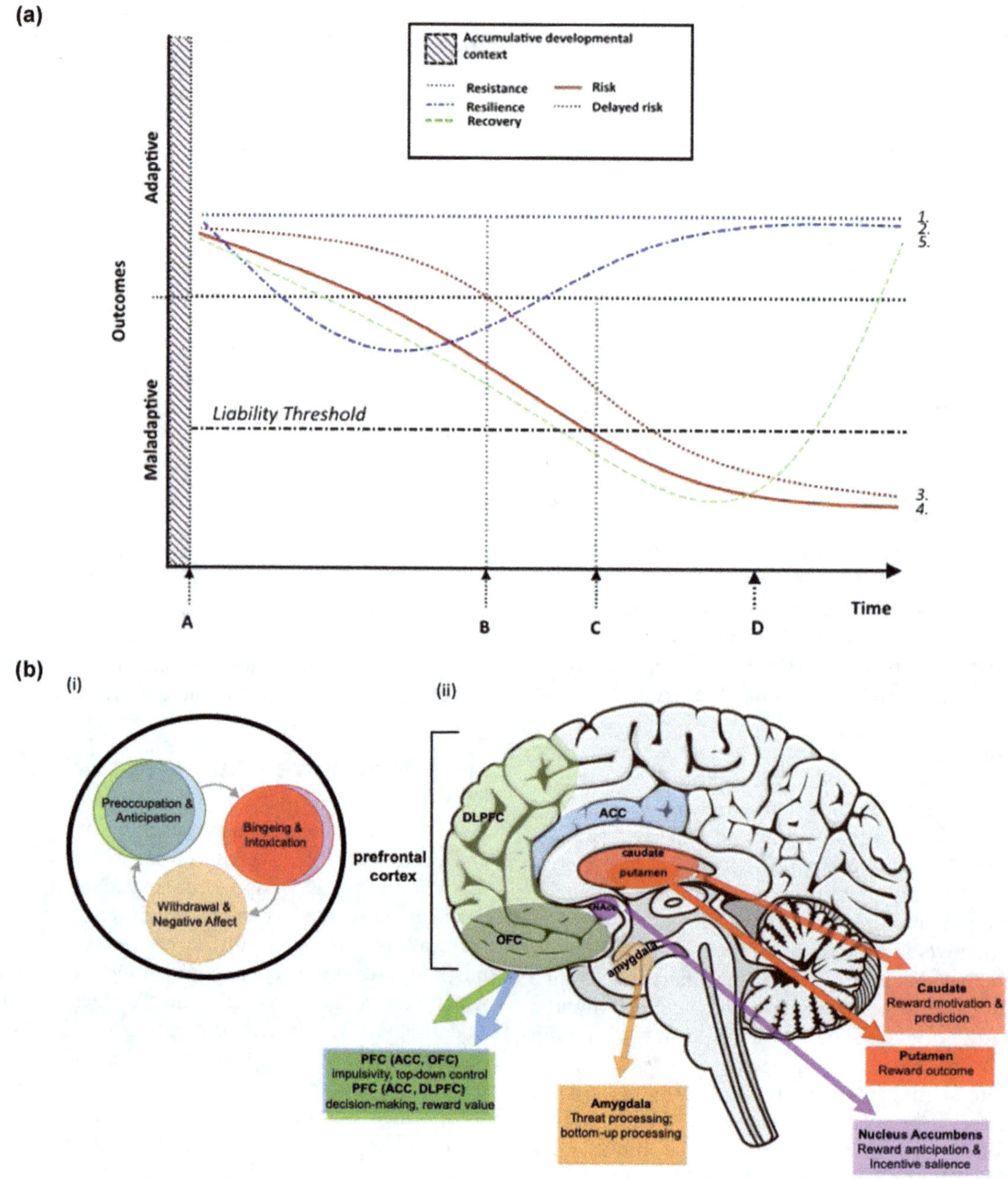

FIGURE 2 | (a) Theoretical neurodevelopmental trajectories corresponding to adaptive and maladaptive outcomes. **(1)** *Resistance*: absence of change in the developmental trajectory despite exposure to adversity; **(2)** *Resilience*: initial reaction followed by gradual degradation of the response to adversity and eventual restoration of an adaptive developmental trajectory; **(3)** *Delayed risk*: apparent early resistance to adversity but eventual decline toward maladaptive outcomes/risk; **(4)** *Risk*: initial and continued reaction to adversity, resulting in maladaptive outcomes, and **(5)** *Recovery*: a shift in neurodevelopmental trajectory back toward adaptive outcomes, following disease onset/crossing the liability threshold for a disorder, and corresponding to intervention (i.e., treatment) onset. Critical time points in delineating those factors that contribute to risk or resistance and resilience include **(A)** the initial departure in neurodevelopmental trajectories, perhaps corresponding to adversity or other stressors, **(B)** the time point at which trajectories may deviate from initial direction (i.e. resilience and delayed risk), **(C)** the time beyond which specific risk outcomes (e.g., substance abuse) are highly probable and beyond which individuals with high levels of risk are likely to have crossed the liability threshold, and **(D)** intervention/treatment onset. Note: "outcomes" includes all relevant intermediate phenotypes consisting of or related to neurodevelopment (e.g., brain structure and function, cognition, behavior, affect, etc.). The "accumulative developmental context" refers to the combined genetic and environmental context that drives brain development (as depicted in **Figure 1**), and although this context is critical to neurodevelopment it precedes observable distinctions between neurodevelopmental trajectories; this includes those factors that may be considered to be detrimental or protective. **(b) (i)** Key stages in the cycle of addiction (after 22) and **(ii)** brain regions that these key stages map to and putative functions of each region that are relevant to the development of SUD. Included here are critical regions in which functional and structural deficits have been shown to be associated with at least one of the stages in the cycle of addiction. Functional variability in these regions in response to the characteristics of the accumulative developmental context (i.e., key genetic, environmental, and psychosocial influences on neurodevelopment) likely underlie the likelihood of which trajectory (i.e., from 2a.) an individual follows. If so, these same regions and the cognitive, behavioral, and affective functions they support have considerable potential to serve as targets for preventive interventions.

nicotine/cholinergic receptor genes; opiates/opioid receptor mu genes). However, individual gene variants do not necessarily increase risk of using or abusing *specific* substances and, indeed, there is evidence that certain genes impact neurobiological systems and phenotypic traits in a manner that may directly influence pathways toward or away from substance use more *generally* (27). This includes genes that are involved in stimulus-reward processing pathways in dopaminergic (e.g., *DRD2, MAOA, COMT*), serotonergic (e.g., *HTR3A, HTR1B, HTR3B*), GABAergic (e.g., *GABRA1, GABRA2, GAD1, KCNJ9/GIRK3*), and glutamatergic neurotransmission systems [e.g., *GRIN2C*; see Ref. (28) for a review]. The phenotypic traits that are associated with these types of "risk" genotypes (e.g., high reward sensitivity, high impulsivity, low risk aversion, a tendency toward compulsive drug seeking) fundamentally interact with stress exposures that, when repeated and/or severe, have potential to compromise the development of neural systems that underlie social, behavioral, cognitive, and emotional functioning in profound and enduring ways (29, 30).

Genetic vulnerabilities in combination with the developmental stage(s) of exposure are critical to the differential effects that the exposure to stress can have on social, psychological, and neural functioning and, in turn, risk for substance abuse (31, 32). Genetic variations contribute an individual's response to existing social influences; thus, genetic influences on propensity to substance abuse and dependence are thought to mediate or moderate the impact of environmental factors on individual characteristics that are associated with risk, with stress exposures being particularly impactful (33). At the core of the gene-by-environment interaction are epigenetic modifications that occur at the level of gene functionality in response to changes in the environment. Adverse experiences, especially in early life, have potential to modify gene expression or suppression with important implications for phenotypic impact on stress hormones and behavior (34, 35). Ongoing environmental change can further modify epigenetic processes, for better or for worse, helping to explain individual differences in response to stress as well as the potential for positive environmental change (e.g., intervention) to reverse earlier negative modifications. Thus, as indicated in our conceptual model (**Figure 1**), not all who are exposed to stress and/or trauma will exhibit maladaptive physiological and psychological stress responses that affect substance abuse liability; differential susceptibility to this outcome is a function of the complex interrelationships among genetic, environmental, and epigenetic factors that individuals dynamically experience.

Environmental Influences

As noted in **Figure 1**, there are a variety of environmental factors that can influence developmental trajectories in a manner that increases the risk for substance misuse. Of particular relevance here are those factors that we know promote adaptations of relevant neurodevelopmental pathways such that an individual's liability for substance abuse and/or dependence are substantially increased. Contextual factors known to interact with biological factors to increase SUD liability include social and cultural systems, stress, and trauma (36).

Childhood maltreatment (CM) is a particularly potent risk factor for substance abuse and dependence (6). Those who experience CM initiate illicit substance use twice as often as nonmaltreated peers and are more likely to abuse substances earlier in adolescence (5, 37). Moreover, an estimated 40–50% of individuals who experience this type of trauma will develop a substance abuse problem in their lifetime (5). Neurobiological changes at the level of brain structure and function have been shown to underlie both CM and SUD and are often found in overlapping brain regions and networks (38–42). Disentangling the specific contributions of CM *per se*, versus those changes that arise in response to early and sustained abuse of substances, presents an interesting and important challenge. Although more research is needed in this domain to understand the independent, interactive, and potentially synergistic, contributions of CM and SUD to neurodevelopmental trajectories in young people, a recent review of the neurocognitive evidence of neurobiological pathways underlying SUD risk provides support for CM-related alterations in three interconnected systems that may heighten SUD vulnerability (**Figure 2b**), (1) *reward processing*—ventral striatum, anterior cingulate cortex (ACC), mPFC (including OFC) and amygdala; (2) *executive cognitive function (ECF)*—prefrontal cortex (PFC), including dlPFC and mPFC; and (3) *threat processing*—medial temporal lobe, in particular the amygdala (43).

Poverty is another common and particularly potent environmental influence to consider when delineating the neural pathways underlying SUD risk. There is consistent evidence to suggest that a child's socioeconomic status (SES) is predictive of neurocognitive trajectories across development and longer-term outcomes, such as academic achievement (44), with lower SES children experiencing suboptimal or maladaptive developmental trajectories, including neurodevelopmental pathways (32, 45–48). The most consistent *structural* impacts of poverty/low SES are seen in brain areas and processes that are sensitive to the effects of stress, including those that are relevant for SUD risk (e.g., hippocampus/memory; amygdala and medial temporal lobe/emotional regulation and threat processing; ACC/reward and decision-making) (44). Moreover, children in lower SES groups also show a range of *functional* deficits, including in brain regions that support ECF, such as prefrontally-mediated attentional focus (49–51), and in prefrontal and parietal regions supporting working memory (52, 53). Lower SES is also associated with greater amygdala responsivity to threatening and fearful stimuli (e.g., faces) in adolescence (54). Interestingly, the functional networks between these cortical and subcortical regions appear to be disrupted by the experience of poverty, with low SES children showing reduced functional connectivity between cortical and subcortical regions during both task-oriented (i.e., emotional processing) and resting-state imaging paradigms (55–57). A recent analysis of the structural connectome in healthy children (6–11 years) found that lower income-to-needs ratios were predictive of greater network inefficiency, particularly for girls, in a range of SUD-relevant regions (e.g., cingulate, insula, amygdala), further supporting the notion that childhood poverty leads to widespread disruption of brain networks (58) and suggesting at least one potential environmental factor that may differentially contribute to risk between males and females. Collectively, these studies, while not explicitly considering substance use or misuse as an outcome, all point to a disruption of structural and functional neurodevelopmental trajectories for those who are economically disadvantaged in regions that are considered relevant for neurocognitive functions related to the extent of SUD liability. Importantly, the impacts of poverty are inextricably linked to the influences of stress and trauma on neurodevelopmental pathways that underlie the risk for substance abuse, since these experiences often occur in concert with one another. However, from a prevention perspective, it may be particularly advantageous to consider poverty as a key factor underlying a maladaptive risk pathway, since economic disadvantage can be more clearly—albeit not more simply—targeted via widely scaling appropriate, evidence-based interventions and policies.

As noted above, it is likely that a key factor underlying the impact of these types of environmental factors (i.e., CM, poverty) on SUD risk are epigenetic modifications that mediate gene-by-environment interactions, specifically those epigenetic factors involved in altering gene regulation of neurobiological systems that are relevant for maladaptive pathways that lead to SUD (59). Of note in the relationship between stress/trauma, neurodevelopment, and substance abuse liability is the role of micro RNAs (MiRNAs) (60). MiRNAs are short noncoding RNAs that epigenetically modulate gene expression. They also regulate central nervous system physiology and have the potential to contribute to alterations in complex systems, including dopaminergic and glutamatergic systems, which are both implicated in SUD (60). A particularly intriguing observation from preclinical studies of SUD-related behaviors is the phenomena of transgenerational epigenetic effects. For example, in rat models, adult drug taking that precedes conception appears to influence reward-related behavior and drug self-administration in first-generation offspring (61, 62). While these types of transgenerational impacts of SUD are potentially highly relevant for those families and communities that are at highest risk for SUD and for which effective prevention is most urgently needed, further study is required to demonstrate similar transgenerational mechanisms in humans. If such effects are found, this information may offer a particularly novel opportunity for cross-generational preventive interventions for SUD.

Neurological Development

The role of deviations or delays in neurodevelopmental pathways underlying problem (especially high risk) behaviors that often precede substance use has been increasingly recognized in studies of SUD risk. As in our Accumulative Risk Model, perturbations in brain structure and function are commonly viewed as critical mediators between the developmental context (i.e., relevant genetics and environmental factors) and the cognitive, behavioral, and affective phenotypes that precede problematic substance use. Understanding the neurobiological contribution to the etiology of substance use involves characterization of brain maturational processes that underlie neurocognitive development during critical periods of development, such as adolescence, that are associated with substance use (e.g., reduced inhibitory control and increased reward sensitivity).

While substance abuse is the result of maladaptive developmental trajectories with their roots in the prenatal period and lasting until the mid to late 20s, substance use initiation is most typical in early to mid-adolescence and, for the subgroup that escalates, substance abuse peaks during the transition into emerging adulthood (63). Critically, new social challenges facing adolescents (e.g., increased autonomous decision-making) coincide with complex changes in brain function and connectivity taking place throughout this time, which have implications for adaptive decision-making and the ability to self-regulate behavior and emotion (64, 65). In effect, some degree of impulsivity, risk-taking, and sensation seeking is normative during adolescence, as indicated above; however, a heightened level of risk-taking may extend from a combination of social circumstances and nonnormative neurodevelopmental immaturity or dysfunction.

Neurobiological development during adolescence occurs transitionally rather than as a single snapshot in time (66). The PFC, which is responsible for ECFs, such as decision-making, impulse control, and working memory, undergoes prolonged development and is still largely under construction during adolescence. A central role of ECFs is to promote behaviors that shield long-term goals from the temptations afforded by short-term benefits that often lead to negative consequences (67). Prefrontal "top-down" neurocognitive regulation over subcortical regions that support affective processes (e.g., emotion regulation, affective decision-making) is somewhat functionally disconnected throughout adolescence (68), translating into a natural bias in adolescents toward acting on emotional stimuli with relatively little cognitive control over those actions. Through both the natural course of development and environmental experience, connections between these regions are strengthened, providing a mechanism for increasing top-down regulation of emotional brain systems and improved behavioral outcomes (69, 70).

In addition, brain circuits involved in reward processing (e.g., the mesocorticolimbic pathway that involves typical reward-related regions, such as the ventral striatum) show rapid maturation during the adolescent years (71–73), which can have the effect of heightening sensitivity to rewarding experiences (i.e., making adolescents typically more reward sensitive and less risk averse). Paralleling this increase in reward sensitivity during this developmental period is a greater tendency toward sensation/novelty seeking (74). The developmental trajectory of reward circuitry likely plays a critical role in substance use initiation rates in early to mid-adolescence and may be especially pronounced in the subgroup that escalates use. Moreover, subsequent use of substances has the potential to exacerbate an already heightened reward sensitivity in some adolescents, resulting in a strengthening of the drug's reinforcing properties (75).

Compounding these neurological liabilities (i.e., reduced ECF and heightened reward sensitivity) are early puberty and erratic hormone levels, as well as the potential to experience detrimental environmental conditions, such as stress, adversity, maltreatment, and other negative experiences that compromise neurodevelopment and can cause measurable dysfunction in these systems. Thus, regardless of the source of delayed or deficient neurodevelopment, the imbalance between increasing social demands and emergent neurobiological systems during adolescence may lead to heightened vulnerability to substance use and escalation (76). This evidence has direct implications for attempts to parse the developmental trajectories that give rise to SUD and the design of intervention components that effectively target this period of development.

Stress Exposures and Physiological Reactivity

"Stress" refers to processes involving perception, appraisal, and response to harmful, threatening, or challenging external events or conditions, known as "stressors," such as poverty, prenatal exposures, child maltreatment, divorce, and bereavement (77). It is a major common denominator across the neurobiological and psychological domains discussed above and is a ubiquitous factor in susceptibility to substance use, escalation, relapse, and treatment resistance (78, 79). There is substantial evidence to support the role of stress in substance use trajectories [e.g., Refs. (6, 80)]; early life adversity is markedly associated with increased risk for substance use, abuse, and dependence (5, 81, 82).

Chronic and/or severe stress early in life alter emergent stress signaling pathways that, in effect, impair the ability of the PFC to exert cognitive control over more reflexive responses. For example, studies have shown neurodevelopmental deficits or delays in mesocorticolimbic circuits in adults who were maltreated as children, suggesting that functional aberrations may be due, in part, to dysregulation in this network of prefrontal and limbic regions (83, 84). Stress exposures also disrupt both hormonal and physiological systems that regulate these functions at the level of brain and peripheral nervous system, thereby impairing learning, memory, decision-making, and other functions that normally support self-regulation of behavior (85–87). Alterations in hormonal systems (e.g., cortisol) that modulate these functions (85) occur with chronically elevated levels of stress hormones which can reduce hippocampal volume, impair memory, and decision-making (2, 87). Psychophysiological studies also show effects of stress on autonomic responses such as heart rate that, when perturbed, are associated with psychopathology (88–90). In general, greater levels of stress alter brain circuitry, largely impacting the ability of the PFC to maintain behavioral and cognitive control over affective responses (91). These biological stress responses activate the same neural systems found altered in many mental health disorders and that underlie the rewarding effects of drugs (e.g., dopaminergic mesocorticolimbic circuitry), potentially reinforcing drug-taking behaviors (92, 93). As a result, when an individual experiences a great deal of stress or adversity, these stress responses affect brain function, leading to poor decision-making and other executive cognitive skills; thus, drug taking may occur as a maladaptive response to stressful experiences.

Adversity and stress have been inextricably linked to risk for substance abuse throughout adolescence (5, 6) possibly via effects on neurocognitive development in a way that predisposes individuals to impulsivity and externalizing behaviors (94, 95). In fact, numerous studies have demonstrated associations between increasing levels of emotional and physiological stress and decreases in behavioral control, heightened impulsivity, and greater incidence of maladaptive behaviors [e.g., Refs. (96–98)]. Moreover, a growing body of evidence suggests that impulsivity and externalizing behaviors may, in particular, mediate the association between adversity and risk for later substance abuse (99). These behaviors have also been consistently associated with deficits in ECFs (15, 100–102) and reportedly develop in response to exposure to early adversity [for review, see Ref. (43)]. As such, there is a plausible confluence of factors at play, corresponding to the Accumulative Risk Model, which may shed light on the delayed development of adverse outcomes; specifically, pathways from early adversity that interact with risk genotypes to impact emergent neural circuits and, in turn, externalizing and impulsive behaviors, thereby increasing propensity to substance misuse.

These findings suggest that very early development sets the stage for a heightened response to substances through primary biological, psychological, and social systems. Andersen and Teicher (103) provide evidence that early life stress predisposes individuals to abuse substances later via alterations in immature neurophysiological systems that have yet to come on board. In adolescence, when these emergent systems become increasingly functional, the damage is expressed in heightened risk for psychopathology. If the behavioral effects of early childhood stress are not observable until neural connections begin to onboard during adolescence (103, 104), implications for prevention are intriguing. For example, a few studies are now suggesting that training to reduce impulsivity, improve ECF, and integrate components that focus on "top-down" cognitive control has potential to reduce substance use initiation *and* escalation (105). Recognizing the increased risk for substance use in people who have experienced early life stressors is critical to guide prevention efforts designed to both prevent the exposure and counteract the potential subsequent negative consequences.

Cognitive and Behavioral Phenotypes

Externalizing disorders are consistently implicated in the use and abuse of a range of substances (106). The neurocognitive characteristics of children and adolescents with externalizing behaviors include heightened reward sensitivity, poor inhibitory control, aggression, and novelty seeking (107, 108). Variation in these dimensions, particularly impulsivity and reward seeking, contributes to the likelihood of substance use initiation as well as the transitions from initial to intermittent to regular substance use, the transition from abuse to addiction, and the propensity for repeated relapse after achieving abstinence (109). Individuals who measure highly on these traits tend to seek highly stimulating and risky situations and show less anxiety in anticipation of the consequences of their behavior (109, 110). Importantly, these cognitive and behavioral predispositions have differential impacts on substance use patterns at different developmental stages (111, 112). Normative development during adolescence is typified by heightened levels of impulsivity and novelty seeking, in part due to dramatic fluctuations in hormone levels that affect brain development and other systems modulating neurocognition (113). However, the subgroup of adolescents that exhibit heightened impulsivity and sensation seeking are at elevated risk to abuse substances (4, 114). These characteristics may, in effect, contribute to individual differences in the reinforcing effects of substances (115).

Psychopathology in many forms [e.g., posttraumatic stress disorder (PTSD), depression, anxiety, conduct disorder (CD), attention deficit hyperactivity disorder (ADHD), oppositional defiant disorder (ODD), antisocial personality disorder (ASPD)] is strongly and consistently related to the risk of substance abuse [for review, see Ref. (116)]. Individuals with these disorders are more likely to use/abuse substances and at an earlier age than those without such disorders (117, 118). They are also more likely to be resistant to substance abuse treatment (119). In general, individuals afflicted with mental health problems are often compromised in their ability to effectively meet social task challenges, as doing so requires intact neurocognitive functions, which are often compromised in psychiatric disorders (120, 121). Further compounding the risk, the development of mental health disorders increases use in an effort to manage symptoms and this association is likely to vary as a function of the type of mental health disorder. Mood and anxiety disorders, for example, double the risk for SUDs (122). Relatedly, alexithymia (i.e., an emotional processing deficit, whereby one experiences difficulty identifying or describing one's emotions), has been identified as a pertinent risk factor for SUD (e.g., up to 2/3 of patients with SUD exhibit alexithymia) (123) and may increase the risk of negative outcomes such as suicide and self-harm in those who develop SUD (124–126). Since alexithymia predicts poor emotional regulation (127), which in turn predicts poor response to intervention [e.g., Ref. (128)], along with other forms of psychopathology that predict SU liability, it may be an important phenotypic characteristic to consider in the context of the differential trajectories highlighted here.

Gender is also an important factor in the association between SUD and other types of psychopathology. For example, males more often exhibit antisocial personality and conduct disorders (129), while females often have higher rates of mood and anxiety disorders (130); as a result of these gender-specific differences in prevalence of certain psychopathologies and their differential associations with substance misuse, these disorders confer differential gender-related risks for substance abuse (131).

Delayed Risk for Substance Misuse

The second maladaptive pathway toward substance misuse that is theorized here and conceptualized in our model is characterized as *delayed risk*: i.e., individuals who either initiate in adolescence but do not escalate until early/emerging adulthood, or who initiate and develop substance-related problems in late adolescence or early adulthood [e.g., Ref. (132)]. While understudied, delayed risk is also seen in those who do not develop SUD until middle or late adulthood [e.g., Ref. (133)], although the critical factors (especially environmental influences) that underlie such trajectories later in life may be distinct from those that drive misuse and escalation in earlier developmental periods.

Longitudinal studies have distinguished delayed risk in late adolescence/emerging adulthood by histories of externalizing behaviors, child maltreatment, and being bullied by peers, whereas other patterns of use (e.g., limited use) have been characterized by family instability and anxiety disorders (134). However, a nonlongitudinal study of men with substance abuse reported nearly identical childhood and adolescent risk factors (135), while another longitudinal study (136) found similar factors to be predictive of adolescent and adult illicit drug use, with the addition of early cannabis use as a significant catalyst for both groups, thus complicating our ability to disentangle which factors may be more closely coupled with delayed vs. early risk.

It may also be the case that the social transitions into emerging adulthood represents a significant risk factor for substance abuse in those who have difficulty with the novel demands of this developmental period. Though social role transitions (e.g., stable employment, marriage/cohabitation, parenthood) are typically associated with decreases in substance use (137), timing of, preparedness for, and adjustment to these transitions may be critical in predicting delayed risk for substance abuse. For example, in a longitudinal study of 18–33 year olds, an earlier transition into parenthood (i.e., late teens, early 20s) was associated with an increased rate of tobacco misuse (138). Likewise, high school seniors making the transition into early adulthood who have no plans for college are more likely to misuse prescription opioids compared to their peers who did have such plans (139). It is possible that the stress of newfound social demands and responsibilities for which some individuals are not developmentally prepared provides a generative context for substance abuse (138). In other words, there may be a developmental mismatch between expectations in adolescence for mature, autonomous behavior and their neurological, psychological, and social capacity for taking on a significantly greater level of responsibility during this transitional period. This mismatch may be an important predictor of delayed substance abuse, both during emerging adulthood and in later adulthood (140). Interestingly, the discordance between demands and abilities as adolescents approach adulthood may actually predict substance misuse later in adulthood. For instance, Green and colleagues (133) reported that individuals who were unmarried, unemployed, and had lower social integration during young adulthood were more likely to have delayed onset SUDs during middle adulthood. Taken together, these results suggest that individuals who experience difficulty adapting to developmentally normative social transitions, particularly during emerging adulthood, when there is less parental support, greater opportunities to engage in risky behaviors, and more access to substances, may be at increased risk for developing SUDs.

Resilience and Resistance to Substance Misuse

Trajectories of *resilience* (i.e., rebounding from adversity after an initially altered trajectory or decline in functioning) and *resistance* (i.e., maintenance of adaptive functioning, despite adversity) are less well characterized than risk in the existing literature, for several reasons. First, since adversity and its negative consequences are major public health concerns, there has historically been a strong emphasis on deleterious sequelae of developmental adversity and stress, to the relative neglect of positive outcomes. Second, resilience and resistance are often not delineated as separate processes in the literature; that is, some proportion of those who are operationally defined as resilient may more aptly be defined as resistant. While studies typically characterize "resilience" as the absence of behavioral health or psychiatric disorders in adulthood, the majority do not track fluctuations in pathways over time and, thus, are unable to distinguish subgroups that sustain mental and behavioral health from childhood into adulthood relative to subgroups that respond to adversity with a decline in function but eventually improve; both classes will appear similar when outcomes are measured in adulthood. Thus, conceptualizing resilience as a single-end point (e.g., lack of psychopathology) may be misleading and prohibits the differentiation of subgroups that have followed pathways that may have diverged at various points in development. Finally, resistance is not often considered explicitly in the SUD literature. This is likely because characterizing subgroups *not* engaging in high-risk behaviors has been less of a priority and possibly also because this subgroup—which does not misuse substances or exhibit other forms of psychopathology—is not readily discernable, particularly in nonlongitudinal, cross-sectional studies. Consequently, the concept of resistance has largely not been in the SUD research lexicon, and has thus been almost entirely overlooked. A notable exception is a study by Hobfoll and colleagues (141) where they contrasted between resistance and resilience, both behaviorally and biologically, in individuals who experienced significant trauma and, yet, ultimately followed different pathways. These trajectories were identified and characterized in individuals who experienced ongoing terrorism. The authors suggested that resistance and resilience differ in terms of impact (resist vs. absorb), function (continue vs. gradually degrade), resumption of function (immediate vs. delayed), as well as overall response to adversity (defeat vs. limit).

While the conceptual model presented in this paper is focused on differentially characterizing trajectories on the basis of neurocognitive evidence, the paucity of literature clearly distinguishing resilience from resistance precludes such a review specifically for outcomes that are overall adaptive. Therefore, to explore the distinction between resilience and resistance further, we instead describe the few existing studies that delineate some of the relevant factors that likely contribute to and distinguish these two positive developmental pathways. Given associations between these influential factors, neurocognitive development, and functioning across the lifespan, we rely on these findings to formulate hypotheses regarding how these positive pathways may operate.

Neurocognitive Factors Relating to Adaptive Pathways

Despite overwhelming evidence of early stress and trauma's adverse influences on adult outcomes, many individuals exposed to trauma exhibit healthy adult functioning [e.g., Refs. (142–144)]. Some studies have begun to highlight the potential of strengthening cognitive and emotion regulatory skills to act in a protective capacity in those who have experienced trauma. For example, in a study of highly traumatized urban adults compared those who did or did not exhibit psychopathology, those who did not develop psychopathology had better nonverbal memory than those who did, despite similar levels of CM and trauma (145). Other work has suggested that emotion regulation, which is related to impulsivity and subsequent substance use patterns (146), is predictive of extent of adaptive coping in maltreated children (147). Moreover, in children exposed to political violence, higher levels of cognitive flexibility has been shown to moderate the relationship between violence exposure and psychological well-being (148). Though these studies did not explicitly measure substance use, it is possible that having well-developed neurocognitive skills (e.g., memory, cognitive flexibility, emotion regulation) enables individuals who have experienced trauma to adaptively navigate their environments and avoid substance misuse and eventual dependence, despite a history of adverse experiences. Indeed, deficits in these neurocognitive skills are related to substance abuse (149–151), providing further support for the inverse relationship, with more robust neurocognitive skills predicting a decreased likelihood of developing SUDs.

Interestingly, a few studies suggest that early adversity may drive neurocognitive adaptation in some individuals in ways that enables them to outperform healthy controls or those who have had fewer adverse experiences. For example, Nolin and Ethier (152) reported that children who had a history of neglect evinced better planning and problem-solving skills than children without histories of abuse. There are also similar findings from research with older adults (i.e., 50 years and older) who have experienced CM, providing additional evidence of preserved cognitive functioning in spite of adverse experiences (e.g., visual memory, verbal memory, executive functioning, attention, processing speed) (153, 154). For example, Feeney and colleagues reported that older adults who had experienced childhood sexual abuse had better executive functioning, attention, and processing speed than those without maltreatment history (153). Similarly, another study demonstrated that, compared to those with moderate levels of CM, individuals with severe levels of maltreatment had lower risk of cognitive impairment (i.e., visual memory, executive functioning, and verbal memory) later in life (154).

Taken together, this work supports the concept of a subset of individuals who may have protective assets, particularly in neurocognitive domains of functioning, that enable them to thrive despite experiences of adversity, trauma, and stress. The extent to which their adaptation corresponds to resilience vs. resistance pathways in patterns of substance use remains to be explored. However, we posit that, based on indices of neurocognitive functioning, classes of individuals may be more aptly characterized by longitudinal investigations that aid in the delineation of critical time points corresponding to these divergent developmental pathways. In particular, a clearer understanding of adaptations to adversity will emerge with further investigation into resilient and resistant trajectories that correspond to the behavioral and mental health endpoints of interest. Longitudinal observations will allow us to more fully characterize adaptations, which are important predictors of ultimate outcomes (adaptive vs. maladaptive) and that may fluctuate or be sustained at particular developmental time points. As such, future work characterizing these different developmental pathways is critical for understanding the precursors of these trajectories and how they unfold *and* to identify and bolster neurocognitive factors that confer resilience or resistance.

Neuroimaging Correlates of Adaptive Pathways

A few recent neuroimaging studies have begun to pinpoint brain regions that differentiate trauma exposed individuals who do or do not exhibit adaptive outcomes (e.g., based on psychopathology or adaptive functioning status). For example, compared to those who experienced maladaptive outcomes, trauma-exposed youths who exhibit adaptive functioning have been found to have lower resting-state functional connectivity (rsFC) within default mode, salience, and executive control networks (155). Interestingly, all of these networks have been shown to be disrupted in substance-abusing samples (156, 157). Other rsFC studies have highlighted the dorsal ACC (dACC) as a region showing distinguishable patterns of connectivity in adaptive vs. maladaptive outcomes for those who have experienced early life stress and/or trauma (158, 159). For example, Philip and colleagues found increased rsFC between the thalamus and dACC in adults who experienced early adversity *without* psychiatric disorders compared to those with psychiatric disorders (158). These findings are intriguing with respect to potential neural correlates of resilient and resistant pathways pertaining to substance use, given that previous work has reported diminished activation and connectivity patterns in the dACC in substance-dependent individuals, particularly when processing rewards (160, 161).

Findings from several other neuroimaging studies suggest that the structure and function of the frontal lobe (e.g., volume, activation, connectivity) is implicated in adaptive functioning following adversity (162–164). Specifically, one study found that adaptive adolescents who had experienced early adversity had increased middle frontal and superior frontal gyri volumes compared to maladaptive adolescents who had experienced early adversity as well as those who had not experienced adversity (163). Moreover, the same study reported that middle frontal gyrus volume negatively correlated with problematic drinking in adolescents who were deemed adaptive but experienced early adversity (163). Another study found that compared to individuals with PTSD, those who were also trauma exposed but did not have any psychiatric disorders showed enhanced ability to recruit frontal regions associated with top-down attentional control during an emotional Stroop Task (165). Similarly, patterns of increased frontolimbic connectivity seem to distinguish maltreated individuals from healthy controls who were comparable in adaptive functioning, including a lack of substance abuse (164). Although these studies did not all measure substance use or neurocognitive functioning, they do provide initial support for increased volume and functional recruitment of frontal regions as being a neuroprotective factor in individuals who have experienced early adversity. Such findings are promising in their ability to distinguish neural profiles of adaptive and maladaptive traumatized populations; however, they also evoke many questions about how frontal lobe development progresses in individuals who follow resilient or resistant pathways in response to adversity. For instance, future studies could probe how specific neuroprotective factors (e.g., increased or decreased frontal lobe activation and connectivity) interact with other factors (e.g., genetic or environmental liabilities) to confer a likelihood of following a resilient or resistant pathway subsequent to early adversity.

Delineating Resilience and Resistance: Future Work

By and large, the literature points to several neurocognitive factors that likely contribute to resilience or resistance pathways subsequent to adversity. However, as noted, prior research has not made concerted attempts to disentangle these pathways, their precursors, and their trajectories. Therefore, many open questions remain as to how subgroups who attain successful outcomes following trauma, maltreatment, or other environmental adversities rebound from or, in contrast, resist engaging in substance misuse. Since not all survivors of adversity develop SUDs or other forms of psychopathology, it is critical for future work to pinpoint and characterize these subgroups. Moreover, the preliminary evidence cited above suggests that individual differences in neurocognitive skills or patterns of connectivity in regions of interest for SUDs may differ across development but may still ultimately predict similar adaptive outcomes. For instance, it is plausible that individuals who are less adept at regulating emotions and engaging executive functions (i.e., regulating top-down processes) may experience initial developmental disruptions that lead to substance use that they rebound from (i.e., resilience trajectory). In contrast, those who are more adept at these neurocognitive skills may resist substance use altogether (i.e., resistance trajectory). As others have suggested in the literature, resilience to adversity is a dynamic, state-like process, not simply a trait, and individuals who appear adaptive later in life may or may not have experienced initial maladaptive pathways from which they have rebounded. Recent studies have also proposed novel models [e.g., the *Resilience Portfolio Model* (165) or the *Diversity Portfolio Model* (166)] that conceptualize "resilience" as an arsenal of protective factors associated with healthier outcomes following trauma. Accordingly, the density and/or diversity of available protective resources and assets may shape their long-term capacity to adapt and thrive despite adverse experiences. As such, future studies that thoroughly characterize neurocognitive profiles, across the developmental timeline, and which delineate how such profiles interact with other factors known to bolster adaptive functioning, may be able to meaningfully distinguish those who are resilient and rebound from those who are resistant. This distinction in pathways is crucial, as those who are resilient may be categorized by particular vulnerabilities during specific windows of time that may serve as critical opportunities to successfully intervene with prevention programs. In summary, delineating the neurocognitive profiles of individuals who exhibit resistant vs. resilient pathways may be critical for identifying novel ways to bolster functioning in those who experience maladaptive pathways/outcomes.

METHODOLOGICAL APPROACHES TO DISTINGUISH TRAJECTORIES

While there is convincing evidence for distinctions between risk, resistance, and resilience trajectories based on phenotypic presentations, studies have yet to effectively delineate the possible neurocognitive correlates or underpinnings that support their distinctions. This information may have important implications for more precision-based, developmentally sensitive intervention targeting. It is reasonable to surmise that environmental risk and protective factors may impact neurocognitive development in unique ways across individuals and/or subgroups, leading to different phenotypic outcomes. With respect to positive outcomes such as resilience, resistance, and recovery, this assumption is supported by the equifinality of the result—i.e., a similarly adaptive outcome profile across these different trajectories—and thus may be logistically difficult to differentiate. Cross-sectional research designs are inadequate in this endeavor; they may be able to confirm that various outcomes are predicted by the level of neurocognitive functioning at a single time point but they are unable to chart the dynamic interplay of risk and protective factors that impact the course of neurodevelopment and its relationship to final outcomes. In contrast, by establishing temporal ordering within subjects, longitudinal research designs are uniquely positioned to pinpoint developmental phenomena and their divergent pathways. Thus, a longitudinal approach is able to model the experiential and contextual impact on neurobiological factors across development to understand the nature of the various pathways that lead to eventual maladaptive versus adaptive outcomes. Pinpointing neural markers that distinguish individuals who move along these distinct pathways will help us to identify novel targets for intervention. By fully characterizing and differentiating these trajectories, longitudinal studies have the potential to aid in the delineation of the precise nature of influential factors at optimal time points along their development (e.g., adversity onset, treatment onset, redirection) and, in doing so, to identify malleable targets that exist along these trajectories, which will serve to maximize the translational potential of this research.

Latent class modeling has the potential to substantially aid in the determination and delineation of unique pathways that underlie SUD liability, including risk, resilience, and resistance. Latent class modeling refers to a group of statistical methods aimed at identifying unobservable (*latent*) subgroups within a particular population. It includes latent class analysis (LCA), which considers outcomes at a particular time point (e.g., adolescence), and a related methodology, latent transition analysis (LTA), which facilitates estimation of transition between subgroups over time. An application of LCA that includes consideration of the types of risk- and resilience/resistance-relevant factors outlined in the Accumulative Risk Model (**Figure 1**) and, especially, pertinent neurodevelopmental factors (e.g., neurocognitive processes, variation in brain structure, function, and connectivity) will facilitate the determination of which specific constellations of factors give rise to which intermediate phenotypes and associated pathways. Moreover, an LTA approach will allow us to determine which factors are particularly relevant at the time points where we see real or apparent shifts in developmental trajectories, either toward or away from increased liability and adverse outcomes.

These latent class approaches hold considerable potential for determining opportunities and methods to optimize preventive interventions. However, to-date, there is a relative paucity of research using latent class modeling in the context of risk for substance abuse and dependence that has focused on neuro-related factors and/or on the types of longitudinal approaches to SUD liability that we are suggesting here. Nonetheless, application of latent class models to substance abuse risk and treatment have revealed some interesting outcomes regarding how patterns of use may impact substance use behaviors or brain activity [e.g., Refs. (167–169)] and support the appropriateness of these methods in the context of SUD liability pathways.

THE POTENTIAL FOR PREVENTION

Based on a burgeoning body of evidence, brain development and function are, for better or for worse, clearly experience dependent. For worse, adversity in its many forms has the potential to impact neurodevelopmental trajectories in ways that undermine emergent self-regulatory mechanisms, increasing risk for psychopathology, including eventual SUD. However, for the better, the brain's substantial plasticity translates to the potential for well-conceived prevention strategies to improve behavioral and mental health outcomes by positively impacting the same neurodevelopmental pathways. Although most prevention science studies do not attempt to elucidate the neural mediators of intervention responses, a considerable number of prevention programs have been shown to reliably reduce risk for substance abuse. Research to enhance our understanding of the neurodevelopmental effects of prevention programming has potential to further differentiate the pathways involved in the relationship between risk factors and behavioral outcomes and, in doing so, will identify mediating mechanisms that explain outcome heterogeneity. This argument is particularly compelling given that, at present, the evidence-based programs that have emerged from various disciplinary perspectives produce only small to modest effects on the phenotypes predictive of SUD risk and resilience/resistance pathways, as well as SUD itself. More comprehensive and in depth information is needed to advance predictive analytics and increase the precision with which we target programmatic components.

It is likely that evidence-based programs work at the level of the brain, driving adaptive changes in brain structure, function, and connectivity. Programs that focus on socioemotional and cognitive functioning are strong candidates in this regard. Development of these skills, both behaviorally and neurobiologically, are particularly vulnerable to adverse psychosocial and environmental influences. Programs that redirect and possibly normalize these specific dimensions of a child's developmental pathway may exert a potent impact on corresponding behavioral, emotional, mental, and physical (e.g., brain function and fitness) domains. The effects of appropriately targeted interventions may be particularly remarkable for children who are disadvantaged by poverty and other social ills. Research that integrates multiple disciplines to better understand influences and outcomes related to substance abuse have directed us toward solutions for these problems that target underlying mechanisms and not solely the distal outcome of substance abuse, *per se*. In other words, it is vital that we address the factors that eventually lead to drug abuse prior to its development, the key principle behind prevention science.

The integrity of the way in which the brain develops in children is a prerequisite for adaptive responses to socioenvironmental challenges and thus, to favorable responses to intervention [e.g., Ref. (170)]. Thanks to the vast brain plasticity throughout childhood and adolescence, there is a great deal of variability in the way children develop in response to environmental inputs, including the divergent pathways under discussion here. This plasticity throughout early childhood and adolescence offers several optimal windows of opportunity for intervention. When neurodevelopment is on course or shows a trend toward improvement, overall intervention outcomes are likely to be favorable. In contrast, existing or emergent neurodevelopmental deficits or delays may compromise intervention effects, potentially explaining differential outcomes in response to even the most highly regarded and efficacious programs. A comprehensive evidence-based set of solutions (programs and policies) to prevent psychopathology and eventual drug abuse that operates to enhance developmental indicators of brain function in multiple domains are needed. This approach will, in turn, improve the ability to self-regulate behavior and reduce the risk for developing SUDs.

Applying this integrative and developmental perspective will lead to significant advancements in our ability to prevent substance use and the eventuality of SUD for some. Indeed, SUD intervention researchers have begun to incorporate cognitive training, mindfulness approaches, behavioral and environmental modifications, and other innovative strategies that target malleable neurodevelopmental processes that contribute to substance abuse (171, 172). Determining which early influences are particularly relevant will be critical to designing interventions that target the underlying generators of SUDs, before behavioral problems and substance use patterns become entrenched. And while there are many outstanding questions in this line of research, we do know enough about prevailing conditions that influence risk for SUDs to exert a positive impact now.

CONCLUSIONS

Studies on the successes and failures in the treatment of SUDs are benefitting from the inclusion of neuroimaging, leading to the identification of biomarkers of SUDs and increasing our understanding of variability in treatment outcomes. Proximal biomarkers in prevention studies are similarly needed to provide targets for intervention, detect differentially receptive subgroups, predict intervention response, and broadly improve outcomes. This technique could be particularly promising for "proven" prevention strategies with protective longitudinal results from early childhood through adolescence and adulthood, but were created before the explosion of biomarker research. Important advances in studies including neuroimaging and other biomarkers have revealed activity within relevant neural circuits in association with behavioral change reflective of protection from substance abuse. The application of early neuroimaging to well-established prevention strategies has potential to elucidate the neural correlates of dimensions of functioning commonly implicated in substance use and related disorders, such as impulsivity, reward sensitivity, and cognitive control, among others. While these dimensions of functioning have been related to substance misuse, SUD treatment outcomes, and relapse, a better understanding of these dimensions and their neural correlates and how they correspond to the distinct adaptive and maladaptive developmental trajectories considered here (i.e., *risk, delayed risk, resilience,* and *resistance*) could identify malleable brain–behavior biomarkers for improving preventive intervention effects. Extending models from treatment research to prevention is sorely needed by identifying functional, malleable mediators, and moderators of well-established prevention programs. Indeed, this line of research—to identify biomarkers and conditions within which they interact that distinguish between developmental pathways—has potential to identify novel targets for intervention. Such information will provide curriculum developers with data critical to optimizing programs and compelling public, mental health, and educational policies to further scale effective prevention strategies. In effect, improving our ability to disrupt pathways to SUD would constitute a significant public health advancement with potential for population level effects.

AUTHOR CONTRIBUTIONS

DF initiated the concept for the paper. DF and ER conceived of the framework and ER elaborated on a proposed new model for understanding distinctive pathways to substance misuse and addiction, including pathways that eventually diverge and lead to positive outcomes despite prevailing risks. By and large, DF and ER framed and wrote the majority of the paper. ER and GP constructed the figures. GP contributed to the writing, referencing, and reviewing/editing of the paper.

REFERENCES

1. Conway KP, Swendsen J, Husky MM, He JP, Merikangas KR. Association of lifetime mental disorders and subsequent alcohol and illicit drug use: results from the National Comorbidity Survey–Adolescent Supplement. *J Am Acad Child Adolesc Psychiatry* (2016) 55(4):280–8. doi: 10.1016/j.jaac.2016.01.006
2. Nelson SE, Van Ryzin MJ, Dishion TJ. Alcohol, marijuana, and tobacco use trajectories from age 12 to 24 years: demographic correlates and young adult substance use problems. *Dev Psychopathol* (2015) 27(1):253–77. doi: 10.1017/S0954579414000650
3. Behrendt S, Wittchen HU, Höfler M, Lieb R, Beesdo K. Transitions from first substance use to substance use disorders in adolescence: is early onset associated with a rapid escalation? *Drug Alcohol Depend* (2009) 99(1–3):68–78. doi: 10.1016/j.drugalcdep.2008.06.014
4. Quinn PD, Harden KP. Differential changes in impulsivity and sensation seeking and the escalation of substance use from adolescence to early adulthood. *Dev Psychopathol* (2013) 25(1):223–39. doi: 10.1017/S0954579412000284
5. Dube SR, Felitti VJ, Dong M, Chapman DP, Giles WH, Anda RF. Childhood abuse, neglect, and household dysfunction and the risk of illicit drug use: the adverse childhood experiences study. *Pediatrics* (2003) 111(3):564–72. doi: 10.1542/peds.111.3.564
6. Edalati H, Krank MD. Childhood maltreatment and development of substance use disorders: a review and a model of cognitive pathways. *Trauma, Violence Abuse* (2016) 17(5):454–67. doi: 10.1177/1524838015584370
7. Asberg K, Renk K. Substance use coping as a mediator of the relationship between trauma symptoms and substance use consequences among

incarcerated females with childhood sexual abuse histories. *Subst Use Misuse* (2012) 47(7):799–808. doi: 10.3109/10826084.2012.669446

8. Fenton MC, Geier T, Keyes K, Skodol AE, Grant BF, Hasin DS. Combined role of childhood maltreatment, family history, and gender in the risk for alcohol dependence. *Psychol Med* (2013) 43(5):1045–57. doi: 10.1017/S0033291712001729
9. Klanecky A, McChargue DE, Bruggeman L. Desire to dissociate: implications for problematic drinking in college students with childhood or adolescent sexual abuse exposure. *Am J Addict* (2012) 21(3):250–6. doi: 10.1111/j.1521-0391.2012.00228.x
10. Elton A, Smitherman S, Young J, Kilts CD. Effects of childhood maltreatment on the neural correlates of stress- and drug cue-induced cocaine craving. *Addict Biol* (2015) 20(4):820–31. doi: 10.1111/adb.12162
11. Huang H, Gundapuneedi T, Rao U. White matter disruptions in adolescents exposed to childhood maltreatment and vulnerability to psychopathology. *Neuropsychopharmacology* (2012) 37(12):2693–701. doi: 10.1038/npp.2012.133
12. Van Dam NT, Rando K, Potenza MN, Tuit K, Sinha R. Childhood maltreatment, altered limbic neurobiology, and substance use relapse severity via trauma-specific reductions in limbic gray matter volume. *JAMA Psychiatry* (2014) 71(8):917–25. doi: 10.1001/jamapsychiatry.2014.680
13. Cicchetti D. Annual research review: resilient functioning in maltreated children—past, present, and future perspectives. *J Child Psychol Psychiatry* (2013) 54(4):402–22. doi: 10.1111/j.1469-7610.2012.02608.x
14. Cowell RA, Cicchetti D, Rogosch FA, Toth SL. Childhood maltreatment and its effect on neurocognitive functioning: timing and chronicity matter. *Dev Psychopathol* (2015) 27(2):521–33. doi: 10.1017/S0954579415000139
15. McLaughlin KA, Peverill M, Gold AL, Alves S, Sheridan MA. Child maltreatment and neural systems underlying emotion regulation. *J Am Acad Child Adolesc Psychiatry* (2015) 54(9):753–62. doi: 10.1016/j.jaac.2015.06.010
16. Evans GW, Li D, Whipple SS. Cumulative risk and child development. *Psychol Bull* (2013) 139(6):1342–96. doi: 10.1037/a0031808
17. Jonson-Reid M, Kohl PL, Drake B. Child and adult outcomes of chronic child maltreatment. *Pediatrics* (2012) 129(5):839–45. doi: 10.1542/peds.2011-2529
18. Stone AL, Becker LG, Huber AM, Catalano RF. Review of risk and protective factors of substance use and problem use in emerging adulthood. *Addict Behav* (2012) 37(7):747–75. doi: 10.1016/j.addbeh.2012.02.014
19. Wingo AP, Ressler KJ, Bradley B. Resilience characteristics mitigate tendency for harmful alcohol and illicit drug use in adults with a history of childhood abuse: a cross-sectional study of 2024 inner-city men and women. *J Psychiatr Res* (2014) 51(1):93–9. doi: 10.1016/j.jpsychires.2014.01.007
20. Mayes LC, Suchman NE. Developmental pathways to substance abuse. In: Cicchetti D, Cohen DJ, editors. *Developmental psychopathology: volume three: risk, disorder, and adaptation.* John Wiley & Sons, Inc. Hoboken, New Jersey. (2015). p. 599–619. doi: 10.1002/9780470939406.ch16
21. Sroufe LA. Pathways to adaptation and maladaptation: psychopathology as developmental deviation. In: Cicchetti, D, editors. The emergence of a discipline. Hillsdale, New Jersey: Psychology Press (2013). p. 27–54. doi: 10.4324/9780203771990-6
22. Volkow ND, Koob GF, McLellan AT. Neurobiologic advances from the brain disease model of addiction. *N Engl J Med* (2016) 374(4):363–71. doi: 10.1056/NEJMra1511480
23. Schulte MH, Cousijn J, den Uyl TE, Goudriaan AE, van den Brink W, Veltman DJ, et al. Recovery of neurocognitive functions following sustained abstinence after substance dependence and implications for treatment. *Clin Psychol Rev* (2014) 34(7):531–50. doi: 10.1016/j.cpr.2014.08.002
24. Charney DA, Zikos E, Gill KJ. Early recovery from alcohol dependence: factors that promote or impede abstinence. *J Subst Abuse Treat* (2010) 38(1):42–50. doi: 10.1016/j.jsat.2009.06.002
25. Garland EL, Roberts-Lewis A, Kelley K, Tronnier C, Hanley A. Cognitive and affective mechanisms linking trait mindfulness to craving among individuals in addiction recovery. *Subst Use Misuse* (2014) 49(5):525–35. doi: 10.3109/10826084.2014.850309
26. Zheng Y, Cleveland HH, Molenaar PC, Harris KS. An alternative framework to investigating and understanding intraindividual processes in substance abuse recovery: an idiographic approach and demonstration. *Eval Rev* (2015) 39(2):229–54. doi: 10.1177/0193841X14567313
27. Palmer RH, Brick L, Nugent NR, Bidwell LC, McGeary JE, Knopik VS, et al. Examining the role of common genetic variants on alcohol, tobacco, cannabis and illicit drug dependence: genetics of vulnerability to drug dependence. *Addiction* (2015) 110(3):530–7. doi: 10.1111/add.12815
28. Prom-Wormley EC, Ebejer J, Dick DM, Bowers MS. The genetic epidemiology of substance use disorder: a review. *Drug and Alcohol Depend* (2017) 180:241–59. doi: 10.1016/j.drugalcdep.2017.06.040
29. Davidson RJ. Asymmetric brain function, affective style, and psychopathology: the role of early experience and plasticity. *Dev Psychopathol* (1994) 6(4):741–58. doi: 10.1017/S0954579400004764
30. Pechtel P, Pizzagalli DA. Effects of early life stress on cognitive and affective function: an integrated review of human literature. *Psychopharmacology* (2011) 214(1):55–70. doi: 10.1007/s00213-010-2009-2
31. Andersen SL. Trajectories of brain development: point of vulnerability or window of opportunity? *Neurosci Biobehav Rev* (2003) 27(1-2):3–18. doi: 10.1016/S0149-7634(03)00005-8
32. Johnson SB, Riis JL, Noble KG. State of the art review: poverty and the developing brain. *Pediatrics* (2016) 137(4):e20153075. doi: 10.1542/peds.2015-3075
33. Enoch MA. The influence of gene–environment interactions on the development of alcoholism and drug dependence. *Curr Psychiatry Rep* (2012) 14(2):150–8. doi: 10.1007/s11920-011-0252-9
34. Szyf M, Tang YY, Hill KG, Musci R. The dynamic epigenome and its implications for behavioral interventions: a role for epigenetics to inform disorder prevention and health promotion. Translational Behavioral Medicine (2016) 6(1):55–62.
35. Szyf M. The early-life social environment and DNA methylation. *Clin Genet* (2012) 81(4):341–9. doi: 10.1111/j.1399-0004.2012.01843.x.
36. Volkow ND, Boyle M. Neuroscience of addiction: relevance to prevention and treatment. *Am J Psychiatry* (2018) 175(8):729–40. doi: 10.1176/appi.ajp.2018.17101174
37. Pirard S, Sharon E, Kang SK, Angarita GA, Gastfriend DR. Prevalence of physical and sexual abuse among substance abuse patients and impact on treatment outcomes. *Drug Alcohol Depend* (2005) 78(1):57–64. doi: 10.1016/j.drugalcdep.2004.09.005
38. Dannlowski U, Stuhrmann A, Beutelmann V, Zwanzger P, Lenzen T, Grotegerd D, et al. Limbic scars: long-term consequences of childhood maltreatment revealed by functional and structural magnetic resonance imaging. *Biol Psychiatry* (2012) 71(4):286–93. doi: 10.1016/j.biopsych.2011.10.021
39. Ersche KD, Jones PS, Williams GB, Turton AJ, Robbins TW, Bullmore ET. Abnormal brain structure implicated in stimulant drug addiction. *Science* (2012) 335(6068):601–4. doi: 10.1126/science.1214463
40. Hanson JL, Chung MK, Avants BB, Shirtcliff EA, Gee JC, Davidson RJ, et al. Early stress is associated with alterations in the orbitofrontal cortex: a tensor-based morphometry investigation of brain structure and behavioral risk. *J Neurosci* (2010) 30(22):7466–72. doi: 10.1523/JNEUROSCI.0859-10.2010
41. Robbins TW, Gillan CM, Smith DG, de Wit S, Ersche KD. Neurocognitive endophenotypes of impulsivity and compulsivity: towards dimensional psychiatry. *Trends Cognit Sci* (2012) 16(1):81–91. doi: 10.1016/j.tics.2011.11.009
42. Teicher MH, Samson JA. Childhood maltreatment and psychopathology: a case for ecophenotypic variants as clinically and neurobiologically distinct subtypes. *Am J Psychiatry* (2013) 170(10):1114–33. doi: 10.1176/appi.ajp.2013.12070957
43. Puetz VB, McCrory E. Exploring the relationship between childhood maltreatment and addiction: a review of the neurocognitive evidence. *Curr Addict Rep* (2015) 2(4):318–25. doi: 10.1007/s40429-015-0073-8
44. Leijser LM, Siddiqi A, Miller SP. Imaging evidence of the effect of socio-economic status on brain structure and development. *Semin Pediatr Neurol* (2018) 27(1):26–34. doi: 10.1016/j.spen.2018.03.004
45. Brito NH, Noble KG. Socioeconomic status and structural brain development. *Front Neurosci* (2014) 8(276):1–12. doi: 10.3389/fnins.2014.00276
46. Farah MJ, Shera DM, Savage JH, Betancourt L, Giannetta JM, Brodsky NL, et al. Childhood poverty: specific associations with neurocognitive development. *Brain Res* (2006) 1110(1):166–74. doi: 10.1016/j.brainres.2006.06.072
47. Noble KG, McCandliss BD, Farah MJ. Socioeconomic gradients predict individual differences in neurocognitive abilities. *Dev Sci* (2007) 10(4):464–80. doi: 10.1111/j.1467-7687.2007.00600.x
48. Noble KG, Norman MF, Farah MJ. Neurocognitive correlates of

socioeconomic status in kindergarten children. *Dev Sci* (2005) 8(1):74–87. doi: 10.1111/j.1467-7687.2005.00394.x
49. D'angiulli A, Herdman A, Stapells D, Hertzman C. Children's event-related potentials of auditory selective attention vary with their socioeconomic status. *Neuropsychology* (2008) 22(3):293–300. doi: 10.1037/0894-4105.22.3.293
50. Kishiyama MM, Boyce WT, Jimenez AM, Perry LM, Knight RT. Socioeconomic disparities affect prefrontal function in children. *J Cognit Neurosci* (2009) 21(6):1106–15. doi: 10.1162/jocn.2009.21101
51. Stevens C, Lauinger B, Neville H. Differences in the neural mechanisms of selective attention in children from different socioeconomic backgrounds: an event-related brain potential study. *Dev Sci* (2009) 12(4):634–46. doi: 10.1111/j.1467-7687.2009.00807.x
52. Finn AS, Minas JE, Leonard JA, Mackey AP, Salvatore J, Goetz C, et al. Functional brain organization of working memory in adolescents varies in relation to family income and academic achievement. *Dev Sci* (2017) 20(5):e12450. doi: 10.1111/desc.12450
53. Sheridan MA, Fox NA, Zeanah CH, McLaughlin KA, Nelson CA. Variation in neural development as a result of exposure to institutionalization early in childhood. *Proc Nat Acad Sci* (2012) 109(32):12927–32. doi: 10.1073/pnas.1200041109
54. Muscatell KA, Morelli SA, Falk EB, Way BM, Pfeifer JH, Galinsky AD, et al. Social status modulates neural activity in the mentalizing network. *Neuroimage* (2012) 60(3):1771–7. doi: 10.1016/j.neuroimage.2012.01.080
55. Barch D, Pagliaccio D, Belden A, Harms MP, Gaffrey M, Sylvester CM, et al. Effect of hippocampal and amygdala connectivity on the relationship between preschool poverty and school-age depression. *Am J Psychiatry* (2016) 173(6):625–34. doi: 10.1176/appi.ajp.2015.15081014
56. Gianaros PJ, Horenstein JA, Hariri AR, Sheu LK, Manuck SB, Matthews KA, et al. Potential neural embedding of parental social standing. *Soc Cognit Affect Neurosci* (2008) 3(2):91–6. doi: 10.1093/scan/nsn003
57. Javanbakht A, King AP, Evans GW, Swain JE, Angstadt M, Phan KL, et al. Childhood poverty predicts adult amygdala and frontal activity and connectivity in response to emotional faces. *Front Behav Neurosci* (2015) 9(154):1–8. doi: 10.3389/fnbeh.2015.00154
58. Kim DJ, Davis EP, Sandman CA, Glynn L, Sporns O, O'donnell BF, et al. Childhood poverty and the organization of structural brain connectome. *NeuroImage* (2019) 184(1):409–16. doi: 10.1016/j.neuroimage.2018.09.041
59. Nestler EJ. Epigenetic mechanisms of drug addiction. *Neuropharmacology* (2014) 76(B):259–68. doi: 10.1016/j.neuropharm.2013.04.004
60. Doura MB, Unterwald EM. MicroRNAs modulate interactions between stress and risk for cocaine addiction. *Front Cell Neurosci* (2016) 10(125):1–10. doi: 10.3389/fncel.2016.00125
61. Vassoler FM, Oliver DJ, Wyse C, Blau A, Shtutman M, Turner JR, et al. Transgenerational attenuation of opioid self-administration as a consequence of adolescent morphine exposure. *Neuropharmacology* (2017) 113(B):271–80. doi: 10.1016/j.neuropharm.2016.10.006
62. Watson CT, Szutorisz H, Garg P, Martin Q, Landry JA, Sharp AJ, et al. Genome-wide DNA methylation profiling reveals epigenetic changes in the rat nucleus accumbens associated with cross-generational effects of adolescent THC exposure. *Neuropsychopharmacology* (2015) 40(13):2993–3005. doi: 10.1038/npp.2015.155
63. Substance Abuse and Mental Health Services Administration. *2015 National survey on drug use and health: summary of the effects of the 2015 NSDUH Questionnaire redesign: implications for data users.* Rockville (MD): Substance Abuse and Mental Health Services Administration (US) (2016).
64. Crone EA, Dahl RE. Understanding adolescence as a period of social-affective engagement and goal flexibility. *Nat Rev Neurosci* (2012) 13(9):636–50. doi: 10.1038/nrn3313
65. Marek S, Hwang K, Foran W, Hallquist MN, Luna B. The contribution of network organization and integration to the development of cognitive control. *PLoS Biology* (2015) 13(12):e1002328. doi: 10.1371/journal.pbio.1002328
66. Casey BJ, Jones RM, Hare TA. The adolescent brain. *Ann N Y Acad Sci* (2008) 1124(1):111–26. doi: 10.1196/annals.1440.010
67. Kharitonova M, Munakata Y. The role of representations in executive function: investigating a developmental link between flexibility and abstraction. *Front Psychol* (2011) 2(347):1–12. doi: 10.3389/fpsyg.2011.00347
68. Somerville LH, Casey BJ. Developmental neurobiology of cognitive control and motivational systems. *Curr Opin Neurobiol* (2010) 20(2):236–41. doi: 10.1016/j.conb.2010.01.006
69. Casey BJ, Jones RM, Somerville LH. Braking and accelerating of the adolescent brain. *J Res Adolesc* (2011) 21(1):21–33. doi: 10.1111/j.1532-7795.2010.00712.x
70. Tottenham N, Hare TA, Casey BJ. Behavioral assessment of emotion discrimination, emotion regulation, and cognitive control in childhood, adolescence, and adulthood. *Front Psychol* (2011) 2(39):1–9. doi: 10.3389/fpsyg.2011.00039
71. Geier CF, Terwilliger R, Teslovich T, Velanova K, Luna B. Immaturities in reward processing and its influence on inhibitory control in adolescence. *Cereb Cortex* (2009) 20(7):1613–29. doi: 10.1093/cercor/bhp225
72. Padmanabhan A, Geier CF, Ordaz SJ, Teslovich T, Luna B. Developmental changes in brain function underlying the influence of reward processing on inhibitory control. *Dev Cognit Neurosci* (2011) 1(4):517–29. doi: 10.1016/j.dcn.2011.06.004
73. Somerville LH, Jones RM, Casey BJ. A time of change: behavioral and neural correlates of adolescent sensitivity to appetitive and aversive environmental cues. *Brain Cogn* (2010) 72(1):124–33. doi: 10.1016/j.bandc.2009.07.003
74. Steinberg L. A dual systems model of adolescent risk-taking. *Dev Psychobiol* (2010) 52(3):216–24. doi: 10.1002/dev.20445
75. Hardin MG, Ernst M. Functional brain imaging of development-related risk and vulnerability for substance use in adolescents. *J Addict Med* (2009) 3(2):47–54. doi: 10.1097/ADM.0b013e31819ca788
76. Casey BJ, Jones RM. Neurobiology of the adolescent brain and behavior: implications for substance use disorders. *J Am Acad Child Adolesc Psychiatry* (2010) 49(12):1189–201. doi: 10.1097/00004583-201012000-00005
77. Levine S. Developmental determinants of sensitivity and resistance to stress. *Psychoneuroendocrinology* (2005) 30(10):939–46. doi: 10.1016/j.psyneuen.2005.03.013
78. Najman JM, Clavarino A, McGee TR, Bor W, Williams GM, Hayatbakhsh MR. Timing and chronicity of family poverty and development of unhealthy behaviors in children: a longitudinal study. *J Adolesc Health* (2010) 46(6):538–44. doi: 10.1016/j.jadohealth.2009.12.001
79. Preston KL, Epstein DH. Stress in the daily lives of cocaine and heroin users: relationship to mood, craving, relapse triggers, and cocaine use. *Psychopharmacology* (2011) 218(1):29–37. doi: 10.1007/s00213-011-2183-x
80. Lee CM, Neighbors C, Woods BA. Marijuana motives: young adults' reasons for using marijuana. *Addict Behav* (2007) 32(7):1384–94. doi: 10.1016/j.addbeh.2006.09.010
81. Chapman DP, Whitfield CL, Felitti VJ, Dube SR, Edwards VJ, Anda RF. Adverse childhood experiences and the risk of depressive disorders in adulthood. *J Affect Disord* (2004) 82(2):217–25. doi: 10.1016/j.jad.2003.12.013
82. Anda RF, Brown DW, Felitti VJ, Dube SR, Giles WH. Adverse childhood experiences and prescription drug use in a cohort study of adult HMO patients. *BMC Public Health* (2008) 8(1):198–206. doi: 10.1186/1471-2458-8-198
83. Davidson RJ, Sutton SK. Affective neuroscience: the emergence of a discipline. *Curr Opin Neurobiol* (1995) 5(2):217–24. doi: 10.1016/0959-4388(95)80029-8
84. Dichter GS, Damiano CA, Allen JA. Reward circuitry dysfunction in psychiatric and neurodevelopmental disorders and genetic syndromes: animal models and clinical findings. *J Neurodev Disord* (2012) 4(1):19–52. doi: 10.1186/1866-1955-4-19
85. Hüther G. Stress and the adaptive self-organization of neuronal connectivity during early childhood. *Int J Dev Neurosci* (1998) 16(3–4):297–306. doi: 10.1016/S0736-5748(98)00023-9
86. Lovallo WR, Farag NH, Sorocco KH, Cohoon AJ, Vincent AS. Lifetime adversity leads to blunted stress axis reactivity: studies from the Oklahoma Family Health Patterns Project. *Biol Psychiatry* (2012) 71(4):344–9. doi: 10.1016/j.biopsych.2011.10.018
87. Nelson CA, Carver LJ. The effects of stress and trauma on brain and memory: a view from developmental cognitive neuroscience. *Dev Psychopathol* (1998) 10(4):793–809. doi: 10.1017/S0954579498001874
88. Gunnar MR, Nelson CA. Event-related potentials in year-old infants: relations with emotionality and cortisol. *Child Dev* (1994) 65(1):80–94. doi: 10.1111/j.1467-8624.1994.tb00736.x
89. Sinha R, Robinson J, O'Malley S. Stress response dampening: effects of gender and family history of alcoholism and anxiety disorders. *Psychopharmacology* (1998) 137(4):311–20. doi: 10.1007/s002130050624
90. Szabo A. The combined effects of orthostatic and mental stress on heart rate, T-wave amplitude, and pulse transit time. *Eur J Appl Physiol Occup Physiol* (1993) 67(6):540–4. doi: 10.1007/BF00241651

91. Teicher MH, Rabi K, Sheu YS, Seraphin SB, Andersen SL, Anderson CM, et al. Neurobiology of childhood trauma and adversity. In: Lanius RA, editor. *The impact of early life trauma on health and disease: the hidden epidemic.* Cambridge University Press, Cambridge, UK (2010). 112–22. doi: 10.1017/CBO9780511777042.014
92. Belujon P, Grace AA. Regulation of dopamine system responsivity and its adaptive and pathological response to stress. *Proc R Soc B* (2015) 282(1805): 20142516. doi: 10.1098/rspb.2014.2516
93. Koob GF, Le Moal M. Drug abuse: hedonic homeostatic dysregulation. *Science* (1997) 278(5335):52–8. doi: 10.1126/science.278.5335.52
94. Breslau J, Miller E, Chung WJJ, Schweitzer JB. Childhood and adolescent onset psychiatric disorders, substance use, and failure to graduate high school on time. *J Psychiatr Res* (2011) 45(3):295–301. doi: 10.1016/j.jpsychires.2010.06.014
95. Lovallo WR. Early life adversity reduces stress reactivity and enhances impulsive behavior: implications for health behaviors. *Int J Psychophysiol* (2013) 90(1):8–16. doi: 10.1016/j.ijpsycho.2012.10.006
96. Greco B, Carli M. Reduced attention and increased impulsivity in mice lacking NPY Y2 receptors: relation to anxiolytic-like phenotype. *Behav Brain Res* (2006) 169(2):325–34. doi: 10.1016/j.bbr.2006.02.002
97. Hatzinger M, Brand S, Perren S, von Wyl A, von Klitzing K, Holsboer-Trachsler E. Hypothalamic–pituitary–adrenocortical (HPA) activity in kindergarten children: importance of gender and associations with behavioral/emotional difficulties. *J Psychiatr Res* (2007) 41(10):861–70. doi: 10.1016/j.jpsychires.2006.07.012
98. Hayaki J, Stein MD, Lassor JA, Herman DS, Anderson BJ. Adversity among drug users: relationship to impulsivity. *Drug Alcohol Depend* (2005) 78(1):65–71. doi: 10.1016/j.drugalcdep.2004.09.002
99. Oshri A, Carlson MW, Kwon JA, Zeichner A, Wickrama KK. Developmental growth trajectories of self-esteem in adolescence: associations with child neglect and drug use and abuse in young adulthood. *J Youth Adolesc* (2017) 46(1):151–64. doi: 10.1007/s10964-016-0483-5
100. DePrince AP, Weinzierl KM, Combs MD. Executive function performance and trauma exposure in a community sample of children. *Child Abuse Negl* (2009) 33(6):353–61. doi: 10.1016/j.chiabu.2008.08.002
101. Mueller SC, Maheu FS, Dozier M, Peloso E, Mandell D, Leibenluft E, et al. Early-life stress is associated with impairment in cognitive control in adolescence: an fMRI study. *Neuropsychologia* (2010) 48(10):3037–44. doi: 10.1016/j.neuropsychologia.2010.06.013
102. Nikulina V, Widom CS. Child maltreatment and executive functioning in middle adulthood: a prospective examination. *Neuropsychology* (2013) 27(4):417. doi: 10.1037/a0032811
103. Andersen SL, Teicher MH. Desperately driven and no brakes: developmental stress exposure and subsequent risk for substance abuse. *Neurosci Biobehav Rev* (2009) 33(4):516–24. doi: 10.1016/j.neubiorev.2008.09.009
104. Walsh ND, Dalgleish T, Lombardo MV, Dunn VJ, Van Harmelen AL, Ban M, et al. General and specific effects of early-life psychosocial adversities on adolescent grey matter volume. *Neuroimage Clin* (2014) 4:308–18. doi: 10.1016/j.nicl.2014.01.001
105. Pentz MA, Riggs NR, Warren CM. Improving substance use prevention efforts with executive function training. *Drug Alcohol Depend* (2016) 163(1):S54–S59. doi: 10.1016/j.drugalcdep.2016.03.001
106. Elkins IJ, McGue M, Iacono WG. Prospective effects of attention-deficit/hyperactivity disorder, conduct disorder, and sex on adolescent substance use and abuse. *Arch Gen Psychiatry* (2007) 64(10):1145–52. doi: 10.1001/archpsyc.64.10.1145
107. Frank MJ, Moustafa AA, Haughey HM, Curran T, Hutchison KE. Genetic triple dissociation reveals multiple roles for dopamine in reinforcement learning. *Proc Natl Acad Sci* (2007) 104(41):16311–6. doi: 10.1073/pnas.0706111104
108. Klein TA, Neumann J, Reuter M, Hennig J, von Cramon DY, Ullsperger M. Genetically determined differences in learning from errors. *Science* (2007) 318(5856):1642–5. doi: 10.1126/science.1145044
109. Kreek MJ, Nielsen DA, Butelman ER, LaForge KS. Genetic influences on impulsivity, risk taking, stress responsivity and vulnerability to drug abuse and addiction. *Nat Neuroscie* (2005) 8(11):1450. doi: 10.1038/nn1583
110. Jutras-Aswad D, Jacobs MM, Yiannoulos G, Roussos P, Bitsios P, Nomura Y, et al. Cannabis-dependence risk relates to synergism between neuroticism and proenkephalin SNPs associated with amygdala gene expression: case-control study. *PloS One* (2012) 7(6):e39243. doi: 10.1371/journal.pone.0039243
111. Kendler KS, Prescott CA, Myers J, Neale MC. The structure of genetic and environmental risk factors for common psychiatric and substance use disorders in men and women. *Arc Gen Psychiatry* (2003) 60(9):929–37. doi: 10.1001/archpsyc.60.9.929
112. Li JJ, Savage JE, Kendler KS, Hickman M, Mahedy L, Macleod J, et al. Polygenic risk, personality dimensions, and adolescent alcohol use problems: a longitudinal study. *J Stud Alcohol Drugs* (2017) 78(3):442–51. doi: 10.15288/jsad.2017.78.442
113. Dahl RE. Adolescent brain development: a period of vulnerabilities and opportunities. Keynote address. *Ann N Y Acad Sci* (2004) 1021(1):1–22. doi: 10.1196/annals.1308.001
114. Fernie G, Peeters M, Gullo MJ, Christiansen P, Cole JC, Sumnall H, et al. Multiple behavioural impulsivity tasks predict prospective alcohol involvement in adolescents. *Addiction* (2013) 108(11):1916–23. doi: 10.1111/add.12283
115. Lerman C, Niaura R. Applying genetic approaches to the treatment of nicotine dependence. *Oncogene* (2002) 21(48):7412–20. doi: 10.1038/sj.onc.1205801
116. Armstrong TD, Costello EJ. Community studies on adolescent substance use, abuse, or dependence and psychiatric comorbidity. *J Consult Clin Psychol* (2002) 70(6):1224–39. doi: 10.1037//0022-006X.70.6.1224
117. De Bellis MD. Developmental traumatology: a contributory mechanism for alcohol and substance use disorders. *Psychoneuroendocrinology* (2002) 27 (1–2):155–70. doi: 10.1016/S0306-4530(01)00042-7
118. Rowe CL, Liddle HA, Greenbaum PE, Henderson CE. Impact of psychiatric comorbidity on treatment of adolescent drug abusers. *J Subst Abuse Treat* (2004) 26(2):129–40. doi: 10.1016/S0740-5472(03)00166-1
119. Tomlinson KL, Brown SA, Abrantes A. Psychiatric comorbidity and substance use treatment outcomes of adolescents. *Psychol Addict Behav* (2004) 18(2):160–9. doi: 10.1037/0893-164X.18.2.160
120. Kovacs M, Goldston D. Cognitive and social cognitive development of depressed children and adolescents. *J Am Acad Child Adolesc Psychiatry* (1991) 30(3):388–92. doi: 10.1097/00004583-199105000-00006
121. Millan MJ, Agid Y, Brüne M, Bullmore ET, Carter CS, Clayton NS, et al. Cognitive dysfunction in psychiatric disorders: characteristics, causes and the quest for improved therapy. *Nat Rev Drug Discov* (2012) 11(2):141–68. doi: 10.1038/nrd3628
122. Quello SB, Brady KT, Sonne SC. Mood disorders and substance use disorder: a complex comorbidity. *Sci Pract Perspect* (2005) 3(1):13–21. doi: 10.1151/spp053113
123. Thorberg FA, Young RM, Sullivan KA, Lyvers M. Alexithymia and alcohol use disorders: a critical review. *Addict Behav* (2009) 34(3):237–45. doi: 10.1016/j.addbeh.2008.10.016
124. Evren C, Evren B, Dalbudak E, Ozcelik B, Oncu F. Childhood abuse and neglect as a risk factor for alexithymia in adult male substance dependent inpatients. *J Psychoact Drugs* (2009) 41(1):85–92. doi: 10.1080/02791072.2009.10400677
125. Evren C, Evren B. Self-mutilation in substance-dependent patients and relationship with childhood abuse and neglect, alexithymia and temperament and character dimensions of personality. *Drug Alcohol Depend* (2005) 80(1):15–22. doi: 10.1016/j.drugalcdep.2005.03.017
126. Sakuraba S, Kubo M, Komoda T, Yamana JI. Suicidal ideation and alexithymia in patients with alcoholism: a pilot study. *Subst Use Misuse* (2005) 40(6):823–30. doi: 10.1081/JA-200030702
127. Stasiewicz PR, Bradizza CM, Gudleski GD, Coffey SF, Schlauch RC, Bailey ST, et al. The relationship of alexithymia to emotional dysregulation within an alcohol dependent treatment sample. *Addict Behav* (2012) 37(4):469–76. doi: 10.1016/j.addbeh.2011.12.011
128. Berking M, Margraf M, Ebert D, Wupperman P, Hofmann SG, Junghanns K. Deficits in emotion-regulation skills predict alcohol use during and after cognitive–behavioral therapy for alcohol dependence. *J Consult Clin Psychol* (2011) 79(3):307–18. doi: 10.1037/a0023421
129. Compton WM, Conway KP, Stinson FS, Colliver JD, Grant BF. Prevalence, correlates, and comorbidity of DSM-IV antisocial personality syndromes and alcohol and specific drug use disorders in the United States: results from the national epidemiologic survey on alcohol and related conditions. *J Clin Psychiatry* (2005) 66(6):677–85. doi: 10.4088/JCP.v66n0602
130. Merikangas KR, He JP, Burstein M, Swanson SA, Avenevoli S, Cui L, et al. Lifetime prevalence of mental disorders in US adolescents: results from

the National Comorbidity Survey Replication–Adolescent Supplement (NCS-A). *J Am Acad Child Adolesc Psychiatry* (2010) 49(10):980–9. doi: 10.1016/j.jaac.2010.05.017
131. Chen P, Jacobson KC. Developmental trajectories of substance use from early adolescence to young adulthood: gender and racial/ethnic differences. *J Adolesc Health* (2012) 50(2):154–63. doi: 10.1016/j.jadohealth.2011.05.013
132. McCambridge J, McAlaney J, Rowe R. Adult consequences of late adolescent alcohol consumption: a systematic review of cohort studies. *PLoS Med* (2011) 8(2):e1000413. doi: 10.1371/journal.pmed.1000413
133. Green KM, Doherty EE, Reisinger HS, Chilcoat HD, Ensminger M. Social integration in young adulthood and the subsequent onset of substance use and disorders among a community population of urban African Americans. *Addiction* (2010) 105(3):484–93. doi: 10.1111/j.1360-0443.2009.02787.x
134. Hill S, Shanahan L, Costello EJ, Copeland W. Predicting persistent, limited, and delayed problematic cannabis use in early adulthood: findings from a longitudinal study. *J Am Acad Child Adolesc Psychiatry* (2017) 56(11):966–74. doi: 10.1016/j.jaac.2017.08.012
135. Kendler KS, Ohlsson H, Edwards AC, Sundquist J, Sundquist K. A developmental etiological model for drug abuse in men. *Drug Alcohol Depend* (2017) 179(1):220–8. doi: 10.1016/j.drugalcdep.2017.06.036
136. Fergusson DM, Boden JM, Horwood LJ. The developmental antecedents of illicit drug use: evidence from a 25-year longitudinal study. *Drug Alcohol Depend* (2008) 96(1-2):65–77. doi: 10.1016/j.drugalcdep.2008.03.003
137. Staff J, Schulenberg JE, Maslowsky J, Bachman JG, O'Malley PM, Maggs JL, et al. Substance use changes and social role transitions: proximal developmental effects on ongoing trajectories from late adolescence through early adulthood. *Dev Psychopathol* (2010) 22(4):917–32. doi: 10.1017/S0954579410000544
138. Oesterle S, Hawkins JD, Hill KG. Men's and women's pathways to adulthood and associated substance misuse. *J Stud Alcohol Drugs* (2011) 72(5):763–73. doi: 10.15288/jsad.2011.72.763
139. McCabe SE, Schulenberg JE, O'malley PM, Patrick ME, Kloska DD. Nonmedical use of prescription opioids during the transition to adulthood: a multi-cohort national longitudinal study. *Addiction* (2014) 109(1):102–10. doi: 10.1111/add.12347
140. Schulenberg JE, Maggs JL. A developmental perspective on alcohol use and heavy drinking during adolescence and the transition to young adulthood. *J Stud Alcohol Suppl* (2002) 14(Suppl):54–70. doi: 10.15288/jsas.2002.s14.54
141. Hobfoll SE, Palmieri PA, Johnson RJ, Canetti-Nisim D, Hall BJ, Galea S. Trajectories of resilience, resistance, and distress during ongoing terrorism: the case of Jews and Arabs in Israel. *J Consult Clin Psychol* (2009) 77(1):138–48. doi: 10.1037/a0014360
142. Bonanno GA. Loss, trauma, and human resilience: have we underestimated the human capacity to thrive after extremely aversive events? *Am Psychol* (2004) 59(1):20–8. doi: 10.1037/0003-066X.59.1.20
143. Bonanno GA, Wortman CB, Nesse RM. Prospective patterns of resilience and maladjustment during widowhood. *Psychol Aging* (2004) 19(2):260–71. doi: 10.1037/0882-7974.19.2.260
144. Masten AS. Ordinary magic: resilience processes in development. *Am Psychol* (2001) 56(3):227–38. doi: 10.1037//0003-066X.56.3.227
145. Wingo AP, Fani N, Bradley B, Ressler KJ. Psychological resilience and neurocognitive performance in a traumatized community sample. *Depress Anxiety* (2010) 27(8):768–74. doi: 10.1002/da.20675
146. Schreiber LR, Grant JE, Odlaug BL. Emotion regulation and impulsivity in young adults. *J Psychiatr Res* (2012) 46(5):651–8. doi: 10.1016/j.jpsychires.2012.02.005
147. Cicchetti D, Rogosch FA. Adaptive coping under conditions of extreme stress: multilevel influences on the determinants of resilience in maltreated children. In: Skinner EA, Zimmer-Gembeck MJ, editors. *Coping and the development of regulation. New directions for child and adolescent development.*, vol. 124 Jossey-Bass (2009). p. 47–59. doi: 10.1002/cd.242
148. Qouta S, El-Sarraj E, Punamäki RL. Mental flexibility as resiliency factor among children exposed to political violence. *Int J Psychol* (2001) 36(1):1–7. doi: 10.1080/00207590042000010
149. Lisdahl KM, Gilbart ER, Wright NE, Shollenbarger S. Dare to delay? The impacts of adolescent alcohol and marijuana use onset on cognition, brain structure, and function. *Front Psychiatry* (2013) 4(53):1–18. doi: 10.3389/fpsyt.2013.00053
150. Naim-Feil J, Fitzgerald PB, Bradshaw JL, Lubman DI, Sheppard D. Neurocognitive deficits, craving, and abstinence among alcohol-dependent individuals following detoxification. *Arch Clin Neuropsychol* (2013) 29(1):26–37. doi: 10.1093/arclin/act090
151. Winhusen TM, Somoza EC, Lewis DF, Kropp FB, Horigian VE, Adinoff B. Frontal systems deficits in stimulant-dependent patients: evidence of pre-illness dysfunction and relationship to treatment response. *Drug Alcohol Depend* (2013) 127(1–3):94–100. doi: 10.1016/j.drugalcdep.2012.06.017
152. Nolin P, Ethier L. Using neuropsychological profiles to classify neglected children with or without physical abuse. *Child Abuse Negl* (2007) 31(6):631–43. doi: 10.1016/j.chiabu.2006.12.009
153. Feeney J, Kamiya Y, Robertson IH, Kenny RA. Cognitive function is preserved in older adults with a reported history of childhood sexual abuse. *J Trauma Stress* (2013) 26(6):735–43. doi: 10.1002/jts.21861
154. Ritchie K, Jaussent I, Stewart R, Dupuy AM, Courtet P, Malafosse A, et al. Adverse childhood environment and late-life cognitive functioning. *Int J Geriatr Psychiatry* (2011) 26(5):503–10. doi: 10.1002/gps.2553
155. Iadipaolo AS, Marusak HA, Paulisin SM, Sala-Hamrick K, Crespo LM, Elrahal F, et al. Distinct neural correlates of trait resilience within core neurocognitive networks in at-risk children and adolescents. *NeuroImage Clin* (2018) 20(1):24–34. doi: 10.1016/j.nicl.2018.06.026
156. Liang X, He Y, Salmeron BJ, Gu H, Stein EA, Yang Y. Interactions between the salience and default-mode networks are disrupted in cocaine addiction. *J Neurosci* (2015) 35(21):8081–90. doi: 10.1523/JNEUROSCI.3188-14.2015
157. Weiland BJ, Sabbineni A, Calhoun VD, Welsh RC, Bryan AD, Jung RE, et al. Reduced left executive control network functional connectivity is associated with alcohol use disorders. *Alcohol Clin Exp Res* (2014) 38(9):2445–53. doi: 10.1111/acer.12505
158. Philip NS, Tyrka AR, Albright SE, Sweet LH, Almeida J, Price LH, et al. Early life stress predicts thalamic hyperconnectivity: a transdiagnostic study of global connectivity. *J Psychiatr Res* (2016) 79(1):93–100. doi: 10.1016/j.jpsychires.2016.05.003
159. van der Werff SJ, Pannekoek JN, Veer IM, van Tol MJ, Aleman A, Veltman DJ, et al. Resilience to childhood maltreatment is associated with increased resting-state functional connectivity of the salience network with the lingual gyrus. *Child Abuse Negl* (2013) 37(11):1021–9. doi: 10.1016/j.chiabu.2013.07.008
160. Fishbein DH, Eldreth DL, Hyde C, Matochik JA, London ED, Contoreggi C, et al. Risky decision making and the anterior cingulate cortex in abstinent drug abusers and nonusers. *Cognit Brain Res* (2005) 23(1):119–36. doi: 10.1016/j.cogbrainres.2004.12.010
161. Motzkin JC, Baskin-Sommers A, Newman JP, Kiehl KA, Koenigs M. Neural correlates of substance abuse: reduced functional connectivity between areas underlying reward and cognitive control. *Human Brain Map* (2014) 35(9):4282–92. doi: 10.1002/hbm.22474
162. Burt KB, Whelan R, Conrod PJ, Banaschewski T, Barker GJ, Bokde AL, et al. Structural brain correlates of adolescent resilience. *J Child Psychol Psychiatry* (2016) 57(11):1287–96. doi: 10.1111/jcpp.12552
163. Demers LA, McKenzie KJ, Hunt RH, Cicchetti D, Cowell RA, Rogosch FA, et al. Separable effects of childhood maltreatment and adult adaptive functioning on amygdala connectivity during emotion processing. *Biol Psychiatry Cognit Neurosci Neuroimaging* (2018) 3(2):116–24. doi: 10.1016/j.bpsc.2017.08.010
164. Banyard V, Hamby S, Grych J. Health effects of adverse childhood events: identifying promising protective factors at the intersection of mental and physical well-being. *Child Abuse Negl* (2017) 65(1):88–98. doi: 10.1016/j.chiabu.2017.01.011
165. Blair KS, Vythilingam M, Crowe SL, McCaffrey DE, Ng P, Wu CC, et al. Cognitive control of attention is differentially affected in trauma-exposed individuals with and without post-traumatic stress disorder. *Psychol Med* (2013) 43(1):85–95. doi: 10.1017/S0033291712000840
166. Chandra S, Leong FT. A diversified portfolio model of adaptability. *Am Psychol* (2016) 71(9):847–62. doi: 10.1037/a0040367
167. Jacquart J, Papini S, Davis ML, Rosenfield D, Powers MB, Frierson GM, et al. Identifying attendance patterns in a smoking cessation treatment and their relationships with quit success. *Drug Alcohol Depend* (2017) 174(1):65–9. doi: 10.1016/j.drugalcdep.2017.01.007

168. Lichenstein SD, Musselman S, Shaw DS, Sitnick S, Forbes EE. Nucleus accumbens functional connectivity at age 20 is associated with trajectory of adolescent cannabis use and predicts psychosocial functioning in young adulthood. *Addiction* (2017) 112(11):1961–70. doi: 10.1111/add.13882
169. Ramirez JJ, Fairlie AM, Olin CC, Lindgren KP. Implicit and explicit drinking identity predict latent classes that differ on the basis of college students' drinking behaviors. *Drug Alcohol Depend* (2017) 178(1):579–85. doi: 10.1016/j.drugalcdep.2017.06.010
170. Blair C, Raver CC. Child development in the context of adversity: experiential canalization of brain and behavior. *Am Psychol* (2012) 67(4):309–18. doi: 10.1037/a0027493
171. Bryck RL, Fisher PA. Training the brain: practical applications of neural plasticity from the intersection of cognitive neuroscience, developmental psychology, and prevention science. *Am Psychol* (2012) 67(2):87–100. doi: 10.1037/a0024657
172. Twamley EW, Savla GN, Zurhellen CH, Heaton RK, Jeste DV. Development and pilot testing of a novel compensatory cognitive training intervention for people with psychosis. *Am J Psychiatr* Rehabil (2008) 11(2):144–63. doi: 10.1080/15487760801963678

10

Heterogeneity in Disordered Gambling: Decision-Making and Impulsivity in Gamblers Grouped by Preferred Form

Steve Sharman[1,2], Luke Clark[2,3], Amanda Roberts[4], Rosanna Michalczuk[2,5], Rachel Cocks[2,6] and Henrietta Bowden-Jones[7,8]*

[1] School of Psychology, College of Applied Health and Communities, University of East London, London, United Kingdom, [2] Department of Psychology, University of Cambridge, Cambridge, United Kingdom, [3] Centre for Gambling Research at UBC, Department of Psychology, University of British Columbia, Vancouver, BC, Canada, [4] School of Psychology, College of Social Science, University of Lincoln, Lincoln, United Kingdom, [5] South London and Maudsley Trust, Bethlem Royal Hospital, London, United Kingdom, [6] Royal Holloway, University of London, London, United Kingdom, [7] National Problem Gambling Clinic, London, United Kingdom, [8] Faculty of Medicine, Faculty of Medicine Centre, Imperial College London, London, United Kingdom

***Correspondence:**
Steve Sharman
ssharman@uel.ac.uk

Background: Previous research has indicated that disordered gamblers display deficits in impulsivity and risky decision-making, compared to healthy control groups. However, disordered gamblers are not a homogenous group, and differences in performance on neurocognitive tasks may be related to the form of gambling in which an individual chooses to engage. The present study used neurocognitive tasks and questionnaire measures to ascertain group differences in gamblers grouped by preferred form of gambling.

Method: Treatment-seeking pathological gamblers from the National Problem Gambling Clinic, London (n = 101), completed a neurocognitive assessment comprising the Cambridge gamble task (CGT), the stop-signal task (SST), a probabilistic reversal learning task (PRL), and the Kirby Monetary Choice Questionnaire, as well as questionnaire measures of gambling severity, impulsivity, depression, and anxiety. Analyses compared gamblers who favored fixed-odds betting terminals (FOBTs) (the modal form) to gamblers who preferred other forms of gambling (non-FOBT).

Results: The FOBT group showed impaired decision-making under risk on the CGT compared to the non-FOBT group, choosing the likely option less on more uncertain decisions. The FOBT group made fewer perseverative errors on the PRL task, had lower depression and anxiety scores, and were less likely to have a family history of problem gambling than the non-FOBT group.

Discussion: Decision-making and cognitive flexibility differences between gamblers grouped by gambling type supports preferred form as an important source of heterogeneity in gambling disorder. Decision-making strategies and risk attitudes should be considered when approaching cognition-focused treatment strategies, allowing interventions to be targeted at specific cognitive deficits.

Keywords: gambling, impulsivity, decision-making, disordered gambling, heterogeneity

INTRODUCTION

Pathological gambling was re-classified from an impulse control disorder to an addictive disorder in the most recent versions of the Diagnostic and Statistical Manual of Mental Disorders (DSM-5) (1) and the International Classification of Diseases and Related Health Problems (11th edition) (ICD-11) (2) in acknowledgement of the parallels between behavioral and substance addictions (3). The term "disordered gambling" is used hereafter as an umbrella term for people experiencing gambling-related harm.

Disruption of executive functions has been identified as being important in the development and maintenance of addictive behaviors (4). More specifically, risky decision-making and low self-control (i.e., impulsivity) are markers that cut across different forms of addiction, through the interaction of impulsive and reflective systems for assessing reward options (5, 6). As in substance addictions, groups of pathological gamblers display statistically significant impairments in decision-making using the Iowa gambling task (IGT), selecting more cards from the disadvantageous decks (7). Pathological gamblers also show deficits in risky decision-making using the Cambridge gamble task (CGT) (8, 9), the Information Sampling Test (IST) (8), and the game of dice task (10). Brevers et al. (11) found that problem gamblers perform worse than controls on tasks assessing decision-making under both explicit risk (where the odds are known) and decisions under ambiguity (where the probabilities are unknown).

Similarly, impulsivity has been seen to be elevated in both substance addictions (12) and disordered gambling (13). Impulsivity can be measured with delay discounting tasks (i.e., impulsive choice) (14–16) as well as tests of response inhibition (i.e., impulsive action) on tasks including the stop-signal task (17), the Go–No Go task (18), and the Stroop test (19). Additionally, disordered gamblers display increased response perseveration and compulsivity on reversal learning tasks (20), although Boog et al. (21) suggest these deficits may arise as a function of reward motivation rather than cognitive inflexibility *per se*. Nevertheless, the multi-dimensional nature of impulsivity has not been fully parsed in disordered gambling. Using a thorough assessment with both neurocognitive tasks and questionnaire measures, Billieux et al. found that disordered gamblers exhibited higher urgency, lower premeditation, impairment in prepotent inhibition, and lower tolerance of delayed rewards than a control group. However, they also observed considerable heterogeneity in the impulsivity profiles of the gamblers: although disordered gamblers reported elevated impulsivity at an overall level, individual gamblers displayed atypical scores on different UPPS subscales, and the disordered gamblers were not reliably impaired across all inhibition tasks, indicating that impulsivity is not universally present in disordered gamblers (22).

In comparing problem gamblers to healthy controls, an alcohol dependent group and a Tourette syndrome group on four impulsivity-related dimensions (self-reported impulsivity, prepotent response impulsivity, choice impulsivity, and motor impulsivity), Kräplin et al., (23) found that gamblers were more impulsive than the healthy control group across all dimensions, and the problem gamblers were the only group that differed on choice impulsivity, indicating some dimensions of impulsivity although a key feature in gambling disorders, are not disorder specific (23).

Traditional models of sub-typing problem gamblers primarily rely on personality traits and clinical characteristics (24–26). Three dominant subtypes of gambler are proposed, termed "behaviorally conditioned," "emotionally vulnerable," and "antisocial impulsivist," with impulsivity emphasized as a dispositional factor in the third pathway. However, approaches to subtyping gamblers to date have rarely consider the form(s) of gambling the individual engages in. The level of skill, or strategy involved in different forms of gambling, can vary: lotteries are chance games, where no single outcome is more likely than any other, whereas gambling forms such as poker offer far greater potential for experienced players to develop successful strategies (27). Studies that utilize preferred form as a source of heterogeneity commonly use a dichotomy of strategic (e.g., sports, cards) *versus* non-strategic (e.g., slots, lotteries) games, describing differences in demographic variables (28–30), personality traits (31), and gambling severity (32).

Preferred form of gambling has also been investigated preliminarily in relation to neurocognitive performance. After characterizing group deficits in pathological gamblers on the IGT and a reversal learning task, Goudriaan et al. (33) separated gamblers based on their preferred forms (slot machine gamblers and casino gamblers); the slot machine gamblers displayed greater impairments in decision-making than the casino gamblers. Using a computational model to decompose performance on the IGT, Lorains et al. (34) found that strategic gamblers were significantly influenced by both gains and losses but demonstrated an inconsistent choice style, where non-strategic gamblers were less sensitive to losses and exhibited poor learning during decision-making. Navas et al. identified non-strategic gamblers displayed higher delay discounting whereas strategic gamblers reported higher cognitive distortions and self-reported reward sensitivity (35). However, in a study by Grant et al. (36), both strategic and non-strategic gamblers were impaired compared to healthy controls on tests of cognitive flexibility or motor impulsivity, but the subgroups did not differ from each other.

In the UK, fixed-odds betting terminals (FOBTs) are a form of electronic gaming machine (EGM) located in high-street betting shops and casinos. These terminals offer multiple games with "fixed odds," including electronic roulette as a popular form. FOBTs appear to be a particularly problematic form of gambling. Disordered gamblers are estimated to account for over 22% of money and over 25% of time spent on FOBTs in the UK (37). In a small sample of treatment-seeking pathological gamblers from the London National Problem Gambling Clinic, FOBTs were the preferred form of gambling in 60% of the sample (16). Subsequent analyses found that FOBT preference is associated with increased gambling severity (38), and that use of "gaming machines" was a significant predictor of pre-treatment dropout (39). Furthermore, in data collected from gamblers seeking residential treatment in the UK, FOBTs were the most common and fastest increasing form of gambling identified by those clients as problematic (40).

Recent meta-analyses have confirmed robust differences on neurocognitive tasks in groups with disordered gambling compared to healthy comparison groups (7, 13, 20, 41). The present study focuses specifically on disordered gamblers, by exploring heterogeneity on neurocognitive and questionnaire measures of impulsivity and risky choice. A moderately large sample of treatment-seeking pathological gamblers were grouped as a function of preferred form of gambling, distinguishing FOBTs as the modal form against a non-FOBT group comprising all other preferred forms. Considering the heterogeneity in previous studies explained by strategic *vs.* non-strategic form preferences, we predicted that FOBT preferences would also predict neurocognitive performance.

METHODS

Participants

Treatment-seeking pathological gamblers were recruited from the National Problem Gambling Clinic, London (NPGC). Inclusion criteria were a current diagnosis of pathological gambling using the Massachusetts Gambling Screen (MAGS) (42), a 12-item gambling screen based on the DSM-IV pathological gambling criteria. This was corroborated by scores indicating problem gambling on the Problem Gambling Severity Index (PGSI > 7) (43). Exclusion criteria were the presence of neurological disorders, previous serious head injury or history of psychotic disorder, leading to exclusion of nine participants. This resulted in a final sample of 101 pathological gamblers (92 male; age M = 37.6, SD = 11.3).

The study protocol was approved by Cambridge South Research Ethics Council, Ref: 09/H0305/77. Participants gave written informed consent in accordance with the Declaration of Helsinki and were reimbursed for time and travel expenses. Participants completed a general screening questionnaire to collate demographic data including age, gender, nationality, ethnicity, education level, employment status, relationship status, and handedness. This questionnaire recorded participants' preferred form of gambling, and family history of disordered gambling.

Participants were grouped based on their stated preferred form of gambling. The modal preferred form was FOBTs in 43 participants (age M = 36.9, SD = 11.7, 41 male). Other forms (n = 58; age M = 38.1, SD = 11; 51 male) comprised sports betting (n = 14), fruit machines (n = 13), betting on horses (n = 10), poker (n = 6), casinos (n = 6), blackjack (n = 4), online casinos (n = 2), stocks and shares (n = 2), and betting shops (n = 1). Smoking status was measured by the Fagerstrom Test for Nicotine Dependence (FTND) (44). IQ estimates were obtained from two measures, the National Adult Reading Test (NART) (45) and the composite of the Matrix Reasoning and Vocabulary tests on the Wechsler Abbreviated Scale of Intelligence (46). All participants were recruited following initial assessment at the NPGC and were either awaiting treatment (FOBT n = 27; non-FOBT n = 38), receiving psychological treatment (FOBT n = 11; non-FOBT n = 14), or had completed a course of CBT (FOBT n = 5; Non-FOBT n = 6). Groups did not differ on treatment stage distributions (χ^2 (2) = .33, p = .85).

Neurocognitive Assessment

Kirby Monetary Choice Questionnaire (Kirby MCQ) (44)

Delay discounting was measured using the Kirby MCQ (47), a temporal discounting task involving 27 binary choices between an immediate smaller reward *versus* a larger reward available following a delay. All rewards were hypothetical monetary rewards. Larger rewards varied across three levels of magnitude (low, medium, and high). The indifference points at each magnitude are used to derive a hyperbolic k value, where higher k values indicate steeper discounting of delayed rewards and thus higher impulsivity. k Values are log transformed to reduce skew and averaged over the three magnitudes to calculate the overall discounting rate.

Cambridge Gamble Task (CGT) (45)

Risky decision-making was examined using the Cambridge gamble task (48). On each trial, 10 boxes are presented that are colored red or blue. The ratio of colors varies from trial to trial (9:1, 8:2, 7:3, and 6:4). The participant is instructed that a token has been hidden under one box. Each trial involves two responses. First, the participant makes a decision regarding which box color the token is hidden, and second, they place a bet of some points on their color choice. Across two conditions (in counterbalanced order), bets are offered in either an ascending or descending sequence, in fixed proportions of the current tally (5, 25, 50, 75, and 95%). Participants complete four blocks of nine trials in each of two conditions; at the start of each block the participant is endowed with 100 points. Key measures were proportion of choice of most likely outcome, deliberation time, and proportion of points bet.

Stop-Signal Task (SST) (46)

Response inhibition was measured using the stop-signal task (49). This is a two-choice response task, where participants are presented with a "Go" stimulus that requires a rapid response (left response key for an arrow pointing left, and right response key for an arrow pointing right). Participants were instructed to inhibit the Go response if an auditory stop signal was presented (a 300-Hz tone). These stop signals occurred on 25% of trials, a short delay after the Go stimulus. This delay was adjusted over successive stop trials using a staircase procedure, to identify a point at which the participant successfully inhibited on 50% of stop trials. The task contained five blocks of 64 trials, resulting in 80 stop trials over the task. Key measures were the median Go reaction time and the stop-signal reaction time.

Probabilistic Reversal Learning Task (PRL) (47)

Perseverative responding was measured with a probabilistic reversal learning task (50). This is a two-choice visual discrimination, with a red and a green stimulus randomly displayed in two of four screen locations. Selection of one stimulus is positively reinforced on 80% of trials (by the word "CORRECT" appearing on the screen); the other stimulus is incorrect ("WRONG") on 80% of trials. After 40 trials for learning the initial discrimination, the contingencies reverse for 40 trials, such that the previously incorrect stimulus is now correct on 80% of selections. Key measures are the number of errors made in the two stages, the number of consecutive errors following the reversal (i.e., perseveration), and the number of response switches following the misleading (probabilistic) feedback.

Self-Report Measures

Anxiety was measured using the Beck Anxiety Inventory (BAI) (51), a 21-item questionnaire measuring anxiety symptoms in the past month on a scale from 0 (not at all) to 3 (severely). Scores of less than 21 indicated low anxiety, scores of 21–35 indicate moderate anxiety, and scores of ≥36 indicated severe anxiety. Depression was measured using the Beck Depression Inventory II (BDI-II, 52), a 21-item scale with scores ranging from 0 to 3. A total BDI-II score of 0–13 indicated minimal depression, scores of 14-19 indicate mild depression, 20–28 indicate moderate depression, and scores of 29–63 indicate severe depression. Impulsivity was measured using the UPPS-S (53), a 59-item self-report scale designed to measure five subscales of impulsivity. Items are answered on a Likert scale, anchored at 1 (agree strongly) to 4 (disagree strongly). The five subscales are negative urgency, positive urgency, (lack of) planning, (lack of) perseveration, and sensation seeking. Gambling cognitions were measured using the Gambling-Related Cognitions Scale (GRCS) (54), a 23-item scale where items are presented as statements, and participants are required to respond on a Likert scale anchored at 1 (strongly disagree) and 7 (strongly agree). The GRCS can be divided in to subscales of inability to stop (five items), interpretative bias (four items), illusion of control (four items), gambling expectancies (four items), and predictive control (six items).

Data Analysis

The neurocognitive tests that involved repeated-measures factors (Kirby MCQ: reward magnitude; CGT: color ratio and ascend/descend condition; PRL: stage) were analyzed with a mixed-factorial ANOVA with group as the between-subject factor. *Post hoc* analysis utilized *t* tests where appropriate. All data were checked for homogeneity of variance, and Greenhouse–Geisser was corrected where p > .05. Group differences on the scores on the questionnaire measures between the FOBT and non-FOBT gambling groups were analyzed using independent samples *t* tests. Chi-squared analyses were used for categorical data. Error bars represent the standard error of the mean. Data from the Kirby MCQ was log transformed prior to analysis.

RESULTS

The two subgroups did not differ significantly on age, gambling severity [(MAGS, (42); PGSI, (43))], IQ estimates, or nicotine dependence (**Table 1**). Although the non-FOBT group showed a trend toward having a greater proportion of females, the groups did not differ significantly on gender distribution (χ^2 (1) = 3.15, p = .06). The non-FOBT group (38.6%) were more likely to have a family history of problem gambling than the FOBT group (23.8%; $\chi^2(1)$ = 5.21, p = .02). The FOBT group scored significantly lower than the non-FOBT group on the BDI (*t* (99) = 2.16, p = .03) and BAI (*t* (97) = 2.87, p = .005). Groups did not differ on scores on any of the UPPS-P or GRCS subscales (**Table 2**).

Kirby MCQ: The ANOVA indicated a significant main effect of magnitude (F(1.8,173) = 52.91, p < .001), such that the k values were lower for delayed rewards of larger absolute magnitude, with significant differences between each of the three levels (lowest *t* = 5.43, all tests p < .001). The main effect of group (F(1,94) = .043, p = .84) and the magnitude x group interaction (F(1.8,173) = .051, p = .94) were not significant.

Cambridge Gamble Task: On quality of decision-making, the ANOVA for proportion of trials on which the participant chose the more likely option showed a significant ratio x group interaction (F(1.6,121.4) = 4.78, p = .016), as well as significant main effects of ratio (F(1.6,121.4) = 43.84, p < .001) and group (F(1,76) = 9.1, p = .003). The FOBT group were less likely to choose the favorable option, and especially so at the more uncertain box ratios (6:4 ratio: *t* (56.8) = 2.84, p = .006; 7:3 *t* (52.8) = 2.13, p = .05). The 8:2 and 9:1 ratios were non-significant (lowest *t* = 1.47, p > .05), **Figure 1**.

An equivalent model for deliberation times indicated a significant ratio x group interaction (F(2.7,247.7) = 3.86, p = .02). The non-FOBT group demonstrated the expected pattern of longer deliberation times when the box color ratio was more evenly distributed (e.g., 6:4), than when the odds were greater (e.g., 9:1). The FOBT group demonstrated the opposite pattern, but analysis of simple effects indicated that the two groups did not differ significantly at any individual ratio (lowest *t* = .29, all

TABLE 1 | Group differences.

Questionnaire/test		Group				Test statistics		
		FOBT (n = 43)		Non-FOBT (n = 58)		T	df	p
		Mean	*Sd*	Mean	*Sd*			
Age		36.86	*11.73*	38.1	*11*	0.55	99	0.59
FTND	44	.77	*1.86*	1.46	*2.46*	1.59	98	0.11
MAGS	42	7.19	*2.04*	7.21	*1.5*	0.06	73.4	0.96
PGSI	43	18.59	*4.5*	19.16	*4.4*	0.63	96	0.53
NART	45	115.7	*6.54*	116.13	*6.58*	0.30	92	0.76
WASI	46	103.7	*17.4*	106.3	*13.34*	0.81	72.1	0.42

TABLE 2 | Questionnaire measures.

Questionnaire/test	Group				Test statistics		
	FOBT (n = 43)		Non-FOBT (n = 58)		t	df	P
	Mean	Sd	Mean	Sd			
GRCS							
Gambling experiences	12.79	*6.17*	13.6	*7*	.61	99	.55
Illusion of control	9.6	*5.51*	7.84	*4.89*	1.69	99	.09
Predictive control	17.67	*8.53*	15.16	*7.39*	1.59	99	.12
Inability to stop	18.98	*7.69*	18.79	*8.11*	.12	99	.91
Interpretive bias	15.26	*6.21*	15.52	*6.79*	.2	99	.84
Beck Depression Inventory	17.51	*10.1*	21.86	*9.86*	2.16	98	0.03*
Beck Anxiety Inventory	11.19	*8.88*	17.37	*11.68*	2.87	97	0.005*
UPPS-P							
Positive urgency	33.74	*9.17*	34.4	*9.62*	0.35	98	0.73
Negative urgency	34.91	*5.74*	36.05	*6.23*	0.94	98	0.35
Lack of perseverance	22.88	*4.74*	23.67	*5.54*	0.74	98	0.46
Lack of premeditation	26	*5.31*	26.91	*5.5*	0.83	98	0.41
Sensation seeking	34.81	*8.08*	32.04	*7.5*	1.77	98	0.08
Kirby MCQ (ln k)							
Magnitude—small	−3.46	*1.31*	−3.48	*1.27*	0.1	94	0.92
Magnitude—medium	−3.9	*1.27*	−3.98	*1.26*	0.32	94	0.75
Magnitude—large	−4.4	*1.5*	−4.44	*1.32*	0.16	94	0.88

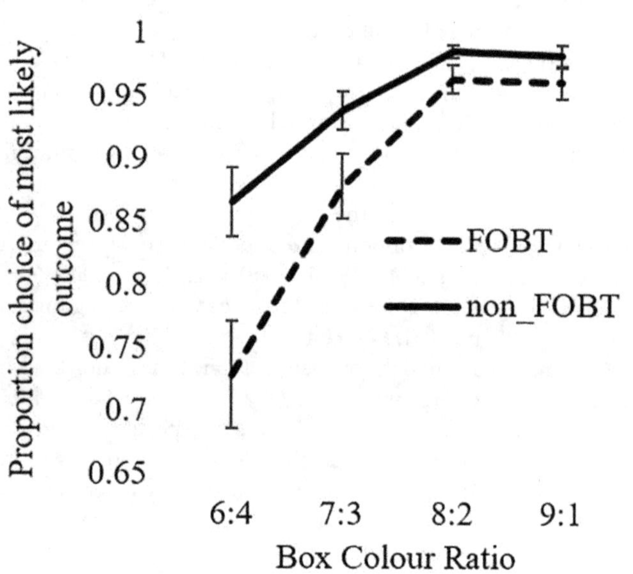

FIGURE 1 | Likely outcome choice as a function of ratio.

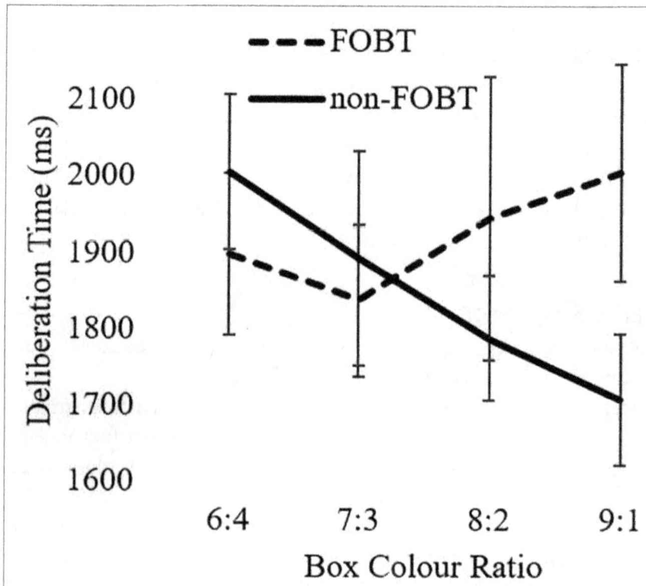

FIGURE 2 | Deliberation time as a function of ratio.

p > .05). Main factors of ratio (F(2.7,247.7) = .88, p = .44) and group (F(1,93) = .243, p = .62) were not significant (**Figure 2**).

For the analysis of betting behavior, the model shows significant main effects for ratio (F(1.6,150.3) = 256.6, p < .001) and condition (F(1,93) = 129.4, p < .001). The ratio x condition interaction was also significant (F(2.1,194) = 8.04, p < .001). Both groups bet more points in the descending condition than the ascending condition across all ratios. The main effect of group and the condition x group, ratio x group, and condition x group x ratio interactions were all non-significant (**Figure 3**). The number of "bankruptcies" (i.e., losing all points within a block, *t* (96) = .15, p = .88) and total points accrued across all trials (*t* (96) = .06, p = .95) did not differ between groups.

Stop-Signal Task: The groups did not differ on the stop-signal reaction time (FOBT M = 142.99ms, SD = 47.88; non-FOBT M = 131.86ms, SD = 41.21; *t* (80) = 1.13, p = .26). The median reaction time on "Go" trials did not differ between groups (FOBT: M = 469.93ms, SD = 113.91, non-FOBT M = 444.59ms, SD = 105.73; *t* (80) = .92, p = .36) indicating the groups did not differ in overall reaction time to go trials. In accordance with the SSD adjustment

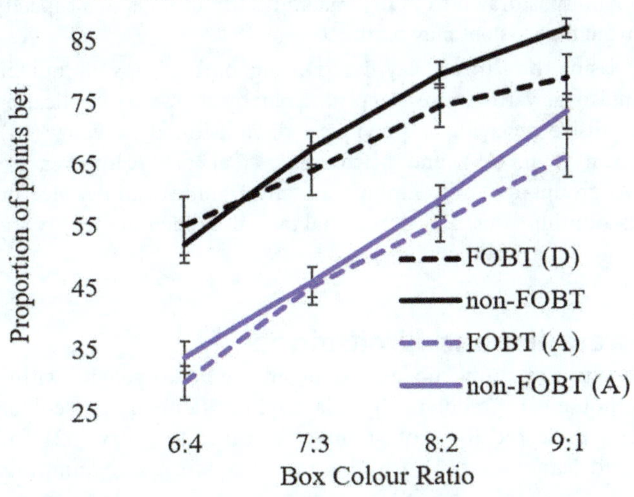

FIGURE 3 | Proportion of points bet as a function of ratio.

procedure, the proportion of successful stop inhibitions was close to 50% and not significantly different between groups (FOBT M = .51, SD = .06; non-FOBT M = .51, SD = .06; t (80) = .095, p = .92).

Probabilistic Reversal Learning: The ANOVA for errors by stage indicated a significant main effect of stage (F(1,87) = 36.63, p < .001), with both groups making more errors in stage 2 (**Figure 4**). The main effect of group (F(1,87) = 1.08, p = .30) and the stage x group interaction (F(1,87) = 1.57, p = .21) were non-significant. However, the groups differed significantly on perseverative errors specifically (t (85.9) = 2.27, p = .03); the non-FOBT group perseverated longer following the reversal switch (M = 5.43, SD = 4.8) than the FOBT group (M = 3.39, SD = 2.9) (**Figure 5**).

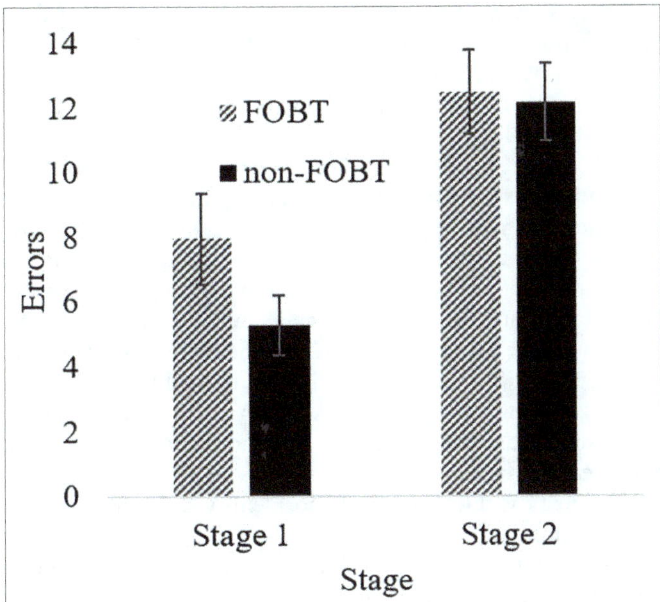

FIGURE 4 | PRL errors by task stage.

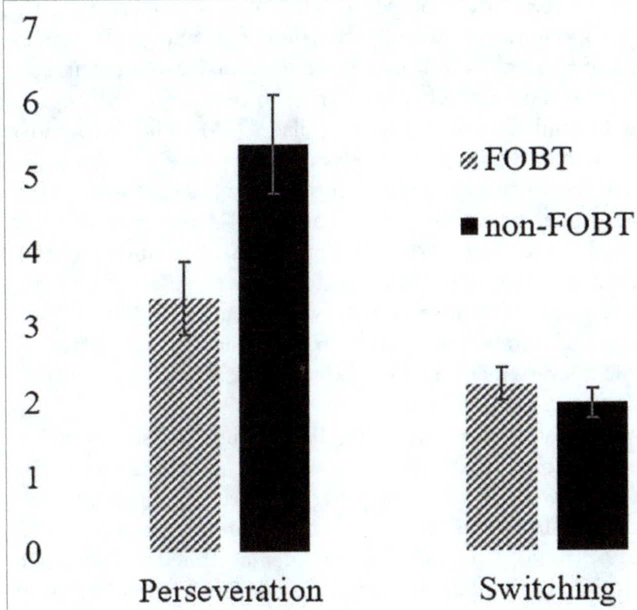

FIGURE 5 | Perseveration and switching by group.

The groups did not differ on the number of times they switched choice following misleading feedback (t (87) = .60, p = .55).

DISCUSSION

The key aim of this study was to explore the heterogeneity within a group of pathological gamblers using a psychological assessment focused on neurocognitive measures of decision-making, and questionnaire measures of impulsivity and common clinical comorbidities. Due the consistently high prevalence of FOBT gambling in UK treatment-seeking samples (including the present sample), our analyses compared FOBT gamblers against a mixed group of non-FOBT-preferring gamblers. The groups were comparable in terms of demographics and gambling severity. Analysis indicated both cognitive strengths and weaknesses in the FOBT gamblers. On the Cambridge gamble task, the FOBT group made fewer "rational" choices (i.e., of the majority color) on decisions with more uncertain odds. However, on the probabilistic reversal learning task, the FOBT group demonstrated lower levels of perseveration, potentially indicative of enhanced cognitive flexibility following the rule switch.

The CGT is a test of decision-making under risk (the odds are explicit) rather than under ambiguity. In prior research, individuals with pathological gambling differed from healthy comparison groups in terms of elevated betting and poorer quality of decision-making (8, 23). In the present study, the FOBT and non-FOBT groups did not differ in betting as a measure of impulsive and risky decision-making. However, differences were observed on decision quality, measured by the proportion of trials where the participant chooses the more likely outcome. Choice was also highly sensitive to the box ratio, with a stepwise increase in advantageous decisions as the ratios became more certain. The FOBT group made a lower proportion of advantageous choices, and this difference was strongest at the 6:4 and 7:3 ratios, where the outcomes were most uncertain. This choice of the unlikely option could be linked to the "gambler's fallacy" (55), a classic cognitive distortion in which gamblers expect the opposite outcome to the recent sequence. On the CGT, if the token has appeared several times under the more likely color, a participant may feel that the unlikely option is "due" and opt against the rational choice. Indeed, this type of gambling distortion is prevalent in roulette, where tables often display history information regarding "hot" and "cold" numbers and colors to emphasize the recent history. FOBT players may therefore be more susceptible to gambler's fallacy-type risky decisions.

Deliberation times to the CGT color choices also differed by preferred form, as an interaction with box ratio. The non-FOBT group showed the expected pattern whereby deliberation times became faster as the decisions became more certain (i.e., toward the 9:1 ratio). The FOBT group demonstrated the opposite pattern, with a trend toward *longer* deliberation at the more certain (9:1) color ratios. Notably, the two groups did not differ significantly at any individual box ratio. This pattern could also be explained by the conflict invoked by cognitive distortions such as the gambler's fallacy at the most certain ratios. Anticipatory regret may be a further influence on these decisions. Regret is a powerful emotion associated with counterfactual thinking ("what might have been") (56), and regret may increase if people do not win in a situation where they can easily imagine themselves winning (57)—for example, when choosing the majority color on the CGT. The pattern of decision latencies in the FOBT group supports the notion that probability is not the sole factor driving their color choice. This may be further expounded by gamblers who exhibit deficient emotion regulation (58).

The probabilistic reversal learning task showed that both groups made more errors in the second stage of the task, indicating increased perseveration and cognitive inflexibility. However, the results demonstrate a difference in perseveration between the two groups following the rule switch; the non-FOBT group perseverated significantly more than the FOBT group, demonstrating lower cognitive flexibility. The higher cognitive flexibility demonstrated by the FOBT group could be reflective of the cognitions associated with the different forms of gambling; the non-FOBT group contained a large number of sports and fruit machine gamblers, forms of gambling that either have relatively long outcome resolution (sports), or do not require any variation in the gambling mechanism (fruit machines), therefore do not require a great deal of quick-fire "switching" between win opportunities. Roulette on an FOBT requires the gambler to process the outcome in a number of different ways (color, odd/even, row, etc.) and then assimilate this outcome in to the decision-making process for subsequent bets, which on an FOBT can occur within 20 s. The continual updating of information requires cognitive flexibility. However, it is unclear from the current study whether a gambler with increased cognitive flexibility is drawn to FOBT machines or develops this capacity through persistent play on the terminals.

Using the Kirby Delay Discounting, both groups discounted smaller rewards more steeply than larger rewards, replicating impulsive behavior as previously demonstrated by Petry (14), Dixon et al. (15), and Michalczuk et al. (16). However, the two groups did not demonstrate any significant difference on discounting rates. The stop-signal task also failed to identify any group differences.

Strengths and Limitations

The current study chose to focus on the heterogeneity within pathological gamblers by classifying gamblers based on their preferred form of gambling, similar to Petry (32) and Goudriaan et al. (33). Although electronic roulette and other games available on FOBTs are primarily non-strategic forms, gamblers often believe they have a strategy, or a winning formula, and will therefore often erroneously believe there are elements of skill in chance games (e.g., fruit machines) (59). This complicates the traditional strategic/non-strategic dichotomy used by Grant et al. (36) and others, as some gamblers will likely play non-strategic games in a strategic manner. In addition, the strategic/non-strategic dichotomy can be dominated by certain specific games, such as Navas et al. (35) whose "type II non-strategic gamblers" were almost exclusively slot machine gamblers. However, for the classification used in the present study, it should be noted that EGM gamblers are present in both subgroups, given that FOBTs and slot machines are both types of EGMs. These forms do differ by gambling environment: FOBTs are housed specifically in gambling facilities (bookmaker's shops) while slot machines are also available in non-gambling venues such as pubs. The influence of these environmental factors on the cognitive differences we have observed is unclear and warrants further investigation. Furthermore, our method for categorizing gamblers was based on their stated single preferred form, but it is acknowledged that many participants also engaged in other forms of gambling.

Although the two groups did not differ on gender distribution, the sample was heavily male dominated (nine females), which prevented analyses of gender within the gambling subgroups. Our sample was treatment seeking with some variability in relation to stage of treatment (waiting list, during treatment or post-treatment). Our results may not be generalizable to the larger numbers of "at risk" gamblers. Therefore, results should be interpreted with caution. Additionally, this study did not have a non-gambling control group; differences in neurocognitive performance between gamblers and non-gamblers are well documented; the aim of this study was to better understand heterogeneity within gamblers who identify different forms as problematic.

Results indicate cognitive differences between pathological gamblers grouped by preferred form, indicating that problem gamblers are a heterogeneous group. This result should be considered when comparing gamblers as a single group to control groups, as the preferred form distribution of the gamblers could influence results.

AUTHOR CONTRIBUTIONS

SS was responsible for data collection, data analysis, and manuscript preparation. LC was responsible for study design,

REFERENCES

1. American Psychiatric Association. *Diagnostic and statistical manual of mental disorders.* 5th ed. Arlington, VA: American Psychiatric Publishing (2013). doi: 10.1176/appi.books.9780890425596
2. World Health Organization. (2018). *International statistical classification of diseases and related health problems* (11th Revision). Retrieved from https://icd.who.int/browse11/l-m/en#/http://id.who.int/icd/entity/1041487064.
3. Grant JE, Potenza MN, Weinstein A, Gorelick DA. Introduction to behavioral addictions. *Am J Drug Alcohol Abuse* (2010) 36(5):233–41. doi: 10.3109/00952990.2010.491884
4. Verdejo-Garcia A, Manning V. Executive functioning in gambling disorder: cognitive profiles and associations with clinical outcomes. *Curr Addict Rep* (2015) 2(3):214–9. doi: 10.1007/s40429-015-0062-y
5. Bechara A. Decision making, impulse control and loss of willpower to resist drugs: a neurocognitive perspective. *Nat Neurosci* (2005) 8(11):1458–63. doi: 10.1038/nn1584
6. Verdejo-Garcia A, Chong TTJ, Stout JC, Yücel M, London ED. Stages of dysfunctional decision-making in addiction. *Pharmacol Biochem Behav* (2017)164:99–105. doi: 10.1016/j.pbb.2017.02.003
7. Kovács I, Richman MJ, Janka Z, Maraz A, Andó B. Decision making measured by the Iowa gambling task in alcohol use disorder and gambling disorder: a systematic review and meta-analysis. *Drug Alcohol Depend* (2017) 181:152–61. doi: 10.1016/j.drugalcdep.2017.09.023
8. Lawrence AJ, Luty J, Bogdan NA, Sahakian BJ, Clark L. Problem gamblers share deficits in impulsive decision-making with alcohol-dependent individuals. *Addiction* (2009) 104(6):1006–15. doi: 10.1111/j.1360-0443.2009.02533.x
9. Kräplin A, Dshemuchadse M, Behrendt S, Scherbaum S, Goschke T, Bühringer G. Dysfunctional decision-making in pathological gambling: pattern specificity and the role of impulsivity. *Psychiatry Res* (2014b) 215(3):675–82. doi: 10.1016/j.psychres.2013.12.041
10. Brand M, Kalbe E, Labudda K, Fujiwara E, Kessler J, Markowitsch HJ. Decision-making impairments in patients with pathological gambling. *Psychiatry Res.* (2005) 133(1):91–9. doi: 10.1016/j.psychres.2004.10.003
11. Brevers D, Cleeremans A, Goudriaan AE, Bechara A, Kornreich C, Verbanck P, et al. Decision making under ambiguity but not under risk is related to problem gambling severity. *Psychiatry Res* (2012) 200(2):568–74. doi: 10.1016/j.psychres.2012.03.053
12. Verdejo-García A, Lawrence AJ, Clark L. Impulsivity as a vulnerability marker for substance-use disorders: review of findings from high-risk research, problem gamblers and genetic association studies. *Neurosci Biobehav Rev* (2008) 32(4):777–810. doi: 10.1016/j.neubiorev.2007.11.003
13. Chowdhury NS, Livesey EJ, Blaszczynski A, Harris JA. Pathological gambling and motor impulsivity: a systematic review with meta-analysis. *J Gambl Stud* (2017) 33(4):1213–39. doi: 10.1007/s10899-017-9683-5
14. Petry NM. Pathological gamblers, with and without substance abuse disorders, discount delayed rewards at high rates. *J Abnorm Psychol* (2001) 110(3):482. doi: 10.1037//0021-843X.110.3.482
15. Dixon MR, Marley J, Jacobs EA. Delay discounting by pathological gamblers. *J Appl Behav Anal* (2003) 36(4):449–58. doi: 10.1901/jaba.2003.36-449
16. Michalczuk R, Bowden-Jones H, Verdejo-Garcia A, Clark L. Impulsivity and cognitive distortions in pathological gamblers attending the UK National Problem Gambling Clinic: a preliminary report. Psychol Med (2011) 41(12):2625–35.
17. Goudriaan AE, Oosterlaan J, De Beurs E, Van Den Brink W. Neurocognitive functions in pathological gambling: a comparison with alcohol dependence, Tourette syndrome and normal controls. *Addiction* (2006) 101(4):534–47. doi: 10.1111/j.1360-0443.2006.01380.x
18. Fuentes D, Tavares H, Artes R, Gorenstein C. Self-reported and neuropsychological measures of impulsivity in pathological gambling. *J Int Neuropsychol Soc* (2006) 12(06):907–12. doi: 10.1017/S1355617706061091
19. Kertzman S, Lowengrub K, Aizer A, Nahum ZB, Kotler M, Dannon PN. Stroop performance in pathological gamblers. *Psychiatry Res* (2006) 142(1): 1-10. doi: 10.1016/j.psychres.2005.07.027
20. Van Timmeren T, Daams JG, Van Holst RJ, Goudriaan AE. Compulsivity-related neurocognitive performance deficits in gambling disorder: a systematic review and meta-analysis. *Neurosci Biobehav Rev* (2018) 84:204– 17. doi: 10.1016/j.neubiorev.2017.11.022
21. Boog M, Höppener P, Goudriaan AE, Boog MC, Franken IH. Cognitive inflexibility in gamblers is primarily present in reward-related decision making. *Front Hum Neurosci* (2014) 8:569. doi: 10.3389/fnhum.2014.00569
22. Billieux J, Lagrange G, Van der Linden M, Lançon C, Adida M, Jeanningros R. Investigation of impulsivity in a sample of treatment-seeking pathological gamblers: a multidimensional perspective. *Psychiatry Res* (2012) 198(2):291–6. doi: 10.1016/j.psychres.2012.01.001
23. Kräplin A, Bühringer G, Oosterlaan J, Van Den Brink W, Goschke T, Goudriaan AE. Dimensions and disorder specificity of impulsivity in pathological gambling. *Addict Behav* (2014a) 39(11):1646–51. doi: 10.1016/j.addbeh.2014.05.021
24. Blaszczynski A, Nower L. A pathways model of problem and pathological gambling. *Addiction* (2002) 97(5):487–99. doi: 10.1046/j.1360-0443.2002.00015.x
25. Ledgerwood DM, Petry NM. Subtyping pathological gamblers based on impulsivity, depression, and anxiety. *Psychol Addict Behav* (2010) 24(4):680. doi: 10.1037/a0019906
26. Jiménez-Murcia S, Granero R, Stinchfield R, Fernández-Aranda F, Penelo E, Savvidou LG, et al. Typologies of young pathological gamblers based on sociodemographic and clinical characteristics. *Compr Psychiatry* (2013) 54(8):1153–60. doi: 10.1016/j.comppsych.2013.05.017
27. Croson R, Fishman P, Pope DG. Poker superstars: Skill or luck? Similarities between golf—thought to be a game of skill—and poker. Chance (2008) 21(4):25–8.
28. Bonnaire C, Kovess-Masfety V, Guignard R, Richard JB, du Roscoät E, Beck F. Gambling type, substance abuse, health and psychosocial correlates of male and female problem gamblers in a nationally representative French sample. *J Gambl Stud* (2017) 33(2):343–69. doi: 10.1007/s10899-016-9628-4
29. Odlaug BL, Marsh PJ, Kim SW, Grant JE. Strategic vs nonstrategic gambling: characteristics of pathological gamblers based on gambling preference. *Ann Clin Psychiatry* (2011) 23(2):105.
30. Potenza MN, Steinberg MA, McLaughlin SD, Wu R, Rounsaville BJ, O'Malley SS. Gender-related differences in the characteristics of problem gamblers using a gambling helpline. *Am J Psychiatr* (2001) 158(9):1500–5. doi: 10.1176/appi.ajp.158.9.1500
31. Moragas L, Granero R, Stinchfield R, Fernández-Aranda F, Fröberg F, Aymamí N, et al. Comparative analysis of distinct phenotypes in gambling disorder based on gambling preferences. *BMC Psychiatry* (2015) 15(1):86. doi: 10.1186/s12888-015-0459-0
32. Petry NM. A comparison of treatment-seeking pathological gamblers based on preferred gambling activity. *Addiction* (2003) 98(5):645–55. doi: 10.1046/j.1360-0443.2003.00336.x
33. Goudriaan AE, Oosterlaan J, de Beurs E, van den Brink W. Decision making in pathological gambling: a comparison between pathological gamblers, alcohol dependents, persons with Tourette syndrome, and normal controls. *Cogn Brain Res* (2005) 23(1):137–51. doi: 10.1016/j.cogbrainres.2005.01.017
34. Lorains FK, Dowling NA, Enticott PG, Bradshaw JL, Trueblood JS, Stout JC. Strategic and non-strategic problem gamblers differ on decision-making

under risk and ambiguity. *Addiction* (2014) 109(7):1128–37. doi: 10.1111/add.12494
35. Navas JF, Billieux J, Perandrés-Gómez A, López-Torrecillas F, Cándido A, Perales JC. Impulsivity traits and gambling cognitions associated with gambling preferences and clinical status. *International Gambling Studies* (2017) 17(1):102–24. doi: 10.1080/14459795.2016.1275739
36. Grant JE, Odlaug BL, Chamberlain SR, Schreiber L. Neurocognitive dysfunction in strategic and non-strategic gamblers. *Prog Neuropsychopharmacol Biol Psychiatry* (2012) 38(2):336–40. doi: 10.1016/j.pnpbp.2012.05.006
37. Orford J, Wardle H, Griffiths M. What proportion of gambling is problem gambling? Estimates from the 2010 British Gambling Prevalence Survey. Int Gambl Stud (2013) 13(1):4–18.
38. Ronzitti S, Soldini E, Lutri V, Smith N, Clerici M, Bowden-Jones H. Types of gambling and levels of harm: a UK study to assess severity of presentation in a treatment-seeking population. *J Behav Addict* (2016) 5(3):439–47. doi: 10.1556/2006.5.2016.068
39. Ronzitti S, Soldini E, Smith N, Bayston A, Clerici M, Bowden-Jones H. Are treatment outcomes determined by type of gambling? A UK Study. *J Gambl Stud* (2018) 34(3):987–97. doi: 10.1007/s10899-018-9752-4
40. Sharman S, Murphy R, Turner JJ, Roberts A. Trends and patterns in UK treatment seeking gamblers: 2000–2015. *Addict Behav* (2019) 89:51–6. doi: 10.1016/j.addbeh.2018.09.009
41. MacKillop J, Amlung MT, Few LR, Ray LA, Sweet LH, Munafò MR. Delayed reward discounting and addictive behavior: a meta-analysis. *Psychopharmacology* (2011) 216(3):305–21. doi: 10.1007/s00213-011-2229-0
42. Shaffer HJ, LaBrie R, Scanlan KM, Cummings TN. Pathological gambling among adolescents: Massachusetts gambling screen (MAGS). *J Gambl Stud* (1994) 10(4):339–62. doi: 10.1007/BF02104901
43. Ferris J, Wynne H. The Canadian problem gambling index. *Ottawa, ON: Canadian Centre on Substance Abuse.* (2001).
44. Heatherton TF, Kozlowski LT, Frecker RC, FAGERSTROM KO. The Fagerström test for nicotine dependence: a revision of the Fagerstrom Tolerance Questionnaire. *Br J Addict* (1991) 86(9):1119–27. doi: 10.1111/j.1360-0443.1991.tb01879.x
45. Nelson HE, Willison J. *National Adult Reading Test (NART).* Windsor: Nfer-Nelson (1991).
46. Wechsler D (1999). *Wechsler abbreviated scale of intelligence.* Psychological Corporation. doi: 10.1037/t15170-000
47. Kirby KN, Petry NM, Bickel WK. Heroin addicts have higher discount rates for delayed rewards than non-drug-using controls. *J Exp Psychol Gen* (1999) 128(1):78. doi: 10.1037//0096-3445.128.1.78
48. Rogers RD, Everitt BJ, Baldacchino A, Blackshaw AJ, Swainson R, Wynne K, et al. Dissociable deficits in the decision-making cognition of chronic amphetamine abusers, opiate abusers, patients with focal damage to prefrontal cortex, and tryptophan-depleted normal volunteers: evidence for monoaminergic mechanisms. *Neuropsychopharmacology* (1999) 20(4):322–39. doi: 10.1016/S0893-133X(98)00091-8
49. Logan GD (1994). On the ability to inhibit thought and action: a users' guide to the stop signal paradigm.
50. Swainson R, Rogers RD, Sahakian BJ, Summers BA, Polkey CE, Robbins TW. Probabilistic learning and reversal deficits in patients with Parkinson's disease or frontal or temporal lobe lesions: possible adverse effects of dopaminergic medication. *Neuropsychologia* (2000) 38(5):596–612. doi: 10.1016/S0028-3932(99)00103-7
51. Beck AT, Steer RA (1990). Manual for the Beck Anxiety Inventory.
52. Beck AT, Steer RA, Brown GK (1996). Beck Depression Inventory. The psychological corporation. *San Antonio, TX.* doi: 10.1037/t00742-000
53. Cyders MA, Smith GT, Spillane NS, Fischer S, Annus AM, Peterson C. Integration of impulsivity and positive mood to predict risky behavior: development and validation of a measure of positive urgency. *Psychol Assess* (2007) 19(1):107. doi: 10.1037/1040-3590.19.1.107
54. Raylu N, Oei TP. The Gambling Related Cognitions Scale (GRCS): Development, confirmatory factor validation and psychometric properties. *Addiction* (2004) 99(6):757–69. doi: 10.1111/j.1360-0443.2004.00753.x
55. Ayton P, Fischer I. The hot hand fallacy and the gambler's fallacy: two faces of subjective randomness? *Mem Cognit* (2004) 32(8):1369–78. doi: 10.3758/BF03206327
56. Kahneman D, Varey CA. Propensities and counterfactuals: the loser that almost won. *J Pers Soc Psychol* (1990) 59(6):1101. doi: 10.1037//0022-3514.59.6.1101
57. Holtgraves T, Skeel J. Cognitive biases in playing the lottery: estimating the odds and choosing the numbers. *J Appl Soc Psychol* (1992) 22(12):934–52. doi: 10.1111/j.1559-1816.1992.tb00935.x
58. Maniaci G, Picone F, Dimarco T, Lipari A, Brancato A, Cannizzaro C. Psychodiagnostic assessment of pathological gamblers: a focus on personality disorders, clinical syndromes and alexithymia. *Int J Ment Health Addict* (2015) 13(6):728–39. doi: 10.1007/s11469-015-9550-5
59. Griffiths MD. The role of cognitive bias and skill in fruit machine gambling. *Br J Psychol* (1994) 85(3):351–69. doi: 10.1111/j.2044-8295.1994.tb02529.x

11

Bias Toward Drug-Related Stimuli is Affected by Loading Working Memory in Abstinent Ex-Methamphetamine Users

*Zoha Deldar[1], Hamed Ekhtiari[1,2], Hamid Reza Pouretemad[3] and Ali Khatibi[4,5]**

[1] Institute for Cognitive Science Studies, Tehran, Iran, [2] Iranian National Center for Addiction Studies, Tehran University of Medical Sciences, Tehran, Iran, [3] Institute for Cognitive and Brain Sciences (ICBS), Shahid Beheshti University, Tehran, Iran, [4] Department of Neurology and Neurosurgery, McGill University, Montreal, QC, Canada, [5] Centre of Precision Rehabilitation for Spinal Pain (CPR Spine), School of Sport, Exercise and Rehabilitation Sciences, University of Birmingham, Birmingham, AL, United States

***Correspondence:**
Ali Khatibi
ali.khatibi@gmail.com

Background: There is a trade-off between drug-related impulsive process and cognitive reflective process among ex-drug abusers. The present study aimed to investigate the impulsive effects of methamphetamine-related stimuli on working memory (WM) performance by manipulating WM load in abstinent ex-methamphetamine users.

Methods: Thirty abstinent ex-methamphetamine users and 30 nonaddict matched control participants were recruited in this study. We used a modified Sternberg task in which participants were instructed to memorize three different sets of methamphetamine-related and non–drug-related words (three, five, or seven words) while performing a secondary attention-demanding task as an interference.

Results: Repeated-measures ANOVA revealed that reaction times of abstinent ex-methamphetamine users increased during low WM load (three words) compared to the control group ($p = 0.01$). No significant differences were observed during high WM loads (five or seven words) (both p's > 0.1). Besides, reaction times of the experimental group during trials with high interference (three, five, or seven words) were not significantly different compared to the control group ($p > 0.2$).

Conclusion: These findings imply that increasing WM load may provide an efficient buffer against attentional capture by salient stimuli (i.e., methamphetamine-related words). This buffer might modify the effect of interference bias. Besides, presenting methamphetamine-related stimuli might facilitate the encoding phase due to bias toward task-relevant stimuli. This finding has an important implication, suggesting that performing concurrent demanding tasks may reduce the power of salient stimuli and thus improve the efficiency of emotional regulation strategies.

Keywords: addiction, dual-process models, working memory bias, working memory interference bias, working memory capacity, abstinent ex-methamphetamine users

INTRODUCTION

Methamphetamine, which is an extremely addictive neurotoxic drug, is the second most used illegal drug after cannabis (1). Prevalence of methamphetamine abuse is 1.2 million people in the United States and 17.2 million people around the world (2). Chronic use of methamphetamine has been associated with multiple physical health problems (e.g., cardiovascular disease), mental health problems (e.g., depression) (3–5), and daily functioning problems (e.g., impulsivity) (6, 7), which can also affect the brain and neurocognitive functions (8–10).

Addiction to methamphetamine—similar to addiction to other substances—is often resistant to conventional interventions (11). Therefore, a critical need exists to address additional and appropriate interventions such as nonpharmacological approaches. In line with this, theoretical models and empirical evidence support a role for the modulation of addiction with cognitive-based approaches (11–17). For example, dual-process models of addiction suggest that addictive behaviors are affected by the dominance of drug-related impulsive processes over the reflective processes (13, 18, 19). Several studies have shown that the drug-related impulsive process is spontaneous, fast, and relatively unconscious, while the reflective process is deliberate, slow, and conscious (13, 18, 19).

There is a trade-off between the drug-related impulsive process and reflective process (11, 13, 15). The drug-related impulsive process is affected by the repeated abuse of drugs (20). Impulsive behaviors in addiction are referred to as behaviors that are associated with selecting an immediate reward, making risky decisions (21), generating memory impairment (22), and showing bias toward salient drug stimuli (12, 23, 24). For example, methamphetamine-related stimuli can involuntarily catch the attention of methamphetamine users (i.e., attentional bias). Attentional bias toward methamphetamine-related stimuli can increase the effect of subjective craving, which may contribute to relapse (25, 26). However, the drug-related impulsive process can be modulated by the reflective system (14, 26). Working memory (WM), which is considered as the main part of the reflective process, can modulate the drug-related impulsive process (14, 26, 27). WM is a temporary storage system that can actively maintain information and manipulate stored information (28). WM is involved in the modulation of the processing of irrelevant information by attentional mechanisms (i.e., the reflective process) (29). However, WM processes can negatively be influenced by emotionally salient stimuli like those related to drugs (18). As a result, the bias toward emotionally salient stimuli can lead to deficits in WM performance (18). Therefore, it is important to understand how WM can modulate the attention given to methamphetamine-related stimuli and vice versa.

Given that WM performance might be impaired in methamphetamine users (10, 30) and in abstinent methamphetamine users, it is plausible that the ability to apply attentional control over methamphetamine-related stimuli is reduced as a result of impaired WM performance. For example, a systematic review on methamphetamine use and cognitive function reported that cognitive domains (e.g., WM performance, attention, cognitive flexibility, inhibitory control, decision making) in methamphetamine users were decreased compared to the control group (31). This reduced cognitive performance was associated with deficits in the brain measures, including lower metabolism, gray matter density, fractional anisotropy, and activation (31). For example, the study of abstinent methamphetamine users showed that WM performance (during a one-back cued response, one- back, two-back, and one-increment tasks) is decreased in abstinent methamphetamine users compared to control group (32). In this study, abstinent methamphetamine users showed increased brain activity in left occipital and right posterior parietal lobe compared to control group, while they showed decreased activity in bilateral putamen/insular cortex and right lateral compared to control group (32). Another study showed a correlation between performance on the delayed recall and increased metabolism in the thalamus in abstinent methamphetamine users compared to the control group (33). Another study also reported a correlation between performance on the word-recall task and hippocampal volume, which was smaller in the abstinent methamphetamine users than in the control group (34). These studies have indicated a decreased cognitive function in methamphetamine users in several domains, including WM performance (31).

Effective cognitive control over addiction encompasses more than simply disengaging attention from methamphetamine stimuli; it is also necessary to maintain attention toward nonmethamphetamine information (14, 35). WM allows us to maintain and prioritize relevant information in the face of irrelevant information (28). Evidence supported the role of WM, and the corresponding processes, in the control of attention (29). To understand effective cognitive control over addiction to methamphetamine, we first need to know the trade-off between the top-down effect of WM in attentional control (reflective process) over methamphetamine-related stimuli and the bottom-up effect of attentional bias in WM (impulsive process) (18).

Studies revealed that automatic attentional mechanisms (i.e., impulsive processes) are not independent of the available processing resources (29, 36). However, investigating the effect of WM capacity (i.e. the ability to actively store information despite ongoing processing, which is an indicator of limited cognitive resources) on the interaction between the reflective process and drug-related impulsive processes is a missing piece in the literature (37–43). Many studies have examined the effect of attentional bias in drug-dependent populations versus control groups (23–24, 25, 44–47). However, according to our knowledge, no study to date has investigated the interactive effect of both bias and WM capacity in abstinent ex-methamphetamine users versus a control group. Therefore, the current study investigated the effect of bias and load on WM maintenance in different ways: first, by showing drug-related words, which are task-relevant stimuli that can facilitate the encoding process; next, by applying an interference task, which can disturb the process of rehearsal and needs to be inhibited; and finally, by increasing WM loads, which can result in greater rehearsal demands. Investigating the effect of these WM manipulations independently in combination with WM load can help determine factors that might contribute

Abbreviations: WM, Working Memory; RTs, Reaction Times.

to dual-process models of methamphetamine addiction and may lead to the development of effective assessment tools and interventions.

METHODS

Ethics Approval

All experimental procedures corresponded to the standards set by the latest revision of the Declaration of Helsinki and were approved by the ethical committee of the Institute for Cognitive Sciences Studies, Tehran, Iran. All participants provided written informed consent, acknowledging their right to withdraw from the experiment without prejudice.

Showing methamphetamine cues to participants may increase the possibility of relapse. Concerning this important ethical issue, we used methamphetamine-related words instead of real substances. In addition, participants were monitored in the following weeks for any signs of drug craving, and they also had access to psychological interventions to manage potential drug cravings.

Participants

Thirty abstinent ex-methamphetamine users (all men, 20–47 years old, experimental group) and 30 participants without a history of addiction or drug abuse (all men, 20–50 years old, control group) were recruited in the current study (**Table 1**). The experimental group was recruited from former methamphetamine-dependent users who were admitted to Vardij Abstinence-Based Residential Centre, Karaj, Iran. This treatment center specializes in amphetamine-type stimulant dependence and is located in a rural area near Tehran—a part of the therapeutic network belonging to Rebirth Society Organization (a nonprofit charity). The abstinent ex-methamphetamine users in this center were relatively homogeneous, and only men were admitted. Participants in the control group (all males) were recruited from employees of Shahid Beheshti University, Tehran, Iran. They reported no history of drug abuse. Both groups were right-handed and were matched for age (20–50 years) and educational level (<12 years of school. Inclusion criteria for the experimental group included having a history of methamphetamine abuse in the past 12 months prior to entering the treatment center (methamphetamine dependence based on *Diagnostic and Statistical Manual of Mental Disorders, Fifth Edition* criteria). The most common mean of drug administration was smoking. Subjects had to be abstinent from any drugs except cigarettes for at least a week before the experiment, with confirmation by urine testing.

TABLE 1 | Demographic and substance abuse characteristics.

Descriptive	Experimental group	Control group
Gender (men)	30	30
Age (years)	31.5 ± 1.22	28.07± 1.42
Education (years)	11.97 ± 0.47	12.78 ± 0.5
Duration of meth abstinence (day)	17.26 ± 1.43	–
Duration of meth dependence (months)	45.2 ± 4.87	–

Values are reported as mean ± SEM.

Exclusion criteria for both the experimental group and the control group included any current or past major clinical neurological disorders, central nervous system–effective medication intake, or any major clinical psychiatric disorders (in Axis I, except substance-related disorders). We excluded data of two participants from the experimental group and data of two participants from the control group because of their inaccurate responses to the cognitive task.

The Modified Sternberg Task With Interference

To test WM performance of participants, we adopted a modified Sternberg task with interference. The task was designed with MATLAB (The MathWorks, Inc., Natick, MA, United States) and used the Psychtoolbox ran on a Microsoft Windows 7 operating system. The modified Sternberg task fits in the category of a complex span task. It consisted of three steps: memorizing a list of words (encoding step), performing a secondary task (as an interference step), and selecting the memorized word among presented words (retrieval step). In order to obtain different levels of WM load, the Sternberg task included a list of either three, five, or seven words (**Figure 1**) (19).

We selected a list of words, that were validated in a previous study based on their mean of craving and emotional valence (49). This list consisted of 24 Persian words: 12 were selected randomly from a list of methamphetamine-related words (i.e., experimental; ex: methamphetamine, drugs), and 12 were selected randomly from a list of non-drug-related words (i.e., neutral; ex: scissors, carriage). All words had two syllables with a maximum of four letters. They were presented with the same font in white color on a black background screen.

Proceeding of the Modified Sternberg Task With Interference

The first step (i.e., WM set) consisted of the presentation of a list of three, five, or seven words (encoding step). Participants had to memorize the presented word list. Words were presented randomly according to methamphetamine-related or non-drug-related content. For example, in the 3-word memory set, there were either two methamphetamine-related words and one non-drug-related word or vice versa. In the 5-word WM set, there were either three methamphetamine-related words and two non-drug-related words or three non-drug-related stimuli and two methamphetamine-related words. Each word was presented for 750 ms with an interstimulus interval of 500 ms. Two fixation crosses (++) were presented in the center of the screen to signal the end of this step (**Figure 1**, left panel).

The second step consisted of a secondary task (as an interference step). In this step, four words were presented one after the other. Two of these four words were methamphetamine-related words, and two were non-drug-related. These words were new and different from the words used in the memory set step. Each word was presented for 500 ms, after which time the font

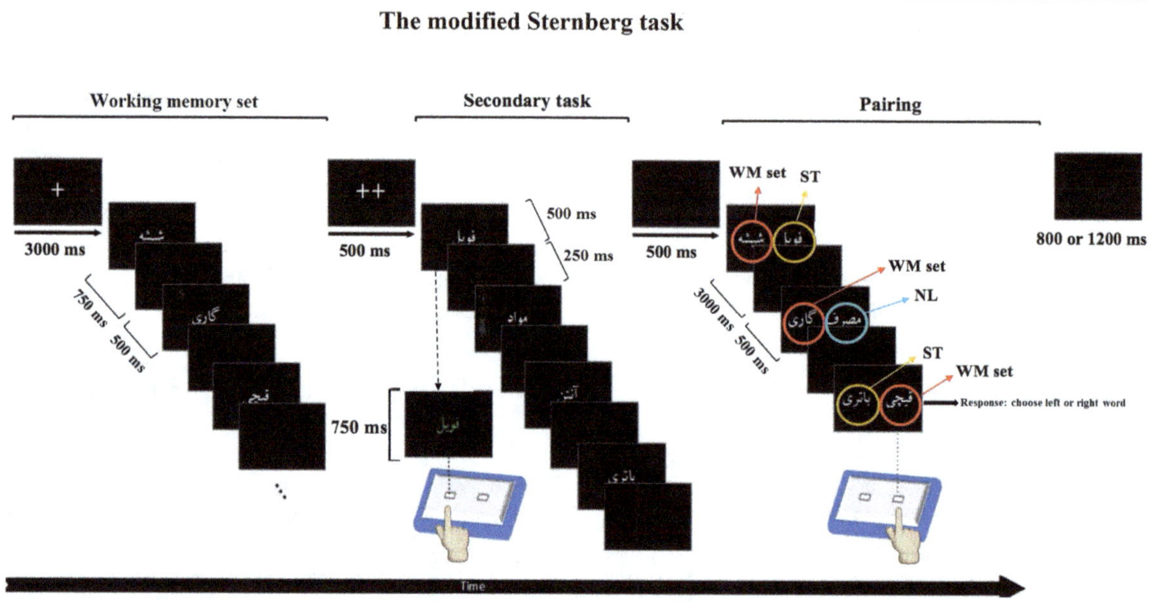

FIGURE 1 | Modified Sternberg task with interference.This Figure is an example of one trial with different responses at different steps of the modified Sternberg task with interference. The modified Sternberg task with interference consisted of three steps. The first step shows a working memory set with three Persian words, out of which one is a methamphetamine-related word (e.g., methamphetamine) and two are non–drug-related words (e.g., cart and scissors). This step is considered as an encoding step. The second step illustrates the secondary task in which the color of the words can change to green or blue (interference step). Subjects have to respond to the color of the word by pressing the corresponding button on the response box (e.g., left for green, right for blue). During the last step, called the pairing step, the participants have to choose the correct word from the working memory set by using the response box (according to their position on the screen; recall step). Numbers represent the display time of the words on the screen (Figure is modified from (48).

color was changed randomly to either blue or green (750 ms). Participants were asked to indicate which font color was used for the words by pressing the corresponding button on the response box (left button for green, right for blue). After the participant's response, a black slide was presented for 250 ms, and the next word appeared. One-third of the trials were null; instead of word stimuli, an empty black screen was presented. The total duration of the secondary task was 6 seconds (**Figure 1**, middle panel).

In the third step (i.e., pairing step), each word from the first step was presented once along with a word from the secondary task (ST trial) or a novel list (NL) of methamphetamine-related and non–drug-related words, which had not been presented in that trial, for 3,000 ms. The participant's task was to choose the word that was presented in the memory set by pressing the corresponding key on the response box (i.e., right button for the word on the right side of the screen, and left button for the word on the left) as fast and as accurate as possible. After the presentation of each pair and response by the participant, the screen was replaced by a black slide for 500 ms, and the next pair appeared on the screen. After all words from the memory set were presented, a single fixation cross was presented in the center of the screen, and the next trial was started. The intertrial time interval was set to be between 800 and 1,200 ms (**Figure 1**, right panel). This pairing step is referred to as retrieval step. A black screen was presented for 500 ms after each probe. At the end of the three probes, a black screen was presented randomly for 800 or 1,200 ms (**Figure 1**, right panel).

Second words (i.e., incorrect words) during the pairing step were selected randomly considering the following restrictions: at least one methamphetamine-related word and one non–drug-related word were required to be among the words. Second words in each probe had a 50% chance of being randomly selected from the ST step of its respective trial (i.e., high interference trials). The remaining second words were again randomly selected among methamphetamine-related and non–drug-related words (NL) not previously presented in its respective trial (i.e., low interference trials).

Regarding the mentioned rules for the presentation of both words, the display in the pairing step included the situations as below:

(A) methamphetamine-related words (WM set) + methamphetamine-related words (ST);
(B) methamphetamine-related words (WM set) + methamphetamine-related words (NL);
(C) methamphetamine-related words (WM set) + non–drug-related words (ST);
(D) methamphetamine-related words (WM set) + non–drug-related words (NL);
(E) non–drug-related words (WM set) + methamphetamine-related words (ST);
(F) non–drug-related words (WM set) + methamphetamine-related words (NL);
(G) non–drug-related words (WM set) + non–drug-related words (ST);
(H) non–drug-related words (WM set) + non–drug-related words (NL).

Experimental Procedure

All subjects participated in one session. The experimental procedure was explained clearly to them at the beginning of the session. Basic demographic information, drug abuse, treatment history, and high-risk behaviors of each subject were recorded during a structured interview by an expert drug counselor. After signing the consent form, participants sat in front of a 13-inch laptop screen at a 60-cm viewing distance in a room with dimmed light to increase their focus on the screen.

The experimental procedure had two different phases: a training phase and a test phase. The goal of the training phase was to learn how to perform the Sternberg task. The training task was designed similarly to the main one, but with different words compared to the main experiment (all of them non–drug-related). After it was sure that participants knew how to perform the task, they proceeded to the testing phase.

Overall, participants performed three conditions, including a condition of three WM words consisting of 72 trials, a condition of five WM words also consisting of 72 trials, and a condition of seven WM words consisting of 72 trials (**Figure 1**). All 24 words appeared equally in the probe; they were also paired with second words (incorrect words) in all types of pairings (i.e., methamphetamine-related words, non–drug-related words, and non–drug-related words from the NL). Each of the 24 words was repeated 27 times during 72 trials. The sequence of words was counterbalanced between participants.

Statistical Analysis

Data analysis was conducted using SPSS 21 and Statistica v13 (Dell Inc., Tulsa, OK, USA). All results are expressed as the mean ± standard error of the mean, and the statistical threshold was set to $p \leq 0.05$. A priori hypotheses were tested with *post hoc* analysis (Tukey test) and planned contrasts. The data from trials with null stimuli were excluded from all statistical tests. To analyze the reaction time (RT), trials with incorrect responses were excluded from relevant statistical tests.

Bias Caused by Difference Sources

Potential bias, caused by the methamphetamine-related words on the performance of experimental participants, was from different sources and should be separated in the current task paradigm.

i. The first bias we considered was the summation of WM interference bias and WM bias during different WM loads (three, five, or seven words). This score was defined as 1/2 * (RT (E − G) + RT (F − H) + RT (G − C) + RT (H − D)). Repeated-measures ANOVA was used to calculate this first bias: the three first bias scores during the different WM loads (three, five, or seven words) were considered as a within-subject factor, and subject group (experimental, control) was considered as the between-subject factor.
ii. The second bias we referred to was the WM interference bias. This score was defined as (RT(E) + RT(F))/2 − (RT(G) + RT(H)/2. Repeated-measures ANOVA tests were used to obtain this second score; three second bias scores during the different WM loads (three, five, or seven words) were considered as a within-subject factor, and subject group (experimental, control) was considered as the between-subject factor.
iii. The third bias we referred to was the WM bias. This score was defined as (RT(G) + RT(H)/2 − (RT(C) + RT(D))/2. Repeated-measures ANOVA tests were used in order to calculate this score: three third bias scores during the different WM loads (three, five, or seven words) were considered as a within-subject factor, and subject group (experimental, control) was considered as the between-subject factor.

The Effect of Different WM Loads on the Performance of Participants During High Interference Trials

The performance of participants during high interference trials (i.e. the high interference effect caused by the words from the secondary task) was measured during different WM loads (three, five, or seven words). High interference trials included trials from A, C, E, and G conditions. To test the effect of presenting different WM loads (three, five, or seven words) on the performance of participants, two separate repeated-measures ANOVA tests were performed on RTs and accuracy of participants during high interference trials. In this analysis, RTs and accuracy during different WM loads (three, five, or seven words) were considered as a within-subject factor, and subject group (experimental, control) was considered as the between-subject factor.

RESULTS

Bias Caused by Difference Sources

The First Bias

Repeated-measures ANOVA test showed a significant interaction effect between WM load and subject group on the first bias of RTs ($F(2, 116) = 3.76$, $p = 0.02$). Planned contrasts analysis revealed that mean scores for the first bias RTs of the methamphetamine user group significantly increased during the performance of the 3-word WM compared to the control group ($p = 0.01$). However, no significant difference was observed in mean RTs during the 5- and 7-word WM sets (both p's > 0.1) (**Figure 2**).

Planned comparisons based on our priory hypothesis revealed that mean scores for the first bias RTs of the control group were significantly increased during the performance of the 3-word WM set compared to the 5- and 7-word memory sets (both p's < 0.001). However, no significant difference was observed in mean scores for the first bias RTs of the control group when comparing the 5-word WM sets to the 7-word sets ($p > 0.2$). Additionally, no significant difference was observed in mean scores for the first bias RTs of the experimental group during the 3-word WM set compared to the 5- and 7-word memory sets (p's > 0.2) (**Figure 2**).

The Second Bias

Repeated-measures ANOVA test showed no significant interaction effect between WM load and subject group on the second bias of RTs of the experimental group compared to the control group ($F(2, 116) = 1.97$, $p = 0.14$). Planned comparisons

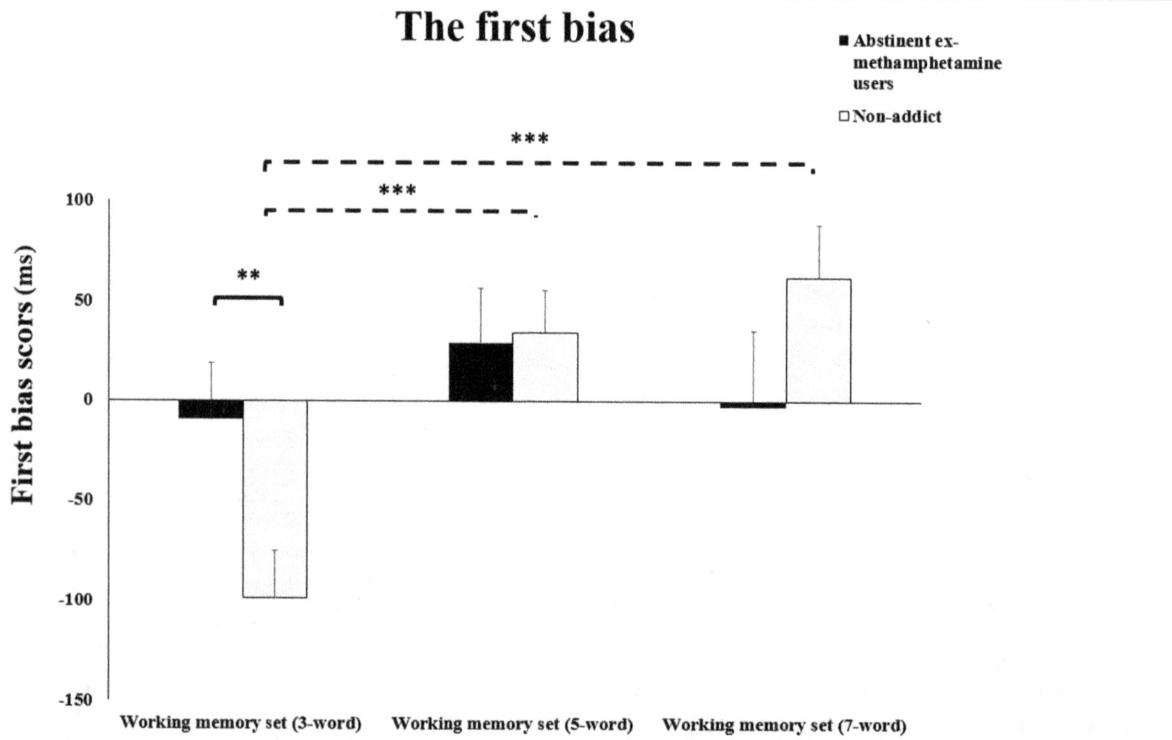

FIGURE 2 | The first bias.The summation of reaction times of working memory interference bias and working memory bias during different working memory loads (three, five, or seven words). Error bars indicate standard error of the mean $^{**}p \le 0.01$; $^{***}p \le 0.01$.

based on our priory hypothesis revealed that mean scores for the second bias RTs of the control group were not significantly changed during the performance of the 3-word WM set compared to the 5- and 7-word memory sets (both *p*'s > 0.2). No significant difference was observed in mean scores for the second bias RTs of the control group when comparing the 5-word WM sets to the 7-word sets (*p* > 0.2). Additionally, mean scores for the second bias RTs of the experimental group were not significantly changed during the performance of the 3-word WM set compared to the 5- and 7-word memory sets (both *p*'s > 0.1). No significant difference was observed in mean scores for the second bias RTs of the experimental group when comparing the 5-word WM sets to the 7-word sets (*p* > 0.05).

The Third Bias

Repeated-measures ANOVA test showed no significant interaction effect between WM load and subject group on the third bias RTs of the experimental group compared to the control group ($F(2, 116) = 0.81$, $p = 0.44$). Planned contrasts analysis revealed that mean scores for the third bias RTs of the control group were not significantly changed during the performance of the 3-word WM set compared to the 5- and 7-word memory sets (both *p*'s > 0.1). No significant difference was observed in mean scores for the third bias RTs of the control group when comparing the 5-word WM sets to the 7-word sets (*p* > 0.2). Additionally, mean scores for the third bias RTs of the experimental group were not significantly changed during the performance of the 3-word WM set compared to the 5- and 7-word memory sets (both *p*'s > 0.2). No significant difference was observed in mean scores for the second bias RTs of the experimental group when comparing the 5-word WM sets to the 7-word sets (*p* > 0.05).

The Effect of Different WM Loads on the Performance of Participants During High Interference Trials

Reaction Times During Trials With High Interference

Repeated-measures ANOVA test showed no significant interaction effects between WM load and subject group on the RT of high interference condition ($F(2, 116) = 0.47$, $p = 0.62$). However, priori hypotheses were tested with planned contrasts, and the type I error rate was controlled for using the Bonferroni correction for multiple comparisons. Planned contrasts analysis revealed that the mean RTs of the methamphetamine user group significantly decreased during the performance of the 3-word WM set compared to performing the 5- and 7-word WM sets (*p*'s < 0.001). However, no significant difference was observed in mean RTs during the 5-word WM set compared to mean RTs when performing the 7-word WM sets (*p* > 0.2). The same results were also found in the control group. Mean RTs of the control group during performance of the 3-word WM set compared to the 5- and 7-word memory sets were significantly decreased (*p*'s < 0.001), but no significant difference was observed in mean RTs when comparing the 5-word WM sets to the 7-word sets (*p* > 0.2) (**Figure 3**).

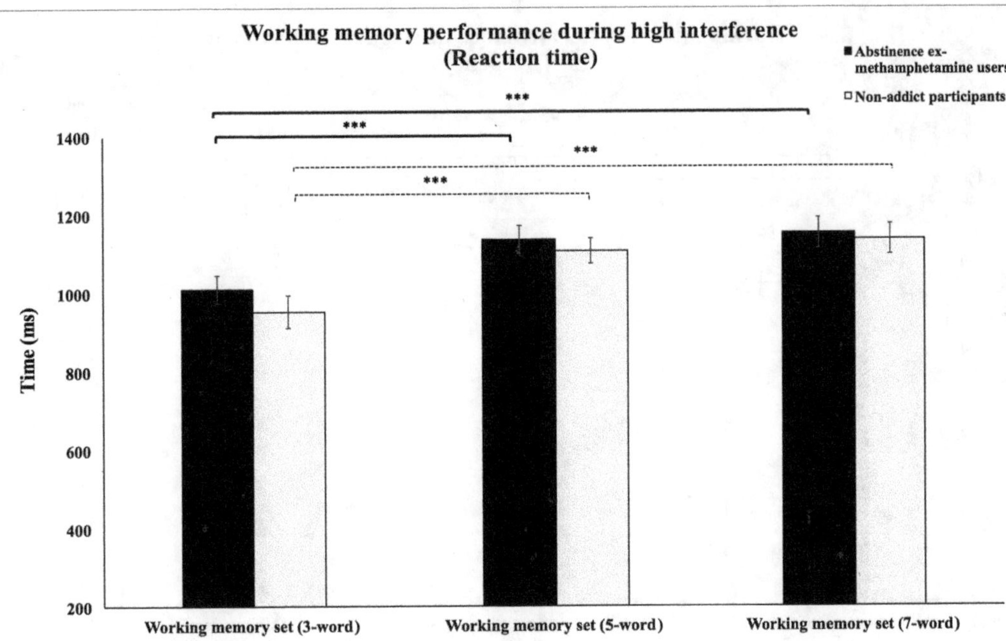

FIGURE 3 | Working memory performance during high interference (reaction times).Mean reaction times of abstinent ex-methamphetamine users and nonaddict control group for the recognition of words from the 3-word working memory sets were compared to the 5- and 7-word working memory sets during trials with high interference. Error bars indicate standard error of the mean ***$p \leq 0.001$.

Accuracy During Trials With High Interference

Repeated-measures ANOVA test showed no significant interaction effects between WM load and subject group on the accuracy of high interference condition ($F(2, 116) = 2.91$, $p = 0.058$). However, priori hypotheses were tested with planned contrasts, and the type I error rate was controlled for using the Bonferroni correction for multiple comparisons. Planned contrasts analysis revealed that the mean accuracy of the methamphetamine user group significantly increased during the performance of the 3-word WM set compared to performing the 5- and 7-word WM sets (p's < 0.001). However, no significant difference was observed in mean accuracy during the 5-word WM set compared to mean accuracy when performing the 7-word WM sets ($p > 0.2$). Mean accuracy of the control group during performance of the 3-word WM set compared to the 5- and 7-word memory sets was significantly increased (p's < 0.001). Besides, mean accuracy was significantly increased when comparing the 5-word WM sets to the 7-word sets ($p = 0.03$) (**Figure 4**).

Demographic information is summarized in **Table 1**.

DISCUSSION

The novel finding of the current study is that abstinent ex-methamphetamine users compared to a nonaddict group showed a bias toward methamphetamine-related stimuli only in in low WM load conditions (3-word WM sets). These results suggest that increasing the load of WM might reduce the effect of interference. In addition, there was no statistically significant difference in WM performance between all three WM load conditions during trials with high interference between both groups. These findings suggest that increasing the load of WM shields the effect of interference. Besides, attentional bias toward methamphetamine-related stimuli, which were presented during the encoding phase of WM, may contribute to optimal WM performance and may increase the availability of the shared cognitive resources.

Bias Caused by Difference Sources

The First Bias

The results showed that abstinent ex-methamphetamine users showed a bias (i.e., the summation of WM interference bias and WM bias) during low WM load (three words) task performance but not during high load WM (five and seven words) compared to the nonaddict group. The impulsive process may trigger cognitive biases such as attentional bias for drug-related stimuli (14, 15, 18). Studies showed that the use of drugs develops a specific reward system in the brain by releasing dopamine in mesolimbic brain areas, which in turn enhance learning by conditioning (26, 50–52). Attentional bias toward drug-related stimuli results in prolonging the disengagement of attention from those stimuli, leading to increased RTs (20, 51, 53). However, following the views that WM protects bias toward distractors, we expected to find a modulation over distraction (i.e. methamphetamine words) under higher WM loads (29).

The Second and Third Bias

Results from the current study showed no significant differences between groups for the second and third biases (i.e., WM

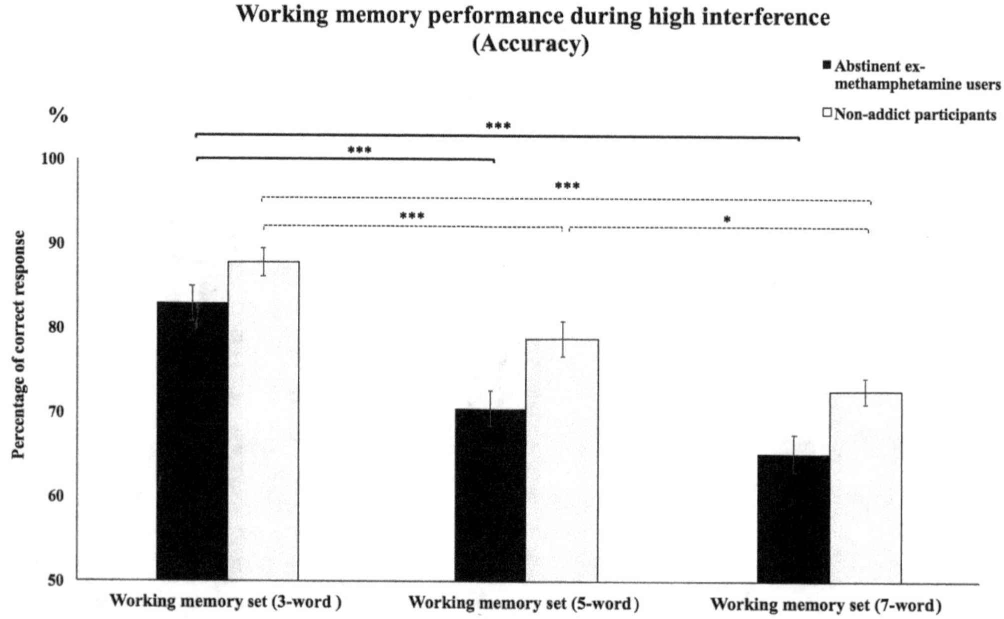

FIGURE 4 | Working memory performance during high interference (accuracy).Mean accuracy of abstinent ex-methamphetamine users and nonaddict control group in recognition of words from the 3-word working memory sets was compared to the five- and seven-word working memory sets during trials with high interference. Error bars indicate standard error of the mean ***$p \leq 0.001$ and *$p \leq 0.05$.

interference bias, WM bias). These results can best be considered with some possible explanations:

i. Abstinent ex-methamphetamine users are probably motivated to quit or stay abstain from drugs (54, 55). This motivation leads individuals to develop avoidance strategies to cope with tempting stimuli, which meanwhile might be effortful for them (54, 56). For example, heavy alcohol drinkers showed an attentional bias toward alcohol-related stimuli, while abstaining alcohol-dependent individuals avoided such stimuli (24, 57, 2, 55). Besides, studies have also indicated that presenting drug-related stimuli long enough (e.g., 500 ms) can give patients enough time to use efficient avoidance strategies; therefore, the effect of attentional bias might be reversed and away from drug-related stimuli (24, 57).
ii. The cognitive effort, which has been closely coupled with concepts of attention, difficulty in concentration, and motivation, can also explain current results (58). Cognitive effort can modulate the cognitive resources dedicated to a particular task (59). Indeed, to accomplish more demanding tasks, we have to exert more effort, which leads to a reduced effect of distractors (59, 60). Although we did not measure cognitive effort during the task, abstinent ex-methamphetamine users might invest more effort to perform WM task.
iii. Drug-related stimuli might elicit an attentional bias toward those stimuli, resulting in an interruption in the performance during the ongoing task. However, it is also possible that drug-related stimuli can elicit a motor response to provide fast and necessary reactions, resulting in avoiding the effect of distractions (61, 62). Besides, according to the literature on anxiety, the shorter RTs for threat stimuli in threat-neutral pairs could indicate an attentional bias away from the threat (61–63). Therefore, it is postulated that salient methamphetamine-related stimuli might lead to increased anxiety, resulting in quicker responses.
iv. The reflective process can moderate the impact of the impulsive process by emphasizing the effect of WM capacity (top-down process) (14, 17, 18, 64–67). For example, studies have supported the moderating effect of WM capacity on alcohol abuse (27, 64). These results indicated that individuals with a lower WM capacity show strong correlations between implicit alcohol associations and the use of alcohol (14, 27, 64). Although traditional models of impulse control have emphasized the adverse effect of increasing cognitive load on self-regulation, emotion-related studies have supported the idea that increased cognitive load can inhibit feelings of temptation (68–71). Regarding this issue, attention toward an emotional target is automatic (i.e., fast and involuntary), but it is also resource-dependent (71–73). It means that an increased cognitive load may lead to a decrease in the motivation to process task-irrelevant stimuli despite their saliency and associated feelings of temptation (71, 74). For example, categorizing the gender of angry faces compared to happy faces—as an index of selective attention to threatening information—was slower during the mental rehearsal of a one-digit number (low cognitive load) compared to the rehearsal of an eight-digit number (high cognitive load) (74). The bottom line is that there is bias variability in the addiction literature, which makes the basic mechanisms still unclear, but this bias might reflect variations in top-down cognitive control (47, 62, 75). In addition to the emotion-related

studies, the WM theory proposed by Andrade et al. (76) also supports the current findings. This theory suggested that retrieving information from WM requires WM capacity, but if the capacity of WM (resource) is occupied during memory reactivation, the emotionality and saliency of new information will be decreased, which will result in updating that information into a less emotional form (67). For example, studies have shown that using a high WM load task (visual-spatial task) during the retrieval of drug-related information could decrease cigarette (77) and food cravings (67, 78).

In summary, studies have indicated that WM and attention processes recruit similar neural networks and share common cognitive resources (79–81). In our case, attentional bias to the methamphetamine-related stimuli, particularly during high WM loads, may bring gain in WM performance (particularly during the encoding phase) and may increase the availability of cognitive resources. The result of the first bias during a task with low WM load indicated that attention was directed toward salient methamphetamine-related stimuli. On the other hand, performing tasks with high WM loads inhibited the effect of bias in abstinent ex-methamphetamine users. Regarding the results of the second and third bias considered, we suggest that presenting methamphetamine-related stimuli and increasing loads of WM were helpful for the experimental group to inhibit the effect of interference. In line with the dual-process models of addiction, which is focused on the trade-off between impulsive and reflective processes, these findings suggest that WM engagement and increased WM load improved avoidance strategy, possibly through reflective processes (71).

The Effect of Different WM Loads on the Performance of Participants During High Interference Trials

Our findings showed that increasing WM load resulted in increased RTs and decreased accuracy in both the abstinent ex-methamphetamine and nonaddict groups. These results were supported by previous studies showing that increasing WM load could decrease WM performance (82–85). However, there was no significant difference between groups, which contradicted our hypothesis.

There are contradictory findings regarding the effect of methamphetamine on WM performance. On the one hand, some studies have revealed overall cognitive deficits in the domains of verbal memory, WM, executive function, and social cognition in methamphetamine users (9, 10, 20, 86–89). For example, one study indicated that chronic methamphetamine users showed a deficit in some CogState battery domains (i.e., evaluated seven cognitive domains including WM) and poor psychological well-being (88). Studies have also revealed that methamphetamine users had deficits in brain function in areas including the dorsolateral prefrontal cortex during performing cognitive tasks that assess executive function (WM) (20, 87). Activity in this brain area can support WM performance and allocation of attentional resources (36, 90, 91).

However, in line with our results, some studies have shown no significant difference in WM performance of abstinent ex-methamphetamine compared to the nonaddict group (30). For example, Boileau et al. (92) asked methamphetamine users and subjects from a control group to perform different cognitive tasks including WM, attention/psychomotor function, and immediate and delayed memory tasks. Their results showed that there was no significant difference in WM performance between both groups, but that in attention/psychomotor function and delayed memory tasks, methamphetamine users showed a deficit. Another study employed attention/psychomotor function tasks (e.g., Stroop), learning/memory tasks, WM tasks, response inhibition tasks, and set-shifting/executive function tasks for both methamphetamine users and a control group (93). The findings indicated no significant difference between groups for all cognitive tasks. Similar results were observed in other studies as well (94, 95); for a review of this topic, see Hart et al. (30).

The use of different kinds of WM tasks in different experiments might explain these contradictory findings. In our study, we utilized the modified Sternberg task, in which methamphetamine-related stimuli were presented during the encoding phase of WM. These salient methamphetamine-related stimuli might cause attentional bias leading to attentional capture and eventually contributing to better performance despite having an interference bias. Indeed, attentional bias to methamphetamine-related stimuli might highlight those stimuli in WM, resulting in enhanced WM performance. Also, type of distractors might be an important factor to explained contradictory findings. For example, the amount of physical separation between targets and distractors might modulate the effects of load on distraction (29).

The availability of cognitive resources for optimal task performance and inhibiting the effect of interference is critical, particularly when WM is highly loaded or saturated (29). Our findings suggest that cognitive resources might be available as they are not dominated by task demands, resulting in optimal performance. Besides, bias toward the methamphetamine-related words (which were task-relevant information) might facilitate the WM process.

Limitations and Future Directions

Only male participants were recruited in the present study to minimize the effect of potentially confounding factors. One noteworthy and currently unexplored direction for future studies might be to examine gender differences. Moreover, participants with the mean of nearly 17-day abstinence from methamphetamine use were recruited. We chose this sample to assess the effect of short time abstinence from methamphetamine on WM performance. However, it is still unclear what may be the effect of long-term abstinence from methamphetamine use on cognitive function. For example, one study revealed that enhanced performance on tests of verbal memory and executive function was observed after approximately 6 months of abstinence from methamphetamine use. In line with this idea, some studies have examined the role of duration of abstinence from methamphetamine use on cognitive function (96, 97). They showed that prolonged greater duration of abstinence from methamphetamine use resulted in better cognitive performance (96–98). Future studies might consider the effect of long-term abstinence from methamphetamine use on WM biases and WM capacity. In addition, this study did not include a sample of active methamphetamine users who do not want to quit drug use, due to the difficulty in performing the modified Sternberg task. Future studies might add this group to compare the effect of motivation to quit on WM performance between abstinent and active groups. Due to the size of the center and the limited-time permission we have for our study, we could not recruit more participants. In several tests, we realized that the power of analysis is below the optimal level, and for some interactions, there was only a trend toward significance. In the future studies hiring complex tasks, more participants should be recruited to have enough power to run all the required analyses properly. This study sought to examine the neurobiological substrates of the interaction between WM bias, WM capacity, and interference effect using a complex span task in methamphetamine users.

CONCLUSION

We investigated the impulsive effects of methamphetamine-related stimuli on WM performance in abstinent ex-methamphetamine users. The experimental group demonstrated bias toward methamphetamine-related stimuli during a task with low WM load (three words) but not while performing tasks with higher WM loads (five and seven words). This result suggests that increasing WM load may provide an efficient buffer against attentional capture by salient stimuli (i.e., methamphetamine-related words). In line with this findings, investigating the effect of increasing WM load on the performance of abstinent ex-methamphetamine users (i.e., WM capacity) showed that increasing WM load had no significant effect on WM performance of abstinent ex-methamphetamine users compared with the control group. These findings suggest that increasing WM loads modified the impact of the interference bias. Besides, presenting methamphetamine-related stimuli facilitated their encoding due to bias toward task-relevant stimuli.

This finding has an important implication, suggesting that performing concurrent demanding tasks may reduce the power of salient stimuli and thus improve the efficiency of emotion regulation strategies. Further investigation on the interactions between WM interference bias, WM bias, and WM capacity may lead to the development of better tools and alternative therapies, including WM training, for the treatment of addiction.

AUTHOR CONTRIBUTIONS

ZD contributed to all aspects of the research. HE contributed to experimental design and data interpretation. HP contributed to experimental design and data interpretation. AK contributed to all aspects of the research.

ACKNOWLEDGMENTS

We would like to thank Dr. Javad Salehi Fadardi for statistical consulting, Mehrshad Golesorkhi for his assistance in data collection, and Drs. Reinout W. Wiers and Thomas E. Gladwin for helpful comments on the manuscript.

REFERENCES

1. Degenhardt L, Hall W. Extent of illicit drug use and dependence, and their contribution to the global burden of disease. *Lancet* (2012) 379(9810):55–70. doi: 10.1016/S0140-6736(11)61138-0
2. Degenhardt L, Mathers B, Guarinieri M, Panda S, Phillips B, Strathdee SA, et al. Meth/amphetamine use and associated HIV: Implications for global policy and public health. *Int J Drug Policy* (2010) 21(5):347–58. doi: 10.1016/j.drugpo.2009.11.007
3. Meredith CW, Jaffe C, Ang-Lee K, Saxon AJ. Implications of chronic methamphetamine use: a literature review. *Harv Rev Psychiatry* (2005) 13(3):141–54. doi: 10.1080/10673220591003605
4. Lecomte T, Mueser KT, MacEwan W, Thornton AE, Buchanan T, Bouchard V, et al. Predictors of persistent psychotic symptoms in persons with methamphetamine abuse receiving psychiatric treatment. *J Nerv Ment Dis* (2013) 201(12):1085–9. doi: 10.1097/NMD.0000000000000059
5. Fassbender C, Lesh TA, Ursu S, Salo R. Reaction time variability and related brain activity in methamphetamine psychosis. *Biol Psychiatry* (2015) 77(5):465–74. doi: 10.1016/j.biopsych.2014.07.028
6. Semple SJ, Patterson TL, Grant I. A comparison of injection and non-injection methamphetamine-using HIV positive men who have sex with men. *Drug Alcohol Depend* (2004) 76(2):203–12. doi: 10.1016/j.drugalcdep.2004.05.003
7. Semple SJ, Zians J, Grant I, Patterson TL. Impulsivity and methamphetamine use. *J Subst Abuse Treat* (2005) 29(2):85–93. doi: 10.1016/j.jsat.2005.05.001
8. Panenka WJ, Procyshyn RM, Lecomte T, MacEwan GW, Flynn SW, Honer WG, et al. Methamphetamine use: A comprehensive review of molecular, preclinical and clinical findings. *Drug Alcohol Depend* (2013) 129(3):167–79. doi: 10.1016/j.drugalcdep.2012.11.016
9. Luo YL, Bian JW, Zheng ZJ, Zhao L, Han S, Sun XH, et al. Effects of methamphetamine abuse on spatial cognitive function. *Sci Rep* (2018) 8(1):5502. doi: 10.1038/s41598-018-23828-y
10. Potvin S, Pelletier J, Grot S, Hebert C, Barr AM, Lecomte T. Cognitive deficits in individuals with methamphetamine use disorder: A meta-analysis. *Addict Behav* (2018) 80:154–60. doi: 10.1016/j.addbeh.2018.01.021
11. Gladwin TE, Wiers CE, Wiers RW. Cognitive neuroscience of cognitive retraining for addiction medicine: From mediating mechanisms to questions of efficacy. *Prog Brain Res* (2016) 224:323–44. doi: 10.1016/bs.pbr.2015.07.021
12. Wiers RW, Cox WM, Field M, Fadardi JS, Palfai TP, Schoenmakers T, et al. The search for new ways to change implicit alcohol-related cognitions in heavy drinkers. *Alcohol Clin Exp Res* (2006) 30(2):320–31. doi: 10.1111/j.1530-0277.2006.00037.x
13. Wiers RW, Bartholow BD, van den Wildenberg E, Thush C, Engels RC, Sher KJ, et al. Automatic and controlled processes and the development of addictive behaviors in adolescents: a review and a model. *Pharmacol Biochem Behav* (2007) 86(2):263–83. doi: 10.1016/j.pbb.2006.09.021
14. Lavigne AM, Wood MD, Janssen T, Wiers RW. Implicit and Explicit Alcohol Cognitions: The Moderating Effect of Executive Functions. *Alcohol Alcohol* (2017) 52(2):256–62. doi: 10.1093/alcalc/agw066
15. Wiers CE, Gladwin TE, Ludwig VU, Gropper S, Stuke H, Gawron CK, et al. Comparing three cognitive biases for alcohol cues in alcohol dependence. *Alcohol Alcohol* (2017) 52(2):242–8. doi: 10.1093/alcalc/agw063
16. Wiers CE, Wiers RW. Imaging the neural effects of cognitive bias modification training. *Neuroimage* (2017) 151:81–91. doi: 10.1016/j.neuroimage.2016.07.041
17. Zerhouni O, Begue L, Comiran F, Wiers RW. Controlled and implicit processes in evaluative conditioning on implicit and explicit attitudes toward alcohol and intentions to drink. *Addict Behav* (2018) 76:335–42. doi: 10.1016/j.addbeh.2017.08.026

18. Stacy AW, Wiers RW. Implicit cognition and addiction: a tool for explaining paradoxical behavior. *Annu Rev Clin Psychol* (2010) 6:551–75. doi: 10.1146/annurev.clinpsy.121208.131444
19. Gladwin T, Wiers RW. How do alcohol cues affect working memory? Persistent slowing due to alcohol-related distracters in an alcohol version of the Sternberg task. *Addict Res Theory* (2012) 20(4):284–90. doi: 10.3109/16066359.2011.614977
20. Hoffman WF, Moore M, Templin R, McFarland B, Hitzemann RJ, Mitchell SH. Neuropsychological function and delay discounting in methamphetamine-dependent individuals. *Psychopharmacology* (2006) 188(2):162–70. doi: 10.1007/s00213-006-0494-0
21. Duarte NA, Woods SP, Rooney A, Atkinson JH, Grant I. Working memory deficits affect risky decision-making in methamphetamine users with attention-deficit/hyperactivity disorder. *J Psychiatr Res* (2012) 46(4):492–9. doi: 10.1016/j.jpsychires.2012.01.006
22. Casaletto KB, Obermeit L, Morgan EE, Weber E, Franklin DR, Grant I, et al. Depression and executive dysfunction contribute to a metamemory deficit among individuals with methamphetamine use disorders. *Addict Behav* (2015) 40:45–50. doi: 10.1016/j.addbeh.2014.08.007
23. Cox WM, Hogan LM, Kristian MR, Race JH. Alcohol attentional bias as a predictor of alcohol abusers' treatment outcome. *Drug Alcohol Depend* (2002) 68(3):237–43. doi: 10.1016/S0376-8716(02)00219-3
24. Field M, Cox WM. Attentional bias in addictive behaviors: a review of its development, causes, and consequences. *Drug Alcohol Depend* (2008) 97(1-2):1–20. doi: 10.1016/j.drugalcdep.2008.03.030
25. Anderson BA. What is abnormal about addiction-related attentional biases? *Drug Alcohol Depend* (2016) 167:8–14. doi: 10.1016/j.drugalcdep.2016.08.002
26. Brooks SJ, Wiemerslage L, Burch KH, Maiorana SA, Cocolas E, Schioth HB, et al. The impact of cognitive training in substance use disorder: the effect of working memory training on impulse control in methamphetamine users. *Psychopharmacology (Berl)* (2017) 234(12):1911–21. doi: 10.1007/s00213-017-4597-6
27. Thush C, Wiers RW, Ames SL, Grenard JL, Sussman S, Stacy AW. Interactions between implicit and explicit cognition and working memory capacity in the prediction of alcohol use in at-risk adolescents. *Drug Alcohol Depend* (2008) 94(1-3):116–24. doi: 10.1016/j.drugalcdep.2007.10.019
28. Baddeley A. Working Memory. In: *Theories, Models, and Controversies.*, vol. 1-29. ANNUAL REVIEWS (2012). doi: 10.1146/annurev-psych-120710-100422
29. SanMiguel I, Corral M-J, Escera C. When Loading Working Memory Reduces Distraction: Behavioral and Electrophysiological Evidence from an Auditory-Visual Distraction Paradigm. *J Cognit Neurosci* (2008) 20(7):1131–45. doi: 10.1162/jocn.2008.20078
30. Hart CL, Marvin CB, Silver R, Smith EE. Is cognitive functioning impaired in methamphetamine users? A critical review. *Neuropsychopharmacology* (2012) 37(3):586–608. doi: 10.1038/npp.2011.276
31. Sabrini S, Wang GY, Lin JC, Ian JK, Curley LE. Methamphetamine use and cognitive function: A systematic review of neuroimaging research. *Drug Alcohol Depend* (2019) 194:75–87. doi: 10.1016/j.drugalcdep.2018.08.041
32. Chang L, Ernst T, Speck O, Patel H, DeSilva M, Leonido-Yee M, et al. Perfusion MRI and computerized cognitive test abnormalities in abstinent methamphetamine users. *Psychiatry Res: Neuroimaging* (2002) 114(2):65–79. doi: 10.1016/S0925-4927(02)00004-5
33. Gene-Jack Wang MD, Nora D. Volkow MD, Linda Chang MD, Miller E, Mark Sedler MD, Hitzemann R, et al. Partial Recovery of Brain Metabolism in Methamphetamine Abusers After Protracted Abstinence. *Am J Psychiatry* (2004) 161(2):242–8. doi: 10.1176/appi.ajp.161.2.242
34. Thompson PM, Hayashi KM, Simon SL, Geaga JA, Hong MS, Sui Y, et al. Structural abnormalities in the brains of human subjects who use methamphetamine. *J Neurosci* (2004) 24(26):6028–36. doi: 10.1523/JNEUROSCI.0713-04.2004
35. Kessler K, Pajak KM, Harkin B, Jones B. A working memory bias for alcohol-related stimuli depends on drinking score. *Psychol Addict Behav* (2013) 27(1):23–31. doi: 10.1037/a0028664
36. Awh E, Vogel EK, Oh SH. Interactions between attention and working memory. *Neurosci* (2006) 139(1):201–8. doi: 10.1016/j.neuroscience.2005.08.023
37. Rosen VM, Engle RW. Working Memory Capacity and Suppression. *J Mem Lang* (1998) 39(3):418–36. doi: 10.1006/jmla.1998.2590
38. Kane MJ, Bleckley MK, Conway AR, Engle RW. A controlled-attention view of working-memory capacity. *J Exp Psychol Gen* (2001) 130(2):169–83. doi: 10.1037//0096-3445.130.2.169
39. Kane MJ, Engle RW. Working-memory capacity and the control of attention: the contributions of goal neglect, response competition, and task set to Stroop interference. *J Exp Psychol Gen* (2003) 132(1):47–70. doi: 10.1037/0096-3445.132.1.47
40. Barrett LF, Tugade MM, Engle RW. Individual differences in working memory capacity and dual-process theories of the mind. *Psychol Bull* (2004) 130(4):553–73. doi: 10.1037/0033-2909.130.4.553
41. Unsworth N, Engle RW. Simple and complex memory spans and their relation to fluid abilities: Evidence from list-length effects. *J Mem Lang* (2006) 54(1):68–80. doi: 10.1016/j.jml.2005.06.003
42. Heitz RP, Schrock JC, Payne TW, Engle RW. Effects of incentive on working memory capacity: behavioral and pupillometric data. *Psychophysiology* (2008) 45(1):119–29. doi: 10.1111/j.1469-8986.2007.00605.x
43. Unsworth N, Redick TS, Heitz RP, Broadway JM, Engle RW. Complex working memory span tasks and higher-order cognition: a latent-variable analysis of the relationship between processing and storage. *Memory* (2009) 17(6):635–54. doi: 10.1080/09658210902998047
44. Townshend JM, Duka T. Attentional bias associated with alcohol cues: differences between heavy and occasional social drinkers. *Psychopharmacology (Berl)* (2001) 157(1):67–74. doi: 10.1007/s002130100764
45. Field M, Wiers RW, Christiansen P, Fillmore MT, Verster JC. Acute alcohol effects on inhibitory control and implicit cognition: implications for loss of control over drinking. *Alcohol Clin Exp Res* (2010) 34(8):1346–52. doi: 10.1111/j.1530-0277.2010.01218.x
46. Miller MA, Fillmore MT. The effect of image complexity on attentional bias towards alcohol-related images in adult drinkers. *Addiction* (2010) 105(5):883–90. doi: 10.1111/j.1360-0443.2009.02860.x
47. Gladwin TE. Attentional bias variability and cued attentional bias for alcohol stimuli. *Addict Res Theory* (2017) 25(1):32–8. doi: 10.1080/16066359.2016.1196674
48. Gladwin TE, den Uyl TE, Fregni FF, Wiers RW. Enhancement of selective attention by tDCS: interaction with interference in a Sternberg task. *Neurosci Lett* (2012) 512(1):33–7. doi: 10.1016/j.neulet.2012.01.056
49. Ekhtiari H, Alam-Mehrjerdi Z, Hassani-Abharian P, Nouri M, Farnam R, Mokri A. Examination and evaluation of craving-inductive verbal cues among Persian-speaking methamphetamine abusers. [Examination and evaluation of craving-inductive verbal cues among Persian-speaking methamphetamine abusers.]. *Adv. Cognit Sci* (2010) 12(2):69–82.
50. Robinson TE, Berridge KC. The neural basis of drug craving: an incentive-sensitization theory of addiction. *Brain Res Brain Res Rev* (1993) 18(3):247–91. doi: 10.1016/0165-0173(93)90013-P
51. Robinson TE, Berridge KC. Addiction. *Annu Rev Psychol* (2003) 54:25–53. doi: 10.1146/annurev.psych.54.101601.145237
52. Smith JL, Mattick RP, Jamadar SD, Iredale JM. Deficits in behavioural inhibition in substance abuse and addiction: a meta-analysis. *Drug Alcohol Depend* (2014) 145:1–33. doi: 10.1016/j.drugalcdep.2014.08.009
53. Petersen SE, Posner MI. The attention system of the human brain: 20 years after. *Annu Rev Neurosci* (2012) 35(1):73–89. doi: 10.1146/annurev-neuro-062111-150525
54. Galla BM, Duckworth AL. More than resisting temptation: Beneficial habits mediate the relationship between self-control and positive life outcomes. *J Pers Soc Psychol* (2015) 109(3):508–25. doi: 10.1037/pspp0000026
55. Brevers D, Bechara A, Kilts CD, Antoniali V, Bruylant A, Verbanck P, et al. Competing motivations: proactive response inhibition toward addiction-related stimuli in quitting-motivated individuals. *J Gambl Stud* (2018) 34(3):785–806. doi: 10.1007/s10899-017-9722-2
56. Hofmann W, Friese M, Strack F. Impulse and self-control from a dual-systems perspective. *Perspect Psychol Sci* (2009) 4(2):162–76. doi: 10.1111/j.1745-6924.2009.01116.x
57. Noel X, Colmant M, Van Der Linden M, Bechara A, Bullens Q, Hanak C, et al. Time course of attention for alcohol cues in abstinent alcoholic patients: the role of initial orienting. *Alcohol Clin Exp Res* (2006) 30(11):1871–7. doi: 10.1111/j.1530-0277.2006.00224.x
58. Westbrook A, Braver TS. Cognitive effort: A neuroeconomic approach. *Cognit Affective Behav Neurosci* (2015) 15(2):395–415. doi: 10.3758/s13415-015-0334-y

59. Lavie N, Hirst A, de Fockert JW, Viding E. Load theory of selective attention and cognitive control. *J Exp Psychol Gen* (2004b) 133(3):339–54. doi: 10.1037/0096-3445.133.3.339
60. Sarter M, Gehring WJ, Kozak R. More attention must be paid: the neurobiology of attentional effort. *Brain Res Rev* (2006) 51(2):145–60. doi: 10.1016/j.brainresrev.2005.11.002
61. Mathews A, Mogg K, Kentish J, Eysenck M. Effect of psychological treatment on cognitive bias in generalized anxiety disorder. *Behav Res Ther* (1995) 33(3):293–303. doi: 10.1016/0005-7967(94)E0022-B
62. Townshend JM, Duka T. Avoidance of alcohol-related stimuli in alcohol-dependent inpatients. *Alcohol Clin Exp Res* (2007) 31(8):1349–57. doi: 10.1111/j.1530-0277.2007.00429.x
63. Brown HM, Eley TC, Broeren S, Macleod C, Rinck M, Hadwin JA, et al. Psychometric properties of reaction time based experimental paradigms measuring anxiety-related information-processing biases in children. *J Anxiety Disord* (2014) 28(1):97–107. doi: 10.1016/j.janxdis.2013.11.004
64. Grenard JL, Ames SL, Wiers RW, Thush C, Sussman S, Stacy AW. Working memory capacity moderates the predictive effects of drug-related associations on substance use. *Psychol Addict Behav* (2008) 22(3):426–32. doi: 10.1037/0893-164X.22.3.426
65. Piechatzek M, Indlekofer F, Daamen M, Glasmacher C, Lieb R, Pfister H, et al. Is moderate substance use associated with altered executive functioning in a population-based sample of young adults? *Hum Psychopharmacol* (2009) 24(8):650–65. doi: 10.1002/hup.1069
66. Boendermaker WJ, Gladwin TE, Peeters M, Prins PJM, Wiers RW. Training working memory in adolescents using serious game elements: pilot randomized controlled trial. *JMIR Serious Games* (2018) 6(2):e10. doi: 10.2196/games.8364
67. Kaag AM, Goudriaan AE, De Vries TJ, Pattij T, Wiers RW. A high working memory load prior to memory retrieval reduces craving in non-treatment seeking problem drinkers. *Psychopharmacology (Berl)* (2018) 235(3):695–708. doi: 10.1007/s00213-017-4785-4
68. Wegner DM. Ironic processes of mental control. *Psychol Rev* (1994) 101(1):34–52. doi: 10.1037//0033-295X.101.1.34
69. Ward A, Mann T. Don't mind if I do: disinhibited eating under cognitive load. *J Pers Soc Psychol* (2000) 78(4):753–63. doi: 10.1037//0022-3514.78.4.753
70. Kim SY, Kim MS, Chun MM. Concurrent working memory load can reduce distraction. *Proc Natl Acad Sci U S A* (2005) 102(45):16524–9. doi: 10.1073/pnas.0505454102
71. Van Dillen LF, Papies EK, Hofmann W. Turning a blind eye to temptation: how cognitive load can facilitate self-regulation. *J Pers Soc Psychol* (2013) 104(3):427–43. doi: 10.1037/a0031262
72. Van Dillen LF, Derks B. Working memory load reduces facilitated processing of threatening faces: an ERP study. *Emotion* (2012) 12(6):1340–9. doi: 10.1037/a0028624
73. Van Dillen LF, van der Wal RC, van den Bos K. On the role of attention and emotion in morality: attentional control modulates unrelated disgust in moral judgments. *Pers Soc Psychol Bull* (2012) 38(9):1222–31. doi: 10.1177/0146167212448485
74. Van Dillen LF, Koole SL. How automatic is "automatic vigilance"? The role of working memory in attentional interference of negative information. *Cogn Emot* (2009) 23(6):1106–17. doi: 10.1080/02699930802338178
75. Iacoviello BM, Wu G, Abend R, Murrough JW, Feder A, Fruchter E, et al. Attention bias variability and symptoms of posttraumatic stress disorder. *J Trauma Stress* (2014) 27(2):232–9. doi: 10.1002/jts.21899
76. Andrade J, Kavanagh D, Baddeley A. Eye-movements and visual imagery: a working memory approach to the treatment of post-traumatic stress disorder. *Br J Clin Psychol* (1997) 36(Pt 2):209–23. doi: 10.1111/j.2044-8260.1997.tb01408.x
77. May J, Andrade J, Panabokke N, Kavanagh D. Visuospatial tasks suppress craving for cigarettes. *Behav Res Ther* (2010) 48(6):476–85. doi: 10.1016/j.brat.2010.02.001
78. Kemps E, Tiggemann M. Hand-held dynamic visual noise reduces naturally occurring food cravings and craving-related consumption. *Appetite* (2013) 68:152–7. doi: 10.1016/j.appet.2013.05.001
79. Fougnie D, Marois R. Attentive tracking disrupts feature binding in visual working memory. *Vis cogn* (2009) 17(1-2):48–66. doi: 10.1080/13506280802281337
80. Kiyonaga A, Egner T. Working memory as internal attention: Toward an integrative account of internal and external selection processes. *Psychon Bull Rev* (2013) 20(2):228–42. doi: 10.3758/s13423-012-0359-y
81. Dowd EW. *Memory-Based Attentional Guidance: A Window to the Relationship between Working Memory and Attention.* Dissertation/Thesis, ProQuest Dissertations Publishing (2016)
82. Lavie N, Hirst A, de Fockert JW, Viding E. Load theory of selective attention and cognitive control. *J Exp Psychol: Gen* (2004a) 133(3):339–54. doi: 10.1037/0096-3445.133.3.339
83. Hester R, Garavan H. Working memory and executive function: The influence of content and load on the control of attention. *Mem Cognit* (2005) 33(2):221–33. doi: 10.3758/BF03195311
84. Klemen J, Buchel C, Buhler M, Menz MM, Rose M. Auditory working memory load impairs visual ventral stream processing: toward a unified model of attentional load. *J Cogn Neurosci* (2010) 22(3):437–46. doi: 10.1162/jocn.2009.21204
85. Simon SS, Tusch ES, Holcomb PJ, Daffner KR. Increasing working memory load reduces processing of cross-modal task-irrelevant stimuli even after controlling for task difficulty and executive capacity. *Front Hum Neurosci* (2016) 10:380–0. doi: 10.3389/fnhum.2016.00380
86. Scott JC, Woods SP, Matt GE, Meyer RA, Heaton RK, Atkinson JH, et al. Neurocognitive effects of methamphetamine: a critical review and meta-analysis. *Neuropsychol Rev* (2007) 17(3):275–97. doi: 10.1007/s11065-007-9031-0
87. Dean AC, Groman SM, Morales AM, London ED. An evaluation of the evidence that methamphetamine abuse causes cognitive decline in humans. *Neuropsychopharmacology* (2012) 38:259. doi: 10.1038/npp.2012.179
88. Zhong N, Jiang H, Du J, Zhao Y, Sun H, Xu D, et al. The cognitive impairments and psychological wellbeing of methamphetamine dependent patients compared with health controls. *Prog Neuropsychopharmacol Biol Psychiatry* (2016) 69:31–7. doi: 10.1016/j.pnpbp.2016.04.005
89. Sabrini S, Wang GY, Lin JC, Ian JK, Curley LE. Methamphetamine use and cognitive function: A systematic review of neuroimaging research. *Drug Alcohol Depend* (2018) 194:75–87. doi: 10.1016/j.drugalcdep.2018.08.041
90. Miller EK, Cohen JD. An integrative theory of prefrontal cortex function. *Annu Rev Neurosci* (2001) 24:167–202. doi: 10.1146/annurev.neuro.24.1.167
91. Barcelo F, Escera C, Corral MJ, Periáñez JA. Task switching and novelty processing activate a common neural network for cognitive control. *J Cognit Neurosci* (2006) 18(10):1734–48. doi: 10.1162/jocn.2006.18.10.1734
92. Boileau I, Rusjan P, Houle S, Wilkins D, Tong J, Selby P, et al. Increased vesicular monoamine transporter binding during early abstinence in human methamphetamine users: Is VMAT2 a stable dopamine neuron biomarker? *J Neurosci* (2008) 28(39):9850–6. doi: 10.1523/JNEUROSCI.3008-08.2008
93. McCann UD, Kuwabara H, Kumar A, Palermo M, Abbey R, Brasic J, et al. Persistent cognitive and dopamine transporter deficits in abstinent methamphetamine users. *Synapse* (2008) 62(2):91–100. doi: 10.1002/syn.20471
94. Johanson CE, Frey KA, Lundahl LH, Keenan P, Lockhart N, Roll J, et al. Cognitive function and nigrostriatal markers in abstinent methamphetamine abusers. *Psychopharmacology (Berl)* (2006) 185(3):327–38. doi: 10.1007/s00213-006-0330-6
95. Silber BY, Croft RJ, Papafotiou K, Stough C. The acute effects of d-amphetamine and methamphetamine on attention and psychomotor performance. *Psychopharmacology (Berl)* (2006) 187(2):154–69. doi: 10.1007/s00213-006-0410-7
96. Salo R, Nordahl TE, Galloway GP, Moore CD, Waters C, Leamon MH. Drug abstinence and cognitive control in methamphetamine-dependent individuals. *J Subst Abuse Treat* (2009) 37(3):292–7. doi: 10.1016/j.jsat.2009.03.004
97. Simon SL, Dean AC, Cordova X, Monterosso JR, London ED. Methamphetamine dependence and neuropsychological functioning: evaluating change during early abstinence. *J Stud Alcohol Drugs* (2010) 71(3):335–44. doi: 10.15288/jsad.2010.71.335
98. van der Plas EAA, Crone EA, van den Wildenberg WPM, Tranel D, Bechara A. Executive control deficits in substance-dependent individuals: A comparison of alcohol, cocaine, and methamphetamine and of men and women. *J Clin Exp Neuropsychol* (2009) 31(6):706–19. doi: 10.1080/13803390802484797

12

Emotion Processing, Reappraisal, and Craving in Alcohol Dependence: A Functional Magnetic Resonance Imaging Study

Jochem M. Jansen[1,2*], *Odile A. van den Heuvel*[3,4], *Ysbrand D. van der Werf*[4], *Stella J. de Wit*[3,4], *Dick J. Veltman*[3,4], *Wim van den Brink*[1] *and Anna E. Goudriaan*[1,5]

[1] *Institute for Addiction Research, Department of Psychiatry, Amsterdam UMC, University of Amsterdam, Amsterdam, Netherlands,* [2] *Institute for Criminal Law & Criminology, Faculty of Law, Leiden University, Leiden, Netherlands,* [3] *Department of Psychiatry, Amsterdam UMC, Vrije Universiteit Amsterdam, Amsterdam, Netherlands,* [4] *Department of Anatomy & Neurosciences, Amsterdam Neuroscience, Amsterdam UMC, Vrije Universiteit Amsterdam, Amsterdam, Netherlands,* [5] *Arkin Mental Health, Amsterdam, Netherlands*

Correspondence:
Jochem Milan Jansen
j.m.jansen@law.leidenuniv.nl or
jochemjansen89@gmail.com

Alcohol dependence has long been related to impaired emotion regulation—including reappraisal—but little is known about the performance and associated neural activity of alcohol-dependent patients (ADPs) on an emotion reappraisal task. This study, therefore, compares reappraisal of negative, positive, neutral, and alcohol-related images at a behavioral and neural level between ADPs and healthy controls (HCs).

Thirty-nine ADPs and 39 age-, gender-, and education-matched HCs performed an emotion reappraisal task during functional magnetic resonance imaging (fMRI), and craving was measured before and after the reappraisal task. During the emotion reappraisal task, participants were instructed to either attend or reappraise positive, negative, neutral, or alcohol-related images, and to indicate their experienced emotion on a visual analogue scale (VAS).

Both ADPs and HCs completed the emotion reappraisal task successfully, showing significant differences in self-reported experienced emotion after attending versus reappraising visual stimuli and in brain activity in emotion processing/reappraisal relevant areas. ADPs were not impaired in cognitive reappraisal at a behavioral or neural level relative to HCs, nor did ADPs indicate any difference in self-reported emotion while attending emotional images. However, ADPs were different from HC in emotion processing: ADPs revealed a blunted response in the (posterior) insula, precuneus, operculum, and superior temporal gyrus while attending emotional images compared neutral images compared to HCs, and in ADPs, higher baseline craving levels were associated with a less blunted response to alcohol-related images than in HCs. These results reveal that ADPs do not show impaired reappraisal abilities when *instructed*, although future studies should assess voluntary reappraisal abilities in alcohol-dependent patients.

Clinical Trial Registration: www.ClinicalTrials.gov, identifier NCT02557815.

Keywords: alcohol dependence, emotion reappraisal, craving, functional magnetic resonance imaging, emotion regulation

INTRODUCTION

The ability to manage emotional information is central to our daily functioning, and adequately managing emotions is achieved through various emotion regulation strategies, including attention shifting and cognitive reappraisal, the process of moderating the emotional impact of a certain thought or stimulus through cognitive reinterpretation (1, 2). Neuroimaging studies using reappraisal tasks in healthy controls (HCs) indicate that the prefrontal cortex, including the dorsolateral prefrontal cortex (dlPFC), is vital for the *regulation* of emotions, whereas the limbic system—including the amygdala and insula—is important for the initial *processing* of emotions (1–4). Other brain areas related to reappraisal include the dorsomedial prefrontal cortex, superior temporal gyrus, dorsal part of the anterior cingulate cortex (ACC), superior parietal lobule, and inferior frontal gyrus (4). These brain regions are part of cognitive–linguistic control networks, associated with effortful (i.e., explicitly applied) reappraisal by cognitively reframing the affective meaning of a negative stimulus in more neutral terms (2, 5).

Impairments in reappraisal are supposed to be related to the development, persistence, and severity of substance dependence (6). Previous studies have indicated that difficulties in coping with negative affect is one of the most prominent clinical factors in substance dependence (7). The induction of negative affect may increase the urge to drink (8, 9), although a recent study failed to show such a relationship between emotional state and craving for alcohol-dependent individuals (10). Impaired emotional reappraisal also predicts negative outcomes, including relapse, in substance use disorder (SUD) patients (11, 12). A recent study showed impaired emotional reappraisal (ER) in Internet gaming disorder patients compared to drug-naïve controls, suggesting that impaired emotion reappraisal might precede neurotoxic effects of alcohol or other substances (13). Together, these studies indicate that emotional reappraisal is central in the etiology of alcohol dependence.

The results from the aforementioned studies on emotional reappraisal in substance dependence are further corroborated by a recent review on the neural circuitry of impaired reappraisal in patients with SUDs compared with HCs. This review showed decreased recruitment of the ACC, dlPFC, and ventromedial prefrontal cortex (vmPFC) during reappraisal, but no differences in amygdala or insular functioning (14). The review therefore concludes that emotion regulation disturbances in substance dependence are related to impaired prefrontal functioning and not to excessive reactivity to emotional stimuli.

Most studies reviewed by Wilcox et al. (14) did not apply an (explicit) reappraisal task, but included emotion reactivity, implicit reappraisal, or behavioral control tasks, and therefore little is known about the neural circuitry of explicit reappraisal in substance use disorders in general and more specifically in alcohol-dependent patients (ADPs). The available studies into emotion regulation in alcohol dependence reveal that impaired emotion regulation is associated with increased craving levels, especially for ADPs who experience increased negative and decreased positive affect (15). Furthermore, interview data demonstrate that ADPs show reduced use of effortful cognitive emotion regulation and tend to apply less beneficial emotion regulation strategies like response modulation and attentional deployment strategies in daily life (16). ADPs also report problems with the identification and regulation of emotions (17), which are linked to the duration of the last heavy drinking episode, as well as higher drinking rates at 1-year follow-up (18). It is currently not clear, however, whether ADPs perform differently on an explicit cognitive reappraisal task and whether related brain activity is different.

The review by Wilcox et al. (14) further concludes that no differences were found in the limbic system, indicating that impaired reappraisal may originate from prefrontal impairments rather than from an excessive response to emotional stimuli. Some studies even point toward lower limbic responsivity to emotional stimuli in SUDs (19, 20), which fits with the findings regarding reduced salience of natural reinforcing stimuli, relative to addiction-relevant stimuli (21).

The current study is the first to assess differences in cognitive reappraisal abilities between ADPs and HCs at the behavioral and the neural level. We hypothesize that ADPs show decreased reappraisal abilities compared to HCs, indicated by self-report scores on a visual analogue scale (state), an emotion regulation questionnaire (trait). Reduced ER-related brain activity in areas such as the dlPFC and ACC is mainly expected for the reappraisal of negative emotion, which has been implicated in substance dependence (22), whereas the ER of alcohol-related images may either result in lower activity [in line with findings from Wilcox et al. (14)] or higher activity (due to increased cognitive load associated with higher salience of these images). We furthermore hypothesize no differences in brain activity during emotional processing of negative and positive images, but greater activations to alcohol-related images in ADPs compared to HCs. Finally, we expect craving levels to increase due to the emotion reappraisal task, and that craving is negatively related to cognitive reappraisal abilities.

METHODS AND MATERIALS

Participants

A total of 39 ADPs (26 males) and 39 HCs (22 males) were included in this between-subjects study and were matched on (mean) age, sex, and education. ADPs were sober for at least 3 weeks and were recruited from addiction treatment centers in the larger city area of Amsterdam, the Netherlands. Sobriety was confirmed with a urine test in the research lab on the test days. None of the participants were active users of psychoactive medication, cannabis, opioids, or stimulants. HCs were recruited through Internet and social media advertisements. All participants were screened for MRI suitability. All subjects were screened (and if positive excluded) for the presence or history of psychiatric disorders, including substance abuse or dependence, using the Composite International Diagnostic Interview (CIDI) (23). The study was approved by the local Medical Ethical Commission of the Academic Medical Center of the University of Amsterdam and participants signed the informed consent form, consistent with the Declaration of Helsinki, before participating in the study. Participants were remunerated for their participation.

Questionnaires

In addition to the CIDI interview, the Alcohol Use Disorder Identification Test (AUDIT) (24), Beck's Depression Inventory (BDI) (25), Beck's Anxiety Inventory (BAI) (26), the Toronto Alexithymia Scale-20 (TAS-20) (27), and the Emotion Regulation Questionnaire (ERQ) (28) were administered to assess levels of depression, anxiety, alexithymia, and emotion regulation, respectively. Finally, craving was assessed with the Alcohol Urge Questionnaire (AUQ) (29) before and after the performance of the emotion reappraisal task.

Emotion Reappraisal Task

Participants viewed 18 negative (e.g., vicious dog, plane crash), 18 positive (e.g., cute puppies, beautiful landscape), 18 neutral (e.g., people at work, neutral landscape), and 18 alcohol-related images (e.g., glass of beer, bottles of wine) on a screen using a mirror attached to the head coil. The negative, positive, and neutral images used in this task were selected from the International Affective Image Set (IAPS) (30). Negative images had a low valence (≤4.0) and high arousal (≥6.0), whereas neutral images had a mildly positive valence ($4.5 < x < 7.0$) and low arousal ($2.0 < x < 4.2$) and positive images had high valence (≥7.0) and arousal (≥5.0), based on the original IAPS scores. The alcohol-related images were selected from Vollstädt-Klein et al. (31) and supplemented by alcohol-related images of popular Dutch alcoholic beverages. All alcohol-related images were separately validated in an independent sample for valence ($3.0 < x < 6.0$) and arousal ($2.0 < x < 4.0$).

The images were paired with one of two different instructions: "attend" and "reappraise." In the attend instruction, participants were told to view and identify themselves with the situation in the image (e.g., "how would you feel in this situation"). In the reappraise condition, participants were told to reappraise their emotions related to these images in such a way that the negative feelings were reduced (e.g., "imagine a less negative outcome or interpretation"). Images were presented in 24 blocks of three images of the same emotion type (negative, positive, neutral, alcohol) with the same instruction (attend, reappraise) and presented in a pseudo-randomized order (see **Figure 1**).

After each image, for both instructions (attend and reappraise), a visual analogue scale (VAS) ranging from 0 to 100 was presented and participants had to rate their emotional state ("How do you feel?" where 0 is very negative, 50 is neutral, and 100 is very positive) by moving a bar to the right or left by pressing a button box multiple times. This moving bar was set in the middle (representing a neutral value of 50) and the range of emotions was indicated by previously validated self-assessment manikins depicting valence (32). Prior to scanning, the assessment was explained and practiced outside the scanner using example stimuli (not used in the experiments) for approximately 5 min. The reappraisal task itself took approximately 25 min.

Analysis

Behavioral Analysis

Data were prepared for analysis by winsorizing extreme values for experienced emotion (mean VAS per condition) and craving

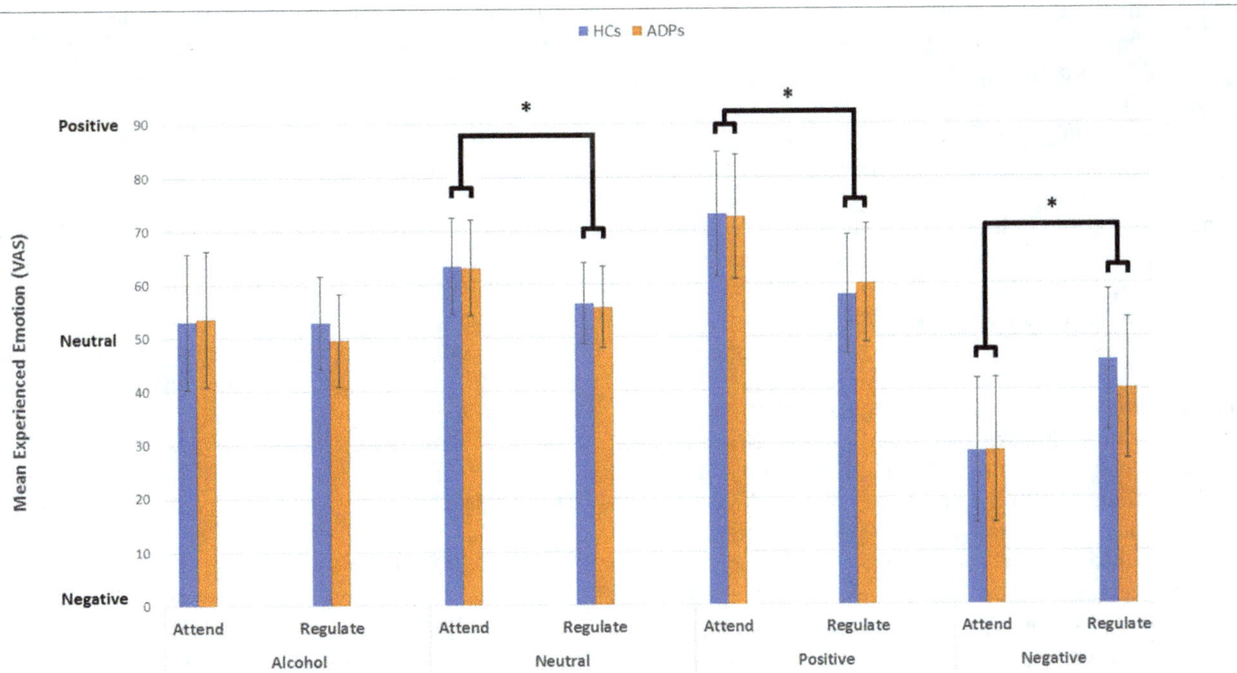

FIGURE 1 | This figure reveals the mean experienced emotion (VAS) per emotion type, instruction, and participant group. Analysis reveals no effect of participant group, but a significant interaction between emotion type and instruction for alcohol-related, neutral, positive, and negative images. Error bars reflect the standard deviation.

(AUQ pre- and post-scores), by replacing values below the 5th and above the 95th percentile by the 5th or 95th percentile, respectively, and by confirming that experienced emotion was normally distributed.

In order to assess effects of emotion type, instruction, and participant group on experienced emotion, a general linear model (GLM) Univariate ANOVA was performed, including experienced emotion (mean VAS) as the dependent variable, and instruction (attend, reappraise), emotion type (alcohol, neutral, positive, negative) and participant group (ADP, HC) as fixed factors. Significant interactions were followed up by Bonferroni-corrected simple effects analyses. Independent sample t tests were performed to assess whether gender influenced experienced emotion per condition with results considered significant at a Bonferroni-corrected $p = .006$ (0.05/8).

The AUQ was administered before (pre) and after (post) the reappraisal task. Due to the many mistakes that were made in the second and seventh question—which are reverse coded and were misinterpreted—these were excluded from the analysis. Both pre and post scores were positively skewed and therefore a $\log(x + 1)$ transformation was applied. A repeated-measures ANOVA was performed including AUQ scores as the dependent variable, time (pre/post) as the within-subjects factor and participant group as the between-group factor. Finally, the increases in craving levels (post- minus pre-AUQ scores) were correlated to the means of experienced emotion per emotion type and instruction.

Functional Magnetic Resonance Imaging Data Acquisition

MRI scanning was performed on a Philips Achieva 3T scanner at the Spinoza Imaging Centre, Amsterdam, the Netherlands. Functional MRI [echo time (TE) = 27.63 ms; repetition time (TR) = 2000 ms; field of view (FOV) = 240 × 240 mm, 37 3-mm slices, 0.3-mm slice gap; 80 × 80 matrix; flip angle = 76.1°] was performed to acquire blood oxygenation level-dependent (BOLD) signals using single-shot multi-echo (33) T2*-weighted echo planar imaging (EPI's). These T2-weighted flow-compensated 8 spin-echo anatomical images were oriented axially along the anterior commissure to the posterior commissure (AC–PC) line. During the baseline session, a T1-weighted 3D data set was obtained for anatomical reference; TR = 8.196 ms, TE = 3.73 ms, field of view (FOV) = 140 × 188 × 220 mm, matrix 240 × 187, flip angle = 8°, slice thickness = 1 mm, number of slices = 220.

Preprocessing and First-Level Analysis

Preprocessing was performed with SPM8 (Wellcome Trust Centre for Neuroimaging, London, United Kingdom) in MATLAB (version 2012b) and included realignment to the first image, slice timing correction to the middle (18th) slice, co-registration of the anatomical T1 of the subject to the mean functional scan, and warping of this co-registered T1 to standard space. Next, the volumes were normalized to the Montreal Neurological Institute (MNI) template and smoothed with a 7-mm Gaussian kernel in order to increase signal-to-noise ratio. To account for low-frequency drifts, a high-pass filter (128 Hz) was applied. Three subjects (two ADP and one HC) were removed due to the low quality of the fMRI data (e.g., scanner artifacts).

In the first-level model regressors of no interest were Instruction and VAS scoring. Instruction was modeled with a boxcar of 3 s, whereas VAS scoring was modeled with a boxcar for the true duration of the scoring process since this was self-paced. The eight regressors of interest included the onsets of the negative, positive, neutral, and alcohol-related images in either attending or reappraising condition, which were modeled as boxcars (duration, 5 s) and convolved with a hemodynamic response function, in the first-level, single-subject, fixed-effects analysis. First-level contrasts for reappraisal [reappraise > attend] were computed per emotion condition (negative, positive, alcohol, and neutral). For emotion processing, separate contrasts were created for attending emotional images (alcohol, positive, or negative) versus neutral images [attend emotion (positive, negative, alcohol) > attend neutral].

Functional Magnetic Resonance Imaging Data Analysis

Separate second-level fMRI analyses were performed for the attend and reappraise conditions. For the attend condition, a 2 × 3 ANOVA was conducted in SPM12, including the [attend emotion > attend neutral] contrast per emotion, in order to assess the interaction between group (ADP, HC) and emotion (alcohol, positive, negative) as well as main effects of group, emotion, and condition. For the reappraise condition, a 2 × 4 ANOVA conducted in SPM12, including the [reappraise > attend] contrasts per emotion, in order to assess the interaction between group (ADP, HC) and emotion (alcohol, neutral, positive, negative) as well as main effects of group, emotion, and condition.

First, the main effects of instruction (attend, reappraise) during the emotion reappraisal task are discussed in order to confirm that the emotion reappraisal task was completed successfully. Then, the group by emotion interactions, as well as the main effects for group and emotion will be discussed. Results are reported at a whole-brain $p < 0.05$ FWE-corrected threshold; furthermore, amygdala Region of Interest (ROI) analyses (based on the BrainMap database) were performed for the attend condition.

In order to assess whether craving is positively correlated to higher brain responsivity during emotion processing and negatively correlated to brain activity during emotion reappraisal, any significant differences in brain activity between ADPs and HCs were followed up by a Pearson correlation analysis, including the extracted individual b values from the peak-voxel coordinate, craving levels before the emotion reappraisal task, and the increase in craving levels due to the emotion reappraisal task.

RESULTS

Demographics

ADPs and HCs were successfully matched on age, gender, and years of education. However, ADPs reported significantly higher levels of depression (BDI), anxiety (BAI), and alexithymia (TAS-20). Analyses were not corrected for these differences, because depression, anxiety, and alexithymia levels are well known to be elevated in alcohol dependence (34–37). There were no group differences in the ERQ scores (**Table 1**).

TABLE 1 | Sample characteristics. This table shows the results for the analyses of the sample characteristics. Values are denoted as mean (standard deviation). Total number of participants per comparison may vary due to a small number of missing values. SD, standard deviation; AUDIT, Alcohol Use Disorders Identification Test; TAS, Toronto Alexithymia Scale; DIDF, difficulties identifying and describing feelings; EOT, externally oriented thinking; ERQ, emotion regulation questionnaire. ERQ Reappraisal and Suppression are subscales of the ERQ.

	Possible range (min–max)	Mean ADP (SD) n = 39	Mean HC (SD) n = 39	Significance
Age		41.64 (8.63)	44.05 (10.52)	t(1,76) = 1.11, p = .27
Years of education		15.31 (3.05)	15.35 (2.98)	t(1,71) = .64, p = .95
Gender		M = 26	M = 22	χ^2(1,78) = .87, p = .35
AUDIT	0–41	22.11 (10.51)	4.17 (2.51)	t(1,71) = 9.97, p < 0.001
TAS-20 total	20–100	51.43 (10.83)	43.06 (8.62)	t(1,67) = 3.54, p = 0.001
TAS-20 DIDF	12–60	31.83 (8.16)	24.86 (7.20)	t(1,68) = 3.79, p < 0.001
TAS-20 EOT	8–40	11.97 (3.30)	11.36 (2.73)	t(1,71) = .86, p = .39
ERQ total	7–70	37.81 (7.95)	36.32 (8.56)	t(1,71) = .77, p = .45
ERQ Reappraisal	6–42	20.22 (5.87)	19.00 (7.80)	t(1,72) = .76, p = .45
ERQ Suppression	4–28	17.72 (5.01)	17.32 (5.10)	t(1,72) = .35, p = .73
Beck Depression Inventory	0–63	10.84 (9.58)	4.27 (6.28)	t(1,72) = 3.39, p = .001
Beck Anxiety Inventory	21–84	30.40 (8.73)	24.18 (4.56)	t(1,74) = 3.89, p < .001

Task Effects and Group Difference (Behavior)

Negative, Positive, Alcohol-Related, and Neutral Images

The three-way repeated-measures ANOVA with experienced emotion (mean VAS per condition) as the dependent variable, emotion type (negative, positive, neutral, alcohol related) and instruction (attend, reappraise) as within-subject factors, and group (ADP, HC) as between-subject factors did not reveal a significant three-way interaction [F(3,624) = 1.06, p = .36, d = .14]. Two-way interactions between participant group and instruction [F(1,624) = .53, p = .47, d = .06] or participant group and emotion type [F(3,624) = .19, p = .90, d = .06] also did not reveal any significant effect.

Results did reveal a significant interaction between emotion type and instruction [F(3,624) = 39.11, p < 0.001, d = .88], indicating that experienced emotion varied between emotion type and instruction. Simple effects analysis for this interaction revealed a significant difference between attending and reappraising neutral [mean difference = 7.66; F(1,624) = 17.06, p < 0.001, d = .33], positive [mean difference = 13.52; F(1,624) = 53.24, p < 0.001, d = .59], and negative images [mean difference = −13.46; F(1,624) = 52.79, p < 0.001, d = .59]. There was no difference between attending and reappraising alcohol-related images [mean difference = 2.59; F(1,624) = 1.96, p = .16, d = .11]. These results indicate that attending neutral [mean = 64.08, SD = 9.84] and positive (mean = 71.10, SD = 11.31) images resulted in the experience of positive emotions, which were reduced during reappraise condition for both neutral (mean = 56.43, SD = 7.58) and positive images (mean = 59.58, SD = 11.41). Attending negative images on the other hand resulted in the experience of negative emotion (mean = 28.13, SD = 13.04), which were reduced (i.e., less negative) in the reappraise condition (mean = 41.60, SD = 12.77; see **Figure 1**).

Independent-sample t tests assessing whether gender influenced experienced emotion during attending revealed no difference in positive, negative, neutral, or alcohol-related images, and also no differences during regulating positive, negative, or neutral images (all p > 0.006). However, female participants experienced more positive emotions during regulating alcohol-related images than male participants [mean = 56.15 (SD = 12.85) vs. mean = 47.27 (SD = 13.01), respectively; t(71) = 2.85, p = .006].

Craving

The repeated-measures ANOVA assessing craving levels revealed no significant interaction between time (pre/post) and participant group [ADP/HC; F(1,71) = .06, p = .81, d = 0.06], but significant main effects for time [F(1,71) = 29.42, p < 0.001, d = 1.29] and group [F(1,71) = 7.57, p < 0.01, d = .65]. These results indicated that the emotion reappraisal task significantly increased craving levels in both ADPs and HCs to an equal extent, but that craving levels in ADPs were overall higher (see **Figure 2**). The increase

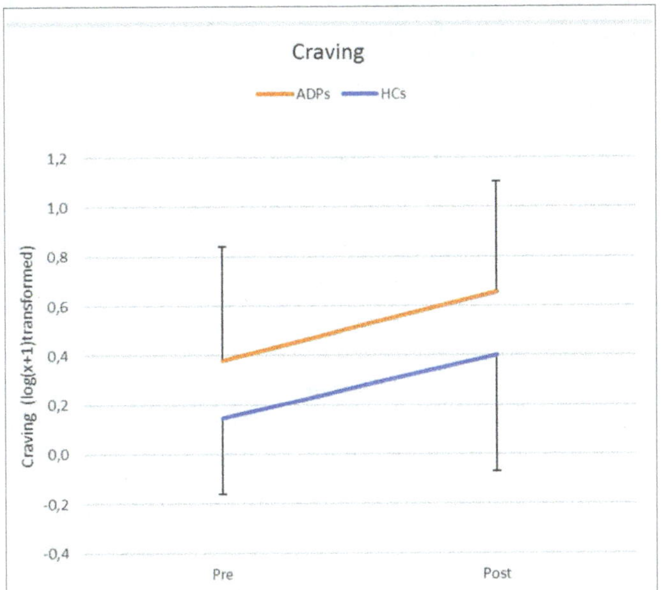

FIGURE 2 | Craving levels per group and time point [pre/post-emotion reappraisal task (ERT)]. Error bars reflect standard deviations. Craving levels were log(x + 1) transformed and refer to self-reported Alcohol Urge Questionnaire (AUQ) scores.

in craving (post/pre) did not correlate with experienced emotion per instruction and emotion type (all *p* values >0.1) in either ADPs, HCs, or over all subjects.

Functional Magnetic Resonance Imaging Results

Main Task Effects

In order to check the experimental manipulation of the emotion reappraisal task, the main effects of task, i.e., attend [attend emotion > attend neutral] and reappraise [reappraise > attend], were assessed for all emotions and both groups combined (see **Figure 3** and **Supplementary Table 1**). Results revealed that attending emotional images (versus neutral images) increased activity in the visual stream and posterior parietal cortex as well as the precentral gyrus. Our ROI analysis revealed no significant activations in the amygdala.

Reappraising images (versus attending) resulted in increased activation in several cortical structures previously implicated in emotion reappraisal, including the interior frontal gyrus, supplementary motor cortex, and middle frontal gyrus (see **Figure 3** and **Supplementary Table 1**). Furthermore, activity in the visual stream and the medial segment of the superior frontal gyrus was significantly higher during the attend relative to the reappraise condition (see **Figure 3** and **Supplementary Table 1**).

Group Differences in Brain Activation

Emotion Processing

The 3 × 2 ANOVA including the [attend emotion > attend neutral] contrasts per emotion (alcohol, positive, negative) and group (ADP, HC) revealed no significant interaction. The main effect of group showed that HCs have higher activity in the bilateral central operculum, precuneus, and superior temporal gyrus during appraising stimuli (see **Table 2** and **Figure 4A**). Furthermore, there was a significant main effect of emotion within the visual stream, but since these effects are not of main interest, they are reported in **Supplementary Information 2**.

Post hoc correlations between the posterior insula (peak voxel), which was significantly more activated during emotion processing (attend emotion > neutral), and both baseline craving levels and the increase in craving levels due to the emotion reappraisal task indicate a significant correlation for baseline craving levels with the posterior insula only for the APDs [$r(37) = .36$, $p = .03$] and not for the HCs [$r(33) = -.05$, $p = .76$]. This correlation seems to be related to the response to alcohol-related images in ADPs [$r(37) = .43$, $p < .01$, see **Figure 4B**], rather than the response to positive [$r(37) = .28$, $p = .09$] or negative images [$r(37) = .21$, $p = .21$].

Emotion Reappraisal

The 4 × 2 ANOVA for including the [reappraise > attend] contrasts per emotion (alcohol, neutral, positive, negative) and

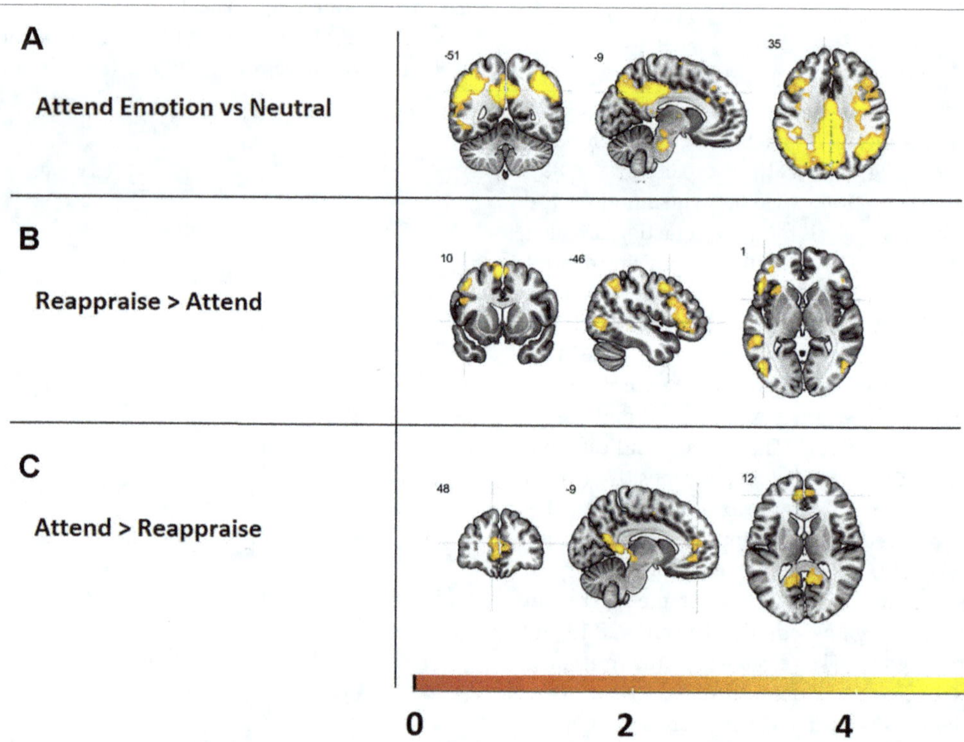

FIGURE 3 | Main effects of the emotion reappraisal task, presented at a threshold of $k > 5$, $p < 0.001$. Top: Brain areas activated while attending emotional images versus neutral images. Middle: activated brain areas during reappraising vs. attending images. Bottom: regions more activated during attending images vs. reappraising images.

TABLE 2 | Main effect of participant group for attending emotional vs. neutral images. *T*, *t* value; *K*, cluster size in voxels; *x*, *y*, *z* are coordinates.

Brain area (attend emotion > neutral)	L/R	*T*	*K*	*x*	*y*	*z*	*p* value (FWE-corrected)
HC > ADP							
Posterior Insula	Left	5.22	70	−36	−10	22	<.001
Parietal Operculum	Right	5.06	100	33	−34	19	0.01
Precuneus	Right	5.00	37	15	−55	28	.013
Central Operculum	Right	4.73	25	42	−7	19	.039
Superior Temporal Gyrus	Right	4.67	18	−21	−7	40	.048
ADP > HC							
n.a.							

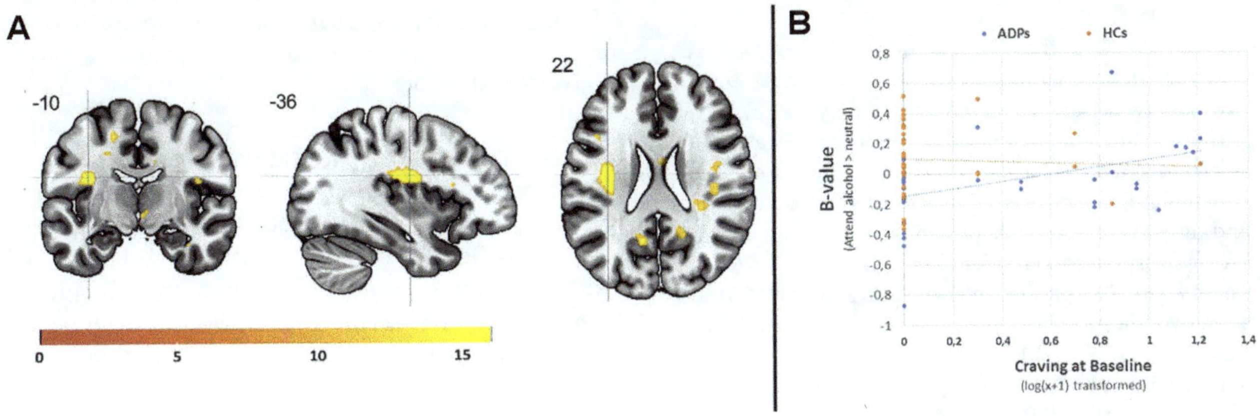

FIGURE 4 | (A) Graphical presentation of the increased activity in healthy controls (HCs) compared to alcohol-dependent patients (ADPs), during emotion processing (attending negative, positive, and alcohol-related images vs. neutral). Crosshair is pointed at the peak voxel in the posterior insula. **(B)** The correlation between the posterior insula and baseline craving levels for the [attend alcohol > neutral] contrast. The threshold for visualization of the results is set at $k > 5$, $p < 0.001$ uncorrected.

group (ADP, HC) revealed no significant interaction or any main effect of group. There was, however, a significant main effect of emotion, indicating a difference in neural response between the neutral, alcohol, positive, and negative images in the visual stream. Since these results are not of main interest, they are reported in **Supplementary Information 2.**

DISCUSSION

This study investigated differences in emotion processing and reappraisal between alcohol-dependent patients (ADPs) and healthy controls (HCs) at the behavioral and the neural level. The emotion reappraisal task was completed successfully as indicated by increased experienced emotion in the attend condition and successful regulation of these emotions in the reappraisal condition. Our results do not show that ADPs have impaired emotion reappraisal based on this paradigm and the emotion regulation questionnaire, nor do they show any difference between ADPs and HCs in neural recruitment during cognitive reappraisal. However, our results do show a reduced neural response to emotional images (in comparison to neutral images) in ADPs versus HCs in the central operculum, precuneus, and superior temporal gyrus. Furthermore, self-reported craving levels increased from pre- to post-testing similarly in both groups, although overall craving levels were significantly higher in ADPs. Finally, self-reported baseline craving levels were correlated to higher neural reactivity to attending alcohol-related images in the ADP group.

The abovementioned results mostly do not correspond with our hypotheses, since we expected reduced emotion regulation ability and decreased associated brain activity in ADPs compared to HCs. These hypotheses were based on a recent review, which indicated reduced emotion regulation abilities and brain function in substance use disorders (14). However, the studies included in this review were mostly studies on emotional reactivity, implicit reappraisal, or behavioral control tasks and are therefore different from our explicit reappraisal paradigm. This may well be a major explanation for our (lack of expected) results, since explicit emotion regulation requires conscious effort, monitoring, and insight, whereas implicit emotion regulation is more automatic. Previous studies also show that ADPs make less use of these effortful emotion regulation strategies in daily life (16). Our results may differ from these previous studies because our participants were actively instructed to regulate their emotions by applying effortful cognitive reappraisal strategies. The fact that we do not show impaired emotion regulation abilities or differences in related brain function when *instructed* to apply these strategies may point to impairments in the selection of the appropriate reappraisal strategy rather than the ability itself. Of note, the ERQ also did not reveal any differences in emotion reappraisal or suppression between ADPs and HCs. This result is surprising, since the ADP group did self-report higher levels of anxiety and depression. Nevertheless, limited availability and access to emotion regulation strategies has been suggested and found by Khosravani et al. (15) and supports the aforementioned explanation. These results may imply that treatment should focus on selecting the right reappraisal strategy, rather than on reappraisal abilities.

In line with our hypothesis, we show that ADPs and HCs score their experienced emotion (using VAS scores) equally during the attend condition for all emotion types. However, ADPs do show significantly lower brain activity during attending the stimuli in several brain areas, including the posterior insula, central operculum, precuneus, and superior temporal gyrus. These findings are in line with previous studies suggesting a blunted neural response to emotional images in APDs (20) and marijuana smokers (19), participants with excess weight (38), and with studies hypothesizing a blunted response to non-addiction-relevant emotional stimuli (21).

In contrast with our hypothesis, the reappraisal task induced craving equally in both ADPs and HCs. This may be explained by a mismatch between specific preferences from the individual ADPs (e.g., someone who only drinks beer) and the diversity of alcohol-related images that were presented (beer, wine, liquor, bar, supermarket), which may have dampened the craving inducing effect. Future studies should consider a personalized approach, matching the presented images to the subject's specific preference.

Comparing our data to data from the Dutch national monitoring system for drug- and alcohol-dependent patients (39), our ADP group was slightly younger (41 years vs. 46 years), but gender distribution was comparable (67% vs. 72% male). Our ADP participants were in treatment for alcohol dependence but were medication free since the use of psychoactive medication was an exclusion criterion. This is atypical for most treatment-seeking alcohol-dependent patients who are often prescribed anti-craving medication. It is possible that patients who are not prescribed any medication (e.g., our participants) experience less craving compared to ADPs who are prescribed medication since severe craving can be an indication to prescribe medication. Possibly the ADPs included in this study experienced less craving than ADPs who are prescribed psychoactive medication, which may explain the similar effects of the emotion regulation task on craving levels for ADPs and HCs in this study. Our *post hoc* correlations in APDs are in line with this explanation, since they reveal that higher baseline craving levels are associated with more activity within the posterior insula while attending alcohol-related images. In other words, ADPs who experience higher baseline craving levels have a stronger neural response to alcohol-related images in a brain region that has previously been implicated in cue-induced craving in alcohol-dependent patients (22).

Together, these results suggest that ADPs show a blunted response to emotional images when compared to HC, but also that within the ADP group, higher craving levels are associated with a "less" blunted neural response to alcohol-related images. Previous studies indicate that reduced responsiveness to emotional cues could be caused by reduced salience of these cues in comparison to addiction-relevant cues (21) and these findings are in line with our results. Another explanation, which we could not confirm with the available data, is that a reduced neural reaction to emotional images may serve as an implicit protective mechanism. Since a higher response to emotional images has been linked to craving (22), reducing this response may lead to less craving. This explanation, however, is speculative and should be investigated further.

Strengths and Limitations

The current study assessed emotion reappraisal as well as emotion processing in alcohol dependence through a comprehensive study, using both questionnaires, behavioral data, as well as fMRI. Despite the strengths of this study, we only studied one form of emotion regulation (reappraisal), and future studies should incorporate multiple emotion regulation strategies, including, e.g., voluntary emotion reappraisal, avoidance, or distraction. Although the reappraisal task induced craving in ADPs and HCs, it is not possible to clarify which images or conditions caused this effect because craving was measured only before and after the reappraisal task, and this may be an explanation why none of the conditions correlated with the increase in craving levels.

The lack of a clear distinction in emotional reappraisal between ADPs and HCs might be explained by insufficient emotional impact of the images that were used in the task. The IAPS database images may lack ecological validity, thus reducing the impact of these images and thus facilitating the emotion reappraisal process. On the other hand, using a comparable task (without the alcohol-related images), we were previously able to differentiate between HCs and patients with obsessive–compulsive disorder during emotion processing, but not during emotional reappraisal (40). Future studies should consider other ways of inducing emotions with higher ecological validity, including personalized scripts, personalized images, or the use of virtual reality. Additionally, future studies should consider incorporating measurements of personality disorders, including borderline personality disorder, that have previously been linked to impaired emotion reappraisal (41), but were not used in the current study.

CONCLUSION

The current study showed neither impaired reappraisal of emotion

ADPs compared to HCs. The results might have been influenced by some methodological limitations, although we did demonstrate a blunted neural response in ADPs while attending emotional (positive, negative, alcohol-related) images. Moreover, baseline craving levels were correlated to a less blunted neural response to alcohol-related images in ADPs. Together, these results may suggest a link between emotional reactivity and craving, and impaired natural emotion processing in alcohol dependence, whereas ADPs show unimpaired reappraisal abilities when explicitly *instructed.* Future studies should assess voluntary reappraisal abilities, more ecologically valid ways of inducing emotions, and compensatory mechanisms in ADPs to further understand the differences during natural (re)appraisal of emotional cues.

AUTHOR CONTRIBUTIONS

All authors made a significant contribution to this article, including acquiring funding (AG and WB), study design (AG and WB), development of the emotion reappraisal task (SW, OH, DV, and YD), data acquisition (JJ), data analysis (JJ, DV, and SW), interpretation of results (JJ, AG, SW, OH, YD, WB, and DV) and contributions to this manuscript (JJ, AG, SW, OH, YD, WB, and DV).

REFERENCES

1. Ochsner KN, Bunge SA, Gross JJ, Gabrieli JDE. Rethinking feelings: an fMRI study of the cognitive regulation of emotion. *J Cogn Neurosci* (2002) 14(8):1215–29. doi: 10.1162/089892902760807212
2. Ochsner KN, Gross JJ. The cognitive control of emotion. *Trends Cogn Sci* (2005) 9(5):242–9. doi: 10.1016/j.tics.2005.03.010
3. Banks SJ, Eddy KT, Angstadt M, Nathan PJ, Phan KL. Amygdala-frontal connectivity during emotion regulation. *Soc Cog Affect Neurosci* (2007) 2(4):303–12. doi: 10.1093/scan/nsm029
4. Buhle JT, Silvers JA, Wager TD, Lopez R, Onyemekwu C, Kober, et al. Cognitive reappraisal of emotion: a meta-analysis of human neuroimaging studies. *Cereb Cortex* (2013) 24(11):2981–90.
5. Dosenbach NU, Fair DA, Miezin FM, Cohen AL, Wenger KK, Dosenbach RA, et al. Distinct brain networks for adaptive and stable task control in humans. *Proc Natl Acad Sci* (2007) 104(26):11073–8. doi: 10.1073/pnas.0704320104
6. Simons JS, Carey KB, Wills TA. Alcohol abuse and dependence symptoms: a multidimensional model of common and specific etiology. *Psychol Addict Behav* (2009) 23(3):415. doi: 10.1037/a0016003
7. Baker TB, Piper ME, McCarthy DE, Majeskie MR, Fiore MC. Addiction motivation reformulated: an affective processing model of negative reinforcement. *Psychol Rev* (2004) 111(1):33. doi: 10.1037/0033-295X.111.1.33
8. Birch CD, Stewart SH, Wall AM, McKee SA, Eisnor SJT, JA. Mood-induced increases in alcohol expectancy strength in internally motivated drinkers. *Psychol Addict Behav* (2004) 18(3):231. doi: 10.1037/0893-164X.18.3.231
9. Sinha R, Fox HC, Hong KA, Bergquist K, Bhagwagar Z, Siedlarz KM. Enhanced negative emotion and alcohol craving, and altered physiological responses following stress and cue exposure in alcohol dependent individuals. *Neuropsychopharmacology* (2008) 34(5):1198–208. doi: 10.1038/npp.2008.78
10. Serre F, Fatseas MD, C.Swendsen J, Auriacombe M. Predictors of craving and substance use among patients with alcohol, tobacco, cannabis or opiate addictions: commonalities and specificities across substances. *Addict Behav* (2018) 83:123–9. doi: 10.1016/j.addbeh.2018.01.041
11. Berking M, Wupperman P, Reichardt A, Pejic T, Dippel A, Znoj H. Emotion-regulation skills as a treatment target in psychotherapy. *Behav Res Therapy* (2008) 46(11):1230–7. doi: 10.1016/j.brat.2008.08.005
12. Sinha R. How does stress lead to risk of alcohol relapse? *Alcohol Res* (2011) 34(4):432–40.
13. Yip SW, Gross JJ, Chawla MM, SS, Shi XH, Liu L, et al. Is neural processing of negative stimuli altered in addiction independent of drug effects? Findings from drug-naïve youth with internet gaming disorder. *Neuropsychopharmacology* (2018) 43(6):1364. doi: 10.1038/npp.2017.283
14. Wilcox CE, Pommy JM, Adinoff B. Neural circuitry of impaired emotion regulation in substance use disorders. *Am J Psychiatry* (2016) 173(3):344–61. doi: 10.1176/appi.ajp.2015.15060710
15. Khosravani V, Bastan FS, Ghorbani F, Kamali Z. Difficulties in emotion regulation mediate negative and positive affects and craving in alcoholic patients. *Addict Behav* (2017) 71:5–81. doi: 10.1016/j.addbeh.2017.02.029
16. Petit G, Luminet O, Maurage F, Tecco J, Lechantre S, Ferauge M, et al. Emotion regulation in alcohol dependence. *Alcohol Clin Exp Res* (2015) 39(12):2471–9. doi: 10.1111/acer.12914
17. Kopera M, Trucco EM, Jakubczyk A, Suszek H, Michalska A, Majewska A, et al. Interpersonal and intrapersonal emotional processes in individuals treated for alcohol use disorder and non-addicted healthy individuals. *Addict Behav* (2018) 79:8–13. doi: 10.1016/j.addbeh.2017.12.006
18. Kopera M, Jakubczyk A, Suszek H, Glass JM, Klimkiewicz A, Wnorowska A, et al. Relationship between emotional processing, drinking severity and relapse in adults treated for alcohol dependence in Poland. *Alcohol Alcohol* (2014) 50(2):173–9. doi: 10.1093/alcalc/agu099
19. Gruber SA, Rogowska J, Yurgelun-Todd DA. Altered affective response in marijuana smokers: an FMRI study. *Drug Alcohol Depend* (2009) 105(1–2):139–53. doi: 10.1016/j.drugalcdep.2009.06.019
20. Marinkovic K, Oscar-Berman M, Urban T, O'Reilly CE, Howard JA, Sawyer K, et al. Alcoholism and dampened temporal limbic activation to emotional faces. *Alcohol Clin Exp Res* (2009) 33(11):1880–92. doi: 10.1111/j.1530-0277.2009.01026.x
21. Verdejo-Garcia APGM, Pérez-García M, Bechara A. Emotion, decision-making and substance dependence: a somatic-marker model of addiction. *Curr Neuropharmacol* (2006) 4(1):17–31. doi: 10.2174/157015906775203057
22. Fox HC, Bergquist KL, Hong KI, Sinha R. Stress-induced and alcohol cue-induced craving in recently abstinent alcohol-dependent individuals. *Alcohol Clin Exp Res* (2007) 31(3):395–403. doi: 10.1111/j.1530-0277.2006.00320.x
23. Wittchen HU. Reliability and validity studies of the WHO-Composite International Diagnostic Interview (CIDI): a critical review. *J Psychiatr Res* (1994) 28(1):57–84.
24. Babor TF, Higgins-Biddle JC, Saunders JB, Monteiro MG. The alcohol use disorders identification test. In Department of Mental Health and Substance Dependence. In: *Guidelines for use in primary care*. Geneva: World Health Organisation (2001).
25. Beck AT, Steer RA, Carbin MG. Psychometric properties of the Beck Depression Inventory: twenty-five years of evaluation. *Clin Psychol Rev* (1988) 8(1):77–100. doi: 10.1016/0272-7358(88)90050-5
26. Beck AT, Epstein N, Brown G, Steer RA. An inventory for measuring clinical anxiety: psychometric properties. *J Consult Clin Psychol* (1988) 56(6):893. doi: 10.1037/0022-006X.56.6.893
27. Kooiman CG, Spinhoven P, Trijsburg RW. The assessment of alexithymia: a critical review of the literature and a psychometric study of the Toronto Alexithymia Scale-20. *J Psychosom Res* (2002) 53(6):1083–90. doi: 10.1016/S0022-3999(02)00348-3
28. Gross JJ, John OP. Individual differences in two emotion regulation processes: implications for affect, relationships, and well-being. *J Pers Soc Psychol* (2003) 85(2):348.
29. Bohn MJ, Krahn DD, Staehler BA. Development and initial validation of a measure of drinking urges in abstinent alcoholics. *Alcohol Clin Exp Res* (1995) 19(3):600–6. doi: 10.1111/j.1530-0277.1995.tb01554.x
30. Lang S, Bradley MM, Cuthbert BN. *International Affective Picture System (IAPS): Technical manual and affective ratings*. Center for research in Psychophysiology. Gainesville: University of Florida (1999).
31. Vollstädt-Klein S, Loeber S, Kirsch M, Bach P, Richter A, Bühler M, et al. Effects of cue-exposure treatment on neural cue reactivity in alcohol dependence: a randomized trial. *Biol Psychiatry* (2011) 69(11):1060–6. doi: 10.1016/j.biopsych.2010.12.016

32. Bradley MM, Lang PJ. Measuring emotion: the self-assessment manikin and the semantic differential. *J Behav Ther Exp Psychiatry* (1994) 25(1):49–59. doi: 10.1016/0005-7916(94)90063-9
33. Choi JS, Kim MJ, Kim JH, Choi JY, Chung YE, Park MS, et al. Comparison of multi-echo and single-echo gradient-recalled echo sequences for SPIO-enhanced Liver MRI at 3 T. *Clin Radiol* (2010) 65(11):916–23. doi: 10.1016/j.crad.2010.07.003
34. Boschloo L, Vogelzangs N, Smit JH, van den Brink W, Veltman DJ, Beekman AT, et al. Comorbidity and risk indicators for alcohol use disorders among persons with anxiety and/or depressive disorders: findings from the Netherlands Study of Depression and Anxiety (NESDA). *J Affect Disord* (2011) 131(1):233–42. doi: 10.1016/j.jad.2010.12.014
35. Davis L, Uezato A, Newell JM, Frazier E. Major depression and comorbid substance use disorders. *Curr Opin Psychiatry* (2008) 21(1):14–8. doi: 10.1097/YCO.0b013e3282f32408
36. Morie KP, Yip SW, Nich C, Hunkele KC, KM, Potenza MN. Alexithymia and addiction: a review and preliminary data suggesting neurobiological links to reward/loss processing. *Curr Addict Rep* (2016) 3(2):239–48. doi: 10.1007/s40429-016-0097-8
37. Stevens, J. *Applied multivariate statistics for the social sciences* (2nd ed.). Hillsdale, NJ, US: Lawrence Erlbaum Associates, Inc. (1992).
38. Steward T, Picó-Pérez M, Mata F, Martínez-Zalacaín I, Cano M, Contreras-Rodríguez O, et al. Emotion regulation and excess weight: impaired affective processing characterized by dysfunctional insula activation and connectivity. *PLoS One* (2016) 11(3):e0152150. doi: 10.1371/journal.pone.0152150
39. Wisselink DJ, Kuijpers WGT, Mol A (2015).Kerncijfers verslavingszorg 2014 (LADIS). http://www.ladis.eu/nl/over-ladis/kerncijfers
40. De Wit SJ, van der Werf YD, Mataix-Cols D, Trujillo JP, van Oppen P, Veltman DJ, et al. Emotion regulation before and after transcranial magnetic stimulation in obsessive compulsive disorder. *Psychol Med* (2015) 45(15):3059–73. doi: 10.1017/S0033291715001026
41. Axelrod SR, Perepletchikova F, Holtzman K, Sinha R. Emotion regulation and substance use frequency in women with substance dependence and borderline personality disorder receiving dialectical behavior therapy. *Am J Drug Alcohol Abuse* (2011) 37(1):37–42. doi: 10.3109/00952990.2010.535582

13

An Examination of Motivation to Change and Neural Alcohol Cue Reactivity Following a Brief Intervention

*Erica N. Grodin[1,2], Aaron C. Lim[1], James MacKillop[3], Mitchell P. Karno[2] and Lara A. Ray[1,2]**

[1] Department of Psychology, University of California, Los Angeles, Los Angeles, CA, United States, [2] Department of Psychiatry and Biobehavioral Sciences, UCLA School of Medicine, University of California, Los Angeles, Los Angeles, CA, United States, [3] Department of Psychiatry and Behavioral Neurosciences, McMaster University, Hamilton, ON, Canada

Correspondence:
Lara A. Ray
lararay@psych.ucla.edu

Background: Brief interventions represent a promising psychological intervention targeting individuals with heavy alcohol use. Motivation to change represents an individual's openness to engage in a behavior change strategy and is thought to be a crucial component of brief interventions. Neuroimaging techniques provide a translational tool to investigate the neurobiological mechanisms underlying potential mediators of treatment response, including motivation to change. Therefore, this study aimed to examine the effect of a brief intervention on motivation to change drinking behavior and neural alcohol taste cue reactivity.

Methods: Non–treatment-seeking heavy drinkers were randomized to receive a brief drinking intervention (n = 22) or an attention-matched control (n = 24). Three indices of motivation to change were assessed at baseline and after the intervention or control session: importance, confidence, and readiness. Immediately following the intervention or control session, participants also underwent an functional magnetic resonance imaging (fMRI) during which they completed an alcohol taste cues paradigm.

Results: There was a significant effect of the brief intervention on increasing ratings of importance of changing drinking behavior, but not on ratings of confidence or readiness to change. Ratings of importance after the intervention or control session were associated with neural alcohol taste cue reactivity, but notably, this effect was only significant for participants who received the intervention. Individuals in the intervention condition showed a positive association between ratings of importance and activation in the precuneus, posterior cingulate, and insula.

Conclusions: The brief drinking intervention was successful at improving one dimension of motivation to change among non–treatment-seeking heavy drinkers. The brief intervention moderated the relationship between ratings of importance and brain activation in circuitry associated with interoceptive awareness and self-reflection. Together, findings represent an initial step toward understanding the neurobiological mechanisms through which a brief intervention may improve motivation to change.

Keywords: brief intervention, mechanisms of behavior change, motivation to change, alcohol, functional magnetic resonance imaging

INTRODUCTION

An increasing number of individuals engage in heavy alcohol use, putting themselves at risk of myriad health, psychological, and social consequences (1). Brief interventions represent a promising psychological intervention targeting individuals with heavy alcohol use who have not yet progressed to moderate or severe alcohol use disorder (AUD). Brief interventions are short (5 to 60 min), traditionally one to five sessions, interventions designed to increase motivation for behavioral change and encourage self-monitoring of high-risk situations for heavy drinking (2). Although specific therapeutic techniques vary, many of these interventions seek to increase motivation by providing individuals normative feedback about individualized risk of developing AUD, inquiring about the desire to change their drinking, and working collaboratively to explore and develop behavior change options (3). Meta-analyses have identified small yet robust effects of brief interventions on alcohol consumption that can be flexibly administered in multiple settings, including hospital emergency departments, primary care, and *via* digital/tele-therapy (2–4). Brief interventions have also been shown to sustain drinking reductions at 12-month follow-up (4).

Motivation for change is conceptualized as a multi-dimensional, dynamic construct representing one's openness to engage in a behavior change strategy (5), and is thought to be a crucial component of brief interventions (6, 7). High levels of motivation for change have been considered a prerequisite for successful treatment response. For instance, among individuals with comorbid substance use disorders and serious mental illness, high motivation was associated with reporting greater cons and fewer benefits to using substances, and taking steps to reduce substance use (8). Motivation for change was also associated with higher client reports of therapeutic alliance with therapists among treatment-seeking problem drinkers (9). Among homeless individuals placed in a housing intervention program, motivation for change was a stronger predictor of alcohol outcomes than treatment attendance (10). Many brief interventions for AUD have, therefore, focused on enhancing motivation for change given its importance in treatment engagement and outcomes.

To advance the literature on behavior change applied to alcohol use, current scientific efforts have focused on elucidating the specific mechanisms of behavior change, including underlying neural-level substrates that subserve changes in alcohol use. To that end, neuroimaging techniques provide a translational tool to investigate the neurobiological mechanisms underlying potential moderators of treatment response. Several studies to date have used neuroimaging to probe the underlying neurobiological mechanisms of psychosocial interventions (11–14). Three studies have examined the mechanisms of motivational interviewing interventions in alcohol-using populations (11, 14, 15). These studies investigated the importance of client and therapist speech as components of motivational interview interventions. The first study found that client change talk was effective in attenuating neural reward response to alcohol cues (11). The second study found that the origin of client change language is crucial for motivational interventions; self-generated change talk and counter-change talk were associated with increased activation in brain regions associated with introspection and self-awareness, when contrasted with experimenter selected language (14). The third study found that therapist statements designed to encourage complex reflections were associated with neural response in brain regions associated with reward and self-reflection, when contrasted with closed questions from therapists (15). Together, these studies provide evidence that neuroimaging can be successfully used to investigate the neurobiological mechanisms of brief interventions for alcohol use.

Although motivation for behavioral change has been identified as a critical component of behavioral interventions, no translational studies have yet explored how the relationship between psychological interventions and motivational change are represented neurobiologically. Identifying a neurobiological substrate of a behavior change target, in this case motivation for change, is critical for understanding the mechanisms of behavior change (16, 17). There are several brain regions that may be involved in these processes, particularly those that are associated with incentive salience and introspection. Brain regions implicated in incentive salience processing in addictive disorders include the ventral striatum (nucleus accumbens), dorsal striatum (caudate and putamen), and the orbitofrontal cortex (18, 19). Brain regions involved in self-reflection and introspection include the posterior cingulate cortex, precuneus, and insula (12, 14).

We recently conducted a study designed to examine the effectiveness of a brief intervention on improving drinking outcomes and modulating neural alcohol cue reactivity (20). This study randomly assigned non–treatment-seeking heavy drinkers to receive a single-session brief intervention or to an attention-matched control condition. The brief intervention was designed to help participants understand their individual level of drinking risk and help initiate changes in their alcohol use. Participants completed an alcohol taste cue reactivity paradigm during a functional magnetic resonance imaging (fMRI) scan immediately following the intervention. Participants completed a follow-up visit one month after the intervention to report on their drinking behavior. There was no significant effect of the brief intervention on drinking outcomes at follow-up or on modulating neural alcohol taste cue reactivity.

A better understanding of the neurobiological mechanisms of how brief interventions work through motivational change may help improve treatments for alcohol using populations. Therefore, this secondary analysis (20) aimed to examine the effect of a brief intervention on motivation to change drinking behavior and neural alcohol taste cue reactivity. To do so, we first tested whether the brief intervention had an effect on proximal outcomes of motivation to change (i.e., readiness rulers). We hypothesized that participants in the brief intervention condition would exhibit greater motivation to change compared to the control group. We also examined the association between motivational readiness and alcohol taste cue reactivity and assessed if the brief intervention moderated this association. We hypothesized motivation to change would be positively related to neural alcohol cue reactivity in circuitry associated with introspection and self-reflection and negatively related to neural alcohol cue reactivity in regions implicated in reward and incentive salience. We further hypothesized that these relationships would be stronger in the intervention condition compared to the control condition.

MATERIALS AND METHODS

Participants and Screening Procedures

The study protocol and all procedures were approved by the Institutional Review Board of the University of California, Los Angeles. Detailed methodology of the general screening and experimental procedures has been published elsewhere (20) and are summarized here. Interested participants completed an initial telephone interview and eligible participants were invited to participate in an in-person screening visit. Upon arrival, all participants read and signed an informed consent form in accordance with the Declaration of Helsinki. During the in-person screening visit, participants completed a psychiatric diagnostic interview and a battery of individual difference measures, including demographics and alcohol and drug use assessments. All participants were required to have a breath alcohol concentration of 0.000 g/dl and to test negative on a urine drug test (except for marijuana, which was allowed to be positive).

Participants were non–treatment-seeking heavy drinkers, indicated by consuming five or more drinks per occasion for men or four or more drinks per occasion for women at least four times in the month preceding study enrollment, and who scored at least an 8 on the Alcohol Use Disorder Identification Test (AUDIT) (21). A total of 120 participants were screened in the laboratory for eligibility; 38 did not meet inclusion criteria, and 12 elected not to participate, leaving 60 participants who were enrolled and randomized. Of the 60 participants randomized, 46 participants completed the entire study. Participants who completed all study visits were compensated US $160.

Study Design

Participants were assessed at three time-points: at baseline, at randomization, and 1-month follow-up. During the randomization visit, participants were randomly assigned to receive a one-session brief drinking intervention or to an attention-matched control condition. Immediately following the intervention or control session, participants completed an fMRI scan to assess brain activity during exposure to alcohol and water taste cues. Participants returned for a follow-up visit approximately 4 weeks after the intervention or control session to assess alcohol use.

The brief intervention consisted of a 30- to 45-min individual face-to-face session based on the principles of motivational interviewing (22, 23) and adhered to the FRAMES model, which includes personal feedback (F), emphasizing personal responsibility (R), providing brief advice (A), offering a menu (M) of change options, conveying empathy (E), and encouraging self-efficacy (S). The aim of the intervention was to help participants understand their level of risk and to help initiate changes in their alcohol use. Participants randomized to the attention-matched control condition viewed a 30-min video about astronomy. In the control condition, there was no mention of alcohol or drug use beyond completion of research assessments.

Individual Difference Measures

The following individual questionnaires and interviews were administered during the study: 1) the 30-day timeline follow-back (TLFB) was administered in interview format to capture daily alcohol use over the 30 days prior to the visit (24), 2) the self-report AUDIT was administered to assess for drinking severity (21), and 3) the Penn Alcohol Craving Scale (PACS) was administered to assess alcohol craving (25). Participants also completed the Fagerstrom Test for Nicotine Dependence (26). The Structured Clinical Interview for DSM-5 (SCID) (27) was administered by a clinician to assess for lifetime and current AUD. Lastly, participants completed a demographics questionnaire reporting, among other variables, age, sex, and level of education.

Motivation to Change Assessment

At each visit, participants also completed three decision rulers designed to measure their motivation to change their drinking behavior [based on Refs. (5, 28)]. Participants were asked to rate on a scale from 1 to 10: "As of now how important is it for you to make a change in your drinking?" (importance ruler), "If you decided to make a change in your drinking how confident are you that you could do it?" (confidence ruler), and "As of now how ready are you to make a change in your drinking?" (readiness ruler).

Neuroimaging Procedures

At the start of the scanning visit, participants were required to have a BrAC of 0.00 g/dl and a urine toxicology screen negative for all drugs (excluding tetrahydrocannabinol). Additionally, female participants were required to have a negative pregnancy test.

Neuroimaging data were acquired on a 3.0T Siemens Prisma scanner at the UCLA Staglin Center for Cognitive Neuroscience. Detailed neuroimaging parameters can be found in Grodin et al. (20). Briefly, the protocol consisted of a high-resolution, matched-bandwidth (MBW) scan and a structural magnetization-prepared rapid-acquisition gradient echo (MPRAGE) scan. This was followed by two runs of a modified version of the Alcohol Cues Task, which involves the delivery of oral alcohol or control (water) tastes to elicit physiological reward responses (29, 30). During the task, participants were presented with a visual cue indicating the trial type (Alcohol Taste or Water Taste), which was followed by a fixation cue and the delivery of the alcohol or water taste (1 ml).

Preprocessing of the neuroimaging data followed conventional procedures implemented in FMRIB's Software Library (FSL 5.0) (www.fmrib.ox.ac.uk/fsl). This included motion correction [Motion Correction Linear Image Registration Tool (McFLIRT, Version 5.0)], high-pass temporal filtering (100-s cutoff) using FSL's FMRI Expert Analysis Tool (FEAT, Version 6.00), and smoothing with a 5-mm full-width at half-maximum Gaussian kernel. FSL's Brain Extract Tool (BET) was used to remove skull and non-brain tissue from both the structural and functional scans. Data were denoised using ICA-AROMA (31) to reduce motion artifacts associated with swallowing.

Data Analysis

General linear models with OLS regression were used to test the main effect of study condition on each of the three motivation-for-change decision rulers (importance, confidence, and readiness). Analyses were adjusted for baseline AUDIT score, age, sex, smoking status, and the baseline ratings from the corresponding decision ruler.

The analysis of the Alcohol Cues Task was conducted using FSL's FEAT as described in Ref. (20). Briefly, alcohol and water taste cues were convolved with a double-gamma hemodynamic response function (HRF). Six motion regressors representing translational and rotational head movement were included as regressors of no interest. Data for each subject were registered to the MBW, followed by the MPRAGE using affine linear transformations, and then were normalized to the Montreal Neurological Institute (MNI avg152) template. Registration was refined using FSL's non-linear registration tool. The primary contrast of interest, the Alcohol Taste Cue > Control Taste Cue contrast, was defined in the first-level models. The second-level model combined the contrast images across the two task runs, within subjects. The third-level model combined the contrast images between subjects. To evaluate if the intervention moderated the association between motivational readiness ratings and brain activation to alcohol taste cues, three interaction models were run with baseline-corrected ratings of importance, confidence, and readiness mean-centered across all subjects. Age, sex, cigarette smoking status, positive urine for tetrahydrocannabinol (THC), and AUD severity were entered as covariates. Z-statistic images were thresholded using a cluster threshold of $Z > 2.3$ and a (corrected) cluster significance threshold of $P < 0.05$ (32). Given the exploratory nature of this study and the dearth of studies on behavioral interventions, neural reactivity to alcohol cues, and mechanisms of motivation to change, we also implemented a more restrictive approach presented in the **Supplementary Materials**. Specifically, we conducted a separate set of analyses using the regions significantly activated in the Alcohol Taste Cue > Water Taste Cue contrast as a mask to investigate if the intervention moderated the association between motivation to change ratings and task-specific brain activation. As the neuroimaging literature has not reached a standard whereby such masks are systematically used to test treatment effects, we provide both approaches in this manuscript (33).

RESULTS

Effect of Brief Intervention on Motivation to Change Ratings

The groups significantly differed on their post-session ratings of importance ($F_{1,40} = 8.77, p = 0.005$), after controlling for age, gender, smoking status, and baseline ratings of importance. Specifically, the intervention group had higher post-session ratings of importance than the control group (intervention group, 6.27 ± 0.39; control group, 4.67 ± 0.37; predicted values). However, there was no significant effect of group on ratings of confidence ($F_{1,40} = 1.35, p = 0.25$; intervention group: 7.13 ± 0.44; control group: 6.25 ± 0.42; predicted values) or readiness ($F_{1,40} = 0.04$; $p = 0.85$; intervention group, 4.73 ± 0.48; control group, 4.62 ± 0.43; predicted values) following the intervention or control sessions (see **Table 1**).

Relationship of Motivation to Change and Neural Alcohol Taste Cue Reactivity

Importance Ruler

Averaging across intervention and control groups, there was no significant association between importance ratings and brain activation to alcohol taste cues. However, consistent with our hypothesis, there was a significant interaction between group and importance ratings on brain activation to alcohol vs. water taste. Specifically, there was a positive association between importance ratings and brain activation in frontal, limbic, and visual regions in the active intervention group ($p < 0.05$ corrected), whereas there was no significant association in the control group (see **Figure 1**, **Table 2**).

For the analyses restricted to the mask representing significant clusters for Alcohol Taste Cue > Control Taste Cue, averaging across intervention, and control groups, there was no significant association between importance ratings and brain activation masked within the alcohol taste cue > water taste cue contrast. There was a significant interaction between group and importance ratings on brain activation to alcohol vs. water taste. Specifically, there was a positive association between importance ratings and brain activation in frontal regions, including the middle and superior frontal gyri and paracingulate, in the active intervention

TABLE 1 | Participant characteristics.

Characteristics	Intervention group (n = 22)	Control group (n = 24)	Statistic	p
Age	36.41 ± 13.56	32.29 ± 9.89	t = 1.18	0.24
Sex (M/F)	13/9	15/9	$\chi^2 = 0.06$	0.81
Cigarette smokers (n)	11	12	$\chi^2 = 0.00$	1
THC positive (n)	6	6	$\chi^2 = 0.04$	0.86
Education (years)	15.45 ± 2.13	15.04 ± 1.78	t = 0.72	0.48
AUDIT total score	17.68 ± 6.49	17.17 ± 7.61	t = 0.25	0.81
PACS score	19.32 ± 6.94	18.79 ± 7.15	t = 0.25	0.80
AUD severity (no diagnosis/ mild/moderate/severe)	1/9/5/7	5/8/5/6	$\chi^2 = 0.95$	0.34
Baseline Visit Motivation Ruler Ratings (T1)				
Importance ruler	4.27 ± 2.53	5.25 ± 2.80	t = 1.21	0.23
Confidence ruler	5.68 ± 2.67	6.08 ± 2.43	t = 0.52	0.60
Readiness ruler	3.23 ± 1.88	3.88 ± 2.01	t = 1.10	0.28

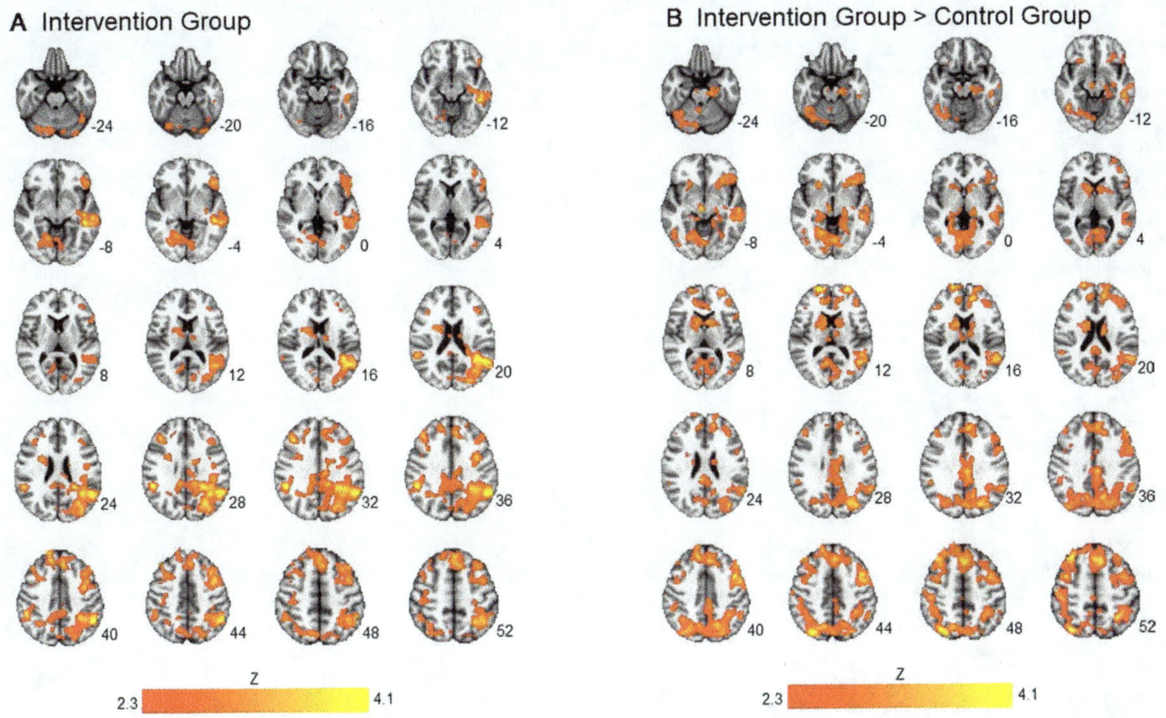

FIGURE 1 | Association between importance ratings and brain activation to alcohol taste cues. The association between ratings of importance of behavioral change and brain activation to alcohol taste cues. **(A)** The intervention group showed a significant positive association between ratings of importance and brain activation in the precuneus, posterior cingulate, and caudate. **(B)** Between groups, the intervention group showed a significant association between importance ratings and brain activation in the posterior cingulate, insula, precuneus, caudate, and anterior cingulate. These associations were not present in the control group. See **Table 2** for a full list of significant regions. Z-statistic maps are whole-brain cluster corrected, $Z > 2.3$, $p < 0.05$. Coordinates are in Montreal Neurological Institute (MNI) space. Brain is displayed in radiological convention (L = R).

group ($p < 0.05$ corrected), whereas there was no significant association in the control group (see **Figure S1**, **Table S1**).

Confidence Ruler

There were no significant associations between ratings of confidence and brain activation to alcohol taste cues across or between groups. There was also no significant interaction between group and confidence ratings on neural alcohol taste cue reactivity.

For the masked analyses, there were no significant associations between ratings of confidence and masked brain activation to alcohol taste cues across or between groups. There was also no significant interaction between group and confidence ratings on masked neural alcohol taste cue reactivity.

Readiness Ruler

Across groups, there was no significant association between readiness ratings and brain activation to alcohol taste cues. There was a significant interaction between group and readiness ratings on neural activation to alcohol taste cues in the temporal lobe. Specifically, the control group showed a negative association between ratings of readiness to change and brain activation in the middle and superior temporal gyrus ($p < 0.05$ corrected). There was no significant association, positive or negative, between ratings of readiness to change and brain activation to alcohol cues in the intervention group (see **Figure 2**, **Table 3**).

For the masked analyses, there were no significant associations between ratings of readiness and masked brain activation to alcohol taste cues across or between groups. There was also no significant interaction between group and confidence ratings on masked neural alcohol taste cue reactivity.

DISCUSSION

This study examined the effect of a brief intervention on motivation to change, as indicated by ratings of importance, confidence, and readiness, in a sample of non–treatment-seeking heavy drinkers. This study also explored the relationship between indices of motivation to change and the neural substrates of alcohol taste cue-reactivity after a brief drinking intervention. We found that the brief intervention was successful in significantly increasing ratings of importance of changing behavior related to alcohol use. However, there was no effect of the intervention on ratings of confidence or readiness to change. Correspondingly, we found that the brief intervention moderated the association between ratings of importance of behavioral change and neural alcohol taste cue reactivity. Specifically, there was a significant positive association between ratings of importance and neural alcohol taste cue reactivity in regions associated with introspection and self-awareness in the intervention group, but not in the control group.

TABLE 2 | association between importance ratings and brain activation to alcohol vs. water taste cues in intervention and control groups.

Brain region	Cluster voxels	Max. Z	x	y	z
Intervention group positive					
L Middle temporal gyrus	10,401	4.34	−46	−36	−10
L Angular gyrus		4.13	−52	−52	36
L Posterior cingulate gyrus		3.55	−14	−40	32
R Posterior cingulate gyrus		3.42	10	−40	28
R Precuneus		3.08	16	−70	50
L Middle frontal gyrus	4,187	3.90	−42	6	46
L Superior frontal gyrus		3.80	−4	24	48
L Cerebellar pyramis	2,374	4.49	−22	−80	−36
R Caudate	1,142	4.31	22	2	20
R Middle frontal gyrus		3.47	42	34	36
Control group positive					
N/A					
Intervention group negative					
N/A					
Control group negative					
N/A					
Intervention group > control group					
R Precuneus	11,068	4.69	32	−72	48
R/L posterior cingulate		3.64	−6	−24	34
L Precuneus		3.76	−14	−64	36
L Caudate		3.23	−10	8	10
R Lateral occipital cortex		3.11	26	−722	34
L middle frontal gyrus	7,647	4.11	−44	10	40
L frontal pole		3.83	−24	62	12
L superior frontal gyrus		3.57	−10	20	56
R/L anterior cingulate		3.46	16	42	10
L insula		3.17	−28	24	−4
R caudate	865	4.43	20	2	20
Control group > intervention group					
N/A					

One goal of this study was to explicitly test if the brief intervention was effective at impacting motivation to change indices, which may serve as mechanism of behavior change (MOBC) (17). As we hypothesized, the brief drinking intervention increased ratings of importance of behavioral change. The intervention did not, however, impact ratings of confidence or readiness. Notably, as reported elsewhere, there was no significant main effect of the intervention on alcohol outcomes in the 4 weeks following the brief intervention (20). Therefore, it may not be surprising that the intervention was also not successful at increasing ratings of confidence or readiness to change. Importance, confidence, and readiness measure different elements of the change process, with each element being necessary, but not sufficient to induce a behavioral change (10, 22, 28). These results are similar to those of a motivational interview study among young adults admitted to an emergency room who reported risky drinking *via* the AUDIT or exhibited elevated blood alcohol content (34). In this study, a motivational interview, relative to personalized feedback alone, increased readiness to change ratings only at a trend level, and readiness to change did not mediate treatment effects on drinking outcomes. By contrast, adult emergency department heavy drinkers randomized to receive brief intervention relative to those receiving standard care reported higher readiness scores at 3 months post-treatment (35), and readiness mediated intervention effects only among those with high baseline motivation to change. Changes in readiness to change have also been shown to mediate brief intervention effects among underage heavy drinkers (36). Overall, these findings corroborate potential mechanisms of action of brief intervention, and may also explain the relatively small effect sizes reported in meta-analyses (2). Further, these results extend the literature by suggesting that neuroimaging tools, and cue reactivity in particular, were sensitive to changes in importance ratings, despite the fact that such changes did not lead to detectable treatment effects on alcohol use.

Notably, there is significant heterogeneity in measures utilized in the literature to capture readiness to change, with varying number of factors included in an instrument [e.g., Contemplation Ladder (37)], without widespread consensus on associations among measures. In light of these differences, studies utilizing the three ladders in this study suggest that baseline importance and confidence rather than readiness predict favorable drinking outcomes at 6 months post-brief intervention (38, 39). However, another study monitoring measures of readiness to change using these ladders found significant effects of confidence and readiness ratings on 12-month alcohol outcomes, with weaker effects of importance of change (40). Other brief intervention studies,

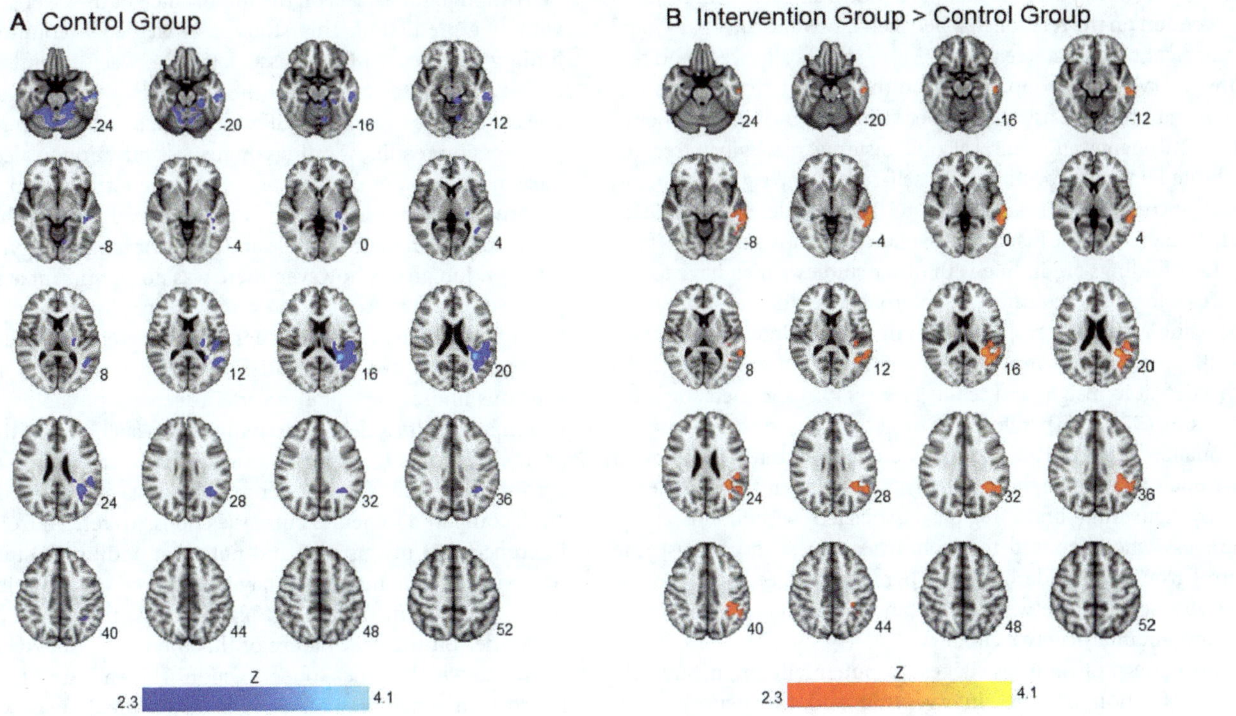

FIGURE 2 | Association between readiness ratings and brain activation to alcohol taste cues. The association between ratings of readiness to change and brain activation to alcohol taste cues. **(A)** The control group showed a significant negative association between ratings of readiness and brain activation in the temporal lobe. **(B)** Between groups, the intervention group showed a significantly greater activation in the temporal lobe due to the negative relationship found in the control group. See **Table 3** for a full list of significant regions. Z-statistic maps are whole-brain cluster corrected, $Z > 2.3$, $p < 0.05$. Coordinates are in MNI space. Brain is displayed in radiological convention (L = R).

TABLE 3 | Association between readiness ratings and brain activation to alcohol vs. water taste cues in intervention and control groups.

Brain region	Cluster voxels	Max. Z	x	y	z
Intervention group positive					
N/A					
Control group positive					
N/A					
Intervention group negative					
N/A					
Control group negative					
R cerebellar tonsil	2,385	3.50	24	−66	−36
L superior temporal gyrus	2,232	3.96	−32	−44	18
L middle temporal gyrus		2.82	−60	−24	−18
Intervention group > control group					
L middle temporal gyrus	2,660	3.78	−66	−36	0
Control group > intervention group					
N/A					

however, have identified that baseline perception of alcohol-related problems is predictive of *greater* drinking 3 months later, whereas "Taking Action" ratings and having a personalized plan for change were significant predictors of reduced drinking 3 and 12 months later, respectively (41, 42). In light of this mixed literature, the findings for the present study may provide evidence for a modest effect of brief interventions on at least one dimension of readiness to change among non–treatment-seeking adult heavy drinkers. Additional research is needed to examine the clinical utility of the importance measure, as well as its overlap with other readiness to change assessments. Within this mixed literature, however, what remains more consistently corroborated is that alterations in importance ratings alone are insufficient to produce behavioral change. Within an MOBC context, the brief intervention within this study was successful at increasing the recognition of the importance of changing drinking behavior, when compared with the attention-matched control. Similarly, as the intervention was not successful in increasing ratings of confidence or readiness or in reducing drinking reported at follow-up, the brief behavioral intervention may need to be better modified to target these motivation to change ladders in efforts to induce reductions in drinking. Furthermore, there is evidence to suggest that during brief interventions, patients who set clear objectives for alcohol use reduction have better alcohol use outcomes over 12 months (43). These individuals also engaged in more change talk during the intervention and had higher ratings of importance and readiness to change (43). These results suggest that targeting patient goals for alcohol reduction may improve outcomes, potentially through motivation to change mechanisms.

The present findings did not support an overall association between motivation to change and neural alcohol taste cue reactivity; however, they did identify a moderating effect of the brief intervention on the relationship between motivation to change and neural alcohol taste cue reactivity. More specifically, we found that in the intervention group, but not in the control group, there was a significant positive association between ratings of importance of behavioral change and neural alcohol taste cue reactivity in regions implicated in introspection and self-reflection, e.g., precuneus, posterior cingulate, insula. Several studies have identified a role for the precuneus and the insula in self-related cognitive processes (44–46). Our findings are in line with other studies which have found increases in the recruitment of interoceptive and self-referential processing regions in response to motivational interventions (14, 47–50). Addictive disorders have been theorized to be associated with a deficit in insight and self-awareness (51) and metacognitive processing (52, 53). Therefore, the brief intervention's emphasis on personalized level of risk and focus on change may have allowed individuals to increase their awareness of their drinking problems, thereby activating brain regions associated with interoceptive awareness when exposed to alcohol taste cues. In contrast, the control group, who did not receive personalized feedback, did not show an association between importance of behavioral change and activation in interoceptive circuitry.

This pattern of findings suggests a potentially important role of self-reflection in brief intervention and the neurobiology of alcohol cue reactivity. To wit, self-reflection during the intervention may have yielded higher problem awareness (i.e., importance for change). This self-reflection generalized to the scanning environment, wherein problem awareness prompted by the intervention was associated with greater introspection in response to alcohol cues. In contrast, participants in the control group did not engage in a self-reflective process about their drinking before the scanning session, and for them, the rating of importance was not associated with greater introspection in response to alcohol cues. These findings imply that it matters how people arrive at varying states of motivational readiness and that people who engage in self-reflection and also rate high on importance for change are the ones most likely to respond to subsequent alcohol cues with introspection. Future analyses should examine how these processes relate to alcohol use.

There was also a significant moderating effect of the brief intervention on the association between importance ratings and neural alcohol taste cue reactivity in regions implicated in incentive reward processing. The intervention group, when contrasted with the control group, showed a significant positive association between importance ratings and neural alcohol taste cue reactivity in the caudate, anterior cingulate, and insula, key regions of the incentive reward network (54). Intriguingly, the anterior cingulate is also implicated in monitoring conflict (55, 56). The activation of the anterior cingulate may represent the conflict between personal realizations of the importance of changing drinking behavior and the alcohol cue-elicited craving responses in incentive reward regions. Notably, the neuroimaging results using the mask-based approach did not fully conform with the pattern of findings from whole brain analyses discussed herein, and more broadly, did not address the study hypotheses given that the task contrast mask did not include brain regions subserving interoception.

Although the effects on the importance ratings were consistent with our prediction, this study also yielded a counterintuitive finding with regard to the association between neural activation to alcohol taste cues and the readiness to change ratings. Specifically, we found a significant interaction between group and post-session readiness ratings on neural activation to alcohol taste cues in the temporal lobe, such that the control group showed a negative association between ratings of readiness to change and brain activation in the middle and superior temporal gyrus. In the intervention group, however, there was no significant association, positive or negative, between ratings of readiness to change and brain activation to alcohol cues. In interpreting these findings, we considered two possibilities. The first is that this may be a spurious finding or type II error. The second possibility is that in fact these results reflect underlying effects such that in the control group, readiness to change was associated with decreased neural activation in the superior temporal gyrus during alcohol taste cues, compared to neural cues. We choose to refrain from reverse inference (57) in this case and note that additional studies and/or advanced data modeling may be required (58) to fully unpack this counterintuitive finding. Nonetheless, this result allows us to ponder on the very nature of this thematic issue, which is the degree to which clinical phenomenon will lend itself to cognitive neuroscience examination. Specifically, by breaking down clinical phenomena too finely we may lose its clinical significance, whereas having "large chunks" of clinical data explained by neuroimaging may lead to inconclusive or unreliable findings (59).

This study represents an initial step toward understanding the neurobiological mechanisms through which a brief intervention may improve motivation to change. Although this study has several strengths, it should be considered in light of its limitations. First, this study has a modest sample size; future studies should recruit larger sample sizes, particularly as the effect sizes of brief interventions are modest (60). Relatedly, this study recruited and enrolled non–treatment-seeking individuals from the community, and therefore, may not have shown the same changes in motivation to change following a psychosocial intervention as a treatment-seeking sample, which in turn may have reduced our power to identify associations between measures of readiness to change and neural alcohol cue reactivity. Additionally, the scanning portion of the study did not employ a pre-/post-treatment design, which may have been more sensitive to the effects of the intervention.

In conclusion, this study sought to identify the neurobiological mechanisms underlying changes in motivation induced by a brief intervention in non–treatment-seeking heavy drinkers. The current study found that a brief intervention increased ratings of importance of behavioral change, but was unsuccessful in impacting ratings of confidence or readiness to change compared to an attention-matched control. The brief intervention also moderated the association between neural alcohol taste cue reactivity and ratings of importance, such that in the intervention condition, there was a significant, positive relationship between ratings of importance and activation in regions associated with interoceptive awareness and self-reflection. This association may provide initial support for the role of interoceptive circuitry subserving increases in understanding of importance of behavioral change.

AUTHOR CONTRIBUTIONS

MK, LR, and JM were responsible for the study concept and design. AL and LR conducted the study. EG analyzed the data. EG and AL wrote the manuscript. MK, LR, and JM provided critical feedback on the manuscript. All authors critically reviewed content and approved the final version for publication.

REFERENCES

1. Grant BF, Chou SP, Saha TD, Pickering RP, Kerridge BT, Ruan WJ, et al. Prevalence of 12-month alcohol use, high-risk drinking, and DSM-IV alcohol use disorder in the United States, 2001–2002 to 2012–2013: results from the National Epidemiologic Survey on Alcohol and Related Conditions. *JAMA Psychiatry* (2017) 74(9):911–23. doi: 10.1001/jamapsychiatry.2017.2161
2. Schmidt CS, Schulte B, Seo HN, Kuhn S, O'Donnell A, Kriston L, et al. Meta-analysis on the effectiveness of alcohol screening with brief interventions for patients in emergency care settings. *Addiction* (2016) 111(5):783–94. doi: 10.1111/add.13263
3. Beyer F, Lynch E, Kaner E. Brief interventions in primary care: an evidence overview of practitioner and digital intervention programmes. *Curr Addict Rep* (2018) 5(2):265–73. doi: 10.1007/s40429-018-0198-7
4. Elzerbi C, Donoghue K, Boniface S, Drummond C. Variance in the efficacy of brief interventions to reduce hazardous and harmful alcohol consumption between injury and noninjury patients in emergency departments: a systematic review and meta-analysis of randomized controlled trials. *Ann Emerg Med* (2017) 70(5):714–23 e713. doi: 10.1016/j.annemergmed.2017.05.004
5. Center for Substance Abuse Treatment. Enhancing motivation for change in substance abuse treatment. Treatment Improvement Protocol (TIP) Series, No. 35. HHS Publication No. (SMA) 13-4212. Rockville, MD: Substance Abuse and Mental Health Services Administration (1999).
6. DiClemente CC, Schlundt D, Gemmell L. Readiness and stages of change in addiction treatment. *Am J Addict* (2004) 13(2):103–19. doi: 10.1080/10550490490435777
7. Heather N, Smailes D, Cassidy P. Development of a readiness ruler for use with alcohol brief interventions. *Drug Alcohol Depend* (2008) 98(3):235–40. doi: 10.1016/j.drugalcdep.2008.06.005
8. Carey KB, Purnine DM, Maisto SA, Carey MP, Barnes KL. Decisional balance regarding substance use among persons with schizophrenia. *Community Ment Health J* (1999) 35(4):289–99. doi: 10.1023/A:1018705722246
9. Cook S, Heather N, McCambridge J, and United Kingdom Alcohol Treatment Trial Research, T. The role of the working alliance in treatment for alcohol problems. *Psychol Addict Behav* (2015) 29(2):371–81. doi: 10.1037/adb0000058
10. Collins SE, Malone DK, Larimer ME. Motivation to change and treatment attendance as predictors of alcohol-use outcomes among project-based Housing First residents. *Addict Behav* (2012) 37(8):931–9. doi: 10.1016/j.addbeh.2012.03.029
11. Feldstein Ewing SW, Filbey FM, Sabbineni A, Chandler LD, Hutchison KE. How psychosocial alcohol interventions work: a preliminary look at what fMRI can tell us. *Alcoholism Clin Exp Res* (2011) 35(4):643–51. doi: 10.1111/j.1530-0277.2010.01382.x
12. Feldstein Ewing SW, McEachern AD, Yezhuvath U, Bryan AD, Hutchison KE, Filbey FM. Integrating brain and behavior: evaluating adolescents' response to a cannabis intervention. *Psychol Addict Behav* (2013) 27(2):510. doi: 10.1037/a0029767
13. Houck JM, Moyers TB, Tesche CD. Through a glass darkly: some insights on change talk via magnetoencephalography. *Psychol Addict Behav* (2013) 27(2):489–500. doi: 10.1037/a0029896
14. Feldstein Ewing SW, Yezhuvath U, Houck JM, Filbey FM. Brain-based origins of change language: a beginning. *Addict Behav* (2014) 39(12):1904–10. doi: 10.1016/j.addbeh.2014.07.035
15. Feldstein Ewing SW, Houck JM, Yezhuvath U, Shokri-Kojori E, Truitt D, Filbey FM. The impact of therapists' words on the adolescent brain: in the context of addiction treatment. *Behav Brain Res* (2016) 297:359–69. doi: 10.1016/j.bbr.2015.09.041
16. Morgenstern J, Naqvi NH, Debellis R, Breiter HC. The contributions of cognitive neuroscience and neuroimaging to understanding mechanisms of behavior change in addiction. *Psychol Addict Behav* (2013) 27(2):336–50. doi: 10.1037/a0032435
17. Nielsen L, Riddle M, King JW, Aklin WM, Chen W, Clark D, et al. The NIH Science of Behavior Change Program: transforming the science through a focus on mechanisms of change. *Behav Res Therapy* (2018) 101:3–11. doi: 10.1016/j.brat.2017.07.002
18. Courtney KE, Schacht JP, Hutchison K, Roche DJ, Ray LA. Neural substrates of cue reactivity: association with treatment outcomes and relapse. *Addict Biol* (2016) 21(1):3–22. doi: 10.1111/adb.12314
19. Olney JJ, Warlow SM, Naffziger EE, Berridge KC. Current perspectives on incentive salience and applications to clinical disorders. *Curr Opin Behav Sci* (2018) 22:59–69. doi: 10.1016/j.cobeha.2018.01.007
20. Grodin EN, Ray LA, MacKillop J, Lim AC, Karno MP. Elucidating the effect of a brief drinking intervention using neuroimaging: a preliminary study. *Alcohol Clin Exp Res* (2019) 43(2):367–77. doi: 10.1111/acer.13941
21. Saunders, JB, Aasland OG, Babor TF, Delafuente JR, Grant M. Development of the alcohol-use disorders identification test (audit)—Who Collaborative Project on early detection of persons with harmful alcohol-consumption. 2. *Addiction* (1993) 88(6):791–804. doi: 10.1111/j.1360-0443.1993.tb02093.x
22. Miller W, Rollnick S. "Motivational interviewing: preparing people for change", 2nd ed. New York, NY, US: The Guilford Press (2002).
23. Miller WR, Rose GS. Toward a theory of motivational interviewing. *Am Psychol* (2009) 64(6):527–37. doi: 10.1037/a0016830
24. Sobell MB, Sobell LC, Klajner F, Pavan D, Basian E. The reliability of a timeline method for assessing normal drinker college students' recent drinking history: utility for alcohol research. *Addict Behav* (1986) 11(2):149–61. doi: 10.1016/0306-4603(86)90040-7
25. Flannery B, Volpicelli J, Pettinati H. Psychometric properties of the Penn alcohol craving scale. *Alcoholism Clin Exp Res* (1999) 23(8):1289–95. doi: 10.1111/j.1530-0277.1999.tb04349.x
26. Heatherton TF, Kozlowski LT, Frecker RC, FAGERSTROM KO. The Fagerström test for nicotine dependence: a revision of the Fagerstrom Tolerance Questionnaire. *Br J Addict* (1991) 86(9):1119–27. doi: 10.1111/j.1360-0443.1991.tb01879.x
27. First MB, Williams JBW, Karg RS, Spitzer RL. Structured clinical interview for DSM-5—research version (SCID-5 for DSM-5, Research Version; SCID-5-RV). Arlington, VA: American Psychiatric Association (2015).
28. Rollnick S. Readiness, importance, and confidence: critical conditions of change in treatment. In: Miller WR, Heather N, eds. *Applied clinical psychology. Treating addictive behaviors.* New York, NY, US: Plenum Press (1998). p. 49–60. doi: 10.1007/978-1-4899-1934-2_4
29. Filbey FM, Claus E, Audette AR, Niculescu M, Banich MT, Tanabe J, et al. Exposure to the taste of alcohol elicits activation of the mesocorticolimbic neurocircuitry. *Neuropsychopharmacology* (2008a) 33(6):1391–401. doi: 10.1038/sj.npp.1301513
30. Filbey FM, Ray L, Smolen A, Claus ED, Audette A, Hutchison KE. Differential neural response to alcohol priming and alcohol taste cues is associated with DRD4 VNTR and OPRM1 genotypes. *Alcohol Clin Exp Res* (2008b) 32(7):1113–23. doi: 10.1111/j.1530-0277.2008.00692.x
31. Pruim RHR, Mennes M, van Rooij D, Llera A, Buitelaar JK, Beckmann CF. ICA-AROMA: a robust ICA-based strategy for removing motion artifacts from fMRI data. *Neuroimage* (2015) 112:267–77. doi: 10.1016/j.neuroimage.2015.02.064
32. Worsley K. *Statistical analysis of activation images. Functional MRI: an introduction to methods* (2001) 14:251–70. doi: 10.1093/acprof:oso/9780192630711.003.0014
33. Langenecker SA, Crane NA, Jenkins LM, Phan KL, Klumpp H. Pathways to neuroprediction: opportunities and challenges to prediction of treatment response in depression. *Curr Behav Neurosci Rep* (2018) 5(1):48–60. doi: 10.1007/s40473-018-0140-2
34. Barnett NP, Apodaca TR, Magill M, Colby SM, Gwaltney C, Rohsenow DJ, et al. Moderators and mediators of two brief interventions for alcohol in

the emergency department. *Addiction* (2010) 105(3):452–65. doi: 10.1111/j.1360-0443.2009.02814.x
35. Stein LAR, Minugh PA, Longabaugh R, Wirtz P, Baird J, Nirenberg TD, et al. Readiness to change as a mediator of the effect of a brief motivational intervention on posttreatment alcohol-related consequences of injured emergency department hazardous drinkers. *Psychol Addict Behav* (2009) 23(2):185–95. doi: 10.1037/a0015648
36. Magill M, Colby SM, Orchowski L, Murphy JG, Hoadley A, Brazil LA, et al. How does brief motivational intervention change heavy drinking and harm among underage young adult drinkers? *J Consult Clin Psychol* (2017) 85(5):447–58. doi: 10.1037/ccp0000200
37. Biener L, Abrams DB. The Contemplation Ladder: validation of a measure of readiness to consider smoking cessation. *Health Psychol* (1991) 10(5):360–5. doi: 10.1037//0278-6133.10.5.360
38. Williams EC, Horton NJ, Samet JH, Saitz R. Do brief measures of readiness to change predict alcohol consumption and consequences in primary care patients with unhealthy alcohol use? *Alcoholism Clin Exp Res* (2007) 31(3):428–35. doi: 10.1111/j.1530-0277.2006.00324.x
39. Bertholet N, Gaume J, Faouzi M, Gmel G, Daeppen JB. Predictive value of readiness, importance, and confidence in ability to change drinking and smoking. *Bmc Public Health* (2012) 12:708. doi: 10.1186/1471-2458-12-708
40. Gaume J, Bertholet N, Daeppen JB. Readiness to change predicts drinking: findings from 12-month follow-up of alcohol use disorder outpatients. *Alcohol Alcohol* (2017) 52(1):65–71. doi: 10.1093/alcalc/agw047
41. Bertholet N, Cheng DM, Palfai TP, Samet JH, Saitz R. Does readiness to change predict subsequent alcohol consumption in medical inpatients with unhealthy alcohol use? *Addict Behav* (2009) 34(8):636–40. doi: 10.1016/j.addbeh.2009.03.034
42. Lee CS, Baird J, Longabaugh R, Nirenberg TD, Mello MJ, Woolard R. Change plan as an active ingredient of brief motivational interventions for reducing negative consequences of drinking in hazardous drinking emergency-department patients. *J Stud Alcohol Drugs* (2010) 71(5):726–33. doi: 10.15288/jsad.2010.71.726
43. Daeppen JB, Bertholet N, Gmel G, Gaume J. Communication during brief intervention, intention to change, and outcome. *Subst Abus* (2007) 28(3):43–51. doi: 10.1300/J465v28n03_05
44. Shad MU, Keshavan MS, Steinberg JL, Mihalakos P, Thomas BP, Motes MA, et al. Neurobiology of self-awareness in schizophrenia: an fMRI study. *Schizophrenia Res* (2012) 138(2–3):113–9. doi: 10.1016/j.schres.2012.03.016
45. Cabanis M, Pyka M, Mehl S, Muller BW, Loos-Jankowiak S, Winterer G, et al. The precuneus and the insula in self-attributional processes. *Cogn Affect Behav Neurosci* (2013) 13(2):330–45. doi: 10.3758/s13415-012-0143-5
46. Ye Q, Zou FT, Lau H, Hu Y, Kwok SC. Causal evidence for mnemonic metacognition in human precuneus. *J Neurosci* (2018) 38(28):6379–87. doi: 10.1523/JNEUROSCI.0660-18.2018
47. Chua HF, Liberzon I, Welsh RC, Strecher VJ. Neural correlates of message tailoring and self-relatedness in smoking cessation programming. *Biol Psychiatry* (2009a) 65(2):165–8. doi: 10.1016/j.biopsych.2008.08.030
48. Chua HF, Polk T, Welsh R, Liberzon I, Strecher V. Neural responses to elements of a web-based smoking cessation program. *Stud Health Technol Inform* (2009b) 144:174–8. doi: 10.3233/978-1-60750-017-9-174
49. Wang AL, Ruparel K, Loughead JW, Strasser AA, Blady SJ, Lynch KG, et al. Content matters: neuroimaging investigation of brain and behavioral impact of televised anti-tobacco public service announcements. *J Neurosci* (2013) 33(17):7420–7. doi: 10.1523/JNEUROSCI.3840-12.2013
50. Wilson SJ, Sayette MA, Fiez JA. Neural correlates of self-focused and other-focused strategies for coping with cigarette cue exposure. *Psychol Addict Behav* (2013) 27(2):466–76. doi: 10.1037/a0027055
51. Moeller SJ, Goldstein RZ. Impaired self-awareness in human addiction: deficient attribution of personal relevance. *Trends Cogn Sci* (2014) 18(12):635–41. doi: 10.1016/j.tics.2014.09.003
52. Balconi M, Finocchiaro R, Campanella S. Reward sensitivity, decisional bias, and metacognitive deficits in cocaine drug addiction. *J Addict Med* (2014) 8(6):399–406. doi: 10.1097/ADM.0000000000000065
53. Wasmuth SL, Outcalt J, Buck K, Leonhardt BL, Vohs J, Lysaker PH. Metacognition in persons with substance abuse: findings and implications for occupational therapists. *Can J Occup Ther* (2015) 82(3):150–9. doi: 10.1177/0008417414564865
54. Koob GF, Volkow ND. Neurobiology of addiction: a neurocircuitry analysis. *Lancet Psychiatry* (2016) 3(8):760–73. doi: 10.1016/S2215-0366(16)00104-8
55. Botvinick MM, Cohen JD, Carter CS. Conflict monitoring and anterior cingulate cortex: an update. *Trends Cogn Sci* (2004) 8(12):539–46. doi: 10.1016/j.tics.2004.10.003
56. Shapira-Lichter I, Strauss I, Oren N, Gazit T, Sammartino F, Giacobbe P, et al. Conflict monitoring mechanism at the single-neuron level in the human ventral anterior cingulate cortex. *NeuroImage* (2018) 175:45–55. doi: 10.1016/j.neuroimage.2018.03.028
57. Poldrack RA. Inferring mental states from neuroimaging data: from reverse inference to large-scale decoding. *Neuron* (2011) 72(5):692–7. doi: 10.1016/j.neuron.2011.11.001
58. Hutzler F. Reverse inference is not a fallacy per se: cognitive processes can be inferred from functional imaging data. *Neuroimage* (2014) 84:1061–9. doi: 10.1016/j.neuroimage.2012.12.075
59. Krakauer JW, Ghazanfar AA, Gomez-Marin A, MacIver MA, Poeppel D. Neuroscience needs behavior: correcting a reductionist bias. *Neuron* (2017) 93(3):480–90. doi: 10.1016/j.neuron.2016.12.041
60. Huh D, Mun EY, Larimer ME, White HR, Ray AE, Rhew IC, et al. Brief motivational interventions for college student drinking may not be as powerful as we think: an individual participant-level data meta-analysis. *Alcohol Clin Exp Res* (2015) 39(5):919–31. doi: 10.1111/acer.12714

14

The Interplay of Inflammatory Processes and Cognition in Alcohol use Disorders

Violette Coppens[1,2†], Manuel Morrens[1,2†], Marianne Destoop[1,3] and Geert Dom[1,3]*

[1] Faculty of Medicine and Health Sciences, Collaborative Antwerp Psychiatric Research Institute (CAPRI), University of Antwerp, Antwerp, Belgium, [2] Scientific Initiative of Neuropsychiatric and Psychopharmacological Studies (SINAPS), University Department of Psychiatry, Duffel, Belgium, [3] Department of Addiction, Psychiatric Hospital Multiversum, Boechout, Belgium

Correspondence:
Geert Dom
geert.dom@uantwerpen.be

†These authors have contributed equally to this work.

Rationale: Of late, evidence emerges that the pathophysiology of psychiatric diseases and their affiliated symptomatologies are at least partly contributable to inflammatory processes. Also in alcohol use disorders (AUD), this interaction is strongly apparent, with severely immunogenic liver cirrhosis being one of the most critical sequelae of chronic abusive drinking. This somatic immune system activation negatively impacts brain functioning, and additionally, alcohol abuse appears to have a direct detrimental effect on the brain by actively stimulating its immune cells and responses. As cognitive decline majorly contributes to AUD's debility, it is important to know to what extent impairment of cognitive functioning is due to these (neuro-)inflammatory aberrations.

Method: We hereby summarize the current existing literature on the interplay between AUD, inflammation, and cognition in a systematic review according to the PRISMA-P guidelines for the systematic review.

Main findings: Although literature on the role of inflammation in alcohol use-related cognitive deficiency remains scarce, current findings indicate that pro-inflammatory processes indeed result in exacerbation of several domains of cognitive deterioration. Interestingly, microglia, the immune cells of the brain, appear to exert initial compensatory neuroprotective functionalities upon acute ethanol exposure while chronic alcohol intake seems to attenuate these responses and overall microglial activity.

Conclusion: As these results indicate inflammation to be of importance in cognitive impairment following alcohol consumption and might as such provide alternate therapeutic avenues, a considerable increase in research efforts in this domain is urgently required.

Keywords: inflammation, alcohol use disorder, cognition, alcohol addiction, psychiatry

INTRODUCTION

Alcohol is the most commonly (ab)used substance worldwide with high-risk drinking occurring in up to 30% in Western populations (1). On a global scale, the WHO estimates the prevalence of alcohol use disorder (AUD) to be as high as 16% (WHO, 2004[1]) being equally present across almost all sociodemographic classes (1) WHO, 2004). Both excessive alcohol use and AUD have a profound (public) health impact as they strongly increase morbidity and mortality through inducing cardiovascular diseases, hypertension, diabetes, liver cirrhosis, and many other somatic comorbidities (1).

AUD is associated to different cognitive deficits, such as abnormalities in working memory, attention, and executive functions like response inhibition (2). As thoroughly investigated in a meta-analysis by Stavro et al. (3), these deficits remain considerable in the first 12 months of sobriety but improve after 1 year of abstinence. Nonetheless, they impact decision making in patients and thus interfere with readiness to change drinking behavior and the ability to attain abstinence (4). Moreover, poorer cognitive functioning predicts increased relapse risk over a 12-month follow-up period (5).

The specific etiopathogenesis of these AUD-related cognitive impairments is rather complex, as it may be an inherent premorbid trait vulnerability, but may also result from alcohol-related brain damage (ARBD). As alcohol has major neurotoxic effects, its abuse is related to mild brain atrophy that seems mostly driven by white matter loss and changes in cortical neuronal dendritic arborization (6). ARBD can either be the consequence of a direct molecular impact of the substance on the brain and/or may result from impaired liver functioning, malnutrition (vitamin B1 deficiency), and risk-taking behavior potentially associated with head injury (7). As such, cognitive alterations in AUD patients result from central as well as peripheral abnormalities (7, 8). Nonetheless, Davies et al. (9) demonstrated in a sample of abstinent (750 days) alcohol-dependent subjects without any hepatic, neurological, or other somatic impairments that deficit in visuospatial scanning, verbal memory, and processing speed were still present. These findings suggest enduring, alcohol-induced cognitive impairments. However, it should be noted that it is very likely that these cognitive impairments can both be the result of chronic alcohol use but can also reflect pre-existing cognitive impairments underlying vulnerabilities for escalating alcohol use and subsequent development of AUD. Parsons' (10) analysis of previous studies on the relationship between alcohol consumption and cognitive deficits showed that increase in alcohol use resulted in more pronounced cognitive impairments, suggestive of a dose–response relation. Finally and most importantly, evidence is growing that not only alcohol use but also alcohol withdrawal is a neurotoxic process. Repeated detoxifications have been associated with progressive cognitive decline and impairments (11). With regard to the underlying processes responsible for the many cognition-related dysfunctions following alcohol abuse, cerebral edema, neuronal cell loss, and dysfunction of the blood–brain barrier (BBB) have been demonstrated in the brain of deceased AUD patients (12). These physiological abnormalities have further been linked to a higher concentration of CNS ammonia, mitochondrial damage, and oxidative stress caused by increased levels of reactive oxygen species (ROS) in relevant brain regions (13–15). Recently, also neuroinflammation gains more attention as to playing a role in the above neurodetrimental effects. In the last few years, neuroinflammation has been associated to cognitive decline in several pathological situations, including old age (16, 17), Alzheimer's disease (18), schizophrenia (De Picker et al., 2018, submitted), and bipolar disorder (Van den Ameele et al., submitted). Also in AUD patients, increasing evidence points toward an aberrantly activated immune system. Excessive production of cytokines and chemokines and altered activation of microglial cells—the immune cells of the brain—have been documented in both acute and chronic phases of AUD (7, 8).

As changes in immune system activation may result in cytotoxic effects, thereby impacting neurotransmission, neuroendocrine function, and neural plasticity (19, 20), neuroinflammation presumably also at least partly contributes to cognitive deficits linked to alcohol exposure.

These findings are supported by animal studies linking inflammation to alcohol disorders and related cognitive dysfunctioning. For instance, elevated levels of the pro-inflammatory cytokines interleukin 6 (IL-6), IL-1b, and tumor necrosis factor alfa (TNF-a) have been found in the rodent brain after chronic alcohol consumption (21, 22).

Moreover, Marshall et al. (23) demonstrated (chronic) ethanol exposure in the rat to activate microglia, the brain's most prominent immune cells, and to induce a 26% increase in anti-inflammatory cytokine IL-10 and an even larger increase (38%) in the neurotrophic factor transforming growth factor beta (TGF-b1) up to 7 days after exposure. Finally, the cellular and molecular immune system alterations induced by ethanol consumption are primarily found in the prefrontal cortex and the hippocampus of the rats; these brain regions are known to play a substantial role in several cognitive functions like memory and executive functioning (24, 25).

With this systematic review, we document the influence of AUD-related inflammation on decreased cognitive functioning observed in AUD patients.

METHOD

This systematic review was conducted and reported according to the PRISMA-P (preferred reporting items for systematic review and meta-analysis protocols) guideline (26). We aimed to investigate all types of cognitive aberrations in individuals consuming any amount of alcohol units provided that the study discussed any type of inflammatory mediation in relation to cognition. In order to obtain original studies investigating the impact of the immune system on cognitive functioning of alcohol use and AUD, a PubMed search (January 1946–October 2018) for English language articles was conducted using the following search terms: (alcohol* OR ethyl* OR ethanol) AND (cognit* OR attention OR memory OR "executive function*") AND (immun* OR microglia* OR

[1] http://www.who.int/gho/substance_abuse/burden/alcohol_prevalence/en/

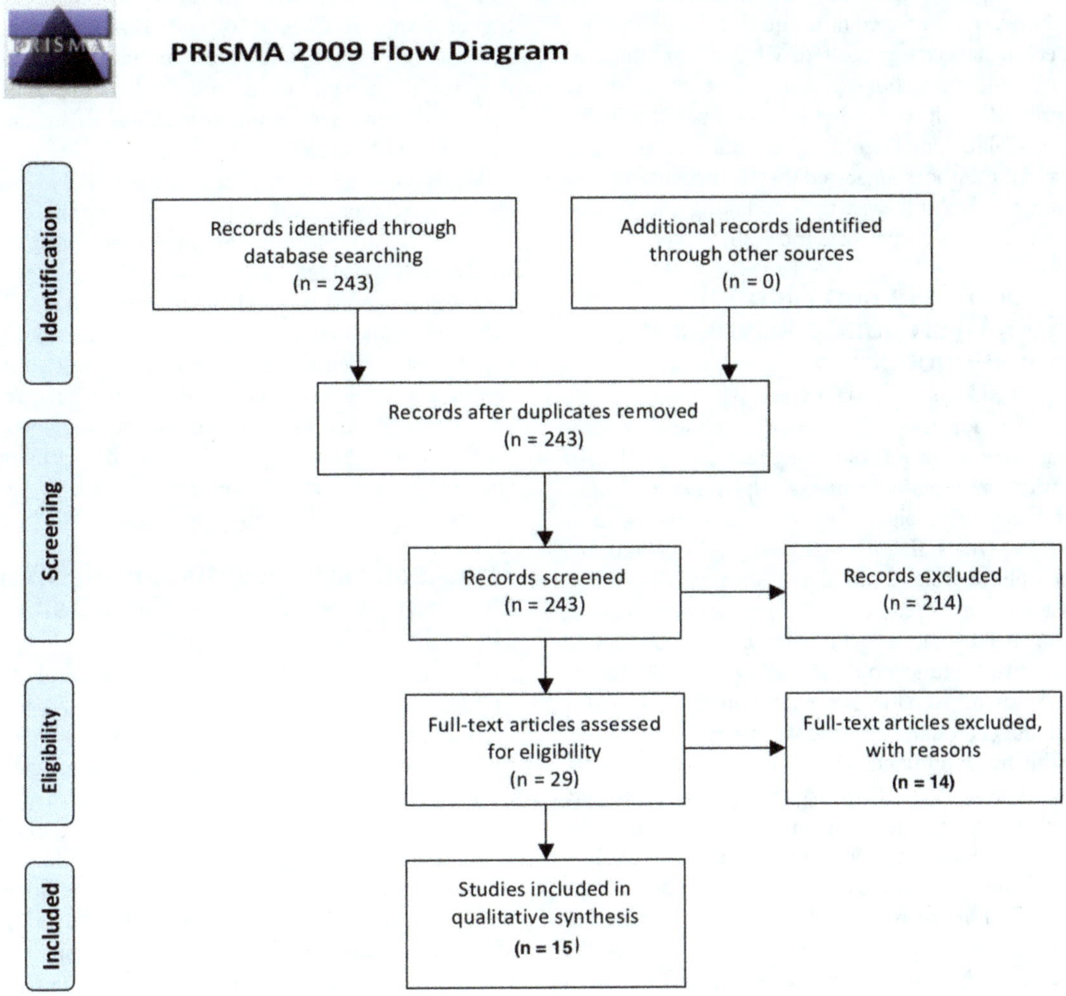

FIGURE 1 | Overview of the selection process of included papers according to PRISMA guidelines (26).

inflamm* OR cytokine* OR kynuren*) NOT review[publication type] AND english[language]. The papers were filtered for human studies exclusively. An overview of the inclusion process can be found in **Figure 1**. Briefly, the above PubMed search yielded 243 results; abstract screening led to exclusion of 214 papers, leaving 29 papers that were read entirely. Of these, 16 manuscripts were deemed eligible for inclusion in the review. Of the 14 papers excluded after full-text analysis, 6 were excluded based on the absence of statistical analyses of the effect ethyl had on cognition/inflammation; 3 studies were not performed in humans; 3 studies did not concern the interaction between the immune system and cognition; 1 paper did not concern alcohol consumption; and 1 paper did not concern cognition.

Of note, the latest edition of DSM (V) refers to the disorder of being dependent on alcohol consumption as "alcohol use disorder, AUD." However, this terminology is rather recent, and literature predating this overarching term mostly refers to this or similar conditions with "alcohol dependence" or related expressions. In order to avoid rephrasing bias in this work, we opted to retain the terminology as applied in the original paper. As such, terminology applied throughout this review remains somewhat heterogeneous in its definition of alcohol consumption disorders.

RESULTS

The PubMed database search resulted in an initial 243 records. Following removal of duplicates and screening of abstracts for relevance, 28 records remained. Eligibility of these 28 records was assessed by detailed evaluation of the full texts. Eight papers were deemed not relevant, and three papers concerned preclinical research, resulting in a final selection of 17 papers included in the current review.

Relation Between the Immune System and Cognitive Functioning

Alcohol abuse has been associated with cognitive impairment in humans, mainly by deleterious effects on memory function and on executive functions including cognitive flexibility and response inhibition (27). In addition, preclinical findings link ethanol consumption to altered immune signaling and to decreased cognitive capabilities (24, 25). Also in humans, a three-way interaction between an affected immune system, alcohol use, and cognitive decline has been suggested: Miguez-Burbano et al. (28) showed that memory functioning is more severely decreased in alcohol abusing HIV-infected individuals compared to sober HIV-infected peers. Hazardous alcohol consumption was related to thymus size, and the authors suggested that the negative impact of alcohol on thymus volume was the mediating mechanism underlying impaired cognitive performance (28).

The Association Between Alcohol Consumption, Dysregulated Cytokines, and Cognitive Functioning

In a large group of alcohol-dependent male patients (n = 78), Yen et al. (29) looked for associations between plasma cytokine concentrations and cognitive functioning. They showed that, at the start of the withdrawal period, patients display elevation of all investigated cytokines [TNF-alpha (TNF-α), interferon gamma (IFN-γ), interleukin 1 (IL-1), IL-2, IL-4, IL-5, IL-6, IL-8, IL-10, and granulocyte-macrophage colony-stimulating factor (GM-CSF)]. Although the patients displayed reduced information processing speed, these abnormalities did not correlate with cytokine levels. Nonetheless, cognitive dysfunctioning improved after 4 weeks of abstinence, which was mirrored by normalization of the cytokine levels. Felipo et al. (17) did demonstrate peripheral levels of IL-6, together with hyperammonemia, to be a driving factor for cognitive impairment, as assessed by a series of tasks addressing psychomotor and processing speed. In this line, Hanak et al. (2) recently investigated the impact of alcohol detoxification on IL-6 in a small group of patients with AUD (n = 27). They showed that when craving is caused by stress, but not when caused by alcohol or mood, IL-6 decreases after 3 weeks of detoxification. Given the small sample size in each group (n = 5) and the suboptimal statistical analysis strategies used (lack of *post hoc* exploratory analyses), these findings need to be confirmed approached with caution. The authors also aimed to find associations with cognitive functioning, and in line with the findings of Felipo et al. (17) results pointed toward more pronounced working memory deficits in the subgroup with highest levels of IL-6. Here again, methodological problems hamper interpretability. These findings thus corroborate with the previous finding that pro-inflammatory cytokines are correlated to craving in alcohol-dependent individuals (n = 52) (30). Moreover, reductions in selective attention as assessed by a self-developed validated computerized task appeared to be inversely related to the anti-inflammatory cytokine IL-10 after 3 weeks of abstinence, suggesting that reductions in protective levels of anti-inflammatory markers may lead to cognitive impairments.

Wilhelm et al. (31) investigated plasma levels of the pro-inflammatory compound tissue inhibitor of metalloproteinases (TIMP-1) and found them to be associated to self-reported memory complaints in a small sample of female (but not male) alcohol-dependent patients.

More indirect findings come from Duivis et al. (32), who demonstrated that cognitive symptoms of depression and anxiety like negative emotional state, concentration/decision making capacity, thoughts of death or suïcide,... correlate with several peripheral markers of inflammation (namely, higher levels of CRP, IL-6, and TNF-α). Interestingly, when controlling for several lifestyle factors including alcohol use, these correlations disappeared, suggesting that, at least partially, alcohol consumption mediates inflammation-associated cognitive deficiencies.

Boyer et al. (33) found a weak correlation between alcohol abuse in schizophrenic patients and cognitive dysfunctioning (mainly attention), but this was not associated to plasma CRP concentrations.

Although only a handful of studies looked into the associations between cytokines and cognitive dysfunctioning in alcohol-dependent patients, early results suggest impairments (in several cognitive domains including attention, processing speed, and memory) are associate to increases in pro-inflammatory markers and reductions in anti-inflammatory cytokines. Alcohol abstinence may partially remediate some of these deficits as mirrored by normalization of cytokines.

The Association Between Alcohol Consumption, Altered Glial Cells, and Cognitive Dysfunctioning

Kalk et al. (34) recently investigated microglial activation *via* PET tracer imaging in newly abstinent (< 1 month) alcohol-dependent patients (n = 9). In contrast to their expectations, they found less microglial activation than healthy controls, which they suggested to be the result of a potential loss of microglia cells. Although microglia appeared to be less activated in patients, tracer binding strongly correlated with delayed verbal memory, pointing toward poor memory performance in those patients with low microglia activation. This would intuitively contrast with the report of Marshall et al. (23), who showed increased PET tracer binding/microglial activation after acute 4-day ethanol administration in rats. However, both findings can be reconciled by indications from Marshall's study suggesting that activated microglia adopt a neuroprotective (the so-called *M2 phenotype*) rather than a neurotoxic (M1) profile in response to ethanol and that chronic alcohol abuse decreases the number of these safeguarders.

The literature investigating the impact of alcohol use and abstinence on glial activation patterns and their functionality is too scarce to be informative. However, the little preliminary data that are available suggest this to be a research avenue of interest for future studies focusing on the role of inflammation on cognitive deterioration by alcohol use.

The Role of the Gastrointestinal System and Liver Pathologies in Inflammation and Cognitive Dysfunction in Alcohol Disorders

Many of the articles included in this review pointed toward an important role of the liver function and gut permeability and its relation with alcohol (ab) use and subsequent inflammatory processes.

Alcohol use has well known pathological effects on the liver; as such, alcoholic liver disease (ALD) is the most prevalent type of chronic liver disease worldwide. ALD is accompanied by an inflammatory presentation characterized by increases in pro-inflammatory cytokines and chemokines (35, 36). Alcohol dependence has also been associated with a leaky gut, resulting in increased permeability, which has been associated to increases in plasma lipopolysaccharides (LPS) levels, which in their turn are known to have a proinflammatory stimulating nature. These gut abnormalities and associated LPS increases normalized after a 3-week abstinence period (30). The neuroinflammation described in patients with AUD therefore results from both direct proinflammatory effects of alcohol on the brain and indirect immunological damage *via* the liver (7, 8).

Hepatic encephalopathy (HE) implies the deterioration of brain functioning arising from acute and chronic liver failure as a result of chronic alcohol abuse (7, 37). This may result in cognitive symptoms such as deficitary judgment, memory impairment, and confusion. Excess brain ammonia levels have been put forward as a strong leading factor, although *postmortem* findings suggest that a pro-inflammatory state, abnormal astrocyte, and microglial activation also seem to be involved (7, 37, 38). Dennis et al. (7) showed that HE is associated to increases in cortical IL-6 levels compared to controls or non-HE alcoholic patients, which was partly associated to microglial proliferation and activation in neuroplasticity associated brain regions (including the subventricular zone). This proinflammatory, cytotoxic environment was reflected in reduced neuronal cell counts (7). Cagnin et al. (39) investigated PK11195-binding, reflecting activated glial cells (microglia and astrocytes), in a very small sample (n = 5) of patients with HE (three of which were alcohol-induced), and found significant increases in glial activation, especially in pallidum, right putamen, and right DLPFC. Of note, the patients with the most severe cognitive impairment had the highest increases in tracer binding (including two of the alcohol-induced HE).

HE has also been shown to increase plasma IL-6 levels (40), but it should be noted that it is not clear to what extent IL-6 is able to pass the blood–brain barrier in normal physiological conditions and in HE brains (7, 41).

Furthermore, the cognitive impairments inversely related to levels of the anti-inflammatory cytokine IL-10 in AD patients as described by Leclercq et al. (30) appeared to be partly associated to increased intestinal permeability.

So, although associations between alcohol-induced immune dysregulations and cognitive dysfunctioning in the absence of liver pathology have been shown, affected liver functioning may further fuel a pro-inflammatory state peripherally and in the CNS, thereby negatively impacting cognitive functioning in AUD patients.

DISCUSSION

The current body of evidence suggests that acute exposure to alcohol leads to an anti-inflammatory response of the immune system (42), while chronic exposure seems to be associated more to pro-inflammatory reactions that remain present during abstinence (30). This seems to point toward an initial protective or homeostatic response of the central immune system to alcohol, whereas chronic alcohol consumption rather induces damaging pro-inflammatory states as reflected by elevation of pro-inflammatory signaling molecules (30, 43). Few studies looked into the associations between immune markers and cognitive dysfunctioning in AUD patients, and while these findings suggest that cognitive impairments (including deficits in attention, processing speed, and memory) are associated to increases in pro-inflammatory markers and reductions in anti-inflammatory cytokines, these findings are rather modest and even contradictory in nature. For example, while Cagnin et al. (38, 39) demonstrated *via* PET imaging an increase in glial cell activation in patients with HE, Kalk et al. (34) found the opposite to be true in newly abstinent alcohol-dependent patients. These discrepant findings might be allocated to the differing pathologies but might also reflect technological variability as the tracer used by Kalk et al. (34) is thought to be more specific for microglia, while that of Cagnin et al. (39) rather binds to all glial cell types in equal proportions. An overview of the findings on the interplay between inflammatory processes, ethanol exposure, and cognitive effects can be found in **Table 1**.

A hypothetical mechanistic link between neuroinflammation and cognitive decline in AUD might stem from the tryptophan catabolism (TRYCAT) pathway. This inflammatory degradation process catabolizes the essential amino acid tryptophan to kynurenine and its metabolites. It mainly occurs in microglia and astrocytes and is activated by pro-inflammatory cytokines (44). Several receptors of neuroactive kynurenine metabolites have been associated to cognitive functioning (45) (Van den Ameele et al., 2018, submitted) and might as such be of hypothetical interest to further explore the relationship between inflammation and cognitive functioning in AUD. A single study investigated the impact of retrospectively established alcohol use before, during, and after pregnancy in mothers on the cytokine and kynurenine levels in children with ADHD (mean age 10.4 +/−2.5 years), but no associations between kynurenine levels in the children on one hand and alcohol use on the other was found (46). Sadly, potential effects or correlations in the mother were not scrutinized, and no additional studies exist so far assessing the potential interaction between kynurenine and/or other TRYCAT metabolites in patients with AUD.

The relationship between immune dysregulation and cognitive deficits in AUD patients seems to be further modulated by hepatic and alcohol use–induced gastro-intestinal pathologies (38, 39), although a direct effect of alcohol on the brain will additionally contribute to this interaction. Further research should elucidate the complex interaction of alcohol use, its central and peripheral effects driving immune dysregulations, and these accumulating effects on cognitive deficits in AUD patients. Moreover, it should be investigated to what extent these effects remain after abstinence, and more importantly, to what extent immune regulatory treatment options may be protective toward cognitive functions or remediate already existing cognitive deficits in chronic users. Finally, future studies need to look into the role of potential confounding or mediating factors. First, chronic tobacco smoking has been on itself related with neuro-inflammatory processes (47). About 60% of

TABLE 1 | Overview of the current literature on the interplay between inflammatory processes, ethanol exposure, and cognitive effects (NM = not mentioned in publication).

Clinical findings				
Reference	**Patient population**	**State of ethanol exposure**	**Type of inflammatory response**	**Effect on cognition**
(29)	Alcohol dependence	Early withdrawal	↑ Pro-inflammatory cytokines in peripheral blood	Reduced information processing speed
		4w abstinence	Normalization of cytokine levels	Improvement in cognitive dysfunctioning
(17)	Liver cirrhosis	NM	↑ Pro-inflammatory cytokines in peripheral blood	Reduced psychomotor and processing speed
(2)	AUD	Alcohol detoxification	↑ Pro-inflammatory cytokines in peripheral blood	Increased working memory deficits
(30)	Alcohol dependence	3-week abstinence	↑ Anti-inflammatory cytokines in peripheral blood	Reduction in selective attention
(31)	Alcohol-dependent women	Current alcohol dependence	↑ Pro-inflammatory TIMP-1	Association with memory complaints
(32)	Depression and anxiety	Alcohol use	↑ Pro-inflammatory cytokines in peripheral blood	Cognitive deficiencies
(33)	Schizophrenia	Alcohol abuse	Pro-inflammatory acute phase protein CRP	No association with attention
(34)	Alcohol dependence	Early abstinence	↓ Microglial activation	Delayed verbal memory
(39)	Cirrhosis	NM	↑ Microglial activation	More severe cognitive impairment

Post-mortem findings				
Reference	**Patient population**	**State of ethanol exposure**	**Type of inflammatory response**	**Effect on brain**
(7)	Hepatic encephalopathy (HE)	Chronic alcohol abuse	↑ Cerebral pro-inflammatory cytokines ↑ Microglial proliferation and activation	Reduced neuronal cell counts

↑, *Increased;* ↓, *Decreased.*

alcohol-dependent individuals are also lifetime (heavy) smokers (48). So, the role of tobacco smoking needs to be differentiated from that of alcohol. Second, comorbidity between AUD and other mental disorders is highly prevalent. Often, these mental disorders themselves are associated with cognitive decline and neuroinflammation. For example, the prevalence of affective disorders in AUD is estimated to be 22.9% (49). Next, the most important metabolite of alcohol, acetaldehyde, has been implicated within inflammatory processes, gut permeability, and liver disease (50, 51). Alcohol metabolization is strongly influenced by genetic differences in acetaldehyde dehydrogenase activity, leaving individuals significant differences in alcohol metabolization (and acetaldehyde accumulation) between individuals and different ethnic groups. These genetic difference may represent an important aspect of the alcohol X inflammation X cognition three-way interaction.

Although we attempted to reflect on the existing literature as accurately as possible, this review contains several study- and review design–inherent limitations.

First, the DSM-V categorizes all alcohol-related disorders under the same flag of "AUD." However, as some literature described in this review predates this novel classification, investigated populations over the included studies are often differentially defined. As such, this literature overview might encompass a heterogeneous population with differing levels of alcohol abuse as papers scrutinize "alcohol dependence" or "chronic alcohol abuse" while data were piled in this work as hallmarking the whole of AUD. Second, in addition to "classical" cognitive functions like working memory and processing speed, alcohol dependence is dependent on more complex cognitive reasonings like the sociocognitive ability to infer other's thoughts (theory of mind). Although we did not ambition to exclude papers on the relation of inflammation with these more complex cognitions, no works were found on this topic. Likewise, although extensive literature is available on the considerable role of different domains of cognitive impairment on patient prognosis, therapeutic outcome, relapse rate,… [for review see Ref. (52)], no reports are available on the role of inflammation in AUD prognosis and outcome. As such, these relevant areas of interest remain a lacunae in this review as well. Additionally, we did not take into account potential differences in the amount of ethyl units consumed. However, we can expect the interaction between different AUD, cognition, and inflammatory parameters to be increasingly affected with increasing alcohol dosage and thus increasing inflammation.

Lastly, while extensive preclinical literature provides strong evidence for this three-way interaction between AUD, its cognitive impairments, and immune system aberrations, the actual number of studies investigating it is surprisingly low.

This evidently renders making hard statements on the nature of the interactions somewhat difficult. However, this review aimed at providing sufficient indications that addressing this research avenue more in depth might vastly elucidate inflammatory pathways to be of importance in cognitive deficits marking AUD.

AUTHOR CONTRIBUTIONS

VC and MM performed literature search and wrote the article. MD and GD acted as advisory board on included papers and reviewed the manuscript.

REFERENCES

1. Grant BF, Chou SP, Tulshi D, Saha RP, Pickering BT, Kerridge W, et al. Prevalence of 12-month alcohol use, high-risk drinking, and DSM-IV alcohol use disorder in the United States, 2001-2002 to 2012-2013: results from the National Epidemiologic Survey on Alcohol and Related Conditions. *JAMA Psychiatry* (2017) 74(9):911–23. doi: 10.1001/jamapsychiatry.2017.2161
2. Hanak C, Benoit J, Fabry L, Hein M, Verbanck P, de Witte P, et al. Changes in pro-inflammatory markers in detoxifying chronic alcohol abusers, divided by Lesch Typology, reflect cognitive dysfunction. *Alcohol Alcohol* (2017) 52(5):529–34. doi: 10.1093/alcalc/agx043
3. Stavro K, Pelletier J, Potvin S. Widespread and sustained cognitive deficits in alcoholism: a meta-analysis. *Addict Biol* (2013) 18(2):203–13. doi: 10.1111/j.1369-1600.2011.00418.x
4. Blume AW, Schmaling KB, Marlatt GA. Memory, executive cognitive function, and readiness to change drinking behavior. *Addict Behav* (2005) 30(2):301–14. doi: 10.1016/j.addbeh.2004.05.019
5. Allsop S, Saunders B, Phillips M. The process of relapse in severely dependent male problem drinkers. *Addiction* (2000) 95(1):95–106. doi: 10.1046/j.1360-0443.2000.9519510.x
6. Harper C, Corbett D. Changes in the basal dendrites of cortical pyramidal cells from alcoholic patients—a quantitative golgi study. *J Neurol Neurosurg Psychiatry* (1990) 53(10):856–61. doi: 10.1136/jnnp.53.10.856
7. Dennis CV, Sheahan PJ, Graeber MB, Sheedy DL, Kril Jillian J., Sutherland Greg T. Microglial proliferation in the brain of chronic alcoholics with hepatic encephalopathy. *Metab Brain Dis* (2014) 29(4):1027–39. doi: 10.1007/s11011-013-9469-0
8. Kelley KW, Dantzer R. Alcoholism and Inflammation: neuroimmunology of behavioral and mood disorders. *Brain Behav Immun* (2011) 25 Suppl 1: June S13–20. doi: 10.1016/j.bbi.2010.12.013
9. Davies SJC, Pandit SA, Feeney A, Stevenson BJ, Kerwin RW, Nutt DJ, et al. Is there cognitive impairment in clinically 'healthy' abstinent alcohol dependence? *Alcohol Alcohol* (2005) 40(6):498–503. doi: 10.1093/alcalc/agh203
10. Parsons OA, Nixon SJ. Cognitive functioning in sober social drinkers: a review of the research since 1986. *J Stud Alcohol* (1998) 59(2):180–90. doi: 10.15288/jsa.1998.59.180
11. Duka T, Townshend JM, Collier K, Stephens DN. Impairment in cognitive functions after multiple detoxifications in alcoholic inpatients. *Alcohol Clin Exp Res* (2003) 27(10):1563–72. doi: 10.1097/01.ALC.0000090142.11260.D7
12. Pratt OE, Rooprai HK, Shaw GK, Thomson AD. The genesis of alcoholic brain tissue injury. *Alcohol Alcohol* (1990) 25(2-3):217–30. doi: 10.1093/oxfordjournals.alcalc.a044995
13. Haorah J, Knipe B, Leibhart J, Ghorpade A, Persidsky Y. Alcohol-induced oxidative stress in brain endothelial cells causes blood-brain barrier dysfunction. *J Leukocyte Biol* (2005) 78(6):1223–32. doi: 10.1189/jlb.0605340
14. Haorah J, Ramirez SH, Schall K, Smith D, Pandya R, Persidsky Y. Oxidative stress activates protein tyrosine kinase and matrix metalloproteinases leading to blood-brain barrier dysfunction. *J Neurochem* (2007) 101(2):566–76. doi: 10.1111/j.1471-4159.2006.04393.x
15. Spanagel R, Siegmund S, Cowen M, Schroff K-C, Schumann G, Fiserova M, et al. The neuronal nitric oxide synthase gene is critically involved in neurobehavioral effects of alcohol. *J Neurosci : Official J Soc Neurosci* (2002) 22(19):8676–83. doi: 10.1523/JNEUROSCI.22-19-08676.2002
16. Teunissen CE, van Boxtel MPJ, Bosma H, Bosmans E, Delanghe J, De Bruijn C, et al. Inflammation markers in relation to cognition in a healthy aging population. *J Neuroimmunol* (2003) 134(1-2):142–50. doi: 10.1016/S0165-5728(02)00398-3
17. Felipo V, Urios A, Montesinos E, Molina I, Garcia-Torres ML, Civera M, et al. Contribution of hyperammonemia and inflammatory factors to cognitive impairment in minimal hepatic encephalopathy. *Metab Brain Dis* (2012) 27(1):51–8. doi: 10.1007/s11011-011-9269-3
18. Kinney JW, Bemiller SM, Murtishaw AS, Leisgang AM, Salazar AM, Lamb BT. Inflammation as a central mechanism in Alzheimer's disease. *Alzheimer's Dementia: J Alzheimer's Assoc* (2018) 4:575–90. doi: 10.1016/j.trci.2018.06.014
19. Beumer W, Gibney SM, Drexhage RC, Pont-Lezica L, Doorduin J, Klein HC, et al. The immune theory of psychiatric diseases: a key role for activated microglia and circulating monocytes. *J Leukocyte Biol* (2012) 92(5):959–75. doi: 10.1189/jlb.0212100
20. Miller AH, Maletic V, Raison Charles L. Inflammation and its discontents: the role of cytokines in the pathophysiology of major depression. *Biol Psychiatry* (2009) 65(9):732–41. doi: 10.1016/j.biopsych.2008.11.029
21. Qin L, He J, Hanes RN, Pluzarev O, Hong J-S, Crews FT. Increased systemic and brain cytokine production and neuroinflammation by endotoxin following ethanol treatment. *J Neuroinflamm* (2008) 5:10. doi: 10.1186/1742-2094-5-10
22. Zhao Y-N, Wang F, Fan Y-X, Ping G-F, Yang J-Y, Wu C-F. Activated microglia are implicated in cognitive deficits, neuronal death, and successful recovery following intermittent ethanol exposure. *Behav Brain Res* (2013) 236(1):270–82. doi: 10.1016/j.bbr.2012.08.052
23. Marshall SA, McClain JA, Kelso ML, Hopkins DM, Pauly JR, Nixon K. Microglial activation is not equivalent to neuroinflammation in alcohol-induced neurodegeneration: the importance of microglia phenotype. *Neurobiol Dis* (2013) 54:239–51. doi: 10.1016/j.nbd.2012.12.016
24. Vetreno RP, Ramos RL, Anzalone S, Savage LM. Brain and behavioral pathology in an animal model of Wernicke's encephalopathy and Wernicke-Korsakoff syndrome. *Brain Res* (2012) 1436:178–92. doi: 10.1016/j.brainres.2011.11.038
25. Oliveira AC, Pereira MC, da Silva Santana LN, Fernandes RM, Teixeira FB, Oliveira GB, et al. Chronic ethanol exposure during adolescence through early adulthood in female rats induces emotional and memory deficits associated with morphological and molecular alterations in hippocampus. *J Psychopharmacol* (2015) 29(6):712–24. doi: 10.1177/0269881115581960
26. Moher D, Shamseer L, Clarke M, Ghersi D, Liberati A, Petticrew M, et al. Preferred Reporting Items for Systematic Review and Meta-Analysis Protocols (PRISMA-P) 2015 Statement. *Syst Rev* (2015) 4:1. doi: 10.1186/2046-4053-4-1
27. Houston RJ, Derrick JL, Leonard KE, Testa M, Quigley BM, Kubiak A. Effects of heavy drinking on executive cognitive functioning in a community sample. *Addict Behav* (2014) 39(1):345–49. doi: 10.1016/j.addbeh.2013.09.032
28. Míguez-Burbano, M. J., Nair M, Lewis JE, Fishman J. The role of alcohol on platelets, thymus and cognitive performance among HIV-infected subjects: are they related? *Platelets* (2009) 20(4):260–67. doi: 10.1080/09537100902964759
29. Yen C-H, Ho P-S, Yeh Y-W, Liang C-S, Kuo S-C, Huang C-C, et al. Differential cytokine levels between early withdrawal and remission states in patients with alcohol dependence. *Psychoneuroendocrinology* (2017) 76:183–91. doi: 10.1016/j.psyneuen.2016.10.015
30. Leclercq S, Cani PD, Neyrinck AM, Stärkel P, Jamar F, Mikolajczak M, et al. Role of intestinal permeability and inflammation in the biological and behavioral control of alcohol-dependent subjects. *Brain Behav Immun* (2012) 26(6):911–18. doi: 10.1016/j.bbi.2012.04.001
31. Wilhelm CJ, Fuller BE, Huckans M, Loftis JM. Peripheral immune factors are elevated in women with current or recent alcohol dependence and associated with altered mood and memory. *Drug Alcohol Depend* (2017) 176:71–8. doi: 10.1016/j.drugalcdep.2017.02.023
32. Duivis HE, Vogelzangs N, Kupper N, de Jonge P, Penninx BW. Differential association of somatic and cognitive symptoms of depression and anxiety with inflammation: findings from the Netherlands Study of Depression and Anxiety (NESDA). *Psychoneuroendocrinology* (2013) 38(9):1573–85. doi: 10.1016/j.psyneuen.2013.01.002

33. Boyer L, Richieri R, Dassa D, Boucekine M, Fernandez J, Vaillant Florence, et al. Association of metabolic syndrome and inflammation with neurocognition in patients with schizophrenia. *Psychiatry Res* (2013) 210(2):381–86. doi: 10.1016/j.psychres.2013.06.020
34. Kalk NJ, Guo Q, Owen D, Cherian R, Erritzoe D, Gilmour A, et al. Decreased hippocampal translocator protein (18 kDa) expression in alcohol dependence: a [C]PBR28 PET Study. *Transl Psychiatry* (2017) 7(1):e996. doi: 10.1038/tp.2016.264
35. Seitz HK, Bataller R, Cortez-Pinto H, Gao B, Gual A, Lackner C, et al. Alcoholic liver disease. *Nat Rev Dis Prim* (2018) 4(1):16. doi: 10.1038/s41572-018-0014-7
36. McClain CJ, Barve S, Deaciuc I, Kugelmas M, Hill D. Cytokines in alcoholic liver disease. *Semin Liver Dis* (1999) 19(2):205–19. doi: 10.1055/s-2007-1007110
37. Zemtsova I, Görg B, Keitel V, Bidmon H-J, Schrör K, Häussinger D. Microglia activation in hepatic encephalopathy in rats and humans. *Hepatol* (2011) 54(1):204–15. doi: 10.1002/hep.24326
38. Görg B, Schliess F, Häussinger D. Osmotic and oxidative/nitrosative stress in ammonia toxicity and hepatic encephalopathy. *Arch Biochem Biophysics* (2013) 536(2):158–63. doi: 10.1016/j.abb.2013.03.010
39. Cagnin A, Taylor-Robinson SD, Forton DM, Banati RB. In vivo imaging of cerebral 'peripheral benzodiazepine binding sites' in patients with hepatic encephalopathy. *Gut* (2006) 55(4):547–53. doi: 10.1136/gut.2005.075051
40. Shawcross DL, Wright G, Olde Damink SWM, Jalan R. Role of ammonia and inflammation in minimal hepatic encephalopathy. *Metab Brain Dis* (2007) 22(1):125–38. doi: 10.1007/s11011-006-9042-1
41. Rangroo Thrane V, Thrane AS, Chang J, Alleluia V, Nagelhus EA, Nedergaard M. Real-time analysis of microglial activation and motility in hepatic and hyperammonemic encephalopathy. *Neuroscience* (2012) 220:247–55. doi: 10.1016/j.neuroscience.2012.06.022
42. Neupane SP, Skulberg A, Skulberg Knut R., Aass HCD, Bramness JG. Cytokine changes following acute ethanol intoxication in healthy men: a crossover study. *Mediators Inflamm* (2016) 2016:3758590. doi: 10.1155/2016/3758590
43. Yen C-H, Shih M-C, Cheng C-Y, Ma K-H, Lu R-B, Huang S-Y. Incongruent reduction of dopamine transporter availability in different subgroups of alcohol dependence. *Medicine* (2016) 95(33):e4048. doi: 10.1097/MD.0000000000004048
44. Campbell BM, Charych E, Lee, A. W., Möller T. Kynurenines in CNS disease: regulation by inflammatory cytokines. *Front Neurosci* (2014) 8:12. doi: 10.3389/fnins.2014.00012
45. De Picker LJ, Morrens M, Chance SA, Boche D. Microglia and brain plasticity in acute psychosis and schizophrenia illness course: a meta-review. *Front Psychiatry/Front Res Found* (2017) 8:238. doi: 10.3389/fpsyt.2017.00238
46. Oades RD. An exploration of the associations of pregnancy and perinatal features with cytokines and tryptophan/kynurenine metabolism in children with attention-deficit hyperactivity disorder (ADHD). *Attent Defic Hyper Disord* (2011) 3(4):301–18. doi: 10.1007/s12402-011-0062-2
47. Brody AL, Hubert R, Enoki R, Garcia LY, Mamoun MS, Okita K, et al. Effect of cigarette smoking on a marker for neuroinflammation: a [C]DAA1106 positron emission tomography study. *Neuropsychopharmacol: Official Pub Ame College Neuropsychopharmacol* (2017) 42(8):1630–39. doi: 10.1038/npp.2017.48
48. Smith PH, Chhipa M, Bystrik J, Roy J, Goodwin RD, McKee SA. Cigarette smoking among those with mental disorders in the US population: 2012-2013 update. *Tob Control* (2018) [Epub ahead of print]. doi: 10.1136/tobaccocontrol-2018-054268
49. Turner S, Mota N, Bolton J, Sareen J. Self-medication with alcohol or drugs for mood and anxiety disorders: a narrative review of the epidemiological literature. *Depression Anxiety* (2018) 35(9):851–60. doi: 10.1002/da.22771
50. Antoniak DT, Duryee MJ, Mikuls TR, Thiele GM, Anderson DR. Aldehyde-modified proteins as mediators of early inflammation in atherosclerotic disease. *Free Radical Biol Med* (2015) 89 409–18. doi: 10.1016/j.freeradbiomed.2015.09.003
51. Malaguarnera G, Bertino G, Vacante M, Malaguarnera M. Hepatocellular carcinoma markers in the omics era: the glycomic analysis. *Hepatobiliary Surg Nutr* (2014) 3(6):407–9. doi: 10.3978/j.issn.2304-3881.2014.07.04
52. Rolland B, D'Hondt F, Montègue S, Brion M, Peyron E, D'Aviau de Ternay J, et al. A patient-tailored evidence-based approach for developing early neuropsychological training programs in addiction settings. *Neuropsychol Rev* (2019) 29(1):103–15. doi: 10.1007/s11065-018-9395-3

15

Dysfunctional Personality Beliefs Linked to Emotion Recognition Deficits in Individuals with Cocaine Addiction and Personality Disorders

Natalia Albein-Urios[1], Jose M. Martinez-Gonzalez[2], Oscar Lozano-Rojas[3,4] and Antonio Verdejo-Garcia[5]*

[1] Cognitive Neuroscience Unit, School of Psychology, Deakin University, Geelong, VIC, Australia, [2] Centro Provincial de Drogodependencias, Diputación de Granada, Granada, Spain, [3] Departamento de Psicología Clínica, Experimental y Social, Universidad de Huelva, Huelva, Spain, [4] Research Center on Natural Resources, Health and Environment, University of Huelva, Huelva, Spain, [5] Turner Institute for Brain and Mental Health, Monash University, Melbourne, VIC, Australia

***Correspondence:**
Antonio Verdejo-Garcia
antonio.verdejo@monash.edu

Background: Facial emotion recognition is impaired in addiction and personality disorders. Dysfunctional personality beliefs reflect negative interpersonal schemas that may underpin emotion recognition deficits. We aimed to examine the association between personality beliefs and emotion recognition among participants with cocaine use disorder including those with comorbid personality disorders.

Methods: We recruited 70 participants with cocaine use disorder aged between 19 and 52 who had used 14 g of cocaine over 4.8 years on average. Thirty-eight participants had an additional personality disorder (11 Borderline, 7 Histrionic, 5 Antisocial, 10 Avoidant, and 5 Obsessive–Compulsive). Dysfunctional beliefs were indicated with the Personality Belief Questionnaire, and facial emotion recognition was indicated with the Ekman's Test. We applied correlations/multiple regressions to test the relationship between beliefs and emotion recognition.

Results: Personality beliefs reflecting paranoid, borderline, and antisocial schemas were negatively associated with emotion recognition. Antisocial beliefs were associated with poorer recognition of fear, and paranoid beliefs with poorer recognition of disgust. Antisocial beliefs were significantly associated with emotion recognition after adjusting for cocaine use.

Conclusion: Dysfunctional personality beliefs are associated with poorer emotion recognition in cocaine addiction. Personality-related negative schemas about the self and others can impact social cognition and interaction during cocaine treatment.

Keywords: emotion recognition, personality disorders, cocaine use disorder, personality beliefs, antisocial beliefs

INTRODUCTION

Facial emotion recognition reflects the ability to identify basic emotions in others and is essential for adaptive social interaction (1, 2). Deficits in facial emotion recognition are a hallmark of substance use disorders (SUD) (3). However, although SUD often co-occur with personality disorders (4), little is known on the relationship between comorbid personality dysfunction and facial emotion recognition. This is important because personality disorders are characterized by difficulties with social interaction and disturbed representations of others (5–7). Individuals with personality disorders have lower facial emotion recognition accuracy than healthy controls (8–10). However, we do not know if the comorbidity between SUD and personality disorders is associated with additive or specific impacts on facial emotion recognition. Unraveling the link between personality dysfunction and facial emotion recognition can contribute to understand social interaction problems and persistence of SUD among individuals with comorbid personality disorders.

In the context of SUD without comorbidities, previous studies have found that individuals with cocaine-SUD have poorer recognition of specific emotions such as anger and fear (11). In the only study comparing individuals with cocaine-SUD with and without personality disorders, Morgan and Marshall (12) found no significant effects of comorbidity on fear recognition. Using psychophysiological measures of fear and arousal reactivity, Baschnagel et al. (13) also failed to find a significant effect of the comorbidity on psychophysiological measures of emotion processing. However, these studies have adopted a categorical approach, by comparing comorbid versus non-comorbid participants (13) or covarying the effect of the comorbid personality diagnosis (12). However, current evidence supports the view that dimensional measures of personality dysfunction are better suited than categorical approaches to gain insight on emotion recognition deficits (14). Dimensional measures of antisociality and anxiety are negatively associated with emotion recognition accuracy, and specifically with poorer recognition of anger and fear among healthy individuals (15).

Personality beliefs are key dimensional features of personality disorders that have been neglected in previous studies of emotion recognition (16, 17). Dysfunctional beliefs reflect deep-rooted negative schemas that can consistently bias cognitive and affective judgments about oneself and others (17). Since these negative schemas are linked to specific personality disorders, the degree of disturbance can be estimated by measuring endorsement of specific sets of beliefs (e.g., antisocial—"I should do whatever I can get away with"; obsessive–compulsive—"Any flaw or defect may lead to a catastrophe") (18). The Personality Belief Questionnaire (PBQ) was originally designed to measure these personality beliefs and has received recent attention and excellent kudos as a dimensional measure of personality dysfunction that is well aligned with contemporary views, as well as reliable and predictive of severity of personality dysfunction (17, 19). Previous studies have shown that individuals with cocaine-SUD have elevated PBQ scores compared to healthy controls (20, 21). Moreover, those with cocaine-SUD and personality disorders exhibit higher scores than controls in antisocial, borderline, histrionic, and narcissistic scales (20). PBQ scores are also elevated among people with other psychiatric disorders (i.e., depression and eating disorders) who have comorbid personality disorders compared to those with single diagnoses (17, 19).

In this study, we aimed to examine the relationship between dimensional estimates of dysfunctional personality beliefs, measured with the PBQ, and emotion recognition, indicated by the gold-standard Ekman facial emotion recognition test, among people with cocaine-SUD including those with comorbid personality disorders. In fitting with previous evidence on dimensional personality correlates of emotion recognition, we hypothesized that dysfunctional beliefs associated with antisocial and anxious-like personality disorders would be linked to lower emotion recognition accuracy and specifically poorer recognition of fear and anger.

METHODS

Participants

The sample comprised 70 participants (11 females) with cocaine use disorder, of whom 38 (54%; consistent with previously reported comorbidity rates) (22) had comorbid personality disorders (11 Borderline, 7 Histrionic, 5 Antisocial, 10 Avoidant, and 5 Obsessive–Compulsive). Participants with and without comorbid personality disorders did not significantly differ on sociodemographic characteristics or cocaine use patterns (**Table 1**).

TABLE 1 | Sociodemographic characteristics, drug use patterns, and personality beliefs and emotion recognition scores in participants with and without personality disorders.

	Whole sample (n = 70)	SUD (n = 32)	SUD + PD (n = 38)	t	p
Age	33.53 (6.84)	32.60 (6.38)	34.32 (7.19)	−1.050	0.297
Education (yrs.)	10.20 (1.77)	10.00 (1.61)	10.37 (1.91)	−0.864	0.391
Cocaine grams/mo.	14.00 (19.92)	14.45 (20.15)	13.63 (20.01)	0.169	0.866
Cocaine duration (mo.)	57.37 (51.32)	55.02 (53.10)	59.29 (50.45)	−0.342	0.734
PBQ Paranoid	19.91 (13.63)	16.56 (12.68)	22.73 (13.92)	−1.925	0.058
PBQ Schizoid	23.04 (10.96)	21.22 (10.45)	24.58 (11.29)	−1.283	0.204
PBQ Antisocial	17.21 (8.51)	15.84 (8.13)	18.37 (8.75)	−1.242	0.219
PBQ Borderline	16.41 (10.29)	12.28 (9.48)	19.89 (9.75)	−3.296	0.002*
PBQ Histrionic	16.66 (8.58)	15.09 (7.18)	17.97 (9.51)	−1.408	0.164
PBQ Narcissistic	12.04 (7.65)	11.75 (8.80)	12.29 (6.62)	−0.294	0.769
PBQ Avoidant	17.44 (9.06)	14.44 (8.89)	19.97 (8.51)	−2.657	0.010
PBQ Dependent	20.26 (10.52)	17.41 (8.94)	22.73 (11.25)	−2.152	0.035
PBQ O–C	25.16 (10.78)	23.41 (11.57)	26.63 (9.98)	−1.252	0.215
Total Emotion Recognition	48.74 (4.94)	49.40 (4.41)	48.18 (5.34)	1.032	0.306

*SUD, substance use disorder (cocaine); PD, personality disorder; yrs., years; mo., months; PBQ, Personality Beliefs Questionnaire; O–C, Obsessive–compulsive. *p < 0.005.*

All participants were recruited from a city-wide public outpatient addiction treatment center in Granada (Spain). Treatment consisted of cognitive behavioral therapy and psychosocial support. The inclusion criteria were as follows: i) meeting Diagnostic and Statistical Manual of Mental Disorders, Fourth Edition, Text Revision (DSM-IV-TR) (23) criteria for cocaine dependence indicated with the Structured Clinical Interview for DSM-IV Disorders–Clinical Version (SCID-CV) (24), ii) being abstinent for at least 2 weeks indicated by self-report and regular urine analyses, and iii) IQ levels ≥80 (to ensure facial emotion recognition was not impacted by general cognitive dysfunction) indicated with the Kaufman Brief Intelligence Test (25). Personality disorders included in the DSM-IV-TR were diagnosed by an accredited clinical psychologist (JM-G) using the International Personality Disorders Examination (26). Participants received personality disorders diagnosis at the same time as cocaine dependence diagnosis. The exclusion criteria were as follows: i) other Axis I comorbid disorders, with the exceptions of alcohol abuse and nicotine dependence, indicated with the SCID-CV; ii) history of head injury and/or neurological, infectious, systemic, or any other diseases affecting the central nervous system, indicated by self-report and clinical records.

Measures

Interview for Research on Addictive Behavior (27): This semi-structured interview collects information about substance use patterns (i.e., dosage, frequency, and duration) and yields two main measures: monthly use of each substance (quantity per month) and total duration of use of each substance (duration in months).

Personality Belief Questionnaire (PBQ) (18): The PBQ was administered to dimensionally measure dysfunctional beliefs or negative schemas associated with personality disorders. It is a 126-item self-report questionnaire that measures the degree of endorsement of dysfunctional beliefs associated with personality disorders, i.e., paranoid, schizoid, antisocial, borderline, histrionic, narcissistic, avoidant, dependent, and obsessive–compulsive beliefs. The Spanish version of the scale that we used in this study has demonstrated sound psychometric characteristics (28).

Ekman Faces Test (EFT): This is a computer task that assesses recognition of facial emotional expressions. The task uses stimuli from the Facial Expressions of Emotion: Stimuli and Tests (FEEST) (29). We presented 60 faces depicting expressions of anger, disgust, fear, happiness, sadness, and surprise (6 emotions, 10 faces each). Each face was presented on a computer monitor for a maximum of 5 s, after which individuals were asked to select the emotion that best described it. The performance measure was the sum score of total correct identifications (total recognition: range, 0–60).

Procedures

The Human Research Ethics Committee of the University of Granada approved the study. All participants provided written informed consent. Participants underwent two assessment sessions: one to diagnose substance use and personality disorders, and a second one to complete personality beliefs and emotion recognition measures, along with other cognitive measures that have been published elsewhere.

Analyses

First, we contrasted emotion recognition scores between participants with and without personality disorders using *t*-tests. Next, we examined the relationship between personality beliefs and total emotion recognition scores using *Spearman* correlation coefficients. When there was a significant association between specific dysfunctional beliefs and total emotion recognition, we run additional correlations between such beliefs and discrete emotions recognition scores (e.g., anger and fear). Finally, we tested if the relationship between dysfunctional beliefs and total emotion recognition scores stood after adjusting for sociodemographic characteristics and lifetime substance use using multiple regression. Results from group contrasts and correlational analyses, involving multiple tests, were considered significant if p values were below 0.005 to protect against Type I error. Results from targeted regression analyses were considered significant at the standard $p < 0.05$ value. Data is available at https://monash.figshare.com/s/f35e993c96fbb2899ecb.

RESULTS

Emotion Recognition in Participants With Versus Without Personality Disorders

We found no significant differences between participants with and without personality disorders in total emotion recognition scores (**Table 1**). As expected, participants with personality disorders had generally higher PBQ scores (reflecting greater endorsement of dysfunctional personality beliefs), but the group differences were only significant for borderline beliefs (**Table 1**).

Relationship Between Emotion Recognition and Dysfunctional Personality Beliefs

We found significant negative associations between the total emotion recognition score and antisocial, borderline, and paranoid beliefs (**Table 2**). Subsequent analyses showed that

TABLE 2 | Correlations between dysfunctional personality beliefs and emotion recognition.

	Emotion recognition total score	
	rho	*p*
PBQ Paranoid	−0.359	0.002*
PBQ Schizoid	−0.186	0.122
PBQ Antisocial	−0.399	0.001*
PBQ Borderline	−0.355	0.003*
PBQ Histrionic	−0.133	0.272
PBQ Narcissistic	−0.212	0.080
PBQ Avoidant	−0.247	0.039
PBQ Dependent	−0.321	0.007
PBQ Obsessive–Compulsive	−0.329	0.005

PBQ, Personality Beliefs Questionnaire. *$p < 0.005$.

TABLE 3 | Multiple regression model entering sociodemographic characteristics, drug use patterns, and dysfunctional beliefs as predictors of emotion recognition.

	Age		Education		Cocaine (gr)		Cocaine (mo)		Paranoid		Antisocial		Borderline	
	β	*p*	*β*	*p*	*β*	*p*	*β*	*p*	*β*	*p*	*β*	*p*	*β*	*p*
Emotion recognition total score	−0.031	0.813	0.139	0.253	−0.021	0.860	−0.070	0.586	0.144	0.482	−0.342	0.019*	−0.322	0.109

*gr, grams; mo, months; O-C. *p < 0.05.*

antisocial beliefs were negatively associated with recognition of fear, $r = -0.376$, $p = 0.001$, whereas paranoid beliefs were negatively associated with recognition of disgust, $r = -0.372$, $p = 0.002$ (**Supplementary Table S1**).

Regression Analyses Adjusted by Sociodemographic and Drug Use Characteristics

After adjusting for age, education, and lifetime drug use, antisocial beliefs were significantly associated with total emotion recognition scores ($F_{\text{full model}} = 3.647$, $Adj\ R^2_{\text{full model}} = 0.214$, $p_{\text{full model}} = 0.002$, $Beta_{\text{antisocial}} = -0.342$, $p_{\text{antisocial}} = 0.019$) (**Table 3**). No other individual predictors were significantly associated with emotion recognition.

DISCUSSION

Our findings show that, although participants *with* and *without* personality disorders did not differ in emotion recognition, the degree of endorsement of dysfunctional personality beliefs was negatively associated with facial emotion recognition accuracy. These results suggest that individuals with more negative schemas associated with personality dysfunction can have greater problems to identify and interpret emotions in others, and ultimately more social interaction problems.

The link between dysfunctional personality beliefs and poorer emotion recognition provides support to the notion that maladaptive personality schemas are associated with social interaction deficits in people with SUD (30, 31). This relationship is acknowledged in modern definitions of personality disorders and stimulant addiction, which refer to disturbances in interpersonal functioning (32, 33). The directionality of the association is unclear. It is possible that emotion recognition deficits predate personality dysfunction and thus contributes to the formation of dysfunctional beliefs *via* early negative social interaction experiences (34). It is also plausible that dysfunctional beliefs cause stable biases in affective judgment that ultimately impact emotion recognition (e.g., "Others will try to use me or manipulate me if I don't watch out") (16). Since participants were in the "craving phase" of their SUD (35), it is also possible that state-related symptoms such as anhedonia modulate the link between personality and emotion recognition (36). Furthermore, the link between emotion recognition and dysfunctional personality beliefs, which are dimensional measures of personality dysfunction, supports the view that dimensional (versus categorical) indices of personality dysfunction can be more tightly aligned with social cognition and interaction phenotypes (37). Although emotion recognition is a well-recognized index of social cognition skills (1, 2), our findings can also stimulate further research on other aspects of social cognition and interaction in the context of addiction and personality disorders.

The link between specific personality beliefs and difficulties to recognize emotions in others has also important clinical value. In fact, we found specific associations between antisocial beliefs and poorer recognition of fear, which is consistent with previous findings among individuals with antisocial personality disorder (38) and align with the "low fear" theory of antisocial personality and psychopathy (39). Since fear recognition is essential to avoid risk (e.g., by recognizing others' appraisal about potentially risky situations such as those conducive to relapse) and harm to others (e.g., by recognizing their fear in response to one's actions), individuals with greater endorsement of antisocial beliefs and poorer emotion recognition might be at particularly high risk of poor clinical outcomes (40). We also found negative associations between paranoid beliefs and poorer recognition of disgust, but this relationship did not survive adjustment for sociodemographic and clinical characteristics. Therefore, these relationships might be conflated with other indicators of severity (e.g., higher levels of drug use) and should be reassessed in future studies. Establishing these links is important, since little is known about the social cognition correlates of personality dysfunctions associated with paranoid schemas compared to antisocial or borderline schemas (38).

Our findings need to be appraised in the context of relevant limitations. First, results are cross-sectional and correlational, meaning that we cannot draw causal conclusions. Second, we focused on two very specific indices of personality dysfunction (beliefs) and social cognition (emotion recognition), and hence, more comprehensive assessments are needed to confirm if the relationship between these constructs stands in the context of other indices of personality dysfunction (e.g., dimensional diagnostic tools) and social cognition (e.g., empathy). Third, according to the cognitive theory of personality disorders (41), participants with personality disorders should have generally elevated dysfunctional beliefs; the fact that we only found differences in borderline beliefs may be due to the small number of cases. Fourth, although we interpret findings mostly in the context of personality dysfunction, other etiological and clinical aspects of cocaine addiction (e.g., genetic vulnerability and cocaine dosage) may also contribute to emotion recognition deficits.

AUTHOR CONTRIBUTIONS

AV-G, JM-G and OL-R designed the study. NA-U and JM-G conducted assessments. OL-R and AV-G conducted statistical analyses. NA-U and AV-G wrote a first draft of the manuscript, which was reviewed by all authors.

REFERENCES

1. Adolphs R, Tranel D, Damasio H, Damasio A. Impaired recognition of emotion in facial expressions following bilateral damage to the human amygdala. *Nature* (1994) 372:669–72. doi: 10.1038/372669a0
2. Corden B, Critchley HD, Skuse D, Dolan RJ. Fear recognition ability predicts differences in social cognitive and neural functioning in men. *J Cogn Neurosci* (2006) 18:889–97. doi: 10.1162/jocn.2006.18.6.889
3. Castellano F, Bartoli F, Crocamo C, Gamba G, Tremolada M, Santambrogio J, et al. Facial emotion recognition in alcohol and substance use disorders: a meta-analysis. *Neurosci Biobehav Rev* (2015) 59:147–54. doi: 10.1016/j.neubiorev.2015.11.001
4. Vergara-Moragues E, Gonzalez-Saiz F, Lozano OM, Verdejo Garcia A. Psychopathological stability of personality disorders in substance abuse patients treated in a therapeutic community. *J Addict Dis* (2013) 32(4):343–53. doi: 10.1080/10550887.2013.854154
5. Arntz A, Veen G. Evaluations of others by borderline patients. *J Nerv Ment Dis* (2001) 189(8):513–21. doi: 10.1097/00005053-200108000-00004
6. Arntz A, Weertman A, Salet S. Interpretation bias in Cluster-C and borderline personality disorders. *Behav Res Ther* (2011) 49(8):472–81. doi: 10.1016/j.brat.2011.05.002
7. Schotte CK, de Doncker D, Vankerckhoven C, Vertommen H, Cosyns P. Self-report assessment of the DSM-IV personality disorders. Measurement of trait and distress characteristics: the ADP-IV. *Psychol Med* (1998) 28(5):1179–88. doi: 10.1017/S0033291798007041
8. Daros AR, Zakzanis KK, Ruocco AC. Facial emotion recognition in borderline personality disorder. *Psychol Med* (2013) 43(9):1953–63. doi: 10.1017/S0033291712002607
9. Dawel A, O'Kearney R, McKone E, Palermo R. Not just fear and sadness: meta-analytic evidence of pervasive emotion recognition deficits for facial and vocal expressions in psychopathy. *Neurosci Biobehav Rev* (2012) 36(10):2288–304. doi: 10.1016/j.neubiorev.2012.08.006
10. Marsh AA, Blair RJ. Deficits in facial affect recognition among antisocial populations: a meta-analysis. *Neurosci Biobehav Rev* (2008) 32(3):454–65. doi: 10.1016/j.neubiorev.2007.08.003
11. Fernandez-Serrano MJ, Lozano O, Perez-Garcia M, Verdejo-Garcia A. Impact of severity of drug use on discrete emotions recognition in polysubstance abusers. *Drug Alcohol Depend* (2010) 109(1–3):57–64. doi: 10.1016/j.drugalcdep.2009.12.007
12. Morgan MJ, Marshall JP. Deficient fear recognition in regular cocaine users is not attributable to elevated impulsivity or conduct disorder prior to cocaine use. *J Psychopharmacol* (2013) 27(6):526–32. doi: 10.1177/0269881113477708
13. Baschnagel JS, Coffey SF, Hawk LW, Jr., Schumacher JA, Holloman G. Psychophysiological assessment of emotional processing in patients with borderline personality disorder with and without comorbid substance use. *Personal Disord* (2013) 4(3):203–13. doi: 10.1037/a0029777
14. Murphy FC, Ewbank MP, Calder AJ. Emotion and personality factors influence the neural response to emotional stimuli. *Behav Brain Sci* (2012) 35(3):156–7. doi: 10.1017/S0140525X11001725
15. Calder AJ, Ewbank M, Passamonti L. Personality influences the neural responses to viewing facial expressions of emotion. *Philos trans R Soc Lond B Biol Sci* (2011) 366(1571):1684–701. doi: 10.1098/rstb.2010.0362
16. Beck AT, Butler AC, Brown GK, Dahlsgaard KK, Newman CF, Beck JS. Dysfunctional beliefs discriminate personality disorders. *Behav Res Ther* (2001) 39(10):1213–25. doi: 10.1016/S0005-7967(00)00099-1
17. Fournier JC, Derubeis RJ, Beck AT. Dysfunctional cognitions in personality pathology: the structure and validity of the personality belief questionnaire. *Psychol Med* (2012) 42(4):795–805. doi: 10.1017/S0033291711001711
18. Beck AT, Beck JS. *The Personality Belief Questionnaire*. Bala Cynwyd, PA: The Beck Institute for Cognitive Therapy and Research (1991).
19. Bhar SS, Beck AT, Butler AC. Beliefs and personality disorders: an overview of the personality beliefs questionnaire. *J Clin Psychol* (2012) 68(1):88–100. doi: 10.1002/jclp.20856
20. Albein-Urios N, Martinez-González JM, Lozano O, Verdejo-Garcia A. Monetary delay discounting in gambling and cocaine dependence with personality comorbidities. *Addict Behav* (2014) 39(11):1658–62. doi: 10.1016/j.addbeh.2014.06.001
21. Albein-Urios N, Martinez-Gonzalez JM, Lozano Ó, Moreno-López L, Soriano-Mas C, Verdejo-Garcia A. Negative urgency, disinhibition and reduced temporal pole gray matter characterize the comorbidity of cocaine dependence and personality disorders. *Drug Alcohol Depend* (2013) 132(1–2):231–7. doi: 10.1016/j.drugalcdep.2013.02.008
22. Arias F, Szerman N, Vega P, Mesias B, Basurte I, Morant C, et al. Cocaine abuse or dependency and other pyschiatric disorders. Madrid study on dual pathology. *Rev Psiquiatr Salud Ment* (2013) 6(3):121–8. doi: 10.1016/j.rpsm.2012.09.002
23. American Psychiatric Association. *Diagnostic and statistical manual of mental disorders*. 4th ed., text rev. Washington, DC: Author (2000).
24. First MB, Spitzer RL, Gibbon M, Williams JBW. *Structured Clinical Interview for DSM-IV Axis I disorders (SCID I)*. New York: Biometric Research Department (1997).
25. Kaufman AS, Kaufman NL. *Kaufman Brief Intelligence Test 1*. Circle Pines, MN: American Guidance Service (1990).
26. Loranger AW, Sartorius N, Andreoli A, Berger P, Buchheim P, Jacobsberg LB, et al. The international personality disorder examination. The world health organization/alcohol, drug abuse, and mental health administration international pilot study of personality disorders. *Arch Gen Psychiatry* (1994) 51:215–24. doi: 10.1001/archpsyc.1994.03950030051005
27. Verdejo-Garcia AJ, Lopez-Torrecillas F, Aguilar de Arcos F, Perez-Garcia M. Differential effects of MDMA, cocaine, and cannabis use severity on distinctive components of the executive functions in polysubstance users: a multiple regression analysis. *Addict Behav* (2005) 30(1):89–101. doi: 10.1016/j.addbeh.2004.04.015
28. Albein-Urios N, Martínez-González JM, Lozano-Rojas OM, Verdejo-García A. Estudio preliminar para la validación de la versión española del Personality Belief Questionnaire (PBQ). *Trastornos Adictivos* (2011) 13:144–50. doi: 10.1016/S1575-0973(11)70030-7
29. Young AW, Perrett D, Calder AJ, Sprengelmeyer R, Ekman P. *Facial emotional expressions: stimuli and tests (FEEST)*. Bury St. Edmunds: Thames Valley Test Company (2002).
30. Quednow BB, Hulka LM, Preller KH, Baumgartner MR, Eisenegger C, Vonmoos M. Stable self-serving personality traits in recreational and dependent cocaine users. *PloS One* (2017) 12(3):e0172853. doi: 10.1371/journal.pone.0172853
31. Verdejo-Garcia A, Verdejo-Roman J, Albein-Urios N, Martinez-Gonzalez JM, Soriano-Mas C. Brain substrates of social decision-making in dual diagnosis: cocaine dependence and personality disorders. *Addict Biol* (2017) 22(2):457–67. doi: 10.1111/adb.12318
32. American Psychiatric Association. *Diagnostic and statistical manual of mental disorders (DSM-5®)*. Arlington, VA: American Psychiatric Pub (2013). doi: 10.1176/appi.books.9780890425596
33. Quednow BB. Social cognition and interaction in stimulant use disorders. *Curr Opin Behav Sci* (2017) 13:55–62. doi: 10.1016/j.cobeha.2016.10.001
34. Hasenfratz L, Benish-Weisman M, Steinberg T, Knafo-Noam A. Temperament and peer problems from early to middle childhood: gene-environment correlations with negative emotionality and sociability. *Dev Psychopathol* (2015) 27(4 Pt 1):1089–109. doi: 10.1017/S095457941500070X
35. Koob GF, Volkow ND. Neurobiology of addiction: a neurocircuitry analysis. *Lancet Psychiatry* (2016) (8), 760–73. doi: 10.1016/S2215-0366(16)00104-8
36. Hatzigiakoumis DS, Martinotti G, Giannantonio MD, Janiri L. Anhedonia and substance dependence: clinical correlates and treatment options. *Front Psychiatry* (2011) 17(2):10. doi: 10.3389/fpsyt.2011.00010

37. DeFife JA, Goldberg M, Westen D. Dimensional assessment of self- and interpersonal functioning in adolescents: implications for DSM-5's general definition of personality disorder. *J Pers Disord* (2015) 29(2):248–60. doi: 10.1521/pedi_2013_27_085
38. Herpertz SC, Bertsch K. The social-cognitive basis of personality disorders. *Curr Opin Psychiatry* (2014) 27(1):73–7. doi: 10.1097/YCO.0000000000000026
39. Patrick CJ, Cuthbert BN, Lang PJ. Emotion in the criminal psychopath: fear image processing. *J Abnorm Psychol* (1994) 103(3):523–34. doi: 10.1037//0021-843X.103.3.523
40. Moeller SJ, Goldstein RZ. Impaired self-awareness in human addiction: deficient attribution of personal relevance. *Trends Cogn Sci* (2014) 18(12):635–41. doi: 10.1016/j.tics.2014.09.003
41. Beck AT, Freeman A, Davis DD, Pretzer J, Fleming B, Beck JS. *Cognitive therapy of personality disorders*. 2nd ed. New York: Guilford Press (2004).

16

Cognitive Function Impairments Linked to Alcohol and Cannabis use during Adolescence: A Study of Gender Differences

*Simasadat Noorbakhsh, Mohammad H. Afzali, Elroy Boers and Patricia J. Conrod**

Département de Psychiatrie, Université de Montréal, Centre de Recherche du CHU Sainte-Justine, Montréal, QC, Canada

***Correspondence:**
Patricia J. Conrod
patricia.conrod@umontreal.ca

Major neurocognitive changes occur during adolescence, making this phase one of the most critical developmental periods of life. Furthermore, this phase in life is also the time in which youth substance use begins. Several studies have demonstrated the differential associations of alcohol and cannabis use concerning the neurocognitive functioning of both males and females. Past and contemporary literature on gender-specific effects in neuroscience of addiction is predominantly based on cross-sectional datasets and data that is limited in terms of measurement variability. Given the importance of gender-specific effects in addiction studies, and in order to address the two above-mentioned gaps in the literature, the present study aimed to compare neurocognitive functioning of male and female adolescents in the context of cannabis and alcohol use, while employing a longitudinal design with multiple repeated measurements. Participants were 3,826 high school students (47% female; mean age, 12.7), who were recruited from 31 high schools in the greater Montreal area. Participants were requested to complete annual surveys for five consecutive years, from 7th to 11th grade, assessing their alcohol/cannabis use and neurocognitive functioning (working memory, delayed recall memory, perceptual reasoning, and inhibition control). The analytical strategy focused on the longitudinal association between each predictor (female, male) and each of the outcomes (domains of neurocognitive functioning). Multilevel linear models assessed the association of alcohol and cannabis consumption and the four domains of neurocognitive functioning. Results revealed a gender by within-subject interaction, suggesting a weaker effect of yearly fluctuation of cannabis use on working memory among males compared to females. Our findings suggest a different pattern of neurocognitive impairment of female and male working memory after using cannabis over the course of adolescence. Early initiation of cannabis use potentially results in more spatial working memory deficits in female adolescents. This may negatively influence young females' capacity in academic settings and lead to significant impairment in adulthood, which critically decreases the individual's quality of life.

Keywords: cognitive function, alcohol, cannabis, gender difference, adolescent

INTRODUCTION

Given the increased rate of substance use from early to late adolescence (Duncan et al., 2006), it is becoming more and more critical to understand the effects of substance use on teens' neurocognitive functioning. Alcohol and cannabis are the most commonly used psychoactive substances in Canada (Statistics Canada, 2015). Heavy drinking during adolescence has been indicated as a significant factor for declined memory (Mahmood et al., 2010) and impaired neurocognitive functioning (Mahmood et al., 2010), while cannabis use has been demonstrated to be associated with short-term and long-term cognitive deficits, such as impaired inhibitory control and working memory (Volkow et al., 2016; Morin et al., 2019). The proportion of males aged 12 years and over using alcohol or cannabis is approximately 5% to 10% higher than that of females in the same age group (Leatherdale and Burkhalter, 2012; Statistics Canada, 2018). Although the rate of substance use is different for male adolescents than for female adolescents, contemporary knowledge concerning gender-specific trajectories of substance use is limited. In particular, research distinguishing between different neurocognitive outcomes attributed to alcohol and cannabis use in adolescence, as well as taking into account potential gender-specific varying effects, is scarce.

The developmental phase of adolescence is, among others, marked by a multitude of neurocognitive and psychosocial changes, making the phase of adolescence one of the most critical developmental periods of life (Giedd, 2015). Furthermore, experimentation with substance use often starts in adolescence and so does the process of addiction (Volkow et al., 2016). For example, more than 90% of people who have an addiction today started to use various substances before they were 18 years old (Public Health Agency of Canada, 2018). This could reflect normal adolescent-specific behaviors (risk-taking, novelty-seeking, response to peer pressure) that increase the probability of someone experimenting with substances, and perhaps could also reflect the incomplete development neurocognitive functioning (Sowell et al., 2004).

The latter has been demonstrated by previous work showing that, relative to young adults and older people, the balance between adolescents' reward motivation and executive control is not fully developed, therefore making adolescents more prone to engaging in health-risk behaviors such as alcohol use and cannabis use (Hammond et al., 2014). This disturbed balance has also been shown to accentuate the difference between adolescents who frequently engage in health-risk behaviors and those who do not (Squeglia et al., 2009). However, this differing balance has not only been found between adolescents and older people, and adolescents who frequently engage in health-risk behavior and those who do not, but also between male and female adolescents, predominantly because male and female adolescents do not share the same brain structure and neurodevelopmental pace (Lenroot and Giedd, 2010). That is, it has been suggested that early exposure to alcohol and cannabis use affects male and female adolescents' neurocognitive development differently. Therefore, identifying gender-specific influences of alcohol and cannabis use separate for male and female adolescents could be beneficial to explain differential proneness to substance use in adolescents. Although, while within the realm of research on substance use, the importance of standard reporting on gender differences has been well acknowledged, only one-fourth of all studies on adolescent substance use have reported on this (Karlsson Lind et al., 2017). Thus, the results of this longitudinal study could potentially contribute in moving a step forward within this specific field of research.

To date, several studies have demonstrated differential associations of alcohol use, brain structure, and neurocognitive functioning for male and female adolescents. Specifically, Medina et al. (2008) examined the role of gender concerning the association of alcohol-use disorder and prefrontal cortex (PFC) morphometry in adolescents. Despite similar patterns of alcohol use, and even after controlling for variables such as conduct disorder and family history of substance-use disorders, Medina and colleagues found that gender moderated the association of alcohol-use disorder and PFC morphometry in adolescents. Also, it was revealed that, compared to same-gender controls, females showed smaller volumes of PFC morphometry, whereas males showed larger volumes (Medina et al., 2008). These findings are in line with previous work on functional neuroimaging, reporting that males suffering from alcohol-use disorder had increased superior frontal activation while female drinkers had limited superior frontal activation during spatial working memory tasks (Caldwell et al., 2005). The latter indicates, and has been supported by other works, that the fronto-parietal network regions could be particularly susceptible to alterations due to alcohol misuse/use, with females portraying greater adverse effects than males (Caldwell et al., 2005; Squeglia et al., 2012). Moreover, it has been proposed that regions in the brain network develop sooner among females than males (Giedd et al., 1996), implying that females may experience a stronger impaired working memory than males, if alcohol use has its onset in early adolescence (Wager and Smith, 2003).

Another brain region that might show a differing developmental trajectory for male and female adolescents when it concerns substance use is the PFC. The PFC has been shown to have protracted development and has been identified to be the last region of the brain to develop in adolescence. Several pre-clinical studies suggested that exposure to cannabis products during adolescence impacts neuromaturational processes in this region (Miller et al., 2019). Furthermore, functional neuroimaging studies found abnormal PFC activation patterns among adolescent marijuana users compared to controls, when it concerned an inhibition related go/no-go task (Tapert et al., 2007), as well as verbal memory (Jacobsen et al., 2007) and spatial working memory (Schweinsburg et al., 2008) tasks. Despite these valuable study results, when it concerns the moderating role of gender on the association of PFC structure and function and cannabis use in adolescents, past and contemporary findings are rather inconsistent. Whereas Pfefferbaum et al. (2002) found increased myelination of the PFC among young women, another study by Nagel et al. (2006) revealed contrasting results. Specifically, Nagel et al. (2006) found that women had reduced PFC white matter volume than men, of which the white matter volume of men remained moderately unaffected. Finally, in a study of PFC morphology, Medina et al. (2009) reported that, after 28 days of abstinence, female cannabis users showed higher volumes of PFC as well as a poorer performance on executive functioning tasks, whereas the control group demonstrated the opposite pattern.

To date, there is a strong body of research on the potential consequences of alcohol and cannabis use on brain structure and cognitive function in clinical, adult populations (Adger and Saha, 2013; Kuntsche and Gmel, 2013; Volkow et al., 2016). However, many previous studies utilized cross-sectional designs, which do not allow for causal modeling of associations (McHugh et al., 2018). However, to our knowledge, there is one notable exception. Using a longitudinal design, Morin et al. (2019) investigated the time-varying association of substance use (cannabis and alcohol) and neurocognitive functioning (inhibition control, perceptual reasoning, working memory, and delayed recall memory). The result of this study demonstrated that cannabis use has potential neurotoxic effects on inhibitory control and working memory of all the participants (Morin et al., 2019). Although, we value the study of Morin et al. (2019), they did not take into account the role of gender, which is rather striking given the previously presented work on the differences concerning neurocognitive functioning between female and male adolescents. Therefore, in extending the work by Morin et al. (2019), the present study aimed to explore potential differences in male and female adolescents concerning the development of neurocognitive functions in the context of alcohol and cannabis use over the course of adolescence.

In doing so, while also extending previous and contemporary cross-sectional works, we developed a longitudinal study in which we compared male and female adolescent neurocognitive functioning (i.e., working memory, recall memory, perceptual reasoning, and inhibitory control) in the context of alcohol and cannabis. We analyzed this prospective data using a multi-level statistical framework allowing for the dissociation of three different, yet potentially additive (or interacting), associations of low neurocognitive functioning and substance use: common vulnerability, time-varying concurrent (same year) relationships, and time-varying lagged relationships. Based on previous works on the different levels of vulnerability of females and males to substance use in samples of adults and adolescents (Medina et al., 2008; Squeglia et al., 2009, 2011, 2012; Alfonso-Loeches et al., 2013; Ewing et al., 2014; McHugh et al., 2018), we hypothesized that there is a difference between neurocognitive functioning of males and females linked to alcohol and cannabis use over the course of adolescence.

MATERIALS AND METHODS

Participants

Participants were 3,826 high school students [47% female; mean age, 12.7 years (SD = 0.5)] from the Co-Venture study (NCT01655615; Landry et al., 2004; O'Leary-Barrett et al., 2017). A more detailed description of this study has been published elsewhere (O'Leary-Barrett et al., 2017). Participants were recruited from 31 public or private (French/English) high schools in the greater Montreal area, and were requested to participate in annual surveys for five consecutive years, from 7th to 11th grade. Among others, those surveyed had their alcohol and drug use, neurocognitive functions, and personality dimensions assessed. Our sample of high school students consisted of 15% of the entire population of 7th grade high school students in the greater Montreal area and they epidemiologically matched the size and socioeconomic status of each school district. Participant inclusion criteria consisted of providing informed assent and parent consent. Participants were excluded if they had unusual response patterns (e.g., same answer, sham drug item) or were reacting faster than usual (Reaction Time). Among the participants who completed the annual surveys, 3,659 (95.6%) of them were included in the analysis based on the minimal response to the questions and demographic information. The Co-Venture study obtained ethical approval from the ethics committee of the Sainte-Justine Hospital and the school boards of the schools that were recruited.

Measures

Substance use and disorders (alcohol and cannabis) were evaluated by the modified version of the "Detection of Alcohol and Drug Problems in Adolescents" questionnaire (Landry et al., 2004). Participants were asked to rate the frequency of their substance consumptions on a scale of 0–5 (never to everyday). There was a specific question for the quantity of alcohol consumed, but not for cannabis consumption. In line with previous studies in the field of substance use, assessing the quantity of used cannabis is still a challenge (Piontek et al., 2008).

More details regarding the frequency and quantity of alcohol use and frequency of cannabis use can be found in **Tables 1**, **2**. Self-reports measuring substance use during adolescence can be more accurate than biological measures (such as urine tests) when the confidentiality is guaranteed (Clark and Winters, 2002), as there is a higher chance of reporting any episodic substance use. In the Co-Venture study, confidentiality was guaranteed unless there was a risk of harm to self or others.

Outcomes

Utilizing a computerized neuropsychological assessment battery, the following cognitive functions were assessed. The detailed description of measures can be found in the original study protocol (O'Leary-Barrett et al., 2017).

Spatial working memory: like the spatial working memory sub-test of the Cambridge Neuropsychological Test Automated Battery (Owen et al., 1990), "Find the Phone" task was the measurement tool for assessing spatial working memory. This task is based on the Self-Order Pointing Task (Cragg and Nation, 2007) and the subjects are asked to search through a number of phones which are supposed to ring. The measure of spatial memory deficit is the number of times that the participant reselects the items that have already rung. The task had good internal reliability, with Cronbach α coefficient of 0.88 (Cragg and Nation, 2007).

Delayed recall memory: to assess the delayed recall memory, the computerized version of the "Dot Location" test as a part of Child Memory Scales (Cohen, 1997) was used. In this task, the participants memorize the location of circles in eight different

TABLE 1 | Frequency distribution for substance use variables in females over 5 years.

Substance and assessment for girls[a]	Frequency or quantity					
Frequency	**Never**	**Occasionally**	**Once a month**	**Once or twice per week**	**Three times or more per week**	**Every day**
Cannabis use						
Year 1	47.19%	1.27%	0.21%	0.11%	0.08%	0.08%
Year 2	37.51%	2.67%	0.82%	0.50%	0.24%	0.16%
Year 3	30.44%	4.45%	1.14%	1.43%	0.42%	0.32%
Year 4	26.39%	6.56%	1.51%	1.11%	0.48%	0.56%
Year 5	21.65%	8.02%	2.09%	1.75%	0.48%	0.42%
Alcohol use						
Year 1	33.35%	13.79%	1.06%	0.66%	0.03%	0.05%
Year 2	20.14%	17.73%	2.86%	1.03%	0.13%	0.00%
Year 3	12.78%	18.08%	4.79%	2.46%	0.05%	0.03%
Year 4	7.89%	17.76%	6.99%	3.79%	0.16%	0.03%
Year 5	5.24%	15.96%	7.62%	5.29%	0.29%	0.00%
	Number of standard drinks on a drinking occasion					
Quantity[b]	**<1**	**1–2**	**3–5**	**6–8**	**>8**	
Alcohol use						
Year 1	2.65%	5.29%	1.27%	0.11%	0.08%	
Year 2	2.49%	9.40%	3.10%	0.50%	0.21%	
Year 3	1.59%	11.86%	5.69%	1.03%	0.40%	
Year 4	1.40%	11.86%	9.11%	2.17%	0.56%	
Year 5	0.85%	11.41%	11.59%	2.33%	0.48%	

[a]Year 1: assessment in 7th grade, year 2: 8th grade, and so on. [b]Alcohol use quantity variables were categorized here for presentation purposes; in the analyses, alcohol use quantity was used as a continuous variable.

TABLE 2 | Frequency distribution for substance use variables in males over 5 years.

Substance and assessment for boys[a]	Frequency or quantity					
Frequency	**Never**	**Occasionally**	**Once a month**	**Once or twice per week**	**Three times or more per week**	**Every day**
Cannabis use						
Year 1	47.41%	1.48%	0.53%	0.34%	0.24%	0.32%
Year 2	38.22%	2.57%	0.50%	0.45%	0.16%	0.16%
Year 3	31.18%	4.95%	0.64%	0.93%	0.45%	0.58%
Year 4	25.36%	6.51%	1.16%	1.43%	0.77%	1.01%
Year 5	19.90%	6.91%	2.22%	1.83%	1.06%	1.24%
Alcohol use						
Year 1	29.27%	18.03%	1.99%	0.74%	0.16%	0.13%
Year 2	20.12%	17.68%	3.18%	0.87%	0.13%	0.08%
Year 3	14.06%	18.10%	4.21%	2.12%	0.16%	0.08%
Year 4	9.16%	15.11%	6.75%	4.61%	0.37%	0.24%
Year 5	6.14%	12.73%	6.70%	6.88%	0.53%	0.19%
	Number of standard drinks on a drinking occasion					
Quantity[b]	**<1**	**1–2**	**3–5**	**6–8**	**>8**	
Alcohol use						
Year 1	4.42%	6.62%	1.16%	0.29%	0.21%	
Year 2	4.02%	8.52%	1.88%	0.42%	0.26%	
Year 3	3.02%	10.01%	4.10%	0.98%	0.48%	
Year 4	1.80%	10.03%	7.41%	2.99%	0.56%	
Year 5	1.14%	8.58%	8.71%	4.16%	1.32%	

[a]Year 1: assessment in 7th grade, year 2: 8th grade, and so on. [b]Alcohol use quantity variables were categorized here for presentation purposes; in the analyses, alcohol use quantity was used as a continuous variable.

colors on the screen. Thirty minutes later, the subjects are asked to relocate the circles as they were placed on the previous image. Test-retest reliability ranged from 0.71 to 0.91 for subscales (Cohen, 1997).

Perceptual reasoning: to measure perceptual reasoning, an abbreviation of the original Cattell's Culture Fair Intelligence Test was used. In this nine-item task, the adolescents were asked to complete a series of puzzles with an increasing level of difficulty (Bilker et al., 2012). The scores from this test are highly correlated with that of Raven's 60-item perceptual reasoning matrices, with the correlation of 0.98 for the short form (Bilker et al., 2012).

Inhibitory control: to assess the cognitive control and response inhibition, an adopted version of Go/No-Go PALP (Passive Avoidance Learning Paradigm), which requires individuals to inhibit a rewarded response in order to prevent further punishment (Newman et al., 1985; Castellanos-Ryan et al., 2011), was used. By trial and error, subjects learn to react to "good" numbers and not react to "bad" numbers. The poorer response inhibition is the number of errors on trials involving a No-Go response. Confirming the previous studies, response inhibition is correlated with other functional imaging measures of PFC activities in Go-No-Go tasks (Whelan et al., 2012).

We controlled for socioeconomic status measured by the family affluence scale (Currie et al., 1997) and school-cluster effects in all of our analysis.

Statistical Analysis

The analytic strategy was focused on the longitudinal association between each predictor (female, male) and each of the outcomes (domains of cognition). Multilevel linear models assessed the association of alcohol (quantity by frequency) and cannabis (frequency) consumption and the four domains of cognition (working memory, delayed recall memory, perceptual reasoning, and inhibitory control). Two separate multilevel linear models were estimated for longitudinal effects of cannabis and alcohol as time-varying predictors of perpetration. The levels were time (nested in individuals) and individuals (nested in schools). The time parameter was coded from one to five (the survey waves). Predictors were person-mean centered. For both outcomes, the predictor terms were as follows: gender, socioeconomic status, linear and quadratic effects of time, between-subject differences in consumption measured by average substance use (alcohol or cannabis) over all waves, within-subject difference in consumption measured by current year change in use with regards to participant's mean use, and lagged within-subject measured by past year change in use with regards to participant's mean use. As the results of these effects were reported in a previous publication (Morin et al., 2019): interaction of gender by average use over all assessments, interaction of gender by change in use current year compared with the participant's mean use, and interaction of gender by past year's substance use compared with the participant's mean use. Between-subject effects were interpreted as a common vulnerability between consumption and poor neurocognitive performance, while within-subject effects were interpreted as potentially neurotoxic effects of substance use. The interaction of gender with within-person effects were interpreted as a potential sensitivity in one gender relative to the other with respect to the neurotoxic effects of substances on cognitive development. The intraclass correlation coefficient (ICC) function from the psych package in the R statistical environment was used to estimate the within-subject stability of cognitive data over time; ICCs were 0.74 for working memory, 0.80 for perceptual reasoning, 0.58 for delayed memory recall, and 0.68 for response inhibition.

RESULTS

Overall, 3,826 students [2,028 boys (53%); mean age, 12.7 years] were involved. Analyses included the interactions of cannabis/alcohol use and gender, time, and SES. For socioeconomic status, the participants with lower SES revealed worse perceptual reasoning. Considering the main variables, the quantity of alcohol use and the frequency of cannabis use increased yearly for both genders (**Tables 1, 2**).

Cannabis Model

Table 3 presents results for the cannabis model. The results indicated a significant between-person effect of cannabis (the general level of cannabis use) on inhibition control (β = 2.10, SE = 0.71, p = 0.001). Furthermore, it was shown that the past year fluctuation in cannabis use was significantly associated with females' perceptual reasoning (β = 0.12, SE = 0.05, p = 0.02). When we included the interaction with male-gender in our model, cannabis use revealed differential association of cannabis use and working memory among

TABLE 3 | Estimated parameters for cannabis model in a school sample of adolescents assessed over 5 years[a].

	Working memory			Perceptual reasoning			Delayed recall memory			Inhibition control		
	Estimate	SE	p	Estimate	SE	p	Estimate	SE	p	Estimate	SE	p
Intercept	21.04	1.50	0.00	15.48	0.42	0.00	17.86	0.48	0.00	34.80	3.00	0.00
Time	−6.76	0.97	0.00	1.25	0.27	0.00	−9.58	0.32	0.00	−8.92	1.96	0.00
Time squared	0.83	0.16	0.00	−0.10	0.04	0.02	2.00	0.05	0.00	0.88	0.33	0.01
SES*	0.10	0.08	0.20	−0.06	0.02	0.03	−0.03	0.02	0.16	0.31	0.15	0.04
Gender (female)	1.22	0.61	0.05	0.07	0.19	0.72	0.10	0.16	0.51	1.93	1.16	0.10
Cannabis, B*	0.23	0.37	0.54	−0.18	0.12	0.11	−0.08	0.10	0.42	**2.10**	**0.71**	**0.00**
Cannabis, W*	0.05	0.18	0.79	0.00	0.05	0.92	−0.09	0.06	0.12	−0.40	0.38	0.29
Cannabis, W (lagged)	−0.23	0.18	0.20	**0.12**	**0.05**	**0.02**	0.11	0.06	0.05	−0.13	0.38	0.73
Gender (male) × cannabis, B	0.25	0.49	0.61	−0.09	0.15	0.56	−0.01	0.13	0.93	−0.35	0.96	0.72
Gender (male) × cannabis, W	**−0.51**	**0.25**	**0.04**	−0.05	0.07	0.52	0.08	0.08	0.32	0.02	0.53	0.97
Gender (male) × cannabis, W (lagged)	0.40	0.25	0.12	0.00	0.07	0.98	−0.09	0.08	0.25	0.22	0.54	0.69

[a]*Significant effects are indicated by boldface. Performance on working memory and inhibitory control tasks was measured by counting number of errors; a lower score indicates a better performance.* **SES, socioeconomic status; B, between-subjects; W, within-subjects. Bold values correspond to significant predictors.*

TABLE 4 | Estimated parameters for alcohol model in a school sample of adolescents assessed over 5 years[a].

	Working memory			Perceptual reasoning			Delayed recall memory			Inhibition control		
	Estimate	SE	*p*	Estimate	SE	*p*	Estimate	SE	*p*	Estimate	SE	*p*
Intercept	21.54	1.49	0.00	15.12	0.42	0.00	17.71	0.48	0.00	37.80	2.97	0.00
Time	−6.50	0.99	0.00	1.18	0.27	0.00	−9.57	0.33	0.00	−9.41	1.98	0.00
Time squared	0.79	0.17	0.00	−0.09	0.05	0.04	2.00	0.05	0.00	0.95	0.33	0.00
SES*	0.12	0.08	0.15	−0.07	0.03	0.01	−0.04	0.02	0.05	0.38	0.16	0.02
Gender (female)	1.74	0.47	0.00	0.24	0.15	0.11	0.23	0.12	0.06	1.21	0.92	0.19
Alcohol, B*	−0.41	0.32	0.20	−0.03	0.10	0.74	0.06	0.08	0.49	0.22	0.61	0.72
Alcohol, W*	−0.20	0.18	0.26	0.08	0.05	0.13	0.03	0.06	0.62	0.28	0.35	0.42
Alcohol, W (lagged)	−0.10	0.18	0.57	0.02	0.05	0.75	−0.03	0.06	0.66	**−0.80**	**0.35**	**0.02**
Gender (male) × alcohol, B	0.62	0.43	0.15	0.00	0.14	0.97	0.00	0.11	0.97	0.28	0.85	0.74
Gender (male) × alcohol, W	0.12	0.24	0.61	−0.12	0.07	0.08	0.00	0.08	0.98	−0.16	0.49	0.75
Gender (male) × alcohol, W (lagged)	0.03	0.24	0.90	0.08	0.07	0.23	0.04	0.08	0.59	0.67	0.50	0.18

[a]*Significant effects are indicated by boldface. Performance on working memory and inhibitory control tasks was measured by counting number of errors; a lower score indicates a better performance. *SES, socioeconomic status; B, between-subjects; W, within-subjects. Bold values correspond to significant predictors.*

TABLE 5 | Estimated parameters for combined alcohol-cannabis model in a school sample of adolescents assessed over 5 years[a].

	Working memory			Perceptual reasoning			Delayed recall memory			Inhibition control		
	Estimate	SE	*p*	Estimate	SE	*p*	Estimate	SE	*p*	Estimate	SE	*p*
Intercept	20.65	1.53	0.00	15.62	0.43	0.00	17.79	0.49	0.00	35.39	3.05	0.00
Time	−6.49	0.99	0.00	1.20	0.27	0.00	−9.56	0.33	0.00	−9.35	1.98	0.00
Time squared	0.80	0.17	0.00	−0.09	0.05	0.04	1.99	0.05	0.00	0.94	0.33	0.00
SES*	0.14	0.08	0.09	−0.08	0.03	0.00	−0.04	0.02	0.04	0.42	0.16	0.01
Gender (female)	0.96	0.67	0.15	0.10	0.21	0.62	0.17	0.17	0.32	1.68	1.29	0.19
Cannabis, B*	0.61	0.45	0.17	−0.27	0.14	0.06	−0.17	0.12	0.15	**3.06**	**0.86**	**0.00**
Cannabis, W*	0.14	0.18	0.45	−0.02	0.05	0.71	−0.11	0.06	0.08	−0.33	0.38	0.39
Cannabis, W (lagged)	−0.31	0.19	0.09	0.13	0.05	0.01	**0.13**	**0.06**	**0.03**	−0.22	0.38	0.57
Alcohol Frequency, B	**−0.94**	**0.38**	**0.01**	0.24	0.12	0.05	0.19	0.10	0.06	**−1.73**	**0.73**	**0.02**
Alcohol Frequency, W	−0.20	0.18	0.26	0.06	0.05	0.19	0.04	0.06	0.51	0.42	0.35	0.23
Alcohol Frequency, W (lagged)	−0.03	0.18	0.88	−0.02	0.05	0.63	−0.05	0.06	0.40	−0.67	0.36	0.06
Gender (male) × Cannabis, B	0.25	0.58	0.67	−0.10	0.18	0.57	0.03	0.15	0.86	−1.08	1.14	0.35
Gender (male) × Cannabis, W	**−0.65**	**0.26**	**0.01**	−0.03	0.07	0.68	0.09	0.08	0.29	−0.15	0.54	0.78
Gender (male) × Cannabis, (lagged)	0.50	0.26	0.06	−0.01	0.07	0.94	−0.10	0.08	0.22	0.33	0.55	0.55
Gender (male) × Alcohol, B	0.49	0.51	0.34	−0.02	0.16	0.89	−0.04	0.13	0.75	1.22	0.99	0.22
Gender (male) × Alcohol, W	0.32	0.24	0.19	−0.12	0.07	0.09	−0.02	0.08	0.84	−0.21	0.50	0.67
Gender (male) × Alcohol (lagged)	−0.09	0.25	0.73	0.09	0.07	0.20	0.06	0.08	0.44	0.64	0.51	0.21

[a]*Significant effects are indicated by boldface. Performance on working memory and inhibitory control tasks was measured by counting number of errors; a lower score indicates a better performance. *SES, socioeconomic status; B, between-subjects; W, within-subjects. Bold values correspond to significant predictors.*

genders ($\beta = -0.51$, SE = 0.25, $p = 0.04$), implying potentially different neurotoxic effects of cannabis use for male and female adolescents. There were no significant interactions between time and gender, or time and gender and cannabis use (**Supplementary Table S1**).

Alcohol Model

Table 4 presents results for the alcohol model. When including the interaction with male-gender, the results indicated that alcohol use did not significantly interact with any of the neurocognitive domains. However, at the lagged-person level, it was shown that past year fluctuations in alcohol use were significantly associated with female adolescents' inhibition control ($\beta = -0.80$, SE = 0.35, $p = 0.02$). Furthermore, at the between-person level, it was shown that alcohol use (general level of alcohol use) was not significantly associated with any of the neurocognitive domains when it concerned female adolescents.

Combined Alcohol-Cannabis Model

Table 5 presents the results of an integrated model of the simultaneous effect of alcohol and cannabis. The results revealed a male-gender by within-subject interaction, suggesting that the effect of yearly cannabis use fluctuation on working memory among males compared to females is weaker ($\beta = -0.65$, SE = 0.26, $p = 0.01$), meaning that females make more errors in working memory task than males. Furthermore, at the between-person level, it was revealed that alcohol use (general level of alcohol use) was significantly associated with perceptual reasoning ($\beta = -0.94$, SE = 0.38, $p = 0.01$) and inhibition control ($\beta = -1.73$, SE = 0.73, $p = 0.02$) of female adolescents only. Regarding the general level of cannabis use, the models revealed significant between-person associations of cannabis use and inhibition control, for female adolescents only ($\beta = 3.06$, SE = 0.86, $p = 0.00$). In addition, the past year fluctuation of cannabis use was shown to be significantly associated with female adolescents' delayed recall memory ($\beta = 0.12$, SE = 0.05, $p = 0.02$).

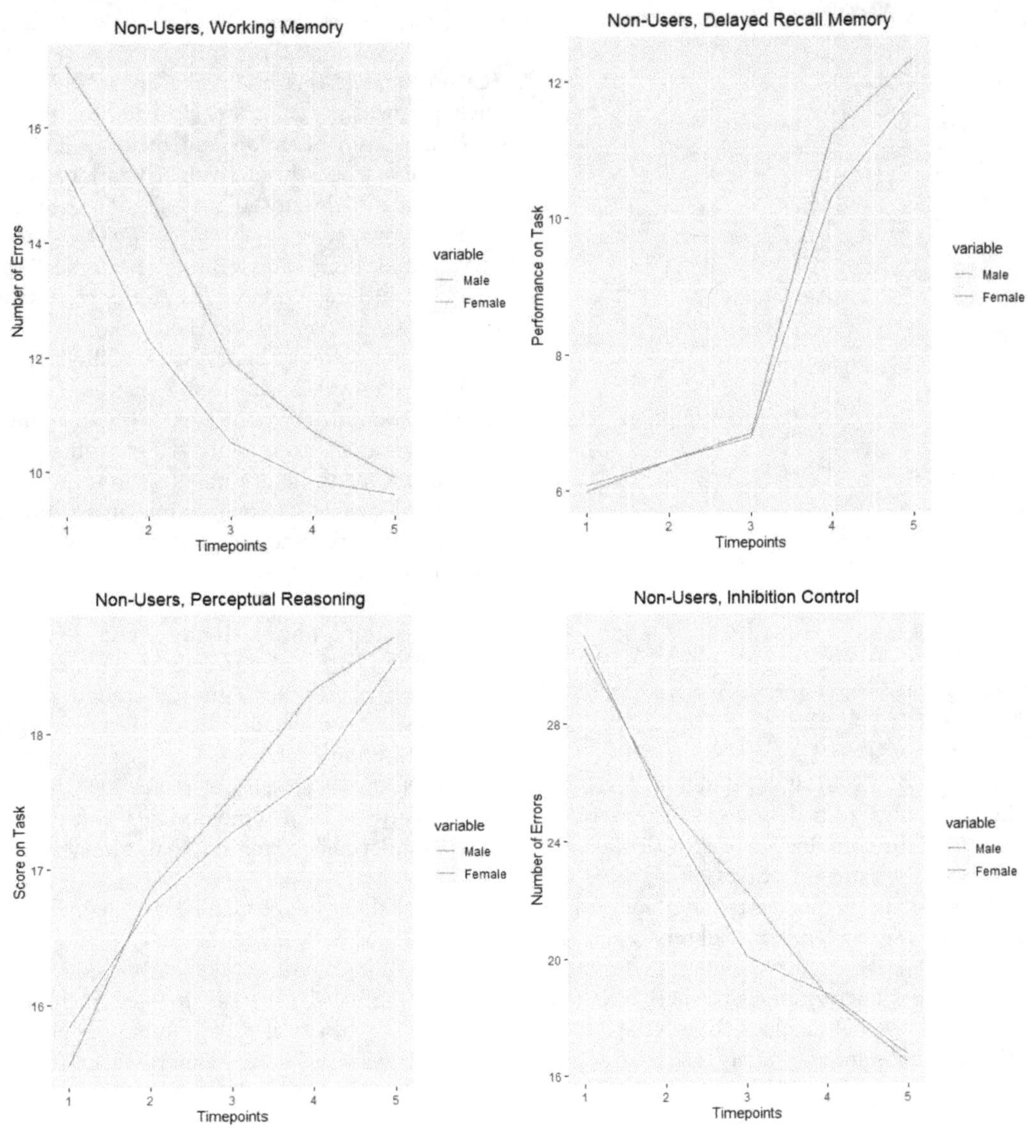

FIGURE 1 | Non-user students' cognitive tasks performance over 5 years (grade 7–11).

To facilitate interpretation of these results, the mean of cognitive tasks performance of non-user adolescents are presented in **Figure 1**. In general, across all time points, non-using female adolescents were making fewer errors than boys during the working memory task. However, when it concerned the other cognitive tasks, no significant differences between male and female adolescents were observed. Furthermore, **Figure 2** represents the working memory performance of those who were cannabis users and who used in a particular year. It was shown that female adolescents using cannabis displayed higher initial levels of errors concerning the working memory task than male adolescents using cannabis across time points 1 and 2, indicating that although non-cannabis using male adolescents made more errors during the working memory task, female cannabis users were shown to be more sensitive to the negative consequences of cannabis on working memory. However, these effects were shown to disappear over time.

DISCUSSION

This study examined the gender differences in female and male adolescents' neurocognitive functioning (working memory, perceptual reasoning, delayed recall memory, and inhibition control) utilizing a longitudinal design among a large sample of nearly 4,000 North-American adolescents, distinguishing between three time-varying effects of predictor variables: between-person effect, within-person effect, and lagged within-person effect. Based on the results, several important conclusions can be drawn. First, among the studied neurocognitive functions,

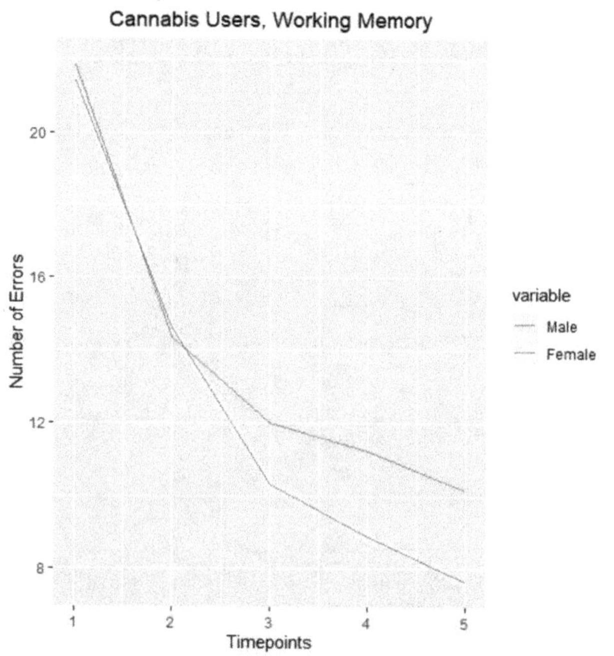

FIGURE 2 | Number of errors on working memory task in male and female cannabis users (once a month and more) measured over 5 years.

female cannabis users had significantly different levels of working memory impairments than males. We also found robust male/female differences in the combined model of alcohol and cannabis use, confirming the different effects of cannabis use on females and males working memory even after controlling for the effect of alcohol use. We did not observe such an effect for alcohol users. While significant alteration in the brain regions responsible for working memory have been reported in previous findings (Kanayama et al., 2004; Jager et al., 2006; Becker et al., 2010), results from this study revealed a new gender-specific developmental effect. Therefore, the gender-specific impairments related to cannabis use in females were limited to early stages of adolescent development, in line with the hypothesis that there are gender differences concerning the effects of cannabis on neurocognitive functioning in early adolescence.

Given the shifting policy of cannabis use laws, the prevalence of adolescents' misuse/use is rising. Meanwhile, having a better understanding of the neurocognitive functions after exposure to cannabis for boys and girls separately is the key to leading future research on the optimal treatment methods for cannabis dependency. The current evidence on gender-specific underlying neurobiological mechanisms of executive functioning and decision making regions of the brain, can be a possible explanation for the "Telescoping" phenomenon, which narrates a faster progression from the first exposure to a substance to the addiction phase in women (Hernandez-Avila et al., 2004). To be more specific, working memory is an essential component in academic success at school (Aronen et al., 2005). At least 10% of females 15 years and above report using cannabis in the past year (Health Canada, 2018) which increases the risk of school drop out up to 2.3 times more than non-user students (Bray et al., 2000). Students' cognitive function level decreases significantly for days after cannabis use (Crean et al., 2011) and for a considerable period, it affects their performance at school. In addition, the long term effects of cannabis on attention and memory are more long-lasting and severe when the individuals start using cannabis during adolescence (Schweinsburg et al., 2008) or are heavy-regular users (Solowij et al., 2002). Consequently, a secondary effect of acute intoxication, cannabis user students fail to learn at school, which in the long term leads to poorer grades and higher school drop out rates (Lynskey and Hall, 2000).

Working memory involves the ability to process and store information over a short time period and has been found to be predominantly associated with PFC and parietal cortex activities (van Asselen et al., 2006). In many studies, cannabis use was related to significant alterations in brain activity during functional magnetic resonance imaging (fMRI) tasks measuring spatial working memory (Jager et al., 2006; Becker et al., 2010). On the other hand, strong evidence on neurodevelopmental trajectories of the PFC shows discrepancy by gender. Due to sexual dimorphism during brain development, the full maturation process of female brain volumes is almost reached at the age of 10–11, while maturation could be as late as 14–15 years for male adolescents (Lenroot et al., 2007). Female PFC maturation peaks size 1 to 2 years earlier than for males (Giedd et al., 1996; Lenroot et al., 2007). As a result, females may experience more impairments in working memory than males, under the condition that cannabis use has its onset in adolescence.

Several studies have highlighted the importance of assessing the interaction between gender and age of onset after exposure to THC. In animal studies, while both male and female adolescent rats had impaired spatial working memory after cannabis exposure (O'Shea et al., 2006; Rubino et al., 2009), it was only the male rats with lasting memory deficit in adulthood (O'Shea et al., 2006). Also, in human subjects, gender can be a moderator in the association of brain structure, cognitive functioning, and cannabis use. For example, a number of studies highlighted that higher executive functioning (Medina et al., 2009) and memory performance impairments were linked to cannabis use (Gruber et al., 1997; Crane et al., 2013) in female adolescents. In contrast, as an acute effect of THC, Makela et al. found improved spatial working memory in young adult females (Makela et al., 2006). Those inconsistencies in the previous studies (Ketcherside et al., 2016) can be the result of differences in developmental stage, design of study (longitudinal/cross-sectional), levels of THC exposure and intoxication (Morin et al., 2019), and age of initiation (Gorey et al., 2019).

When considering gender differences in alcohol and cannabis effects on neurocognition, it is first important to account for the developmental sensitivity in neurocognitive performance. Considering the late maturation of brain substrates related to working memory among boys, there is a neuroplastic effect that decreases cannabis-related impairment among male adolescents compared to female adolescents. In contrast, as the maturation of prefrontal regions related to working memory happens earlier in girls, the negative effects of cannabis on working memory appears to be more pronounced during early adolescence. We can conclude that initiation of cannabis use during early adolescence might effect males and females differently due to these gender-based differences in neuromaturation (Lenroot and Giedd, 2010). Whether these drug-related changes are implicated in females' elevated risk for substance use disorders is a question worthy of further investigation.

The current study has some limitations. First, we looked into the effects of alcohol and cannabis use, but not the substance use disorder as it is defined in the DSM-5 (American Psychiatric Association, 2013), or polysubstance use. As we did not have the clinical substance use data, the results from this study could not be generalized to clinical population. Second, like other studies on cannabis use, we could not identify the cannabis exposure quantity (Piontek et al., 2008). Cannabis legalization in North America might provide the opportunity to use a standard scale for cannabis intake in the future studies. Third, we applied a self-report scale for measuring alcohol and cannabis use and our assessment did not include more objective observation methods such as biological tests. Regarding the sensitive nature of reporting substance use, those behaviors might have been underreported. Fourth, even though cognitive functioning was assessed with valid and reliable instruments, the results could be different in clinical settings due to its limitations (e.g., false-positive/negative results, over-diagnosis; Roebuck-Spencer et al., 2017). As cognitive tests used in the current study were done in school and they were administrated with other tests, fatigue and boredom could affect the students' cognitive functioning and neuropsychological status. In addition, we have not considered possible neurological or neurocognitive disorders of the participants. Finally, although observing the interaction of some other demographic variables such as SES (Johnson and Novak, 2009), sexual orientation (Medley et al., 2016), and racial/ethnic (Guerrero et al., 2014) differences with gender could be significant, this study was not intended to thoroughly explore those effects. Nevertheless, the current study was designed to report the association of gender differences and cognitive impairment due to alcohol and cannabis use during early ages.

In conclusion, the current study carried out one of the first analysis of gender differences in patterns of adolescents' neurocognitive impairments, using a longitudinal design from the Co-Venture study across five consecutive years. The results from this study provide a more detailed understanding of gender-specific processes in addiction vulnerability that could be used to inform public health messaging and targeted drug and alcohol prevention for young people (Conrod, 2016). Spatial working memory deficits could negatively influence young females' capacity in academic settings and could lead to significant impairment in adulthood, which critically decreases the individual's quality of life.

AUTHOR CONTRIBUTIONS

SN and PC conceived the presented idea. MA developed the theory and performed the computations. PC verified the analytical methods. PC encouraged SN to investigate the cognitive developmental trajectories of male and female adolescents and supervised the findings of this work. EB critically reviewed and revised the manuscript. All authors discussed the results and contributed to the final manuscript.

REFERENCES

1. Adger, H. Jr., and Saha, S. (2013). Alcohol use disorders in adolescents. *Pediat. Rev.* 34, 103–113. doi: 10.1542/pir.34-3-103
2. Alfonso-Loeches, S., Pascual, M., and Guerri, C. (2013). Gender differences in alcohol-induced neurotoxicity and brain damage. *Toxicology* 311, 27–34. doi: 10.1016/j.tox.2013.03.001
3. American Psychiatric Association. (2013). *Diagnostic and Statistical Manual of Mental Disorders (DSM-5@).* Arlington, TX: American Psychiatric Publishing.
4. Aronen, E., Vuontela, V., Steenari, M.-R., Salmi, J., and Carlson, S. (2005). Working memory, psychiatric symptoms, and academic performance at school. *Neurobiol. Learn. Mem.* 83, 33–42. doi: 10.1016/j.nlm.2004.06.010
5. Becker, B., Wagner, D., Gouzoulis-Mayfrank, E., Spuentrup, E., and Daumann, J. (2010). The impact of early-onset cannabis use on functional brain correlates of working memory. *Prog. Neuropsychopharmacol. Biol. Psychiatry* 34, 837–845. doi: 10.1016/j.pnpbp.2010.03.032
6. Bilker, W. B., Hansen, J. A., Brensinger, C. M., Richard, J., Gur, R. E., and Gur, R. C. (2012). Development of abbreviated nine-item forms of the Raven's standard progressive matrices test. *Assessment* 19, 354–369. doi: 10.1177/1073191112446655
7. Bray, J. W., Zarkin, G. A., Ringwalt, C., and Qi, J. (2000). The relationship between marijuana initiation and dropping out of high school. *Health Econ.* 9, 9–18. doi: 10.1002/(sici)1099-1050(200001)9:1<9::aid-hec471>3.0.co;2-z
8. Caldwell, L. C., Schweinsburg, A. D., Nagel, B. J., Barlett, V. C., Brown, S. A., and Tapert, S. F. (2005). Gender and adolescent alcohol use disorders on BOLD (blood oxygen level dependent) response to spatial working memory. *Alcohol Alcohol.* 40, 194–200. doi: 10.1093/alcalc/agh134
9. Castellanos-Ryan, N., Rubia, K., and Conrod, P. J. (2011). Response inhibition and reward response bias mediate the predictive relationships between impulsivity and sensation seeking and common and unique variance in conduct disorder and substance misuse. *Alcohol. Clin. Exp. Res.* 35, 140–155. doi: 10.1111/j.1530- 0277.2010.01331.x
10. Clark, D. B., and Winters, K. C. (2002). Measuring risks and outcomes in substance use disorders prevention research. *J. Consult. Clin. Psychol.* 70, 1207–1223. doi: 10.1037/0022-006x.70.6.1207
11. Cohen, M. (1997). *Children's Memory Scale.* San Antonio, TX: Psychological Corporation.
12. Conrod, P. J. (2016). Personality-targeted interventions for substance use and misuse. *Curr. Addict. Rep.* 3, 426–436. doi: 10.1007/s40429-016- 0127-6
13. Cragg, L., and Nation, K. (2007). Self-ordered pointing as a test of working memory in typically developing children. *Memory* 15, 526–535. doi: 10.1080/09658210701390750
14. Crane, N. A., Schuster, R. M., and Gonzalez, R. (2013). Preliminary evidence for a sex-specific relationship between amount of cannabis use and neurocognitive performance in young adult cannabis users. *J. Int. Neuropsychol. Soc.* 19, 1009–1015. doi: 10.1017/s135561771300088x
15. Crean, R. D., Crane, N. A., and Mason, B. J. (2011). An evidence based review of acute and long-term effects of cannabis use on executive cognitive functions. *J. Addict. Med.* 5, 1–8. doi: 10.1097/adm.0b013e31820c23fa

16. Currie, C. E., Elton, R. A., Todd, J., and Platt, S. (1997). Indicators of socioeconomic status for adolescents: the WHO Health Behaviour in School-aged Children Survey. *Health Educ. Res.* 12, 385–397. doi: 10.1093/her/ 12.3.385
17. Duncan, S. C., Duncan, T. E., and Strycker, L. A. (2006). Alcohol use from ages 9 to 16: a cohort-sequential latent growth model. *Drug Alcohol Depend.* 81, 71–81. doi: 10.1016/j.drugalcdep.2005.06.001
18. Ewing, S. W. F., Sakhardande, A., and Blakemore, S.-J. (2014). The effect of alcohol consumption on the adolescent brain: a systematic review of MRI and fMRI studies of alcohol-using youth. *Neuroimage Clin.* 5, 420–437. doi: 10.1016/j.nicl. 2014.06.011
19. Giedd, J. N. (2015). Adolescent neuroscience of addiction: a new era. *Dev. Cogn. Neurosci.* 16, 192–193. doi: 10.1016/j.dcn.2015.11.002
20. Giedd, J. N., Vaituzis, A. C., Hamburger, S. D., Lange, N., Rajapakse, J. C., Kaysen, D., et al. (1996). Quantitative MRI of the temporal lobe, amygdala, and hippocampus in normal human development: ages 4–18 years. *J. Comp. Neurol.* 366, 223–230. doi: 10.1002/(sici)1096-9861(19960304)366:2<223::aid-cne3>3.0.co;2-7
21. Gorey, C., Kuhns, L., Smaragdi, E., Kroon, E., and Cousijn, J. (2019). Age- related differences in the impact of cannabis use on the brain and cognition: a systematic review. *Eur. Arch. Psychiatry Clin. Neurosci.* 269, 37–58. doi: 10.1007/s00406-019-00981-7
22. Gruber, A. J., Pope, H. G. Jr., and Oliva, P. (1997). Very long-term users of marijuana in the United States: a pilot study. *Subst. Use Misuse* 32, 249–264. doi: 10.3109/10826089709055849
23. Guerrero, E. G., Marsh, J. C., Cao, D., Shin, H.-C., and Andrews, C. (2014). Gender disparities in utilization and outcome of comprehensive substance abuse treatment among racial/ethnic groups. *J. Subst. Abuse Treat.* 46, 584–591. doi: 10.1016/j.jsat.2013.12.008
24. Hammond, C. J., Mayes, L. C., and Potenza, M. N. (2014). Neurobiology of adolescent substance use and addictive behaviors: prevention and treatment implications. *Adolesc. Med. State Art Rev.* 25, 15–32.
25. Health Canada. (2018). *Summary of results for the Canadian Student Tobacco, Alcohol and Drugs Survey 2016–17.* Available online at: https://www.canada.ca/ en/health-canada/services/canadian-student-tobacco-alcohol-drugs-survey/. Accessed April 25, 2019.
26. Hernandez-Avila, C. A., Rounsaville, B. J., and Kranzler, H. R. (2004). Opioid-,cannabis-and alcohol-dependent women show more rapid progression to substance abuse treatment. *Drug Alcohol Depend.* 74, 265–272. doi: 10.1016/j. drugalcdep.2004.02.001
27. Jacobsen, L. K., Pugh, K. R., Constable, R. T., Westerveld, M., and Mencl, W. E. (2007). Functional correlates of verbal memory deficits emerging during nicotine withdrawal in abstinent adolescent cannabis users. *Biol. Psychiatry* 61, 31–40. doi: 10.1016/j.biopsych.2006.02.014
28. Jager, G., Kahn, R. S., Van Den Brink, W., Van Ree, J. M., and Ramsey, N. F. (2006). Long-term effects of frequent cannabis use on working memory and attention: an fMRI study. *Psychopharmacology* 185, 358–368. doi: 10.1007/s00213-005- 0298-7
29. Johnson, E. O., and Novak, S. P. (2009). Onset and persistence of daily smoking: the interplay of socioeconomic status, gender and psychiatric disorders. *Drug Alcohol Depend.* 104, S50–S57. doi: 10.1016/j. drugalcdep.2009. 04.007
30. Kanayama, G., Rogowska, J., Pope, H. G., Gruber, S. A., and Yurgelun-Todd, D. A. (2004). Spatial working memory in heavy cannabis users: a functional magnetic resonance imaging study. *Psychopharmacology* 176, 239–247. doi: 10.1007/ s00213-004-1885-8
31. Karlsson Lind, L., von Euler, M., Korkmaz, S., and Schenck-Gustafsson, K. (2017). Sex differences in drugs: the development of a comprehensive knowledge base to improve gender awareness prescribing. *Biol. Sex Differ.* 8:32. doi: 10.1186/ s13293-017-0155-5
32. Ketcherside, A., Baine, J., and Filbey, F. (2016). Sex effects of marijuana on brain structure and function. *Curr. Addict. Rep.* 3, 323–331. doi: 10.1007/ s40429-016- 0114-y
33. Kuntsche, E., and Gmel, G. (2013). Alcohol consumption in late adolescence and early adulthood-where is the problem? *Swiss Med. Wkly.* 143:w13826. doi: 10.4414/smw.2013.13826
34. Landry, M., Tremblay, J., Guyon, L., Bergeron, J., and Brunelle, N. (2004). La Grille de dépistage de la consommation problématique d'alcool et de drogues chez les adolescents et les adolescentes (DEP-ADO): développement et qualités psychométriques. *Drogues Sant. Soci.* 3, 20–37. doi: 10.7202/010517ar
35. Leatherdale, S. T., and Burkhalter, R. (2012). The substance use profile of Canadian youth: exploring the prevalence of alcohol, drug and tobacco use by gender and grade. *Addict. Behav.* 37, 318–322. doi: 10.1016/j. addbeh.2011. 10.007
36. Lenroot, R. K., and Giedd, J. N. (2010). Sex differences in the adolescent brain. *Brain Cogn.* 72, 46–55. doi: 10.1016/j.bandc.2009.10.008
37. Lenroot, R. K., Gogtay, N., Greenstein, D. K., Wells, E. M., Wallace, G. L., Clasen, L. S., et al. (2007). Sexual dimorphism of brain developmental trajectories during childhood and adolescence. *NeuroImage* 36, 1065–1073. doi: 10.1016/j.neuroimage.2007.03.053
38. Lynskey, M., and Hall, W. (2000). The effects of adolescent cannabis use on educational attainment: a review. *Addiction* 95, 1621–1630. doi: 10.1046/j.1360- 0443.2000.951116213.x
39. Mahmood, O. M., Jacobus, J., Bava, S., Scarlett, A., and Tapert, S. F. (2010). Learning and memory performances in adolescent users of alcohol and marijuana: interactive effects. *J. Stud. Alcohol Drugs* 71, 885–894. doi: 10.15288/ jsad.2010.71.885
40. Makela, P., Wakeley, J., Gijsman, H., Robson, P. J., Bhagwagar, Z., and Rogers, R. D. (2006). Low doses of Δ-9 tetrahydrocannabinol (THC) have divergent effects on short-term spatial memory in young, healthy adults. *Neuropsychopharmacology* 31, 462–470. doi: 10.1038/sj.npp.1300871
41. McHugh, R. K., Votaw, V. R., Sugarman, D. E., and Greenfield, S. F. (2018). Sex and gender differences in substance use disorders. *Clin. Psychol. Rev.* 66, 12–23. doi: 10.1016/j.cpr.2017.10.012
42. Medina, K. L., McQueeny, T., Nagel, B. J., Hanson, K. L., Schweinsburg, A. D., and Tapert, S. F. (2008). Prefrontal cortex volumes in adolescents with alcohol use disorders: unique gender effects. *Alcohol. Clin. Exp. Res.* 32, 386–394. doi: 10.1111/j.1530-0277.2007.00602.x
43. Medina, K. L., McQueeny, T., Nagel, B. J., Hanson, K. L., Yang, T. T., and Tapert, S. F. (2009). IMAGING STUDY: prefrontal cortex morphometry in abstinent adolescent marijuana users: subtle gender effects. *Addict. Biol.* 14, 457–468. doi: 10.1111/j.1369-1600.2009.00166.x
44. Medley, G., Lipari, R. N., Bose, J., Cribb, D. S., Kroutil, L. A., and McHenry, G. (2016). *Sexual Orientation and Estimates of Adult Substance Use and Mental Health: Results From the 2015 National Survey on Drug Use and Health.* NSDUH Data Review. Available online at: https://www.samhsa.gov/data/. Accessed November 18, 2017.
45. Miller, M. L., Chadwick, B., Dickstein, D. L., Purushothaman, I., Egervari, G., Rahman, T., et al. (2019). Adolescent exposure to Δ^9-tetrahydrocannabinol alters the transcriptional trajectory and dendritic architecture of prefrontal pyramidal neurons. *Mol. Psychiatry* 24, 588–600. doi: 10.1038/s41380-018- 0243-x
46. Morin, J.-F. G., Afzali, M. H., Bourque, J., Stewart, S. H., Séguin, J. R., O'Leary- Barrett, M., et al. (2019). A population-based analysis of the relationship between substance use and adolescent cognitive development. *Am. J. Psychiatry* 176, 98–106. doi: 10.1176/appi.ajp.2018.18020202
47. Nagel, B. J., Medina, K. L., Yoshii, J., Schweinsburg, A. D., Moadab, I., and Tapert, S. F. (2006). Age-related changes in prefrontal white matter

volume across adolescence. *Neuroreport* 17, 1427–1431. doi: 10.1097/01. wnr. 0000233099.97784.45

48. Newman, J. P., Widom, C. S., and Nathan, S. (1985). Passive avoidance in syndromes of disinhibition: psychopathy and extraversion. *J. Pers. Soc. Psychol.* 48, 1316–1327. doi: 10.1037/0022-3514.48.5.1316
49. O'Leary-Barrett, M., Masse, B., Pihl, R. O., Stewart, S. H., Seguin, J. R., and Conrod, P. J. (2017). A cluster-randomized controlled trial evaluating the effects of delaying onset of adolescent substance abuse on cognitive development and addiction following a selective, personality-targeted intervention programme: the Co-Venture trial. *Addiction* 112, 1871–1881. doi: 10.1111/add.13876
50. O'Shea, M., McGregor, I. S., and Mallet, P. E. (2006). Repeated cannabinoid exposure during perinatal, adolescent or early adult ages produces similar longlasting deficits in object recognition and reduced social interaction in rats. *J. Psychopharmacol.* 20, 611–621. doi: 10.1177/0269881106065188
51. Owen, A. M., Downes, J. J., Sahakian, B. J., Polkey, C. E., and Robbins, T. W. (1990). Planning and spatial working memory following frontal lobe lesions in man. *Neuropsychologia* 28, 1021–1034. doi: 10.1016/0028-3932(90) 90137-d
52. Pfefferbaum, A., Rosenbloom, M., Serventi, K. L., and Sullivan, E. V. (2002). Corpus callosum, pons, and cortical white matter in alcoholic women. *Alcohol. Clin. Exp. Res.* 26, 400–406. doi: 10.1111/j.1530-0277.2002. tb02552.x
53. Piontek, D., Kraus, L., and Klempova, D. (2008). Short scales to assess cannabis- related problems: a review of psychometric properties. *Subst. Abuse Treat. Prev. Policy* 3:25. doi: 10.1186/1747-597x-3-25
54. Public Health Agency of Canada. (2018). *Preventing Problematic Substance Use in Youth.* Available online at: https://www.canada.ca/en/public-health/news/ 2018/10/preventing-problematic-substance-use-in-youth.html. Accessed May 12, 2019.
55. Roebuck-Spencer, T. M., Glen, T., Puente, A. E., Denney, R. L., Ruff, R. M., Hostetter, G., et al. (2017). Cognitive screening tests versus comprehensive neuropsychological test batteries: a national academy of neuropsychology education paper. *Arch. Clin. Neuropsychol.* 32, 491–498. doi: 10.1093/arclin/ acx021
56. Rubino, T., Realini, N., Braida, D., Guidi, S., Capurro, V., Viganò, D., et al. (2009). Changes in hippocampal morphology and neuroplasticity induced by adolescent THC treatment are associated with cognitive impairment in adulthood. *Hippocampus* 19, 763–772. doi: 10.1002/hipo. 20554
57. Schweinsburg, A. D., Brown, S. A., and Tapert, S. F. (2008). The influence of marijuana use on neurocognitive functioning in adolescents. *Curr. Drug Abuse Rev.* 1, 99–111. doi: 10.2174/1874473710801010099
58. Schweinsburg, A. D., Nagel, B. J., Schweinsburg, B. C., Park, A., Theilmann, R. J., and Tapert, S. F. (2008). Abstinent adolescent marijuana users show altered fMRI response during spatial working memory. *Psychiatry Res.* 163, 40–51. doi: 10.1016/j.pscychresns.2007.04.018
59. Solowij, N., Stephens, R. S., Roffman, R. A., Babor, T., Kadden, R., Miller, M., et al. (2002). Cognitive functioning of long-term heavy cannabis users seeking treatment. *JAMA* 287, 1123–1131. doi: 10.1001/jama.287.9.1123
60. Sowell, E. R., Thompson, P. M., Leonard, C. M., Welcome, S. E., Kan, E., and Toga, A. W. (2004). Longitudinal mapping of cortical thickness and brain growth in normal children. *J. Neurosci.* 24, 8223–8231. doi: 10.1523/JNEUROSCI.1798-04.2004
61. Squeglia, L. M., Jacobus, J., and Tapert, S. F. (2009). The influence of substance use on adolescent brain development. *Clin. EEG Neurosci.* 40, 31–38. doi: 10.1177/ 155005940904000110
62. Squeglia, L. M., Schweinsburg, A. D., Pulido, C., and Tapert, S. F. (2011). Adolescent binge drinking linked to abnormal spatial working memory brain activation: differential gender effects. *Alcohol. Clin. Exp. Res.* 35, 1831–1841. doi: 10.1111/j.1530-0277.2011.01527.x
63. Squeglia, L. M., Sorg, S. F., Schweinsburg, A. D., Wetherill, R. R., Pulido, C., and Tapert, S. F. (2012). Binge drinking differentially affects adolescent male and female brain morphometry. *Psychopharmacology* 220, 529–539. doi: 10.1007/ s00213-011-2500-4
64. Statistics Canada. (2015). *Canadian Tobacco Alcohol and Drugs (CTADS): 2015 Summary 2017.* Available online at: https://www.canada.ca/en/health-canada/services/canadian-tobacco-alcohol-drugs-survey/2015-summary.html. Accessed January 7, 2019.
65. Statistics Canada. (2018). *Canadian Health Characteristics, Annual Estimates (Table: 13-10-0096-01).* Available online at: https://www150.statcan.gc.ca/t1/tbl1/en/cv.action?pid=1310009601. Accessed January 12, 2019.
66. Tapert, S. F., Schweinsburg, A. D., Drummond, S. P., Paulus, M. P., Brown, S. A., Yang, T. T., et al. (2007). Functional MRI of inhibitory processing in abstinent adolescent marijuana users. *Psychopharmacology* 194, 173–183. doi: 10.1007/ s00213-007-0823-y
67. van Asselen, M., Kessels, R. P., Neggers, S. F., Kappelle, L. J., Frijns, C. J., and Postma, A. (2006). Brain areas involved in spatial working memory. *Neuropsychologia* 44, 1185–1194. doi: 10.1016/j.neuropsychologia.2005.10.005
68. Volkow, N. D., Swanson, J. M., Evins, A. E., DeLisi, L. E., Meier, M. H., Gonzalez, R., et al. (2016). Effects of cannabis use on human behavior, including cognition, motivation, and psychosis: a review. *JAMA Psychiatry* 73, 292–297. doi: 10.1001/jamapsychiatry.2015.3278
69. Wager, T. D., and Smith, E. E. (2003). Neuroimaging studies of working memory. *Cogn. Affect. Behav. Neurosci.* 3, 255–274. doi: 10.3758/cabn.3.4.255
70. Whelan, R., Conrod, P. J., Poline, J.-B., Lourdusamy, A., Banaschewski, T., Barker, G. J., et al. (2012). Adolescent impulsivity phenotypes characterized by distinct brain networks. *Nat. Neurosci.* 15, 920–925. doi: 10.1038/nn.3092

17

Negative Mood Induction Increases Choice of Heroin Versus Food Pictures in Opiate-Dependent Individuals: Correlation with Self-Medication Coping Motives and Subjective Reactivity

Lee Hogarth[1*], *Lorna Hardy*[1], *Alexandra Bakou*[1], *Justin Mahlberg*[2], *Gabrielle Weidemann*[2,3], *Sharon Cashel*[2] *and Ahmed A. Moustafa*[2,3]

[1] *School of Psychology, University of Exeter, Exeter, United Kingdom,* [2] *School of Social Sciences and Psychology, Western Sydney University, Sydney, NSW, Australia,* [3] *MARCS Institute for Brain, Behaviour and Development, Western Sydney University, Sydney, NSW, Australia*

***Correspondence:**
Lee Hogarth
l.hogarth@exeter.ac.uk

Acute growth in negative affect is thought to play a major role in triggering relapse in opiate-dependent individuals. Consistent with this view, three lab studies have demonstrated that negative mood induction increases opiate craving in opiate-dependent individuals. The current study sought to confirm these effects with a behavioral measure of heroin seeking, and test whether the effect is associated with self-reported opiate use to cope with negative affect and subjective reactivity to mood induction. Participants were heroin-dependent individuals engaged with treatment services (n = 47) and control participants (n = 25). Heroin users completed a questionnaire assessing reasons for using heroin: negative affect, social pressure, and cued craving. Baseline heroin choice was measured by preference to enlarge heroin versus food thumbnail pictures in two-alternative forced-choice trials. Negative mood was then induced by depressive statements and music before heroin choice was tested again. Subjective reactivity was indexed by negative and positive mood reported at the pre-induction to post-test timepoints. Heroin users chose heroin images more frequently than controls overall (p = .001) and showed a negative mood-induced increase in heroin choice compared to control participants (interaction p < .05). Mood-induced heroin choice was associated with self-reported heroin use to cope with negative affect (p < .05), but not social pressure (p = .39) or cued craving (p = .52), and with subjective mood reactivity (p = .007). These data suggest that acute negative mood is a trigger for heroin seeking in heroin-dependent individuals, and this effect is pronounced in those who report using heroin to cope with negative affect, and those who show greater subjective reactivity to negative triggers. Interventions should seek to target negative coping motives to build resilience to affective triggers for relapse.

Keywords: negative mood induction, coping motives, heroin-seeking behavior, opiate dependence, vulnerability

INTRODUCTION

According to negative reinforcement theory, negative affective states act as powerful triggers for drug use behavior, motivating drug use to cope with those states [e.g., Refs. (1–3)]. Evidence for this proposal comes from lab studies where negative mood induction (including stress) increased various metrics of drug motivated behavior, including craving, choice, demand, consumption, and cognitive bias. Such mood induction effects have been extensively demonstrated for alcohol (4–7), tobacco (8–10), and cocaine (11–14). Furthermore, individual sensitivity to negative mood-induced craving predicts relapse in alcohol- (15–18) and cocaine-dependent individuals (19, 20), suggesting this sensitivity is an important risk factor for relapse.

Three studies have tested whether negative mood induction motivates opiate craving in opiate-dependent individuals. The study by Childress and colleagues (21) recruited 10 opiate-dependent clients who had been abstinent for 30 days, exposed them to guided self-hypnosis of a depressive scene, and found that subjective opiate craving increased from pre- to post-induction. The second study by Hyman and colleagues (22) recruited 14 opiate-dependent individuals who had been detoxified and were undergoing naltrexone treatment. Exposure to guided imagery of a personalized stress situation increased subjective opiate craving from baseline, while exposure to neutral imagery had no effect. Positive correlations were found between stress effects on craving and subjective reactivity (anxiety, fear, and sadness). Finally, the third study by Stathopoulou and colleagues (23) recruited 76 opiate-dependent individuals who had been on methadone maintenance for 4 months and exposed them to short video clips to induce sadness. After excluding 10 participants who showed no increase in subjective negative mood, it was found that the increase in craving from pre to post was related to subjective negative mood, and was moderated by anxiety such that this relationship was only significant in those with high anxiety sensitivity. There was no relationship between mood-induced craving and self-reported opiate use to cope with negative affect. Overall, this work provides preliminary support for the notion that acute negative mood is an important trigger for opiate seeking.

One limitation of the existing literature is that there is no demonstration of negative mood induction increasing a behavioral measure of heroin-seeking behavior. The three prior studies all measured opiate craving which has an unknown relationship to behavior (24). To address this limitation, we employed a pictorial choice procedure in which opiate-dependent individuals had the choice to enlarge heroin versus food thumbnail pictures in a series of two-alternative forced choice trials. Prior studies have validated the pictorial drug choice task by demonstrating that percent drug choice was increased in drug users versus non-users, or as a function of dependence level in the drug user group, in cocaine (25, 26), alcohol (27, 28), and tobacco users (28, 29), and was sensitive to the motivating effects of negative mood induction (10, 27, 30). In the current study, opiate users and control participants completed a concurrent pictorial choice task for heroin versus food pictures before and after mood induction. The first prediction was that heroin users would choose heroin images more frequently than control participants, validating the pictorial choice measure as an index of heroin value. The second prediction was that heroin users would show a mood-induced increase in heroin choice whereas control participants would not, suggesting that acute negative affect is an important trigger for heroin-seeking behavior.

The second limitation of the existing literature is that individual sensitivity to mood-induced opiate craving remains obscure. The two studies by Hyman et al. and Stathopoulou et al. (22, 23) found that mood-induced opiate craving was associated with subjective mood reactivity, consistent with a range of other induction studies [e.g., Refs. (27, 31–34), but see Refs. (35, 36)]. Consequently, the third prediction of the study was that mood-induced heroin choice would be associated with subjective mood reactivity. More interestingly, however, Stathopoulou and colleagues (23) found that mood-induced opiate craving was not associated with self-reported opiate use to cope with negative affect. This finding is at odds with multiple studies that show that coping motives are associated with greater sensitivity to mood-induced drug-motivated behavior [Refs. (5, 7, 15, 16, 27, 37–43); but see Refs. (30, 40, 44)]. The fourth prediction of the current study, therefore, was that mood-induced heroin choice behavior would be greater in opiate users who reported using to cope with negative affect. Sensitivity to negative affect-triggered heroin seeking could be an important mechanism driving relapse (45, 46).

METHOD

Participants and Procedures

Participation was open to males and females aged 18–65 being treated for current heroin addiction by opioid medication at the Royal Prince Alfred (RPA) Hospital Drug Health Clinic in Sydney, Australia. Data were collected from 47 opiate-dependent outpatients (male = 32, female = 15) after they received opiate medication. In total, 2 participants (4.3%) were aged 19–24, 14 (29.8%) were 25–39, 16 (34.0%) were 40–49, and 15 participants (31.9%) were 50+ years of age. Thirty-five participants were receiving methadone (mean dose = 79 mg), 2 participants received buprenorphine (mean dose = 6 mg), and 10 participants were receiving suboxone (mean dose = 21 mg). The majority of these participants were currently unemployed, educated to high school level, and single. Eligibility criteria included: 1) current attendance in treatment for heroin addiction, 2) over 18 years of age, 3) English speaking, and 4) receiving opiate medication for the last 30 days. Healthy controls that did not have a history of opiate addiction were recruited *via* word of mouth from the community. Exclusion criteria included history of substance dependence or any other *DSM-IV* axis I disorders. Participants were matched for gender (opiate users = 33% female; controls = 48% female, Fishers exact $p = .21$), and age, $t(34.26) = 1.66$, $p = .11$. A chi-square comparing three categories of educational attainment (below high school, high school, greater than high school achievement) was non-significant, $\chi^2(2, 71) = 4.48$, $p = .11$, suggesting the two groups were matched for educational attainment. One opiate-using participant was excluded for showing an extremely outlying reduction in heroin choice from pre- to post-induction (>3 times the inter quartile range), leaving 46 opiate users and 25 control participants in the analyzed data set. The study was approved by the Western Sydney University Human Research Ethics Committee, and participants provided informed written consent.

Questionnaires

Participants reported gender and age. Heroin users completed the Reasons for Drinking Questionnaire (RFDQ), adapted for heroin use (47). Instructions stated "The following 16 questions are a list of reasons why people take illicit opiates. Please rate each of these reasons on how important each is for you." Within the questionnaire, the word "alcohol" from the original was replaced with the word "heroin." Responses were scored on a 1–10 scale ranging from "not at all important" to "very important." The RFDQ has three subscales reflecting heroin use to cope with negative affect, social pressure, and cued craving, obtained by averaging relevant items, giving a subscale score range of 1–10. We adapted the RFDQ because the drinking to cope subscale in the original version has been shown to be associated with greater sensitivity to negative mood-induced alcohol choice in two of our prior studies with student drinkers in a task similar to the present (27, 37).

Mood-Induced Heroin Picture Choice Task

The trial structure and timings of the heroin picture choice task are shown in **Figure 1**. At baseline, participants freely chose to enlarge a heroin or food thumbnail picture with a left or right key press, over 32 trials. In each trial, a heroin and food thumbnail was presented randomly in the left or right position, sampled from a set of 28 of each image type (obtained online from non-copyrighted images). Following baseline choice, pre-induction subjective mood was measured by participants reporting the extent to which they currently felt five negative (jittery, upset, distressed, sad, irritable) and five positive emotions (enthusiastic, happy, excited, inspired, alert), randomly ordered, on a five-point scale ranging from "not at all" to "extremely." Sad music was then played through headphones (Barber's Adagio for Strings), and participants were instructed to carefully consider 16 negative statements (e.g., "I don't think things are ever going to get better") randomly ordered [for full list, see Ref. (34)]. The heroin choice test comprised 32 trials identical to baseline, except that the sad music continued to play and a negative statement (randomly selected from the set of 16) was presented prior to each choice (the same picture set was used as at baseline). Post-induction subjective mood was then measured in the same way as before.

RESULTS

Heroin Choice

Figure 2A shows the percentage (and SEM) choice of heroin versus food images, in heroin users and controls. ANOVA on these data, with the variables group (heroin users, controls) and block (baseline, test), yielded a significant main effect of group, $F(1,69) = 19.85$, $p = .001$, $\eta_p^2 = .223$, and interaction between group and block, $F(1,69) = 4.04$, $p = .048$, $\eta_p^2 = .055$, and no

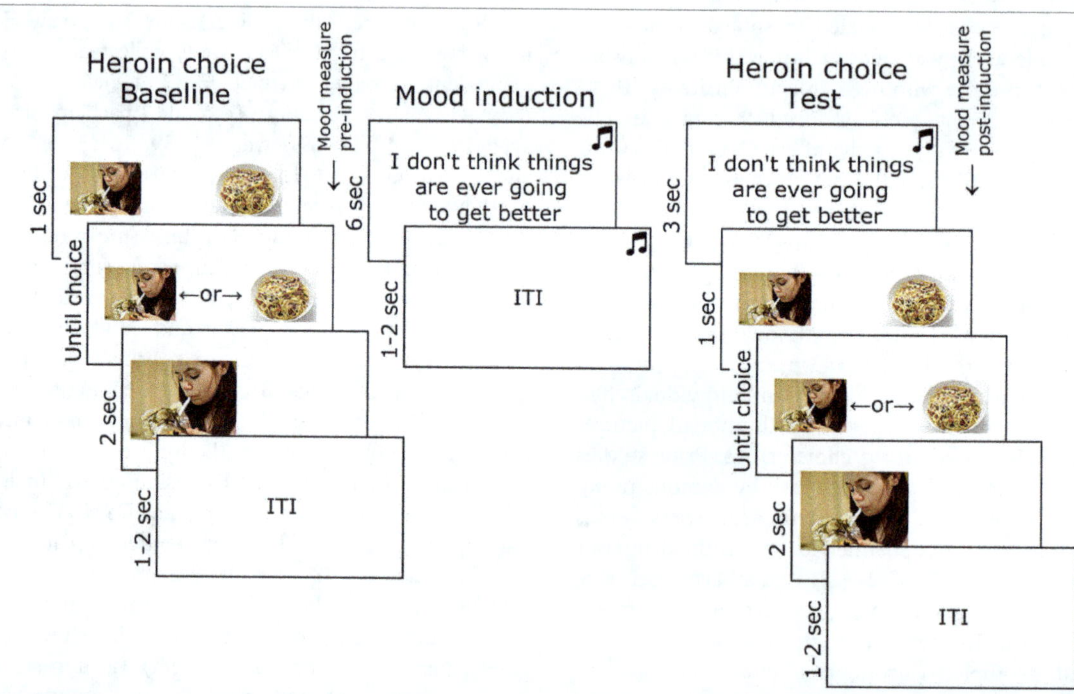

FIGURE 1 | Task used to test the effect of mood induction on heroin choice in opiate-dependent and control participants. Images of heroin and food were obtained online and were not copyrighted.

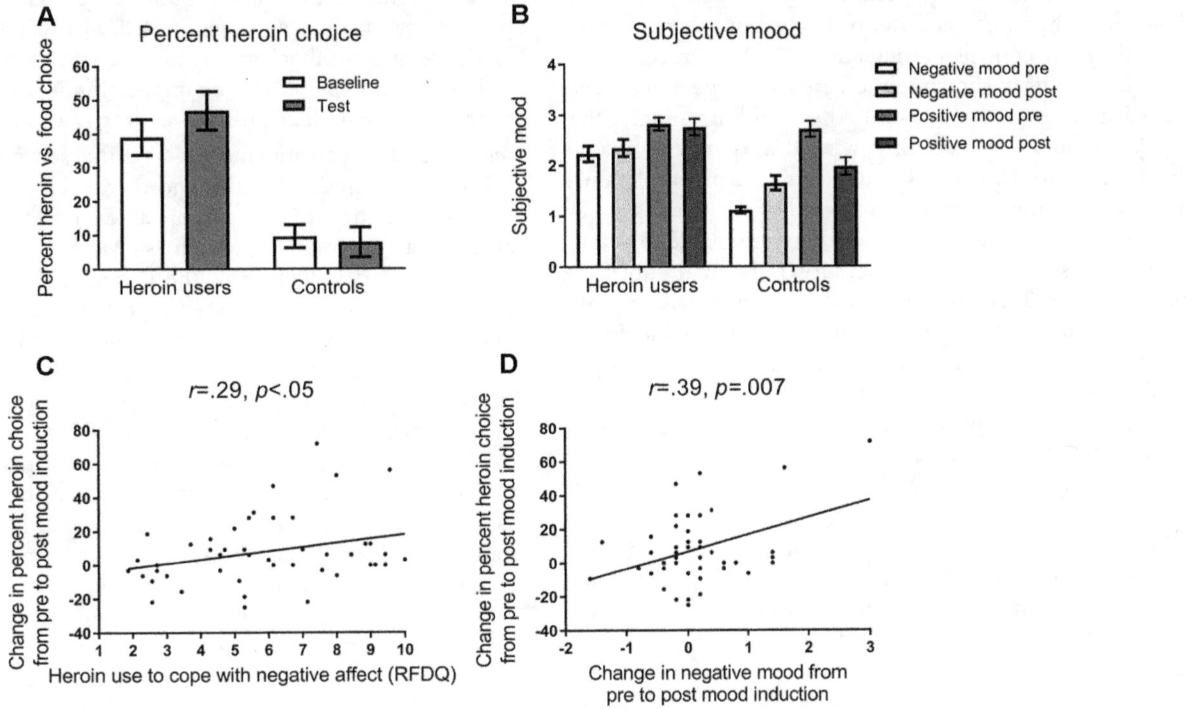

FIGURE 2 | (A) Mean percent (and SEM) choice of heroin versus food pictures in the baseline and test blocks of the task (see **Figure 1**). Opiate-dependent participants showed a higher rate of heroin choice overall compared to control participants, and showed a mood induced increase in heroin choice at test, whereas controls did not. **(B)** Subjective negative and positive mood states reported at pre-induction and post-test timepoints (see **Figure 1**). Opiate-dependent participants showed no overall change in subjective mood states, whereas control participants showed an increase in negative mood and a decrease in positive mood following mood induction. **(C)** Scatterplot and regression slope relating the mood-induced change in percent heroin choice to self-reported opiate use to cope with negative affect in opiate-dependent participants. **(D)** Scatterplot and regression slope relating the mood-induced change in percent heroin choice to self-reported change in negative mood in opiate-dependent participants.

significant main effect of block, $F(1,69) = 1.64, p = .21, \eta_p^2 = .023$. The main effect of block was significant in heroin users, $F(1,45) = 6.96, p = .01, \eta_p^2 = .134$, but not controls, $F(1,24) = .26, p = .62, \eta_p^2 = .011$. These results indicate that heroin users chose heroin images more frequently, and showed increased heroin choice following negative mood induction, compared to controls.

Subjective Mood

Figure 2B shows the mean (and SEM) subjective negative and positive mood reported pre-induction and post-test. ANOVA on these data with the variables group (heroin users, controls), mood state (negative, positive), and timepoint (pre, post) yielded a significant interaction between group, mood state, and timepoint, $F(1,69) = 12.40, p = .001, \eta_p^2 = .152$. In heroin users, there was a significant main effect of mood state, $F(1,45) = 6.06, p = .02, \eta_p^2 = .119$, but no effect of timepoint, $F(1,45) = .12, p = .73, \eta_p^2 = .003$, or interaction between mood state and timepoint, $F(1,45) = .91, p = .34, \eta_p^2 = .020$. By contrast, in controls, there was a significant main effect of mood state, $F(1,24) = 39.22, p < .001, \eta_p^2 = .620$, and a significant interaction between mood state and timepoint, $F(1,24) = 26.79, p < .001, \eta_p^2 = .528$, with negative mood increasing significantly from pre to post, $F(1,24) = 17.23, p < .001, \eta_p^2 = .419$, and positive mood decreasing significantly from pre to post, $F(1,24) = 16.06, p < .001, \eta_p^2 = .401$. Thus, heroin users showed no change in subjective mood following mood induction, whereas controls showed the appropriate change in mood states.

Correlations

As shown in **Figure 2C**, the change in heroin choice from the pre to post mood induction correlated positively with RFDQ heroin use to cope with negative affect, $r = .29, p < .05$, but not with RFDQ heroin use due to social pressure, $r = -.13, p = .39$, or cued craving, $r = .10, p = .52$. Furthermore, as shown in **Figure 2D**, heroin users' change in heroin choice also correlated with the change in negative mood from pre- to post-induction, $r = .39, p = .007$, but not with the change in positive mood $r = -.19, p = .20$. RFDQ heroin use to cope with negative affect did not correlate significantly with the change in negative mood, $r = .28, p < .06$. Thus, heroin users' change in heroin choice from baseline to test was amplified in those who reported heroin use to cope with negative affect, and those who reported the greatest increase in negative mood following induction.

DISCUSSION

The study found that opiate-dependent individuals chose heroin over food images more frequently than control participants. This accords with results from two studies with cocaine-dependent individuals, who chose cocaine over pleasant pictures more frequently than control participants (25, 26). Percent drug choice has also been shown to increase with dependence level within drug user groups (25–29). These findings suggest that the pictorial drug choice task is a valid assay of the relative value ascribed to the drug by drug users. The pictorial choice task may have the advantage over subjective craving as an outcome measure, in being more readily translatable to animal models that also use behavioral measures rather than subjective report (48, 49). This procedure also has an advantage over human concurrent drug self-administration procedures (50–52) in not requiring actual consumption, and so is technically simpler and ethically acceptable for clients who are currently abstinent. Finally, the pictorial drug choice task is superficially similar to attentional bias tasks, but appears more reliable in detecting group differences, and correlations with dependence severity (53).

The second finding was that negative mood induction increased heroin choice in opiate-dependent individuals but not control participants. This extends prior induction studies with opiate users (21–23), by including control participants to demonstrate the specificity of the mood induction effect. The finding also confirms that negative mood acts as a trigger for heroin-seeking behavior (and not just craving), as has been found with other drug classes including alcohol (4–7), tobacco (8–10), and cocaine (11–14).

Sensitivity to mood-induced heroin choice was also found to correlate with subjective changes in negative mood, consistent with two prior opiate studies (22, 23) and induction studies with other drug classes (27, 31–34). These findings accord with the prediction of affective negative reinforcement theory (54) in suggesting that the affective change produced by the induction procedure was responsible for the change in heroin-seeking behavior.

Finally, sensitivity to mood-induced heroin choice was found to correlate with self-reported opiate use to cope with negative affect, but not other opiate use motives (social pressure and cued craving). This finding contradicts the study by Stathopoulou and colleagues (23) which found no association between mood-induced opiate craving and opiate use to cope with negative affect, but corroborates multiple induction studies with other drug classes that have found this same association (5, 7, 15, 16, 27, 37–43). We may therefore accept our association as a true positive. It is possible that coping motives increase the risk of dependence by conferring sensitivity to negative affective triggers for drug-seeking behavior (45, 46).

We might further speculate that individual sensitivity to mood-induced heroin choice is a risk factor for relapse. The basis for this claim is that such sensitivity is associated with relapse risk in alcohol- (15–18) and cocaine-dependent individuals (19, 20). With respect to opiate users, poorer stress tolerance (55) and abnormal cortisol (56) predict poorer treatment engagement or earlier lapse, and preliminary evidence suggests that learning to cope with negative affect may promote abstinence (57). The implication is that sensitivity to negative mood-induced heroin-seeking is also a risk factor for relapse, and that treatments targeting this sensitivity may have efficacy for maintaining abstinence.

One limitation of the current study was that we did not observe an overall change in subjective mood following negative mood induction in the heroin user group, whereas controls did show changes to self-reported positive and negative mood. Despite this, the increase in heroin choice at test for the heroin user group, as well as the correlation between this effect and their change in negative mood, indicated that the mood induction procedure did impact the heroin user group. However, these effects were small and were perhaps reduced by the opiate replacement medications taken shortly before the experiment, similarly to acute alcohol, which has been shown to reduce mood induction effects (58). Future studies may employ a stronger mood induction procedure that produces a reliable change in subjective mood in heroin users, and a larger magnitude of effect on heroin choice behavior.

The second limitation was that we did not employ a control condition to determine whether the change in heroin picture choice was due to the mood induction or time. Previous studies have shown that drug choice remains stable over time then jumps following induction (30). Similarly, percent heroin choice in heroin users of the current study was stable across the two halves of the baseline phase (means = 39% and 39%, respectively), then jumped following induction and was stable across the two halves of the test phase (means = 48% and 46%, respectively). These data, plus the correlation between subjective mood and heroin choice, suggest that the increase in heroin choice was caused by negative mood induction and not by time.

The third limitation was that we could not obtain indices of psychiatric state in the two groups, because we had access to drug-using clients for an extremely short period during their hospital visit. As a consequence, we are unable to test whether the differential mood induction effect between the two groups was due to drug user status, or confounded psychiatric symptoms, such as anxiety or depression, which are known to be associated with greater sensitivity to mood induction effects on alcohol seeking (10, 27).

AUTHOR CONTRIBUTIONS

LHo designed the procedure and wrote the first draft of the manuscript. LHa and AB programmed the task and contributed to the analysis. JM and SC ran the participants and contributed to the analysis. GW and AM oversaw the running of the experiment. All authors contributed to the writing of the manuscript.

REFERENCES

1. Hall FS, Der-Avakian A, Gould TJ, Markou A, Shoaib M, Young JW. Negative affective states and cognitive impairments in nicotine dependence. *Neurosci Biobehav Rev* (2015) 58:168–85. doi: 10.1016/j.neubiorev.2015.06.004

2. Mathew AR, Hogarth L, Leventhal AM, Cook JW, Hitsman B. Cigarette

smoking and depression comorbidity: systematic review and proposed theoretical model. *Addiction* (2017) 112:401–12. doi: 10.1111/add.13604

3. Crum RM, Green KM, Storr CL, Chan YF, Ialongo N, Stuart EA, et al. Depressed mood in childhood and subsequent alcohol use through adolescence and young adulthood. *Arch Gen Psychiatry* (2008) 65:702–12. doi: 10.1001/archpsyc.65.6.702
4. Amlung M, MacKillop J. Understanding the effects of stress and alcohol cues on motivation for alcohol *via* behavioral economics. *Alcohol Clin Exp Res* (2014) 38:1780–9. doi: 10.1111/acer.12423
5. Rousseau GS, Irons JG, Correia CJ. The reinforcing value of alcohol in a drinking to cope paradigm. *Drug Alcohol Depend* (2011) 118:1–4. doi: 10.1016/j.drugalcdep.2011.02.010
6. Zack M, Poulos CX, Fragopoulos F, Woodford TM, MacLeod CM. Negative affect words prime beer consumption in young drinkers. *Addict Behav* (2006) 31:169–73. doi: 10.1016/j.addbeh.2005.04.016
7. Field M, Quigley M. Mild stress increases attentional bias in social drinkers who drink to cope: a replication and extension. *Exp Clin Psychopharmacol* (2009) 17:312–9. doi: 10.1037/a0017090
8. Heckman BW, Carpenter MJ, Correa JB, Wray JM, Saladin ME, Froeliger B, et al. Effects of experimental negative affect manipulations on ad libitum smoking: a meta-analysis. *Addiction* (2015) 110:751–60. doi: 10.1111/add.12866
9. Heckman BW, Kovacs MA, Marquinez NS, Meltzer LR, Tsambarlis ME, Drobes DJ, et al. Influence of affective manipulations on cigarette craving: a meta-analysis. *Addiction* (2013) 108:2068–78. doi: 10.1111/add.12284
10. Hogarth L, Mathew AR, Hitsman B. Current major depression is associated with greater sensitivity to the motivational effect of both negative mood induction and abstinence on tobacco-seeking behavior. *Drug Alcohol Depend* (2017) 176:1–6. doi: 10.1016/j.drugalcdep.2017.02.009
11. Sinha R, Lacadie C, Skudlarski P, Fulbright RK, Rounsaville BJ, Kosten TR, et al. Neural activity associated with stress-induced cocaine craving: a functional magnetic resonance imaging study. *Psychopharmacology* (2005) 183:171–80. doi: 10.1007/s00213-005-0147-8
12. Sinha R, Talih M, Malison R, Cooney N, Anderson G, Kreek M. Hypothalamic–pituitary–adrenal axis and sympatho-adreno-medullary responses during stress-induced and drug cue-induced cocaine craving states. *Psychopharmacology* (2003) 170:62–72. doi: 10.1007/s00213-003-1525-8
13. Sinha R, Fuse T, Aubin LR, O'Malley SS. Psychological stress, drug-related cues and cocaine craving. *Psychopharmacology* (2000) 152:140–8. doi: 10.1007/s002130000499
14. Sinha R, Catapano D, O'Malley S. Stress-induced craving and stress response in cocaine dependent individuals. *Psychopharmacology (Berl)* (1999) 142:343–51. doi: 10.1007/s002130050898
15. Brady KT, Back SE, Waldrop AE, McRae AL, Anton RF, Upadhyaya HP, et al. Cold pressor task reactivity: predictors of alcohol use among alcohol-dependent individuals with and without comorbid posttraumatic stress disorder. *Alcohol Clin Exp Res* (2006) 30:938–46. doi: 10.1111/j.1530-0277.2006.00097.x
16. Cooney NL, Litt MD, Morse PA, Bauer LO, Gaupp L. Alcohol cue reactivity, negative-mood reactivity, and relapse in treated alcoholic men. *J Abnorm Psychol* (1997) 106:243–50. doi: 10.1037/0021-843X.106.2.243
17. Higley A, Crane N, Spadoni A, Quello S, Goodell V, Mason B. Craving in response to stress induction in a human laboratory paradigm predicts treatment outcome in alcohol-dependent individuals. *Psychopharmacology* (2011) 218:121–9. doi: 10.1007/s00213-011-2355-8
18. Sinha R, Fox HC, Hong K, Hansen J, Tuit K, Kreek M. Effects of adrenal sensitivity, stress- and cue-induced craving, and anxiety on subsequent alcohol relapse and treatment outcomes. *Arch Gen Psychiatry* (2011) 68:942–52. doi: 10.1001/archgenpsychiatry.2011.49
19. Sinha R, Garcia M, Paliwal P, Kreek M, Rounsaville BJ. Stress-induced cocaine craving and hypothalamic–pituitary–adrenal responses are predictive of cocaine relapse outcomes. *Arch Gen Psychiatry* (2006) 63:324–31. doi: 10.1001/archpsyc.63.3.324
20. Back SE, Hartwell K, DeSantis SM, Saladin M, McRae-Clark AL, Price KL, et al. Reactivity to laboratory stress provocation predicts relapse to cocaine. *Drug Alcohol Depend* (2010) 106:21–7. doi: 10.1016/j.drugalcdep.2009.07.016
21. Childress AR, Ehrman R, McLellan AT, MacRae J, Natale M, O'Brien CP. Can induced moods trigger drug-related responses in opiate abuse patients? *J Subst Abuse Treat* (1994) 11:17–23. doi: 10.1016/0740-5472(94)90060-4
22. Hyman SM, Fox H, Hong KA, Doebrick C, Sinha R. Stress and drug-cue-induced craving in opioid-dependent individuals in naltrexone treatment. *Exp Clin Psychopharmacol* (2007) 15:134–43. doi: 10.1037/1064-1297.15.2.134
23. Stathopoulou G, Pollack MH, Otto MW. Anxiety sensitivity moderates drug cravings in response to induced negative affect in opioid dependent outpatients. *Addict Behav* (2018) 84:75–8. doi: 10.1016/j.addbeh.2018.03.020
24. Tiffany ST. A cognitive model of drug urges and drug-use behaviour: role of automatic and nonautomatic processes. *Psychol Rev* (1990) 97:147–68. doi: 10.1037/0033-295X.97.2.147
25. Moeller SJ, Beebe-Wang N, Woicik PA, Konova AB, Maloney T, Goldstein RZ. Choice to view cocaine images predicts concurrent and prospective drug use in cocaine addiction. *Drug Alcohol Depend* (2013) 130:178–85. doi: 10.1016/j.drugalcdep.2012.11.001
26. Moeller SJ, Maloney T, Parvaz MA, Dunning JP, Alia-Klein N, Woicik PA, et al. Enhanced choice for viewing cocaine pictures in cocaine addiction. *Biol Psychiatry* (2009) 66:169–76. doi: 10.1016/j.biopsych.2009.02.015
27. Hogarth L, Hardy L, Mathew AR, Hitsman B. Negative mood-induced alcohol-seeking is greater in young adults who report depression symptoms, drinking to cope, and subjective reactivity. *Exp Clin Psychopharmacol* (2018) 26:138–46. doi: 10.1037/pha0000177
28. Hardy L, Parker S, Hartley L, Hogarth L. A concurrent pictorial drug choice task marks multiple risk factors in treatment-engaged smokers and drinkers. *Behav Pharmacol* (2018) 29:716–25. doi: 10.1097/fbp.0000000000000421
29. Miele A, Thompson M, Jao NC, Kalhan R, Leone F, Hogarth L, et al. Cancer patients enrolled in a smoking cessation clinical trial: characteristics and correlates of smoking rate and nicotine dependence. *J Addict* (2018) 2018:7. doi: 10.1155/2018/2438161
30. Hardy L, Hogarth L. A novel concurrent pictorial choice model of mood-induced relapse in hazardous drinkers. *Exp Clin Psychopharmacol* (2017) 25:448–55. doi: 10.1037/pha0000155
31. Owens MM, Ray LA, MacKillop J. Behavioral economic analysis of stress effects on acute motivation for alcohol. *J Exp Anal Behav* (2015) 103:77–86. doi: 10.1002/jeab.114
32. Sinha R, Fox HC, Hong KA, Bergquist K, Bhagwagar Z, Siedlarz KM. Enhanced negative emotion and alcohol craving, and altered physiological responses following stress and cue exposure in alcohol dependent individuals. *Neuropsychopharmacology* (2009) 34:1198–208. doi: 10.1038/npp.2008.78
33. Kelly AB, Masterman PW, Young RM. Negative mood, implicit alcohol-related memory, and alcohol use in young adults: the moderating effect of alcohol expectancy. *Addict Behav* (2011) 36:148–51. doi: 10.1016/j.addbeh.2010.08.025
34. Hogarth L, He Z, Chase HW, Wills AJ, Troisi J, II, Leventhal AM, et al. Negative mood reverses devaluation of goal-directed drug-seeking favouring an incentive learning account of drug dependence. *Psychopharmacology* (2015) 232:3235–47. doi: 10.1007/s00213-015-3977-z
35. Magrys SA, Olmstead MC. Acute stress increases voluntary consumption of alcohol in undergraduates. *Alcohol Alcohol* (2015) 50:213–8. doi: 10.1093/alcalc/agu101
36. McGrath E, Jones A, Field M. Acute stress increases ad-libitum alcohol consumption in heavy drinkers, but not through impaired inhibitory control. *Psychopharmacology* (2016) 233:1227–34. doi: 10.1007/s00213-016-4205-1
37. Hogarth L, Hardy L. Depressive statements prime goal-directed alcohol-seeking in individuals who report drinking to cope with negative affect. *Psychopharmacology* (2018) 235:269–79. doi: 10.1007/s00213-017-4765-8
38. Birch CD, Stewart SH, Wall A, McKee SA, Eisnor SJ, Theakston JA. Mood-induced increases in alcohol expectancy strength in internally motivated drinkers. *Psychol Addict Behav* (2004) 18:231–8. doi: 10.1037/0893-164X.18.3.231
39. Grant VV, Stewart SH, Birch CD. Impact of positive and anxious mood on implicit alcohol-related cognitions in internally motivated undergraduate drinkers. *Addict Behav* (2007) 32:2226–37. doi: 10.1016/j.addbeh.2007.02.012
40. Field M, Powell H. Stress increases attentional bias for alcohol cues in social drinkers who drink to cope. *Alcohol Alcohol* (2007) 42:560–6. doi: 10.1093/alcalc/agm064

41. Zack M, Poulos CX, Fragopoulos F, MacLeod CM. Effects of negative and positive mood phrases on priming of alcohol words in young drinkers with high and low anxiety sensitivity. *Exp Clin Psychopharmacol* (2003) 11:176–85. doi: 10.1037/1064-1297.11.2.176
42. Austin JL, Smith JE. Drinking for negative reinforcement: the semantic priming of alcohol concepts. *Addict Behav* (2008) 33:1572–80. doi: 10.1016/j.addbeh.2008.07.016
43. Woud ML, Becker ES, Rinck M, Salemink E. The relationship between drinking motives and alcohol-related interpretation biases. *J Behav Ther Experimental Psychiatry* (2015) 47:102–10. doi: 10.1016/j.jbtep.2014.11.012
44. Thomas SE, Merrill JE, von Hofe J, Magid V. Coping motives for drinking affect stress reactivity but not alcohol consumption in a clinical laboratory setting. *J Studies Alcohol Drugs* (2014) 75:115–23. doi: 10.15288/jsad.2014.75.115
45. Crum RM, Mojtabai R, Lazareck S, Bolton JM, Robinson J, Sareen J, et al. A prospective assessment of reports of drinking to self-medicate mood symptoms with the incidence and persistence of alcohol dependence. *JAMA Psychiatry* (2013) 70:718–26. doi: 10.1001/jamapsychiatry.2013.1098
46. Crum RM, La Flair L, Storr CL, Green KM, Stuart EA, Alvanzo AAH, et al. Reports of drinking to self-medicate anxiety symptoms: longitudinal assessment for subgroups of individuals with alcohol dependence. *Depress Anxiety* (2013) 30:174–83. doi: 10.1002/da.22024
47. Zywiak WH, Connors GJ, Maisto SA, Westerberg VS. Relapse research and the Reasons for Drinking Questionnaire: a factor analysis of Marlatt's relapse taxonomy. *Addiction* (1996) 91:121–30. doi: 10.1046/j.1360-0443.91.12s1.2.x
48. Russo M, Funk D, Loughlin A, Coen K, Lê AD. Effects of alcohol dependence on discrete choice between alcohol and saccharin. *Neuropsychopharmacology* (2018) 43:1859–66. doi: 10.1038/s41386-018-0101-1
49. Guillem K, Brenot V, Durand A, Ahmed SH. Neuronal representation of individual heroin choices in the orbitofrontal cortex. *Addict Biol* (2018) 23:880–8. doi: 10.1111/adb.12536
50. Bickel WK, DeGrandpre RJ, Higgins ST, Hughes JR, Badger GJ. Effects of simulated employment and recreation on drug taking: a behavioral economic analysis. *Exp Clin Psychopharmacol* (1995) 3:467–76. doi: 10.1037/1064-1297.3.4.467
51. Hart CL, Haney M, Foltin RW, Fischman MW. Alternative reinforcers differentially modify cocaine self-administration by humans. *Behav Pharmacol* (2000) 11:87–91. doi: 10.1097/00008877-200002000-00010
52. Stoops WW, Lile JA, Glaser PEA, Hays LR, Rush CR. Alternative reinforcer response cost impacts cocaine choice in humans. *Prog Neuropsychopharmacol Biol Psychiatry* (2012) 36:189–93. doi: 10.1016/j.pnpbp.2011.10.003
53. Field M, Werthmann J, Franken I, Hofmann W, Hogarth L, Roefs A. The role of attentional bias in obesity and addiction. *Health Psychol* (2016) 35:767–80. doi: 10.1037/hea0000405
54. Baker TB, Piper ME, McCarthy DE, Majeskie MR, Fiore MC. Addiction motivation reformulated: an affective processing model of negative reinforcement. *Psychol Rev* (2004) 111:33–51. doi: 10.1037/0033-295X.111.1.33
55. Strong DR, Brown RA, Sims M, Herman DS, Anderson BJ, Stein MD. Persistence on a stress-challenge task before initiating buprenorphine treatment was associated with successful transition from opioid use to early abstinence. *J Addict Med* (2012) 6:219–25. doi: 10.1097/ADM.0b013e31825d927f
56. Jaremko KM, Sterling RC, Van Bockstaele EJ. Psychological and physiological stress negatively impacts early engagement and retention of opioid-dependent individuals on methadone maintenance. *J Subst Abuse Treat* (2015) 48:117–27. doi: 10.1016/j.jsat.2014.08.006
57. Stein MD, Herman DS, Moitra E, Hecht J, Lopez R, Anderson BJ, et al. A preliminary randomized controlled trial of a distress tolerance treatment for opioid dependent persons initiating buprenorphine. *Drug Alcohol Depend* (2015) 147:243–50. doi: 10.1016/j.drugalcdep.2014.11.007
58. Kushner MG, Mackenzie TB, Fiszdon J, Valentiner DP, Foa E, Anderson N, et al. The effects of alcohol consumption on laboratory-induced panic and state anxiety. *Arch Gen Psychiatry* (1996) 53:264–70. doi: 10.1001/archpsyc.1996.01830030086013

18

Cultural Adaptation and Validation of the Urdu Version of the Cognitive Emotion Regulation Questionnaire (CERQ) in Male Patients with Substance use Disorders (SUDs) in Pakistan

Salman Shahzad[1*], *Nasreen Bano*[1], *Nasreen Begum*[2] *and Hendrée E. Jones*[3]

[1] *Institute of Clinical Psychology, University of Karachi, Karachi, Pakistan,* [2] *Department of Applied Psychology, Virtual University of Pakistan, Lahore, Pakistan,* [3] *Department of Obstetrics & Gynecology, University of North Carolina at Chapel Hill, Chapel Hill, NC, United States*

Correspondence:
Salman Shahzad
shahzad_icp@yahoo.com

Background: Adults with substance use disorders (SUDs) often have co-occurring mental health problems. Emotion regulation may play a vital role in mental health problems. The Cognitive Emotion Regulation Questionnaire (CERQ) is a widely used measure for assessing cognitive emotion regulation. However, it has not been used in Pakistan on patients with co-occurring SUDs and mental health issues. The present study aims to translate and adapt the CERQ into the Urdu language and to determine its reliability and convergent validity in a sample of male patients with SUDs in Pakistan.

Method: Participants completed a demographic information form, the CERQ, the Depression, Anxiety, and Stress Scale Short Form [DASS-21)], and the Rosenberg Self-Esteem Scale [RSES)] in Urdu.

Results: Male participants (N = 237) 18–50 years of age (M = 29.8, SD = 8.1) were recruited from four substance use disorder treatment centers and hospitals in Karachi. The reliability of the Urdu version of the CERQ was based on an examination of its internal consistency reliability (Cronbach's α) and test–retest reliability for both the total scale and its subscales. Internal consistency for the CERQ total ($\alpha = 0.80$) was adequate, as it was for subscales of self-blame, (0.76) acceptance (0.78), rumination (0.72), positive refocusing (0.79), focus on planning (0.89), positive reappraisal (0.81), putting into perspective (0.83), catastrophizing (0.73), and other blame (0.70). The 10–14 day test–retest reliability of the CERQ total score was 0.86. Higher CERQ scores were significantly ($ps < 0.001$) negatively associated with DASS-21depression ($r = -0.24$), anxiety ($r = -0.23$), and stress ($r = -0.27$) subscales, as well as the DASS-21 total score ($r = -0.26$) and positively associated with the RSES self-esteem score ($r = 0.30$).

Conclusion: The Urdu version of the CERQ is a reliable measure for investigating cognitive emotion regulation strategies related to mental health and SUDs in Pakistan.

Keywords: cognitive emotion regulation, self-esteem, substance use, depression, anxiety, stress

INTRODUCTION

In the past two decades, research on the construct of emotion regulation (ER) has grown rapidly. ER is defined as strategies to maintain, increase, or suppress a current affective state and includes the ability to regulate emotions and physiological changes to respond to a situation adequately (1). ER aims to analyze, modify, and control emotional responses, help regulate positive and negative emotions and assess any emotion's severity and extent (2, 3). Researchers have studied ER in different fields, including its application with individuals suffering from various psychopathologies [e.g., (4)].

Disruptions in the ability to regulate emotions have been linked to various psychopathologies, including anxiety and depression (5). Numerous research efforts have identified that ER may become dysfunctional when positive emotions do not balance the regulation of painful emotions. This lack of balance can lead to an inability to cope with unpleasant and persistent negative emotional states (6). These unpleasant and ongoing conditions are disturbing and may easily trigger the development of anxious and depressive symptoms (7). Individuals might try to regulate these undesired states and symptoms with psychoactive substance use and other impulsive and risky behaviors (i.e., non-suicidal self-harm injuries) (8). This emotional dysregulation may impair emotion recognition, which may further increase the risk of impulsive and psychoactive-substance-using behaviors, leading to suicidal ideation and behaviors (9). Moreover, several studies have pointed out that alexithymia (the inability to recognize or describe one's own emotions) may be a risk factor for suicide and self-harm in individuals with substance use disorders (SUDs) (10, 11).

Individuals using maladaptive cognitive emotion regulation strategies (CERs) are prone to risky behavior, including substance use disorder (12). Researchers have found that the lack of ER strategies often leads to risky behaviors and ultimately escalates negative emotions (13). For instance, Froushani and Akrami (14) found that a low ER level resulting from the inability to cope effectively and manage emotions plays a role in the onset of drug use. Shahzad et al. (15) reported that in a sample of male patients with SUDs, emotion regulation strategies predict depression.

Similarly, previous findings have indicated a strong association between mental health issues like anxiety, depression, aggression, and psychological distress with low adaptive coping strategies and the excessive utilization of maladaptive strategies (4, 16). There has been a growing interest in having mental health professionals add emotion regulation as a component of psychotherapy [e.g., (17)]. Garnefski et al. (18) have conceptualized cognitive emotion regulation (CER) as a "conscious, cognitive way of handling the intake of emotionally arousing information." They conceptualized different CER strategies, which include; self-blame, other-blame, rumination, catastrophizing, putting into perspective, positive refocusing, positive reappraisal, acceptance, and planning (18), and have developed the cognitive emotion regulation questionnaire (CERQ) to measure these aspects of CER. Since its development, the CERQ has become a widely used measure for assessing cognitive emotion regulation.

Based on the published literature, CER may have a significant role in mental health and SUDs. It is an essential constituent in assessing patients in clinical research and practice. Researchers have asserted that clinicians must have a reliable and valid tool that can be used in different languages and cultures (19). This goal can be achieved through translating and validating a measure from the original language into other languages (20).

Since its development, the CERQ has been translated into several different languages, including Indonesian (21), Arabic (22), Spanish (23), German (24), Turkish (25), Persian (26), Chinese (27), and French (28). Subsequent research has shown that these translations have excellent psychometric properties, including good reliability and validity. However, studies have yet to examine CERQ reliability and convergent validity in a sample of patients with SUDs. The CERQ has also yet to be translated and adapted into Urdu. In line with previous studies, the present study examined the reliability and convergent validity of the CERQ administered in Urdu, in a sample of adult males with SUD in Pakistan. Construct validity of the CERQ was assessed by investigating its relationships with self-report measures of depression, anxiety and stress, and self-esteem.

MATERIALS AND METHODS

Ethical approval for the study was granted by the Departmental Ethical Review Committee, Institute of Clinical Psychology, University of Karachi, Pakistan. The concerned authorities of substance use treatment and rehabilitation centers/hospitals (i.e., Addicare Center for Treatment for Substance Use and Mental Health Problems, Alhaq Medical Center, Nai Zindagi Welfare Trust, and Parvarish Recovery Center) were approached and provided permission for the study to be conducted in their centers/hospitals. Data were collected from 01 June to 30 December 2019.

Participants

The present study recruited only male patients with a SUD. Although reports of psychoactive substance use among females are also a growing concern in Pakistan, access to this population is challenging due to the extreme stigma and discrimination associated with substance use in females in Pakistan and the fear and shame associated with this problem among women.

Adult male patients diagnosed with SUD were recruited using a purposive sampling technique. A total of 300 participants were initially approached to participate in this study: 5 refused to participate, and 58 did not meet the criteria to participate in the study, leaving a sample of 237 participants. Inclusion criteria were a SUD diagnosis, completion of a minimum of 3 weeks in treatment, detoxification completion, clinically stable, and ability to respond. Exclusion criteria included being unable to comprehend the instructions provided to complete the research questionnaires and being unable to read and write.

Translation Process

The authors obtained permission to translate and adapt the CERQ via email from its copyright owners.

Expert Panel

Experts were selected according to the guidelines provided by the International Test Commission (29). These guidelines state that experts should have sufficient knowledge of both the source and target languages, both source and target cultures, the test content, and general testing principles. All four experts were bilingual with prior experience with translation, and all held a Ph.D. in clinical psychology. Two took part as experts for forward and two for backward translation.

Forward Translation

The instrument was first independently translated into Urdu by the two forward translators. To independently translate the original English CERQ into Urdu, the translators were provided detailed information about the scale's content and the study's objectives, and the sample to be recruited. After independent translation into Urdu, the directions, items, and format of the two different Urdu versions were compared with each other and with the original English version of the scale by the expert panel. The expert panel critically evaluated the translated version to resolve any contradictions and ambiguities in the items. Items of both translations that retained Pakistani culture's conceptual, linguistic, and cultural aspects were merged into a single draft. Substitutes recommended by the experts were also taken into consideration. All the items were retained, and no items were removed in the forward translation process.

Backward Translation

The final forward-translated version was then given to two expert translators for backward translation. These two individuals were not involved in the forward translation and were completely blind to the original version of the CERQ to minimize any bias in back-translation. These two translators independently translated the Urdu version back into English. Each item from the backward translations was analyzed and compared with the original English version of CERQ. Items after backward translation that did not retain the initial concepts were modified and rephrased by the translators. All comments given by the experts were transcribed. After a thorough evaluation of this preliminary version, a final version of the Urdu CERQ was prepared. It was then initially piloted on 30 individuals to determine feasibility. No further revisions were necessary, and the Urdu CERQ was determined to be ready to administer and test.

Measures

Participants completed the Urdu translated version of CERQ, the Depression, Anxiety, and Stress Scale Short Form [DASS-21; (30)], and the Self-Esteem Scale [RSES; (31)]. The DASS-21 and the RSES had previously been translated into Urdu.

Cognitive Emotion Regulation Questionnaire (CERQ)

The CERQ has 36-items, including nine conceptually distinct subscales (32). The nine subscales of the CERQ are self-blame, acceptance, rumination, positive refocusing, focus on planning, positive reappraisal, putting into perspective, catastrophizing, and other blame. Each subscale consists of 4 items, each stating what someone thinks after experiencing threatening or stressful life events. The items are measured on a 5-point Likert-type scale ranging from 1("almost never") to 5 ("almost always"). A CERQ total score is obtained by summing the scores on all 36 items (possible range: 36–180). Subscale scores are obtained by summing the scores of the particular subscale (possible range for each subscale: 4 to 20). Previous research in an English-speaking sample has shown that all subscales have good internal consistencies ranging from 0.68 to 0.86 (32).

Depression Anxiety and Stress Scale, Short Form (DASS-21)

The DASS-21 is a self-report short form of the 42-item DASS (30). It is comprised of three subscales, namely, depression, anxiety, and stress. It contains 21 items measured on a 4-point scale in which "not at all" is scored as 0 and "all the time" as 3.Sample items are: "I couldn't seem to get any enjoyment out of the things I did," "I perspired noticeably (e.g., hands sweaty) in the absence of high temperatures or physical exertion," and "I found myself in situations that made me so anxious I was most relieved when they ended." DASS-21 total score can range from minimum 0 to maximum 63, while scores on each subscale can range from 0 to 21. Reliability studies of the Urdu version of the DASS indicate excellent internal consistency reliability for the total score (Cronbach's $\alpha = 0.93$) and respectable internal consistency reliabilities for the subscales: depression (0.84), anxiety (0.86), and stress (0.83), respectively (33).

The Rosenberg Self Esteem Scale (RSES)

The RSES was developed by Rosenberg (31). It contains 10 self-report 4-point Likert-type items to which respondents indicate "strongly disagree" to "strongly agree." Some items are reverse-scored so that the total score scale ranges from 0 to 30, inclusive, with higher scores indicating higher self-esteem. An Urdu version of the RSES has good internal consistency ($\alpha =$ 0.77) and a 4-week test re-test correlation coefficient of 0.81 (34).

Procedure

Before enrollment in the study, potential participants were provided with an information sheet that shared the study and informed consent procedures. This sheet included the study's objective, voluntary participation, nature of confidentiality, risk, and benefits, and researcher contact details for possible contact after study completion. Data were only collected from those patients who were deemed stable. Participants completed a patient information form at the start of the study. Personal information was obtained regarding age, gender, number of siblings, education, residential area, family structure, number of family members, family income and number of earning members, drug of addiction, history, and the onset of the problem. Researchers ensured test conditions were similar for the instructions and administration of measures at their respective treatment and rehabilitation centers. Out of 237 participants, our Urdu version of the CERQ was re-administered to 47 participants, with a 10–14 days gap. The scores obtained from the same participants on the two different administrations of the test could then be compared be correlated to assess test–retest reliability.

Statistical Analyses

Cronbach's α was used to estimate the internal consistency reliability of the CERQ and its subscales. In contrast, simple Pearson product–moment correlations were used to assess test–retest reliability, calculated for the 47 participants who were re-administered the CERQ. Convergent validity of the CERQ was determined by examining the simple Pearson product-moment correlations of the CERQ total score and subscale scores with the DASS-21 total and subscale scores and with the RSES score. All statistical analyses were conducted with the Statistical Package for Social Sciences (SPSS, V-23.0).

RESULTS

Participant Characteristics

Male patients ($N = 237$) 18–50 years of age (M = 29.8, SD = 8.1) were recruited from different substance use treatment centers and hospitals in Karachi, Pakistan. Regarding marital status, 57.4% reported they were single, 40.9% married, and 1.7% divorced. Their mean years of education completed was (M = 5.3, SD = 5.5) with a monthly income in PKR (M = 24677.2, SD = 31340.5). Regarding work status, 43% were employed, 22.4% were on daily wages and worked as laborers, 14.8% had their own business, and 19.8% were unemployed. In terms of living arrangements, 44.3% lived in a nuclear family setup, and 55.7% were in a joint family setup. Regarding the type of substance use, 44% reported using heroin, 15.6% used cannabis, and 32.9% reported using multiple psychoactive substances. Regarding using psychoactive substances, 32.1% reported such use due to family-related issues (i.e., conflicts). A total of 27.8% reported started using psychoactive substances for experimentation, 27% reported use due to personal psychological issues, and 13.1% reported use due to friends using. Regarding substance use history in their family, 39.2% reported use by their immediate family members. When asked about family history of substance use, 39.2% reported that at least one immediate family member uses drugs.

Table 1 presents descriptive statistics for all self-report measures, including subscales.

TABLE 1 | Descriptive statistics for the Cognitive Emotion Regulation Questionnaire (CERQ) and its subscales, the Depression Anxiety and Stress Scale, Short Form (DASS-21) and its subscales, and the Rosenberg Self-esteem Scale (RSES) ($N = 237$).

Measures	*Min*	*Max*	*M*	*SD*
CERQ Total	112	172	130.2	10.0
Self-blame	11	20	17.8	1.9
Acceptance	15	20	18.5	1.5
Rumination	15	20	18.4	1.5
Positive refocusing	5	20	9.5	2.2
Focus on planning	4	18	9.8	2.7
Positive reappraisal	5	18	9.4	2.3
Putting into perspective	4	16	9.3	2.0
Catastrophizing	15	20	18.5	1.5
Other blame	15	20	18.0	1.5
DASS-21 Total	3	72	43.1	14.3
Depression	0	27	14.6	5.2
Anxiety	0	25	14.0	5.3
Stress	1	23	14.4	4.6
RSES Self-esteem	10	30	15.1	4.9

M, mean; SD, standard deviation; CERQ, Cognitive Emotion Regulation Questionnaire; DASS-21, Depression Anxiety and Stress Scale; Short Form; RSES, Rosenberg Self Esteem Scale. The CERQ total score has a possible range of 36–180, inclusive, while the CERQ subscale scores have a possible range of 4–20, inclusive. The DASS-21 total score has a possible range of 0–63, while the DASS-21 subscale scores have a possible range of 0 to 21. The RSES score has a possible range of 0–30, inclusive.

CERQ Reliability

Our Urdu version of CERQ had good to excellent internal consistency reliability for the total score and subscale scores (see the left-hand section of **Table 2**), with Cronbach's $\alpha = 0.80$ for the total score and subscale reliabilities ranging from $\alpha = 0.70$ (for other blame) to $\alpha = 0.89$ (for focus on planning).

The left-hand section of **Table 2** also lists the test–retest reliabilities for the CERQ total and subscale scores. Of the ten correlations, seven were equal to or >0.9, and the lowest value was 0.76 (for catastrophizing).

CERQ Convergent Validity

Not listed in **Table 2** are the internal consistency reliabilities for the DASS-21 total (Cronbach's $\alpha = 0.95$) and the RSES (Cronbach $\alpha = 0.91$), which were calculated to assess the reliabilities of the convergent validity measures as the indices of reliability of the two respective measures whose correlation is examined sets the lower bound for a validity coefficient. As such, if the reliabilities of the DASS-21 and the RSES were deficient, the convergent validity coefficients would have been adversely impacted, something which did not occur here.

The simple Pearson product-moment correlations of the CERQ total and subscales scores with the DASS-21 total and subscale scores and the RSES score are presented in the right-hand section of **Table 2**. Results for the CERQ total score indicated that it was significantly negatively associated with the DASS-21 total score and the depression, anxiety, and stress subscale scores ($p < 0.001$) and positively associated with self-esteem ($p < 0.001$). There was a clear pattern to the correlations of the CERQ subscale scores with the DASS-21 total and subscale scores and the RSES score, with the CERQ subscales that measure positive characteristics (e.g., focus of planning) showing significant negative associations with the DASS-21 total and subscale scores, and a positive association with the RSES score.

DISCUSSION

The aims and objectives of this study were: (1) to develop a culturally sound Urdu version of CERQ; and to investigate (2)

TABLE 2 | Internal consistency reliabilities (Cronbach's α) and 10–14 day test–retest reliabilities (Pearson Product-Moment Correlations) of the CERQ total and subscale scores, and Pearson Product-Moment Correlations of the CERQ scores with the DASS-21 total and subscale scores and the Rosenberg Self-Esteem Scale ($N = 47$ for test–retest reliability; $N = 237$ otherwise).

	Reliability		Convergent validity				
			DASS-21				RSES
Measures	α	**Test-retest**	**Total Score**	**Depression**	**Anxiety**	**Stress**	
N	237	47	237	237	237	237	237
CERQ Total	0.80	0.86	**−0.26**	**−0.24**	**−0.23**	**−0.27**	**0.30**
Self-blame	0.76	0.85	**0.19**	**0.18**	**0.23**	0.12	**0.14**
Acceptance	0.78	0.92	−0.03	−0.04	−0.02	−0.03	−0.01
Rumination	0.72	0.95	−0.11	−0.10	−0.07	**−0.15**	0.10
Positive refocusing	0.79	0.94	**−0.33**	**−0.29**	**−0.35**	**−0.31**	**0.24**
Focus on planning	0.89	0.98	**−0.30**	**−0.26**	**−0.32**	**−0.28**	**0.19**
Positive reappraisal	0.81	0.97	**−0.23**	**−0.25**	**−0.19**	**−0.21**	**0.22**
Putting into perspective	0.83	0.99	**−0.17**	**−0.20**	**−0.14**	**−0.15**	**0.18**
Catastrophizing	0.73	0.76	−0.01	0.010	0.01	−0.04	0.15
Other blame	0.70	0.90	**0.13**	0.122	0.12	**0.13**	0.00

CERQ, Cognitive Emotion Regulation Questionnaire; DASS-21, Depression Anxiety and Stress Scale, Short Form; RSES, Rosenberg Self Esteem Scale. All test–retest correlations are significant at $p < 0.001$. For the Pearson product-moment correlations (rs) of the CERQ scores with the DASS-21 total and subscale scores and RSES scores, iff $|r| > 0.127$, then r is significant at 0.05, while iff $|r| > 0.212$, then r is significant at $p < 0.001$. The values for those correlations whose $p < 0.05$ are ***bolded***.

the reliability of this Urdu version of the CERQ; and (3) its convergent validity in a sample of male patients with SUD. Convergent validity was examined regarding the relationship of the CERQ total and subscale scores with depression, anxiety, and stress and a measure of self-esteem. No normative data on these measures are available in Pakistan, but the examination of the means in relation to their respective range of scores, as well as their respective standard deviations, would suggest reasonable estimates of DASS-21 and RSES. The overall findings of this study support the strong psychometric properties of the Urdu translated version of CERQ.

The reliability and convergent validity of the Urdu version of the CERQ in a sample of adult males with SUDs would suggest that this translated measure could be used to better understand the CER strategies in this population. This better understanding of cognitive and emotional regulation may then aid in designing and implementing interventions to improve people's coping strategies with substance use disorder. Better interventions for cognitive and emotional regulation may, in turn, help improve treatment adherence, maintain a drug-free status, and overall recovery. Psycho-education of patients with SUDs, their families, and significant others about substance use could also help reduce the stigma and discrimination that creates barriers to recovery.

The present findings show an inverse relationship of CER strategies with depression, anxiety, and stress and a direct relationship with self-esteem. In the context of a substance use disorder, CER strategies, specifically maladaptive strategies, can significantly impair psychosocial functioning. So, it is vital to understand how and when these maladaptive strategies can be detrimental and intervene to overcome these problems. According to a model from Gross (35), emotion regulation plays a crucial role in health outcomes. According to Compare et al. (36), people's strategies to regulate their negative emotions are strongly associated with mental health problems such as depression; emotion dysregulation is more common in depression that impairs an individual's social skills and capacity to identify emotions and quality of life. This study's findings are consistent with previous studies, which found that inappropriate emotion regulation is an integral part of developing and maintaining depression and anxiety disorders (37, 38). Other researchers found that depression is linked with impaired cognitive control, such as difficulty accepting and processing negative material (39). There is research evidence to support this study's findings regarding the role of self-esteem in mental health outcomes (40). Results suggest that low self-esteem can lead to a lack of development and a tendency toward drugs or alcohol consumption (41). Other researchers also found the role of environmental stressors in reducing a person's well-being. Low self-esteem can contribute to various social problems like substance use, and it often plays a vital role in this regard (42).

Individuals use emotion regulation strategies to manage and reduce the consequences of the stressors (43, 44). Some research suggests that reliance on emotion-focused coping (e.g., worry, self-blame) is related to the risk of experiencing mental health issues such as anxiety, depressive symptoms, and drug use (45, 46). A study examining the influence of emotion regulation strategies in depression among male patients with SUDs found that emotion regulation strategies such as affect suppression significantly predicted depression (15). Another study of male patients treated for SUDs concluded that patients with SUDs showed a stronger tendency to use emotion-focused coping efforts, including self-criticism and problem avoidance when facing problems than patients with severe mental illness (47). Thus, patients with SUDs may be using avoidance and disengagement strategies to cope with the difficult situation in an unsuccessful way, which could negatively interfere with treatment adherence and treatment outcome. The relationship between emotion regulation strategies and SUD is necessary for the study reported here. Individuals with adaptive coping strategies respond to challenging situations to reduce the risk of substance use. Those with emotion-focused coping strategies may be less equipped to deal with stressful life situations, leading to higher chances of using drugs. Such a conclusion is consistent with Capella and associates (48) findings that male patients with SUDs who rely on avoidance coping strategies are likely to use drugs. Thus, perhaps individuals depending on emotion-focused coping strategies use drugs to deal with negative emotions and stress.

Limitations

The present study has certain limitations related to the study design. The sample was one of convenience, and data were collected at a single time. However, the relationship of cognitive emotion regulation strategies with depression, anxiety, stress, and self-esteem could operate differently over time. Furthermore, the sample only included male patients receiving treatment for SUD. Thus, generalizability is limited to male patients without a SUD, female patients with or with a SUD, or the non-patient general population. Future research may wish to include a more diverse sample, including non-clinical samples, to understand the role of emotion regulation in improving well-being and mental health outcomes in males and females without a SUD. Future research may also attempt to disentangle the role of emotional regulation as a possible mediator between mental health issues and substance use disorder.

CONCLUSIONS

Existing literature related to cognitive emotion regulation strategies indicates a strong link between cognitive emotion regulation with mental health problems and self-esteem. The present study showed that the Urdu version of the CERQ would be a reliable measure for patients with SUD. Using this measure may help us fill the gap in understanding the emotion regulation strategies and implementing evidence-based practices (EBPs) while linking it with the client's specific problems to improve treatment outcomes. In addition, the Urdu version of the CERQ may be helpful in the identification of adaptive and maladaptive strategies that may constitute the basis for preventive or treatment interventions specifically for patients with SUD aimed at enhancing their well-being.

AUTHOR CONTRIBUTIONS

SS main researcher, design of the research, wrote part of the manuscript, and responsible for the sample selection, data collection, and data analysis. NBa wrote the introduction and discussion. NBe provided data collection, wrote part of the manuscript, and provided statistical analysis. HJ provided manuscript reviews, edits, corrections, and amendments. All authors participated and approved the study design, contributed to manuscript revision, read, and approved the submitted version.

ACKNOWLEDGMENTS

We wish to express our gratitude to all participants for participating in this research.

REFERENCES

1. Thompson RA. Emotion regulation: A theme in search of definition. *Monograph Soc Res Child Develop.* (1994) 59:25–52. doi: 10.1111/j.1540-5834.1994.tb01276.x
2. Gross JJ. The extended process model of emotion regulation: elaborations, applications, and future directions. *Psychol Inq.* (2015) 26:130–7. doi: 10.1080/1047840X.2015.989751
3. Koole SL. The psychology of emotion regulation: an integrative review. *Cogn Emot.* (2009) 23:4–41. doi: 10.1080/02699930802619031
4. Aldao A, Nolen-Hoeksema S, Schweizer S. Emotion-regulation strategies across psychopathology: a meta-analytic review. *Clin Psychol Rev.* (2010) 30:217–37. doi: 10.1016/j.cpr.2009.11.004
5. Young KS, Sandman CF, Craske MG. Positive and negative emotion regulation in adolescence: links to anxiety and depression. *Brain Sci.* (2019) 9:76. doi: 10.3390/brainsci9040076
6. Waugh CE. The roles of positive emotion in the regulation of emotional responses to negative events. *Emotion.* (2020) 20:54–8. doi: 10.1037/emo0000625
7. Van Beveren ML, Goossens L, Volkaert B, Grassmann C, Wante L, Vandeweghe L, et al. How do I feel right now? Emotional awareness, emotion regulation, and depressive symptoms in youth. *Eur Child Adoles Psychiatry.* (2019) 28:389–98. doi: 10.1007/s00787-018-1203-3
8. Nikmanesh Z, Kazemi Y, Khosravy M. Study role of different dimensions of emotional self-regulation on addiction potential. *J Fam Reprod Health.* (2014) 8:69–72. Retrieved from: https://www.ncbi.nlm.nih.gov/pmc/articles/PMC4064769/
9. De Berardis D, Fornaro M, Orsolini L, Valchera A, Carano A, Vellante F, et al. Alexithymia and suicide risk in psychiatric disorders: a mini-review. *Front Psychiatry.* (2017) 8:148. doi: 10.3389/fpsyt.2017.00148
10. Evren C, Evren B, Dalbudak E, Ozcelik B, Oncu F. Childhood abuse and neglect as a risk factor for alexithymia in adult male substance dependent inpatients. *J Psychoactive Drugs.* (2009) 41:85–92. doi: 10.1080/02791072.2009.10400677
11. Sakuraba S, Kubo M, Komoda T, Yamana J. Suicidal ideation and alexithymia in patients with alcoholism: a pilot study. *Subst Use Misuse.* (2005) 40:823–30. doi: 10.1081/JA-200030702
12. Vala M. Comparative study of cognitive regulation between addicted and non-addicted peoples. *Eur J Forensic Sci.* (2016) 3:7–10. doi: 10.5455/ejfs.210576
13. Weiss NH, Sullivan TP, Matthew TT. Explicating the role of emotion dysregulation in risky behaviors: a review and synthesis of the literature with directions for future research and clinical practice. *Curr Opin Psychol.* (2015) 3:22–9. doi: 10.1016/j.copsyc.2015.01.013
14. Parker JDA, Taylor R, Eastabrook J, Schell S, Wood LM. Problem gambling in adolescence: Relationships with internet misuse, gaming

abuse and emotional intelligence. *Pers Individ Differ.* (2008) 45:174–80. doi: 10.1016/J.PAID.2008.03.018

15. Shahzad S, Fatima K, Begum N, Ali M. Emotion regulation strategies as predictors of depression in patients with substance use disorder. *Pakistan J Clin Psychol.* (2020) 19:17–32. Retrieved from: http://www.pjcpku.com/index.php/pjcp/article/view/3
16. Garnefski N, Kraaij V. The cognitive emotion regulation questionnaire: psychometric features and prospective relationships with depression and anxiety in adults. *Eur J Psychol Assess.* (2007) 23:141–9. doi: 10.1027/1015-5759.23.3.141
17. Berking M, Ebert D, Cuijpers P, Hofmann SG. Emotion regulation skills training enhances the efficacy of inpatient cognitive behavioral therapy for major depressive disorder: A randomized controlled trial. *Psychother Psychosom.* (2013) 82:234–45. doi: 10.1159/000348448
18. Garnefski N, Kraaij V, Spinnhoven P. Negative life events, cognitive emotion regulation and emotional problems. *Pers Individ Dif.* (2001) 30:1311–27. doi: 10.1016/S0191-8869(00)00113-6
19. Van Windenfelt BM, Treffers, PDA, de Beurs E, Siebelink BM, Koudijs E. Translation and cross-cultural adaptation of assessment instruments used in psychological research with children and families. *Clin Child Fam Psychol Rev.* (2005) 8:135–47. doi: 10.1007/s10567-005-4752-1
20. Guillemin F, Bombardier C, Beaton D. Cross cultural adaptation of health related quality of life measures: Literature review and proposed guidelines. *J Clin Epidemiol.* (1993) 46:1417–32. doi: 10.1016/0895-4356(93)90142-N
21. Prastuti E, Wagey Tairas MM, Hartini N. Adaptation and validation of cognitive emotion regulation questionnaire (CERQ) in Indonesian version. *J Education Health Comm Psychol.* (2020) 9:132–47.
22. Megreya AM, Latzman RD, Al-Attiyah AA, Alrashidi M. The robustness of the nine-factor structure of the cognitive emotion regulation questionnaire across four arabic-speaking middle eastern countries. *J Cross Cult Psychol.* (2016) 47:875–90. doi: 10.1177/0022022116644785
23. Domínguez-Sánchez FJ, Lasa-Aristu A, Amor PJ, Holgado-Tello FP. Psychometric properties of the Spanish version of the Cognitive Emotion Regulation Questionnaire. *Assessment.* (2011) 20:253–61. doi: 10.1177/1073191110397274
24. Joormann J, Stanton CH. Examining emotion regulation in depression: A review and future directions. *Behav Res Ther.* (2016) 86:35–49. doi: 10.1016/j.brat.2016.07.007
25. Tuna E, Bozo Ö. The cognitive emotion regulation questionnaire: factor structure and psychometric properties of the Turkish version. *J Psychopathol Behav Assess.* (2012) 34:564–70. doi: 10.1007/s10862-012-9303-8
26. Abdi S, Taban S, Ghaemian A. Cognitive emotion regulation questionnaire: validity and reliability of the Persian translation of the CERQ (36-item). *Proc Soc Behav.* (2012) 32:2–7. doi: 10.1016/j.sbspro.2012.01.001
27. Zhu X, Auerbach RP, Yao S, Abela JR, Xiao J, Tong X. Psychometric properties of the cognitive emotion regulation questionnaire: chinese version. *Cogn Emot.* (2008) 22:288–307. doi: 10.1080/02699930701369035
28. Jermann F, Van der Linden M, d'Acremont M, Zermatten A. Cognitive emotion regulation questionnaire (CERQ): confirmatory factor analysis and psychometric properties of the french translation. *Eur J Psychol Assess.* (2006) 22:126–31. doi: 10.1027/1015-5759.22.2.126
29. International Test Commission. (2017). *The ITC Guidelines for Translating and Adapting Tests (Second edition).* [www.InTestCom.org]. Available online at: https://www.intestcom.org/files/guideline_test_adaptation_2ed.pdf
30. Lovibond SH, Lovibond PF. *Manual for the Depression Anxiety and Stress Scales.* 2nd ed. Sydney, NSW: Psychology Foundation (1995).
31. Rosenberg M. *Society and the Adolescent Self-Image.* Princeton, NJ: Princeton University Press (1965).
32. Garnefski N, Kraaij V, Spinhoven P. *Manual for the Use of the Cognitive Emotion Regulation Questionnaire.* Karachi: Leiden University (2002).
33. Kamal A, Aslam N. Translation, Validation, and Effectiveness of Depression, Anxiety and Stress (DASS-21) in assessing the psychological distress among flood affected individuals. *J Pakistan Psychiatr Soc.* (2017) 14:4–20. Available online at: http://www.jpps.com.pk/article/15198028712310-Translation%20Validation%20and%20Effectiveness%20of%20Depression,%20Anxiety%20and%20stress%20scale%20(DASS-21)%20in%20Assessing%20the%20psychological%20Distress%20Among%20Flood%20Affected%20Individuals.pdf
34. Rizwan M, Malik S, Malik JN, Siddiqui RS. Urdu Rosenberg self-esteem scale: an analysis of reliability and validity in Pakistan. *Sociol Int J.* (2017) 1:56–61. doi: 10.15406/sij.2017.01.00010
35. Gross JJ. The emerging field of emotion regulation: an integrative review. *Rev Gen Psychol.* (1998) 2:271–99. doi: 10.1037/1089-2680.2.3.271
36. Compare A, Zarbo C, Shonin E, Gordon WE, and Marconi C. Emotional regulation and depression: A potential mediator between heart and mind. *Cardiovas Psychiatry Neurol.* (2014) 6:324374. doi: 10.1155/2014/324374
37. Barlow DH, Allen LB, Choate ML. Toward a unified treatment for emotional disorders. *Behav Ther.* (2004) 35:205–30. doi: 10.1016/S0005-7894(04)80036-4
38. Mennin DS. Emotion regulation therapy: an integrative approach to treatment-resistant anxiety disorders. *J Contemp Psychother.* (2006) 36:95–105. doi: 10.1007/s10879-006-9012-2
39. Joormann J, Gotlib IH. Emotion regulation in depression: relation to cognitive inhibition. *Cogn Emot.* (2010) 24:281–98. doi: 10.1080/02699930903407948
40. Ali M, Shahzad S. Risk and protective factors for mental health problems in patients with substance use disorder. *Pak J Psychol.* (2020) 50:55–69. Retrieved from: http://www.pjpku.com/index.php/pjp/article/view/24
41. MacArthur JD, MacArthur CT. Self-Esteem. San Francisco, CA: Research Network on Socioeconomic Status and Health. (2004). In Alavi HR. The Role of Self-esteem in Tendency towards Drugs, Theft and Prostitution. *Addict Health.* (2011) 3:119–24. Retrieved from https://www.ncbi.nlm.nih.gov/pmc/articles/PMC3905528/
42. Kahn AP, Fawcett J. *The Encyclopedia of Mental Health (Facts on File Library of Health and Living).* 3rd ed. New York, NY: Facts on File (2007).
43. Skinner EA, Edge K, Altman J, Sherwood H. Searching for the structure of coping: a review and critique of category systems for classifying ways of coping. *Psychol Bull.* (2003) 129:216–69. doi: 10.1037/0033-2909.129.2.216
44. Carver CS, Connor-Smith J. Personality and coping. *Annu Rev Psychol.* (2010) 61:679–704. doi: 10.1146/annurev.psych.093008.100352
45. Dashora P, Erdem G, Slesnick N. Better to bend than to break: coping strategies utilized by substance-abusing homeless youth. *J Health Psychol.* (2011) 16:158–68. doi: 10.1177/1359105310378385
46. Scott RM, Hides L, Allen JS, Lubman DI. Coping style and ecstasy use motives as predictors of current mood symptoms in ecstasy users. *Addict Behav.* (2013) 38:2465–72. doi: 10.1016/j.addbeh.2013.05.005
47. Marquez-Arrico JE, Río-Martínez L, José Francisco Navarro JF, Prat G, Forero DA, Adan A. Coping strategies in male patients under treatment for substance use disorders and/or severe mental illness: influence in clinical course atone-year follow-up. *J Clin Med.* (2019) 8:1972. doi: 10.3390/jcm8111972
48. Capella MM, Benaiges I, Adan A. Neuropsychological performance in polyconsumer men under treatment. Influence of age of onset of substance use. *Sci Rep.* (2015) 5:12038. doi: 10.1038/srep12038

19

Associations among the Big Five Personality Traits, Maladaptive Cognitions and Internet Addiction across Three Time Measurements in 3 Months during the COVID-19 Pandemic

Yu Tian[1]*, Yanli Zhao*[1]*, Fengling Lv*[1]*, Ningbo Qin*[1] *and Peipei Chen*[2*]

[1] *Department of Marxism, Qingdao University of Science and Technology, Qingdao, China,* [2] *Department of Psychology, Shandong Normal University, Jinan, China*

***Correspondence:**
Peipei Chen
690281393@qq.com

The present study examined the longitudinal association among the Big Five personality traits, maladaptive cognitions, and Internet addiction during the COVID-19 pandemic. A total of 481 Chinese university students (247 men; mean age = 20.31 years) were surveyed three times (interval of 1 month) by using the Chinese version of the Big Five Personality Traits Scale, Maladaptive Cognitions Scale, and Internet Addiction Scale. The results of a cross-lagged panel analysis highlighted that (i) extraversion, agreeableness, conscientiousness, and openness were negatively associated with maladaptive cognitions and Internet addiction, whereas neuroticism was found to be positively associated with maladaptive cognitions and Internet addiction across time; (ii) associations among the Big Five personality traits, maladaptive cognitions, and Internet addiction were dynamic and bidirectional; and (iii) maladaptive cognitions played mediating roles in extraversion, agreeableness, conscientiousness, openness, and Internet addiction across time. The Big Five personality traits, maladaptive cognitions, and Internet addiction predicted each other across time, and maladaptive cognitions were likely to be the key mediating factor in the associations between the Big Five personality traits and Internet addiction, which supported and expanded the Davis' cognitive–behavioral model.

Keywords: Internet addiction, maladaptive cognitions, Big Five personality traits, cross-lagged panel design, cognitive–behavioral model

INTRODUCTION

According to the 45th China Statistical Report on Internet Development, more than 904 million Chinese people spent an average of 30.8 h every week on the Internet to shop, play games, communicate with others, and perform other daily life activities (China Internet Network Information Center [CNNIC], 2020). However, spending too much time on the Internet leads to individuals getting affected by Internet addiction [also referred to as pathological Internet use (PIU) in other studies], which has been defined as excessive or compulsive Internet use and preoccupation with and loss of control over this use (Davis, 2001). Numerous recent studies have reported that people, especially university students, have been using the Internet more during the COVID-19 pandemic to mitigate their anxiety levels, resulting in an increased level of Internet addiction (Garcia-Priego et al., 2020; Jiang, 2020; Nagaur, 2020). Previous studies have reported Internet addiction to be positively associated with numerous negative outcomes, including decreased academic achievement (Stavropoulos et al., 2013), emotional disorders (Kim et al., 2017), sleep disorders (Ladner et al., 2010), and even suicidal ideation and behavior in some serious cases (Steinbüchel et al., 2017; Sami et al., 2018). Therefore, a study of factors affecting Internet addiction during the COVID-19 pandemic is warranted to provide implications for the prevention of Internet addiction during this unprecedented time.

Previous studies have suggested that the Big Five personality traits, namely, extraversion, agreeableness, conscientiousness, neuroticism, and openness, are significantly associated with Internet addiction (Zhou et al., 2017; Hou et al., 2018; Kircaburun and Griffiths, 2018; Agbaria and Bdier, 2020; Arpaci and Unver, 2020). Recently, a meta-analysis review study proposed that extraversion, agreeableness, conscientiousness, and openness are negatively associated with Internet addiction, whereas neuroticism is positively associated with Internet addiction (Kayiş et al., 2016). Although previous research has highlighted clear associations between the Big Five personality traits and Internet addiction, several gaps still exist in the relevant literature. First, a majority of studies examining the effects of the Big Five personality traits on Internet addiction had a cross-sectional design, which made it difficult to draw causal inferences. Therefore, more studies with a longitudinal design are warranted to further validate the results of previous studies. Second, the mechanism through which the Big Five personality traits affect Internet addiction has received limited research attention. Although some studies have highlighted coping style (Zhou et al., 2017), self-liking (Kircaburun and Griffiths, 2018), and family function (Hou et al., 2018) to mediate associations between the Big Five personality traits and Internet addiction, more mediating factors should be investigated. Finally, no study has investigated the effects of Internet addiction on the Big Five personality traits; the literature has only suggested that Internet addiction exerts effects on individuals' personality traits, such as shyness and depression (Tian et al., 2017; Soulioti et al., 2018). Therefore, the effects of Internet addiction on individuals' Big Five personality traits merit further research. Considering the aforementioned limitations, the present study provided an in-depth exploration of this topic.

BIDIRECTIONAL ASSOCIATIONS BETWEEN THE BIG FIVE PERSONALITY TRAITS AND INTERNET ADDICTION

Previous studies have reported that extraversion, agreeableness, conscientiousness, and openness are negatively associated with the positive predictors of Internet addictions, such as low self-esteem (Wang et al., 2012), loneliness (Buecker et al., 2020), depression (Bunevicius et al., 2008), and social anxiety (Lee et al., 2014), whereas neuroticism was found to be positively associated with these predictors. Therefore, most studies have suggested that extraversion, agreeableness, conscientiousness, and openness are significantly negative predictors of Internet addiction, whereas neuroticism is a significantly positive predictor of Internet addiction (Kayiş et al., 2016). However, some studies have proposed different conclusions; for example, positive or no associations were found between openness and Internet addiction (Rahmani and Lavasani, 2011; Servidio, 2014) and between extraversion and Internet addiction (Rahmani and Lavasani, 2011; Andreassen et al., 2013). Therefore, further investigation, especially longitudinal studies, on the effects of the Big Five personality traits on Internet addiction is required.

Internet addiction tends to be a predictor of the Big Five personality traits. Although individuals' personality traits are stable, they may fluctuate within a certain range (Asendorpf and Aken, 2010). Numerous studies have demonstrated that Internet addiction may affect individuals' personality traits, such as loneliness (Yao and Zhong, 2014; Tian et al., 2017), depression (Bengü and Ahmet, 2018), and self-esteem issues (Fioravanti et al., 2012). Moreover, the Big Five personality traits have been significantly associated with individuals' loneliness, depression, and self-esteem (Bunevicius et al., 2008; Wang et al., 2012; Buecker et al., 2020), thereby, indicating that the Big Five personality traits can be the outcome variables of Internet addiction. However, an exhaustive review of the relevant literature revealed that the effects of Internet addiction on individuals' Big Five personality traits are yet to be studied; therefore, the present study examined these effects.

THE BIDIRECTIONAL MEDIATING ROLES OF MALADAPTIVE COGNITIONS

The cognitive–behavioral model was employed in our study as the theoretical model to clarify associations and the mechanism through which the Big Five personality traits affect Internet addiction. The model indicated that psychopathology (such as substance dependence, depression, and social anxiety) is a distal necessary cause of symptoms of Internet addiction (Davis, 2001). However, psychopathology alone cannot lead to individuals getting affected by Internet addiction, and it is just a necessary element in the etiology of Internet addiction. Maladaptive cognitions, defined as cognitive distortions about the self (such as "I am good only on the Internet") and the world (such as "The Internet is the only place where I am respected"), are the proximal sufficient causes of Internet addiction. The distal necessary causes may affect Internet addiction through the proximal sufficient causes. Previous studies have highlighted that the Big Five personality traits are significantly associated with depression (Langguth et al., 2007) and social anxiety (Kaplan et al., 2015); therefore, they constitute the distal necessary causes, in turn, suggesting that the Big Five personality traits may also affect Internet addiction through maladaptive cognitions. Although numerous studies have found that individuals' personality traits, such as shyness (Tian et al., 2015), motivation, stress, loneliness, and depression (Lu and Yeo, 2015), can affect Internet addiction through maladaptive cognition, no study has examined the mediating roles of maladaptive cognitions in the associations between the Big Five personality traits and Internet addiction; therefore, this study intends to fill the gaps in research.

The cognitive–behavioral model suggests that the symptoms of Internet addiction could get exhibited through vicious cycles, which can further affect individuals' personality (Davis, 2001). For example, many studies have indicated that Internet addiction can exert a negative effect on individuals' shyness (Tian et al., 2017), self-esteem (Mo et al., 2020), and depression (Soulioti et al., 2018), thereby highlighting that Internet addiction can also exert negative effects on individuals' Big Five personality traits. In addition, the cognitive–behavioral model explained the mechanism through which Internet addiction affects individuals' Big Five personality traits. The model emphasized that the core symptoms of Internet addiction constitute maladaptive cognition, and individuals with Internet addiction are disposed to regard the Internet as the only place where they feel good about themselves (Davis, 2001). More specifically, individuals with maladaptive cognitions tend to spend more time or money on the Internet and less time on activities that they may have found pleasurable before. When an individual reduces face-to-face interactions with their friends or family members, they become socially isolated and experience weak social support and increasing interpersonal issues, which may affect their personality traits (Tian et al., 2017; Soulioti et al., 2018). On the basis of vicious cycles through which Internet addiction operates, maladaptive cognitions also tend to be a key factor determining the effect of Internet addiction on individuals' Big Five personality traits. Therefore, this point of view was also verified in the present study.

THE COVID-19 PANDEMIC

Studies have highlighted that the level of individuals' Internet addiction has increased during the COVID-19 pandemic (Garcia-Priego et al., 2020; Jiang, 2020; Nagaur, 2020). This is because the absence of definite answers to the questions of when the pandemic is going to end and how one can cope with this challenging time may lead individuals to experience more anxiety, depression, and other negative emotions (Özdin and Özdin, 2020). To attenuate the effect of such negative emotions, individuals tend to use the Internet more to release these emotions; however, spending too much time on the Internet may lead to an increased level of Internet addiction (Garcia-Priego et al., 2020; Jiang, 2020). Moreover, prohibitions/recommendations, such as staying at home as much as possible, make it difficult for individuals to have face-to-face communication with each other; therefore, individuals spend more time on the Internet to maintain social ties, which could, in turn, intensify their Internet addiction (Nagaur, 2020). Because of the specific characteristics of this period, the associations between, and the mechanism through which, the Big Five personality traits affect Internet addiction are different. For example, extraversion, agreeableness, conscientiousness, and openness have been found to be negatively associated with anxiety, depression, and other negative emotions (Bunevicius et al., 2008; Wang et al., 2012; Lee et al., 2014), whereas neuroticism is positively associated with these negative emotions. These associations may lead to stronger negative or positive connections between the Big Five personality traits and Internet addiction. Because maladaptive cognitions are the proximal sufficient causes of Internet addiction, stronger associations may be established because of the increased level of maladaptive cognitions. However, these hypotheses required validation in the current study.

THE PRESENT STUDY

The present study examined reciprocal associations among the Big Five personality traits, maladaptive cognitions, and Internet addiction by using a longitudinal design and tested the bidirectional mediating roles of maladaptive cognitions in the association between the Big Five personality traits and Internet addiction. Drawing from the aforementioned literature review, we proposed the following hypotheses: (i) Extraversion, maladaptive cognitions, and Internet addiction can predict each other across time, and maladaptive cognitions play bidirectional mediating roles in the association between extraversion and Internet addiction. (ii) Agreeableness, maladaptive cognitions, and Internet addiction can predict each other across time, and maladaptive cognitions play bidirectional mediating roles in the association between agreeableness and Internet addiction. (iii) Conscientiousness, maladaptive cognitions, and Internet addiction can predict each other across time, and maladaptive cognitions play bidirectional mediating roles in the association between conscientiousness and Internet addiction. (iv) Neuroticism, maladaptive cognitions, and Internet addiction can predict each other across time, and maladaptive cognitions play bidirectional mediating roles in the association between neuroticism and Internet addiction. (v) Openness, maladaptive cognitions, and Internet addiction can predict each other across time, and maladaptive cognitions play bidirectional mediating roles in the association between openness and Internet addiction. The aforementioned hypotheses were tested using a cross-lagged panel design in which three measurement points of each studied variable were employed.

MATERIALS AND METHODS

Participants and Procedure

All students recruited in the present study belonged to the same university, which was located in the northeast of China. Three measurements were conducted during the COVID-19 pandemic at 1-month intervals. During the first measurement, 734 valid questionnaires were collected, of which 390 were completed by male students. During the second measurement, 656 valid questionnaires were collected, of which 345 were completed by male students. During the third measurement, 599 valid questionnaires were collected, of which 304 were completed by male students. A total of 481 students finished all the three measurements, and their responses were utilized for subsequent data analysis. More specifically, the final sample comprised 247 male students and 234 female students, and the mean age of the final sample was 20.31 [standard deviation (SD) = 1.63] years. Some students could not take the surveys because of illness, because they did not receive the message appropriately, or because of the inconvenient network links, which made them give up the survey. A series of independent sample *t*-tests were performed to estimate differences between participating students and non-participating students in the studied variables. No differences were found.

All the three measurements were conducted online because of prohibitions/recommendations to stay at home, and the survey was conducted through three steps. First, teachers sent a message to the students, requesting them to participate in the study's online survey. The students were informed that the survey comprised three measurements that were separated by 1 month each. All the students provided their consent to take part in the survey, and only those who finished all the three measurements were compensated with gifts. Moreover, students were informed that the scores of the survey would not be recorded as their final performance for that term and would be kept confidential. Second, the teachers organized for the students to complete each of the measurements after an online class, and all the students were required to respond to the questionnaires in the time provided. All the teachers were required to be present online during the measurement and answer any questions that came from the students. Third, the teachers briefed the students regarding the primary objective of this survey during the final measurement and distributed gifts among them as rewards.

Measures

Big Five Personality Traits

The Chinese version of the Big Five Inventory was employed to measure the participants' Big Five personality traits (John et al., 1991; Carciofo et al., 2016). The revised questionnaire comprised 44 items, with an eight-item extraversion subscale (e.g., "I am talkative"), a nine-item agreeableness subscale (e.g., "I am helpful and unselfish"), a nine-item conscientiousness subscale (e.g., "I am rigorous and earnest at work"), an eight-item neuroticism subscale (e.g., "I am depressive and melancholy"), and a 10-item openness subscale (e.g., "I am original and constantly coming up with new ideas"). The revised scale employed a five-point Likert from 1 (strongly disagree) to 5 (strongly agree) to estimate the level of each personality trait among the respondents. Cronbach's α values for the extraversion subscale at the three time points in the present study were 0.69, 0.64, and 0.68, respectively. Moreover, the values, respectively, were 0.74, 0.77, and 0.73 for the agreeableness subscale; 0.77, 0.75, and 0.77 for the conscientiousness subscale; 0.70, 0.69, and 0.71 for the neuroticism subscale; 0.73, 0.74, and 0.77 for the openness subscale; and 0.77, 0.79, and 0.81 for the total scale.

Maladaptive Cognitions

The short Chinese version of the Online Cognition Scale (OCS) was utilized to measure individuals' maladaptive cognitions (Davis et al., 2002; Liang, 2008). This scale was related to the degree of comfort they experienced on the Internet (e.g., "I feel very safe when I on the Internet"), their desire and control capability to use the Internet (e.g., "I often use the Internet beyond the limited degree"), and their use of the Internet as an escape from stress (e.g., "I often surf the Internet to avoid doing unpleasant things"). This scale that was used to estimate the level of individuals' maladaptive cognitions comprised 14 items that were responded to on a four-point Likert scale ranging from 1 (strongly disagree) to 4 (strongly agree). Cronbach's α values for the scale at the three time points in the present study were 0.92, 0.95, and 0.95, respectively.

Internet Addiction

The Chinese version of the Internet Addiction Test (IAT) was employed to measure individuals' Internet addiction (Young, 1998; Bai and Fan, 2005), which was related to compulsive Internet access and withdrawal reaction (e.g., "*Irrespective of how tired I am, I always feel energetic when I surf the Internet*"), Internet addiction tolerance (e.g., "*I find myself spending an increasing amount of time on the Internet*"), time management questions (e.g., "*Because of the Internet, my leisure time has been reduced*"), and interpersonal and health problems (e.g., "*I've been told more than once that I spend too much time online*"). The scale comprised 19 items that were responded to on a four-point Likert scale ranging from 1 (strongly disagree) to 4 (strongly agree) that was used to estimate the level of individuals' Internet addiction. Cronbach's α values for the scale at the three time points in the present study were 0.94, 0.96, and 0.97, respectively.

Statistical Analysis

SPSS 20.0 was employed to conduct a correlation analysis (Pearson's correlation) and difference tests (repeated measurement analysis of variance). Additionally, Mplus 7.0 was used to conduct structural equation modeling (SEM) of path analysis (cross-lagged model). More specifically, the total scores of extraversion, agreeableness, conscientiousness, neuroticism, openness, maladaptive cognitions, and Internet addiction were used as observed variables in all the analyses. Within cross-lagged models, the autoregressive effect between time-adjacent measurements was employed to evaluate the stability of the studied variables across time (e.g., T1 extraversion predicts T2 extraversion, and T2 extraversion predicts T3 extraversion); unidirectional effects between the two variables were used as causal associations between the studied variables (e.g., T1 extraversion predicts T2 Internet addiction, and T2 extraversion predicts T3 Internet addiction); and bidirectional effects between the two variables were used as cross-lagged associations between the studied variables (e.g., T1 extraversion predicts T2 Internet addiction, and T1 Internet addiction predicts T2 extraversion). Bootstrapping was conducted with 1,000 bootstrap samples to determine the mediating role of maladaptive cognitions in the association between the Big Five personality traits and Internet addiction. Furthermore, Hu and Bentler's (1999) goodness of fit indices of chi-squared (χ^2) statistic, degree of freedom (df), Tucker–Lewis index (TLI), comparative fit index (CFI), and root-mean-square error of approximation (RMSEA) were used to assess each of the SEMs.

RESULTS

Correlation Analysis and Difference Tests

Table 1 presents the association between all the studied variables across time. The association among T1, T2, and T3 extraversion ranged from 0.64 to 0.68, and that among T1, T2, and T3 agreeableness ranged from 0.55 to 0.65. The association among T1, T2, and T3 conscientiousness ranged from 0.58 to 0.72, and that among T1, T2, and T3 neuroticism ranged from 0.57 to 0.65. The association among T1, T2, and T3 openness ranged from 0.53 to 0.54, and that among T1, T2, and T3 maladaptive cognitions ranged from 0.50 to 0.59. The association among T1, T2, and T3 Internet addiction ranged from 0.53 to 0.63. The associations among the measures of extraversion, agreeableness, conscientiousness, neuroticism, openness, maladaptive cognitions, and Internet addiction were in the expected direction. That is, extraversion, agreeableness, conscientiousness, and openness were negatively associated with maladaptive cognitions and Internet addiction, whereas neuroticism was positively associated with maladaptive cognitions and Internet addiction. Furthermore, maladaptive cognitions and Internet addiction were positively associated with each other.

The results of the repeated measurement analysis of variance indicated a significant difference in Internet addiction across time, and no other differences were revealed. Furthermore, the results of pairwise comparisons indicated no significant difference in extraversion, conscientiousness, and maladaptive cognitions across time; however, agreeableness and openness decreased at T2, neuroticism increased at T2, and Internet addiction increased at T3 (see **Table 2**).

Cross-Lagged Associations Among the Big Five Personality Traits, Maladaptive Cognitions and Internet Addiction

To verify the aforementioned hypothesis, five models (M1–M5) were built to test cross-lagged associations among the Big Five personality traits, maladaptive cognitions, and Internet addiction. First, M1 was built to examine cross-lagged associations among extraversion, maladaptive cognitions, and Internet addiction across time. The results of path analysis highlighted that M1 achieved good model fit indexes (see M1 in **Table 3**). Moreover, the results indicated that T1 extraversion could negatively predict T2 maladaptive cognitions, extraversion could negatively predict Internet addiction across time, maladaptive cognitions and Internet addiction could positively predict each other across time, and all the autoregressive effects of extraversion, maladaptive cognitions, and Internet addiction were significant (see M1 in **Table 3** and **Figure 1**). The bootstrapping results suggested that T1 extraversion could affect T3 Internet addiction through the mediating roles of T2 maladaptive cognitions (95%: −0.031 to −0.002) (see **Table 4**).

Second, M2 was developed to study cross-lagged associations among agreeableness, maladaptive cognitions, and Internet addiction across time. The results of path analysis indicated that M2 achieved good model fit indexes (see M2 in **Table 3**). Moreover, the results highlighted that T2 agreeableness could negatively predict T3 maladaptive cognitions, and agreeableness and Internet addiction could negatively predict each other across time. Additionally, maladaptive cognitions and Internet addiction could positively predict each other across time, and T2 maladaptive cognitions could negatively predict T3 agreeableness. All the autoregressive effects of agreeableness, maladaptive cognitions, and Internet addiction were significant (see M2 in **Table 3** and **Figure 1**). The bootstrapping results have suggested that T1 Internet addiction could affect T3 agreeableness through the mediating roles of T2 maladaptive cognitions (95%: −0.051 to −0.002) (see **Table 5**).

Third, M3 was built to assess cross-lagged associations among conscientiousness, maladaptive cognitions, and Internet addiction across time. The results of path analysis indicated that M3 achieved good model fit indexes (see M3 in **Table 3**). Moreover, the results indicated that T1 conscientiousness could negatively predict T2 maladaptive cognitions, and conscientiousness could negatively predict Internet addiction across time. Maladaptive cognitions and Internet addiction could positively predict each other across time, and T2 maladaptive cognitions could negatively predict T3 conscientiousness. Furthermore, T1 Internet addiction could negatively predict T2 conscientiousness, and all the autoregressive effects of conscientiousness, maladaptive cognitions, and Internet addiction were significant (see M3 in **Table 3** and **Figure 1**). The bootstrapping results revealed that T1 conscientiousness could affect T3 Internet addiction through the mediating roles of T2 maladaptive cognitions (95%: -0.035 to -0.002), and T1 Internet addiction could affect T3 conscientiousness through the mediating roles of T2 maladaptive cognitions (95%: −0.055 to −0.01) (see **Table 6**).

Fourth, M4 was developed to evaluate the cross-lagged associations among neuroticism, maladaptive cognitions, and Internet addiction across time. The results of path analysis revealed that M4 achieved good model fit indexes (see M4 in **Table 3**). Furthermore, the results demonstrated that neuroticism could positively predict Internet addiction across time, maladaptive cognitions and Internet addiction could positively predict each other across time, T2 Internet addiction could positively predict T3 neuroticism, and all the autoregressive effects of neuroticism, maladaptive cognitions, and Internet addiction were significant (see M4 in **Table 3** and **Figure 1**) (see **Table 7**).

Fifth, M5 was built to examine cross-lagged associations among openness, maladaptive cognitions, and Internet addiction across time. The results of path analysis highlighted that M5 achieved good model fit indexes (see M5 in **Table 3**). Furthermore, the results revealed that T2 openness could negatively predict T3 Internet addiction, T2 maladaptive cognitions could negatively predict T3 openness, maladaptive

TABLE 1 | The associations among the Big Five personality traits, maladaptive cognitions, and Internet addiction across time.

Variables	1	2	3	4	5	6	7	8	9	10	11	12	13	14	15	16	17	18	19	20	21
1. T1 extraversion	1																				
2. T1 agreeableness	0.36**	1																			
3. T1 conscientiousness	0.50**	0.52**	1																		
4. T1 neuroticism	−0.47	−0.51**	−0.44**	1																	
5. T1 openness	0.53**	0.49**	0.52**	−0.38	1																
6. T1 MC	−0.21**	−0.39**	−0.36**	0.32**	−0.20**	1															
7. T1 Internet addiction	−0.29**	−0.38**	−0.46**	0.36**	−0.28**	0.67**	1														
8. T2 extraversion	0.68**	0.35**	0.39**	−0.43**	0.39**	−0.25**	−0.30**	1													
9. T2 agreeableness	0.28**	0.61**	0.37**	−0.38**	0.29**	−0.37**	−0.41**	0.51**	1												
10. T2 conscientiousness	0.38**	0.42**	0.65**	−0.39**	0.37**	−0.33**	−0.42**	0.59**	0.58**	1											
11. T2 neuroticism	−0.37**	−0.36**	−0.34**	0.59**	−0.27**	0.30**	0.33**	−0.57**	−0.55**	−0.59**	1										
12. T2 openness	0.38**	0.38**	0.35**	−0.30**	0.53**	−0.20**	−0.26**	0.58**	0.55**	0.55**	−0.34**	1									
13. T2 MC	−0.25**	−0.30**	−0.35**	0.29**	−0.20**	0.59**	0.53**	−0.31**	−0.38**	−0.38**	0.41**	−0.21**	1								
14. T2 Internet addiction	−0.29**	−0.36**	−0.42**	0.36**	−0.25**	0.54**	0.63**	−0.37**	−0.43**	−0.47**	0.44**	−0.30**	0.70**	1							
15. T3 extraversion	0.64**	0.29**	0.38**	−0.36**	0.39**	−0.23**	−0.28**	0.66**	0.36**	0.46**	−0.47**	0.43**	−0.26**	−0.28**	1						
16. T3 agreeableness	0.28**	0.55**	0.38**	−0.33**	0.32**	−0.37**	−0.43**	0.40**	0.65**	0.49**	−0.46**	0.42**	−0.40**	−0.43**	0.55**	1					
17. T3 conscientiousness	0.37**	0.41**	0.58**	−0.33**	0.37**	−0.33**	−0.42**	0.50**	0.48**	0.72**	−0.51**	0.42**	−0.43**	−0.45**	0.63**	0.66**	1				
18. T3 neuroticism	−0.35**	−0.34**	−0.34**	0.57**	−0.25**	0.29**	0.36**	−0.49**	−0.44**	−0.49**	0.65**	−0.36**	0.36**	0.40**	−0.60**	−0.57**	−0.61**	1			
19. T3 openness	0.41**	0.38**	0.41**	−0.28**	0.54**	−0.24**	−0.31**	0.44**	0.41**	0.45**	−0.40**	0.53**	−0.30**	−0.29**	0.63**	0.64**	0.62**	−0.43**	1		
20. T3 MC	−0.19**	−0.25**	−0.28**	0.23**	−0.20**	0.50**	0.49**	−0.28**	−0.39**	−0.32**	0.33**	−0.23**	0.57**	0.53**	−0.30**	−0.47**	−0.45**	0.41**	−0.28**	1	
21. T3 Internet addiction	−0.25**	−0.35**	−0.36**	0.30**	−0.26**	0.46**	0.54**	−0.35**	−0.48**	−0.41**	0.38**	−0.36**	0.54**	0.64**	−0.31**	−0.52**	−0.50**	0.47**	−0.34**	0.73**	1

***p < 0.01. MC, maladaptive cognitions.*

TABLE 2 | Pairwise comparisons of the Big Five personality traits, maladaptive cognitions, and Internet addiction across time.

Variables	T1 ($M \pm SD$)	T2 ($M \pm SD$)	T3 ($M \pm SD$)	F (1, 480)	P
Extraversion	26.01 ± 4.41	26.05 ± 4.25	26.20 ± 4.58	1.09	0.30
Agreeableness	34.45 ± 4.86	33.72 ± 5.14	34.17 ± 4.64	1.75	0.19
Conscientiousness	29.91 ± 5.03	29.76 ± 5.07	30.08 ± 5.33	0.57	0.45
Neuroticism	21.55 ± 4.80	21.99 ± 4.60	21.89 ± 4.84	2.75	0.10
Openness	34.76 ± 4.98	34.19 ± 5.20	34.33 ± 5.47	3.57	0.06
Maladaptive cognitions	33.70 ± 10.15	34.00 ± 11.12	34.69 ± 11.89	3.81	0.05
Internet addiction	37.70 ± 10.80	38.00 ± 11.87	38.90 ± 13.34	4.95	0.03

TABLE 3 | Fit statistics for the model comparison of cross-lagged associations among the Big Five personality traits, maladaptive cognitions, and Internet addiction.

Models	χ^2	df	P	TLI	CFI	RMSEA
M1	98.32	9	<0.001	0.84	0.96	0.14
M2	65.81	9	<0.001	0.90	0.97	0.12
M3	52.07	9	<0.001	0.92	0.98	0.10
M4	83.57	9	<0.001	0.86	0.96	0.13
M5	96.33	9	<0.001	0.82	0.95	0.14

The larger number of the published studies with this method had suggested that the model fit indices of the present study was acceptable (e.g., Hu and Bentler, 1999).

cognitions and Internet addiction could positively predict each other across time, and all the autoregressive effects of openness, maladaptive cognitions, and Internet addiction were significant (see M5 in **Table 3** and **Figure 1**). The bootstrapping results have suggested that T1 Internet addiction could affect T3 openness through the mediating roles of T2 maladaptive cognitions (95%: −0.08 to −0.015) (see **Table 8**).

DISCUSSION

The present study is the first to test bidirectional associations among the Big Five personality traits, maladaptive cognitions, and Internet addiction during the COVID-19 pandemic period by using a longitudinal design. The results suggested that the associations among the Big Five personality traits, maladaptive cognitions, and Internet addiction were dynamic and bidirectional. Moreover, the results indicated that maladaptive cognitions played important mediating roles in the associations among extraversion, agreeableness, conscientiousness, openness, and Internet addiction across time. These results not only verified the conclusions of previous studies through a cross-section design but also tested the mediating roles of maladaptive cognitions in the associations between the Big Five personality traits and Internet addiction. These associations and their influential mechanism were further clarified as follows.

First, the present study demonstrated that extraversion affected individuals' Internet addiction unidirectionally. More specially, extraversion affected not only individuals' Internet addiction directly but also their Internet addiction through maladaptive cognitions indirectly, which supported the study's cognitive–behavioral model. Extraversion has been defined as the intensity and volume of people's social interaction, and it indicates whether people can act with competition and self-confidence (McCrae and Costa, 1997). According to the aforementioned definition of extraversion, individuals with increased social interaction and higher level of competition or self-confidence exhibit a lower level of Internet addiction, which is consistent with previous findings (Baturay and Toker, 2019). Additionally, previous studies have reported that individuals with social problems, which was negatively related with extraversion, demonstrated more maladaptive cognitions with regard to Internet use (Davis, 2001; Tian et al., 2015; Gao et al., 2019). Moreover, the present study found extraversion to negatively predict Internet addiction through maladaptive cognitions, which further verified and expanded the results of previous studies. However, some previous studies have identified no or a positive association between extraversion and Internet addiction (Rahmani and Lavasani, 2011; Andreassen et al., 2013). These inconsistent results can be attributed to the employment of different samples or instruments; for example, one study found that the Chinese population tends to develop a higher level of Internet addiction than people in Western countries (Hu et al., 2012). Therefore, the present study's results should be verified with different samples and instruments by future studies.

Second, agreeableness, maladaptive cognitions, and Internet addiction achieved significant bidirectional associations, which are consistent with the results of previous studies to some degree (Kayiş et al., 2016; Zhou et al., 2017; Hou et al., 2018; Kircaburun and Griffiths, 2018). McCrae and Costa (1997) suggested that agreeable people with characteristics of being highly forgiving and tolerant dislike using force and avoid putting pressure. Previous studies have argued that scores of individuals with Internet addiction are inclined toward using the Internet to avoid negative emotions or relieve stress. Moreover, agreeableness was negatively associated with negative emotions and stress (Suzuki and Matsuda, 2012; Greenidge and Coyne, 2014), which made agreeableness a protective predictor of maladaptive cognitions and Internet addiction.

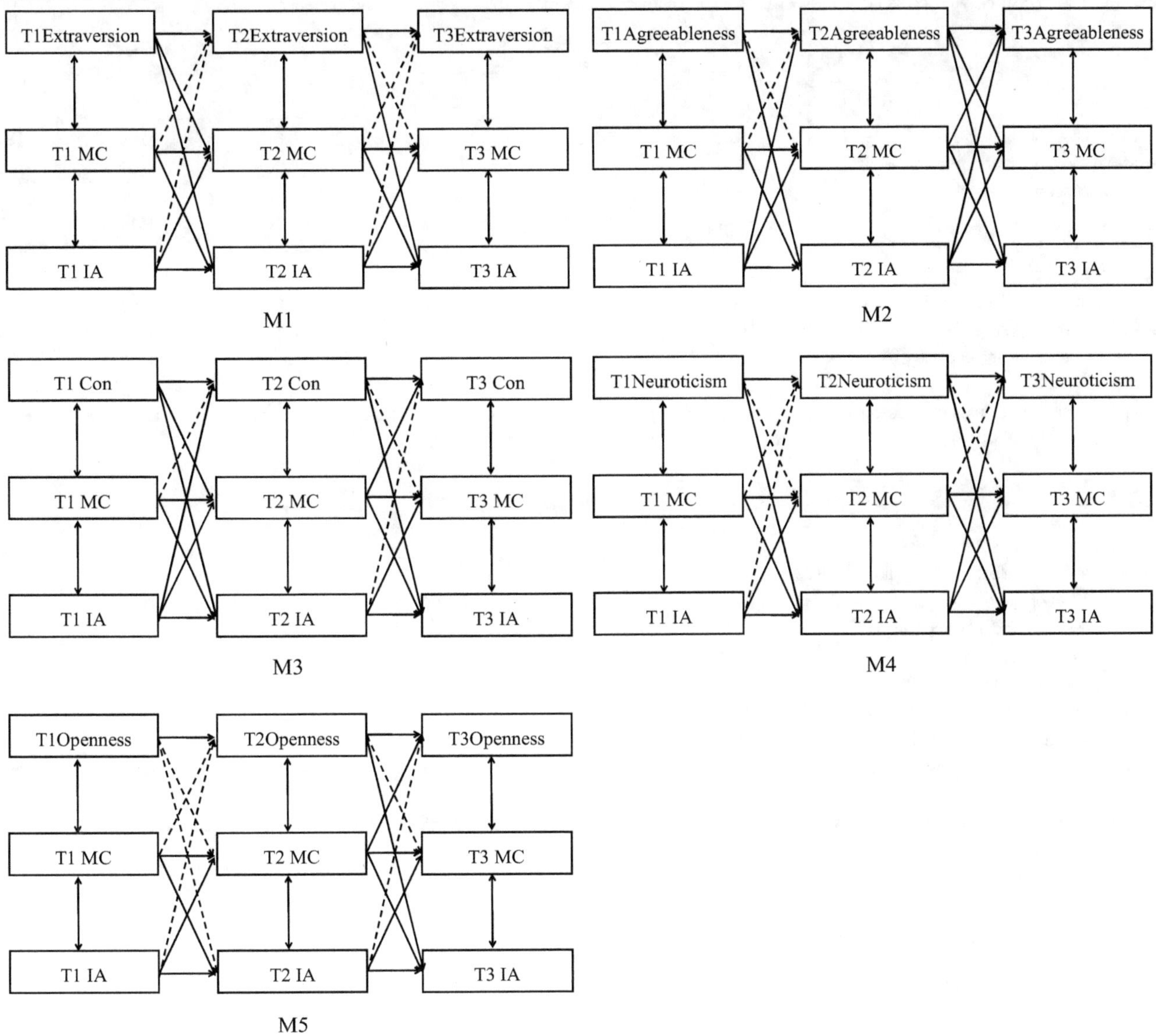

FIGURE 1 | Cross-lagged associations among the Big Five personality traits, maladaptive cognitions, and Internet addiction. Thick lines represent significant paths, and dashed lines represent non-significant paths.

TABLE 4 | Regression coefficients of cross-lagged associations among extraversion, maladaptive cognitions, and Internet addiction within M1.

Items	T1 → T2			T2 → T3		
Paths	**β**	***SE***	***P***	**β**	***SE***	***P***
Autoregressive effect of extraversion	0.65	0.03	<0.001	0.64	0.04	<0.001
Autoregressive effect of maladaptive cognitions	0.42	0.05	<0.001	0.38	0.06	<0.001
Autoregressive effect of Internet addiction	0.45	0.05	<0.001	0.47	0.06	<0.001
Extraversion → maladaptive cognitions	−0.10	0.09	0.008	−0.07	0.11	>0.05
Extraversion → Internet addiction	−0.12	0.10	<0.001	−0.12	0.12	<0.001
Maladaptive cognitions → Internet addiction	0.21	0.06	<0.001	0.17	0.06	<0.001
Internet addiction → maladaptive cognitions	0.23	0.05	<0.001	0.24	0.05	<0.001
Internet addiction → extraversion	−0.06	0.02	>0.05	0.01	0.02	>0.05
Maladaptive cognitions → extraversion	−0.07	0.02	>0.05	−0.07	0.02	>0.05

TABLE 5 | Regression coefficients of cross-lagged associations among agreeableness, maladaptive cognitions, and Internet addiction within M2.

Items	T1 → T2			T2 → T3		
Paths	**β**	***SE***	***P***	**β**	***SE***	***P***
Autoregressive effect of agreeableness	0.53	0.05	<0.001	0.57	0.04	<0.001
Autoregressive effect of maladaptive cognitions	0.41	0.06	<0.001	0.36	0.07	<0.001
Autoregressive effect of Internet addiction	0.46	0.07	<0.001	0.43	0.07	<0.001
Agreeableness → maladaptive cognitions	−0.05	0.12	>0.05	−0.16	0.11	0.001
Agreeableness → Internet addiction	−0.11	0.12	0.020	−0.24	0.12	<0.001
Maladaptive cognitions → Internet addiction	0.19	0.06	<0.001	0.15	0.07	0.017
Internet addiction → maladaptive cognitions	0.24	0.07	<0.001	0.21	0.06	0.001
Internet addiction → agreeableness	−0.18	0.02	<0.001	−0.11	0.02	0.037
Maladaptive cognitions → agreeableness	−0.04	0.03	>0.05	−0.11	0.02	0.028

TABLE 6 | Regression coefficients of cross-lagged associations among conscientiousness, maladaptive cognitions, and Internet addiction within M3.

Items	T1 → T2			T2 → T3		
Paths	**β**	***SE***	***P***	**B**	***SE***	***P***
Autoregressive effect of conscientiousness	0.57	0.05	<0.001	0.64	0.04	<0.001
Autoregressive effect of maladaptive cognitions	0.41	0.06	<0.001	0.38	0.07	<0.001
Autoregressive effect of Internet addiction	0.42	0.07	<0.001	0.46	0.07	<0.001
Conscientiousness → maladaptive cognitions	−0.11	0.09	0.006	−0.06	0.11	>0.05
Conscientiousness → Internet addiction	−0.16	0.08	<0.001	−0.13	0.11	0.002
Maladaptive cognitions → Internet addiction	0.20	0.06	<0.001	0.17	0.08	0.008
Internet addiction → maladaptive cognitions	0.21	0.07	0.001	0.23	0.06	<0.001
Internet addiction → conscientiousness	−0.14	0.02	0.003	−0.04	0.02	>0.05
Maladaptive cognitions → conscientiousness	−0.03	0.02	>0.05	−0.16	0.02	0.001

TABLE 7 | Regression coefficients of cross-lagged associations among neuroticism, maladaptive cognitions, and Internet addiction within M4.

Items	T1 → T2			T2 → T3		
Paths	**β**	***SE***	***P***	**B**	***SE***	***P***
Autoregressive effect of neuroticism	0.54	0.05	<0.001	0.58	0.05	<0.001
Autoregressive effect of maladaptive cognitions	0.41	0.06	<0.001	0.37	0.07	<0.001
Autoregressive effect of Internet addiction	0.45	0.08	<0.001	0.48	0.07	<0.001
Neuroticism → maladaptive cognitions	0.08	0.11	>0.05	0.07	0.13	>0.05
Neuroticism → Internet addiction	0.13	0.11	0.002	0.11	0.13	0.014
Maladaptive cognitions → Internet addiction	0.20	0.06	<0.001	0.16	0.08	0.012
Internet addiction → maladaptive cognitions	0.23	0.07	<0.001	0.24	0.06	<0.001
Internet addiction → neuroticism	0.10	0.02	>0.05	0.11	0.02	0.019
Maladaptive cognitions → neuroticism	0.07	0.02	>0.05	0.04	0.02	>0.05

However, spending too much time or money on the Internet increases the levels of social pressure, academic pressure, and economic pressure (while agreeableness prevented individuals from putting pressure); therefore, maladaptive cognitions and Internet addiction negatively predicted agreeableness. These results expanded the cognitive–behavioral model, which indicated only unidirectional associations among personality, maladaptive cognitions, and Internet addiction, whereas bidirectional associations among them were not found. Moreover, the present study's results suggested that Internet addiction could affect individuals' agreeableness through maladaptive cognitions, indicating that maladaptive cognitions were also critical factors in the effect of Internet addiction on individuals' personality.

Third, conscientiousness, maladaptive cognitions, and Internet addiction also achieved significant bidirectional associations, which are in alignment with the findings of previous studies to some extent (Kayiş et al., 2016; Zhou et al., 2017; Hou et al., 2018; Kircaburun and Griffiths, 2018). Conscientiousness people have the characteristics of being cautious, disciplined, planned, decisive, organized, rule and principle abiding, and hardworking (McCrae and Costa, 1997). Therefore, individuals with a higher level of conscientiousness can hardly spend a large amount of time on

TABLE 8 | Regression coefficients of cross-lagged associations among openness, maladaptive cognitions, and Internet addiction within M5.

Items	T1 → T2			T2 → T3		
Paths	**β**	***SE***	***P***	**β**	***SE***	***P***
Autoregressive effect of openness	0.50	0.04	<0.001	0.49	0.05	<0.001
Autoregressive effect of maladaptive cognitions	0.42	0.06	<0.001	0.39	0.07	<0.001
Autoregressive effect of Internet addiction	0.46	0.07	<0.001	0.45	0.07	<0.001
Openness → maladaptive cognitions	−0.04	0.09	>0.05	−0.09	0.11	>0.05
Openness → Internet addiction	−0.07	0.10	>0.05	−0.18	0.11	<0.001
Maladaptive cognitions → Internet addiction	0.21	0.06	<0.001	0.18	0.07	0.003
Internet addiction → maladaptive cognitions	0.24	0.07	<0.001	0.23	0.07	<0.001
Internet addiction → openness	−0.10	0.03	>0.05	−0.00	0.03	>0.05
Maladaptive cognitions → openness	−0.04	0.03	>0.05	−0.20	0.03	0.001

the Internet because of their traits. However, conscientiousness, maladaptive cognitions, and Internet addiction found execution through vicious circles wherein individuals with higher levels of maladaptive cognitions or Internet addiction were affected by a lower level of conscientiousness, which was an important finding. Moreover, the results suggested that maladaptive cognitions played bidirectional mediating roles in the association between conscientiousness and Internet addiction, indicating that the bidirectional association between conscientiousness and Internet addiction shared the same influential mechanism. These results further expanded the cognitive–behavioral model by demonstrating how maladaptive cognitions are bidirectional mediating factors in the association between personality traits and Internet addiction.

Fourth, neuroticism and Internet addiction also achieved significant bidirectional associations, and no significant associations were found between neuroticism and maladaptive cognitions. Neuroticism has been defined as the loss of emotional balance that is positively associated with negative emotions (such as loneliness and depression; Bunevicius et al., 2008; Buecker et al., 2020). Previous studies have proposed that individuals with negative emotions are more likely to develop Internet addiction than their peers. This is because these individuals tend to use the Internet for relieving negative emotions, obtaining social support, and escaping pressure (Yao and Zhong, 2014; Tian et al., 2017). However, no mediating roles of maladaptive cognitions were found in the association between neuroticism and Internet addiction, indicating that the association between neuroticism and Internet addiction shared different influential mechanisms with other cross-lagged associations in the present study. Different mediating factors may have exerted different effects on the association between the Big Five personality traits and Internet addiction. For example, Zhou et al. (2017) proposed that emotion-focused coping played a greater mediating role in the association between neuroticism and Internet addiction than in the association between other personality traits and Internet addiction. Although the Big Five personality traits were positively related to each other, they exhibited different influential mechanisms on Internet addiction.

Fifth, openness was found to negatively affect individuals' Internet addiction unidirectionally, which is consistent with the findings of previous studies (Kayiş et al., 2016; Zhou et al., 2017; Hou et al., 2018; Kircaburun and Griffiths, 2018). However, some other studies have identified positive or no association between openness and Internet addiction (Rahmani and Lavasani, 2011; Servidio, 2014). For example, Servidio (2014) suggested that individuals with a higher level of openness demonstrate a higher level of novelty seeking and spend more time on the Internet to seek novel information. By contrast, Kayiş et al. (2016) insisted that both virtual and real activities provide individuals with attractive opportunities to satisfy their curiosity and interest, and that open individuals prefer real-life activities as opposed to virtual ones. Although the results of the current study are consistent with Kayiş' study, we would like to explain dissimilarities in their results from a new perspective. First, openness was negatively associated with the positive predictors (such as loneliness, depression, and social anxiety) (Bunevicius et al., 2008; Lee et al., 2014; Buecker et al., 2020) of Internet addiction, thereby indicating that openness had a positive effect on the prevention of Internet addiction in individuals. Second, in addition to being novelty seeking or curious, open individuals are independent, which means that these individuals depend less on external things such as the Internet; therefore, openness was a negative rather than a positive predictor of Internet addiction. Similar with agreeableness, the results of the present study also highlighted that Internet addiction could affect openness through maladaptive cognitions, which further contributed to the cognitive–behavioral model. Spending too much time on the Internet reduces an individual's level of openness, whereas maladaptive cognitions constituted the key driver of this influence.

The present study has several limitations. First, all the studied variables were measured using self-reported questionnaires. Self-reported questionnaires are often associated with measurement errors caused by social desirability and memory recall. Second, the observed variables were used in the study, making it challenging to examine the measurement equivalence of each variable across time. Although the same measurement tools were used to measure the same variables across time, the predictive power of each item and measurement error may have been different across time. Not testing the measurement equivalence of each variable likely introduced more measurement errors in the subsequent data analysis. Third, cross-lagged associations among the Big Five personality traits, maladaptive cognitions, and Internet addiction were examined, which may have introduced the possibility of multicolinearity. Previous studies have examined the association between the Big Five personality traits and Internet addiction by using one model (Zhou et al., 2017; Kircaburun and Griffiths, 2018), whereas the present study examined cross-lagged associations between the studied variables in one model to avoid award excessive complexity to the model. Fourth, because the data were collected after the start of the pandemic, no baseline comparison could be made to support the premise that the present findings constitute unique contributions in this context. Therefore, future studies can compare baseline levels of Big Five personality traits, maladaptive cognitions, and Internet addiction with their corresponding levels during the COVID-19 pandemic. Finally, the present study tested only the bidirectional mediating roles of maladaptive cognitions in the associations between the Big Five personality traits and Internet addiction. Some other studies have found coping style (Zhou et al., 2017), self-liking (Kircaburun and Griffiths, 2018), and family function (Hou et al., 2018) to mediate the association between the Big Five personality traits and Internet addiction; therefore, more mediating factors should be verified through longitudinal studies.

Although this study has several limitations, it makes some critical contributions to relevant research. First, the results of the present study provided important longitudinal evidence to support arguments concerning the association between the Big Five personality traits (especially extraversion and openness) and Internet addiction. The inconsistent conclusions may have been caused by the employment of different samples, different measurement tools, or different data analysis methods. However, both the longitudinal study and meta-analysis provided consistent conclusions that made a difference and suggest that both extraversion and openness were protective factors of Internet addiction. Second, the present study is the first to test the effect of Internet addiction on the Big Five personality traits, suggesting that the association between individuals' personality traits and Internet addiction was executed in vicious circles wherein Internet addiction was also the predictor of the Big Five personality traits. Third, maladaptive cognitions tended to play bidirectional mediating roles in the association between individuals' personality traits (such as conscientiousness) and Internet addiction, further expanding the cognitive–behavioral model. In particular, individuals with personality problems developed Internet addiction through maladaptive cognitions, whereas individuals with Internet addiction developed personality problems by developing maladaptive cognitions. Additionally, to test the longitudinal association among the Big Five personality traits, maladaptive cognitions, and Internet addiction during the COVID-19 pandemic was helpful for the family and school's intervention of Internet addiction during the COVID-19 pandemic. For example, maladaptive cognitions were the key factors in the associations between Big Five personality traits and Internet addiction, which suggested that the family and school could decrease individuals' Internet addiction with different personality traits by decreasing their maladaptive cognitions about the Internet.

AUTHOR CONTRIBUTIONS

YT and YZ wrote the manuscript and data analysis. FL and NQ conducted the data analysis and interpretation of data for the manuscript. PC polished the manuscript and checked the manuscript. All authors contributed to the article and approved the submitted version.

ACKNOWLEDGMENTS

We thank for the insightful and constructive reviews which were provided by the reviewers; we thank for the editor and Frontiers in Psychology to provide us the opportunity to revise our manuscript and publish our manuscript.

REFERENCES

1. Agbaria, Q., and Bdier, D. (2020). The association of big five personality traits and religiosity on internet addiction among israeli-palestinian muslim college students in israel. *Mental Health Relig. Cult.* 22, 1–16. doi: 10.1080/13674676. 2019.1699041
2. Andreassen, C., Griffifiths, M., Gjertsen, S., Krossbakken, E., Kvam, S., and Pallesen, S. (2013). The relationships between behavioral addictions and the five-factor model of personality. *J. Behav. Addict.* 2, 90–99. doi: 10.1556/JBA.2.2013.003
3. Arpaci, I., and Unver, T. K. (2020). Moderating role of gender in the relationship between big five personality traits and smartphone addiction. *Psych. Q.* 91, 577–585. doi: 10.1007/s11126-020-09718-5
4. Asendorpf, J. B., and Aken, M. A. G. V. (2010). Validity of big five personality judgments in childhood: a 9 year longitudinal study. *Eur. J. Personal.* 17, 1–17. doi: 10.1002/per.460
5. Bai, X., and Fan, F. M. (2005). A study on the internet dependence of college students: the revising and applying of a measurement. *Psychol. Devel. Educat.* 4, 99–104. doi: 1001-4918200504-0099-104
6. Baturay, M. H., and Toker, S. (2019). Internet addiction among college students: some causes and effects. *Educat. Inform. Technol.* 24, 1–23. doi: 10.1007/s10639- 019-09894-3
7. Bengü, Y., and Ahmet, U. (2018). The relationship between internet addiction, social anxiety, impulsivity, self-esteem, and depression in a sample of turkish undergraduate medical students. *Psych. Res.* 267, 313–318. doi: 10.1016/j. psychres.2018.06.033
8. Buecker, S., Maes, M., Denissen, J. J. A., and Luhmann, M. (2020). Loneliness and the big five personality traits: a meta-analysis. *Europ. J. Personal.* 34, 8–28. doi: 10.1002/per.2229
9. Bunevicius, A., Katkute, A., and Bunevicius, R. (2008). Symptoms of anxiety and depression in medical students and in humanities students: relationship with big-five personality dimensions and vulnerability to stress. *Int. J. Soc. Psych.* 54, 494–501. doi: 10.1177/0020764008090843
10. Carciofo, R., Yang, J., Song, N., Du, F., and Zhang, K. (2016). Psychometric evaluation of Chinese-language 44-item and 10-item big five personality inventories, including correlations with chronotype, mindfulness and mind wandering. *PLoS One* 11:e0149963. doi: 10.1371/journal.pone.0149963

11. China Internet Network Information Center [CNNIC] (2020). *Statistical report on the development of internet in China*. URL: http://www.cnnic.net.cn/hlwfzyj/ hlwxzbg/hlwtjbg/202004/t20200428_70974.htm (in Chinese)
12. Davis, R. A. (2001). A cognitive-behavioral model of pathological internet use. *Comput. Hum. Behav.* 17, 187–195. doi: 10.1016/S0747-5632(00)00041-8
13. Davis, R. A., Flett, G. L., and Besser, A. (2002). Validation of a new scale for measuring problematic internet use: implications for pre-employment screening. *CyberPsychol. Behav.* 5, 331–345. doi: 10.1089/10949310276 0275581
14. Fioravanti, G., Dèttore, D., and Casale, S. (2012). Adolescent Internet Addiction: testing the Association Between Self-Esteem, the Perception of Internet Attributes, and Preference for Online Social Interactions. *Cyberpsychology* 15, 318–323. doi: 10.1089/cyber.2011.0358
15. Gao, T., Hu, Y., Qin, Z., Cao, R., Liu, S., Mei, S., et al. (2019). The role of school connectedness and maladaptive cognitions in the association between stress and internet addiction: a serial mediation model. *Perspect. Psych. Care* 55, 728–733. doi: 10.1111/ppc.12417
16. Garcia-Priego, B. A., Triana-Romero, A., Samanta Pinto-Galvez, S. M., Duran-Ramos, C., Salas-Nolasco, O., Reyes, M. M., et al. (2020). Anxiety, depression, attitudes, and internet addiction during the initial phase of the 2019 coronavirus disease (COVID-19) epidemic: a cross-sectional study in Mexico. *Preprints medRxiv and bioRxiv* [preprint]. doi: 10.1101/2020.05.10.20095844
17. Greenidge, D., and Coyne, I. (2014). Job stressors and voluntary work behaviours: mediating effect of emotion and moderating roles of personality and emotional intelligence. *Hum. Resour. Manag. J.* 24, 479–495. doi: 10.1111/1748-8583. 12044
18. Hou, J., Fan, N., Qin, H., and Fang, X. Y. (2018). The effect of adolescents' big five personality on internet addiction:the mediating role of family function. *Psychol. Explorat.* 38, 279–288.
19. Hu, J. P., Yan, Z., Yu, C. P., and Zhang, W. (2012). A comparative study of internet addiction of adolescents in china and the united states. *J. South Chin. Norm. Univ.* 5, 54–60.
20. Hu, L. T., and Bentler, P. M. (1999). Cutoff criteria for fit indexes in covariance structural analysis: conventional criteria versus new alternatives. *Struct. Equat. Model.* 6, 1–55. doi: 10.1080/10705519909540118
21. Jiang, L. L. (2020). The Effect of Information Anxiety on Mobile Phone Addiction of College Students in the COVID-19 Epidemic Context: an Mediating Moderating Model. *J. Dalian Univ.* 41, 106–110.
22. John, O. P., Donahue, E. M. Y., and Kentle, R. L. (1991). *The Big Five Inventory-Versions 4a and 54.* Berkeley, CA: University of California.
23. Kaplan, S. C., Levinson, C. A., Rodebaugh, T. L., Menatti, A., and Weeks, J. W. (2015). Social anxiety and the big five personality traits: the interactive relationship of trust and openness. *Cogn. Behav. Ther.* 44, 212–222. doi: 10. 1080/16506073.2015.1008032
24. Kayiş, A. R., Satici, S. A., Yilmaz, M. F., Şimşek, D., Ceyhan, E., and Bakioglu, F. (2016). Big five-personality trait and internet addiction: a meta-analytic review. *Comput. Hum. Behav.* 63, 35–40. doi: 10.1016/j.chb.2016.05.012
25. Kim, D. J., Kim, K., Lee, H. W., Hong, J. P., Cho, M. J., Fava, M., et al. (2017). Internet game addiction, depression, and escape from negative emotions in adulthood. *J. Nerv. Mental Dis.* 205, 568–573. doi: 10.1097/NMD. 0000000000000698
26. Kircaburun, K., and Griffiths, M. D. (2018). Instagram addiction and the big five of personality: the mediating role of self-liking. *J. Behav. Addict.* 7, 158–170. doi: 10.1556/2006.7.2018.15
27. Ladner, J., Villet, H., Tavolacci, M. P., Grigioni, S., and Dechelotte, P. (2010). Internet addiction, mental stress, eating and sleeping disorders: new public health challenges among french university students? *Eur. J. Publ. Health* 20, 28–28.
28. Langguth, B., Kleinjung, T., Fischer, B., Hajak, G., and Sand, P. G. (2007). Tinnitus severity, depression, and the big five personality traits. *Progr. Brain Res.* 166, 221–225. doi: 10.1016/S0079-6123(07)66020-8
29. Lee, S., Tam, C. L., and Chie, Q. T. (2014). Mobile phone usage preferences: the contributing factors of personality, social anxiety and loneliness. *Soc. Indicat. Res.* 118, 1205–1228. doi: 10.1007/s11205-013-0460-2
30. Liang, X. Y. (2008). *A Study on the Effect Mechanism of Online Social Support on Adolescents' Mental Health.* Ph.D. Thesis, Huazhong: Huazhong Normal University.
31. Lu, X., and Yeo, K. J. (2015). Pathological internet use among Malaysia university students: risk factors and the role of cognitive distortion. *Comput. Hum. Behav.* 45, 235–242. doi: 10.1016/j.chb.2014.12.021
32. McCrae, R. R., and Costa, P. T. (1997). Personality trait structure as a human universal. *Am. Psych.* 5, 509–516. doi: 10.1037//0003-066X.52.5.509
33. Mo, P. K. H., Chan, V. W. Y., Wang, X., and Lau, J. T. F. (2020). Gender difference in the association between internet addiction, self-esteem and academic aspirations among adolescents: a structural equation modelling. *Comput. Educat.* 155:103921. doi: 10.1016/j.compedu.2020.103921
34. Nagaur, A. (2020). Internet Addiction and Mental Health among University students during CVOID-19 lockdown. *Mukt Shabd J.* 9, 684–692.
35. Özdin, S., and Özdin, Ş. B. (2020). Levels and predictors of anxiety, depression and health anxiety during covid-19 pandemic in turkish society: the importance of gender. *Int. J. Soc. Psych.* 2020, 1–8. doi: 10.1177/0020764020927051
36. Rahmani, S., and Lavasani, M. G. (2011). The relationship between internet dependency with sensation seeking and personality. *Proc. Soc. Behav. Sci.* 30, 272–277. doi: 10.1016/j.sbspro.2011.10.054
37. Sami, H., Dannielle, L., Lihi, D., and Elena, S. (2018). The effect of sleep disturbances and internet addiction on suicidal ideation among adolescents in the presence of depressive symptoms. *Psych. Res.* 267, 327–332. doi: 10.1016/j.psychres.2018.03.067
38. Servidio, R. (2014). Exploring the effects of demographic factors, Internet usage and personality traits on Internet addiction in a sample of Italian university students. *Comput. Hum. Behav.* 35, 85–92. doi: 10.1016/j.chb.2014.02.024
39. Soulioti, E., Stavropoulos, V., Christidi, S., Papastefanou, Y., and Roussos, P. (2018). The relationship of internet addiction with anxiety and depressive symptomatology. *Psychiatrike* 29, 160–171. doi: 10.22365/jpsych.2018.292.160
40. Stavropoulos, V., Alexandraki, K., and Motti-Stefanidi, F. (2013). Recognizing internet addiction: prevalence and relationship to academic achievement in adolescents enrolled in urban and rural greek high schools. *J. Adolesc.* 36, 565–576. doi: 10.1016/j.adolescence.2013.03.008
41. Steinbüchel, T. A., Herpertz, S., and Külpmann, I. (2017). Internet addiction, suicidality and non-suicidal self-harming behavior—a systematic review. *Psychotherapie* 68, 451–461. doi: 10.1055/s-0043-120448
42. Suzuki, C., and Matsuda, E. (2012). A study of individual differences on dream recall: influence of stressful life events and big five personality traits on dream recall frequency. *Stress Sci. Res.* 27, 71–79. doi: 10.5058/stresskagakukenkyu. 27.71
43. Tian, Y., Bian, Y., Han, P., Gao, F., and Wang, P. (2017). Associations between psychosocial factors and generalized pathological internet use in Chinese university students: a longitudinal crosslagged analysis. *Comput. Hum. Behav.* 72, 178–188. doi: 10.1016/j.chb.2017.02.048
44. Tian, Y., Bian, Y. L., Han, P. G., Wang, P., and Gao, F. Q. (2015). The effect of shyness on Internet addiction: the mediating effects of immersion tendency and network-related maladaptive cognition. *Chin. J. Spec. Educat.* 12, 83–89.
45. Wang, J. L., Jackson, L. A., Zhang, D. J., and Su, Z. Q. (2012). The relationships among the big five personality factors, self-esteem, narcissism, and sensation-seeking to chinese university students' uses of social networking sites (snss). *Comput. Hum. Behav.* 28, 2313–2319. doi: 10.1016/j.chb.2012.07.001
46. Yao, M. Z., and Zhong, Z. (2014). Loneliness, social contacts and Internet addiction: a cross-lagged panel study. *Comput. Hum. Behav.* 30, 164–170. doi: 10.1016/j. chb.2013.08.007
47. Young, K. S. (1998). Internet addiction: the emergence of a new clinical disorder. *Cyberpsychol. Behav.* 1, 237–244. doi: 10.1089/cpb.1998.1.237
48. Zhou, Y. Y., Li, D. P., Li, X., Wang, Y. H., and Zhao, L. Y. (2017). Big five personality and adolescent internet addiction: the mediating role of coping style. *Addict. Behav.* 64, 42–48. doi: 10.1016/j.addbeh.2016.08.009

20

Romantic Love vs. Drug Addiction May Inspire a New Treatment for Addiction

Zhiling Zou[1†], *Hongwen Song*[1,2†], *Yuting Zhang*[3] *and Xiaochu Zhang*[2,3,4,5*]

[1] *Faculty of Psychology, Southwest University, Chongqing, China,* [2] *Center of Medical Physics and Technology, Hefei Institutes of Physical Science, CAS, Hefei, China,* [3] *Chinese Academy of Sciences Key Laboratory of Brain Function and Disease, School of Life Sciences, University of Science and Technology of China, Hefei, China,* [4] *School of Humanities and Social Science, University of Science and Technology of China, Hefei, China,* [5] *Centers for Biomedical Engineering, University of Science and Technology of China, Hefei, China*

Correspondence:

Xiaochu Zhang,
Upon completion of his doctorate in biophysics at the University of Science and Technology of China (USTC) in 2005, he was invited to be a visiting fellow at the National Institute of Drug Abuse in USA where he continued his research about the neural basis of nicotine addiction using multiple neuroimaging tools. In 2010, he joined the faculty at USTC and was invited to be the professor and the PI of the cognitive neuropsychology lab. His current focus is the neural basis of drug and behavior (game or internet) addiction and some related cognitive processes, e.g., love and decision making etc.
zxcustc@ustc.edu.cn

[†] *These authors have contributed equally to this work and shared first authorship.*

Drug addiction is a complex neurological dysfunction induced by recurring drug intoxication. Strategies to prevent and treat drug addiction constitute a topic of research interest. Early-stage romantic love is characterized by some characteristics of addiction, which gradually disappear as the love relationship progresses. Therefore, comparison of the concordance and discordance between romantic love and drug addiction may elucidate potential treatments for addiction. This focused review uses the evidences from our recent studies to compare the neural alterations between romantic love and drug addiction, moreover we also compare the behavioral and neurochemical alterations between romantic love and drug addiction. From the behavioral comparisons we find that there are many similarities between the early stage of romantic love and drug addiction, and this stage romantic love is considered as a behavioral addiction, while significant differences exist between the later stage of romantic love and drug addiction, and this stage of romantic love eventually developed into a prosocial behavior. The neuroimaging comparisons suggest that romantic love and drug addiction both display the functional enhancement in reward and emotion regulation network. Except the similar neural changes, romantic love display special function enhancement in social cognition network, while drug addiction display special dysfunction in cognitive control network. The neurochemical comparisons show that there are many similarities in the dopamine (DA) system, while significant differences in oxytocin (OT) system for romantic love and drug addiction. These findings indicate that the functional alterations in reward and emotion regulation network and the DA system may be the neurophysiological basis of romantic love as a behavioral addiction, and the functional alterations in social cognition network and the OT system may be the neurophysiological basis of romantic love as a prosocial behavior. It seems that the OT system is a critical factor for the development of addiction. So we then discuss strategies to treat drug addiction with OT, and suggest that future research should further investigate OT system interventions aiming to improve cognitive control and/or social cognition functions, in order to develop strategies designed to more effectively treat drug addiction.

Keywords: romantic love, social cognition system, drug addiction, oxytocin, resting-state functional connectivity, drug addiction treatment

INTRODUCTION

Romantic love can be defined as "a state of intense longing for union with another" (Hatfield and Rapson, 1987). The early stage of romantic love is usually characterized by intense emotional responses such as euphoria, intensely focused attention on the preferred individual, obsessive thought about the person, emotional dependency on and craving for emotional union with the beloved person (Hatfield and Rapson, 1987; Aron et al., 2005).

> **KEY CONCEPT 1 | Romantic love**
> Romantic love is defined as "a state of intense longing for union with another" (Hatfield and Rapson, 1987, page 260).

Some researchers regard romantic love as a type of behavioral addiction (Burkett and Young, 2012; Fisher et al., 2016). People who are in the early stage of romantic love express many similar traits with addicts (Liebowitz, 1983; Hatfield and Sprecher, 1986; Meloy and Fisher, 2005; Association, 2013). They focus on their beloved (salience); they yearn for the beloved (craving); they feel a "rush" of exhilaration when seeing or thinking about their beloved (euphoria/intoxication). As their relationship builds the lover seeks to interact with the beloved more (tolerance). If the beloved breaks off the relationship, the lovers experience the common signs of drug withdrawal, such as lethargy, anxiety, insomnia, or hypersomnia, loss of appetite or binge eating, irritability, and chronic loneliness (Fisher et al., 2016).

Our recent study that used resting state functional magnetic resonance imaging (rsfMRI) to study love-related changes in resting state functional connectivity provided some new and important evidences for romantic love related functional alterations in brain network (Song et al., 2015). Combined our previous studies about romantic love (Wang et al., 2016) and addiction (Zhang et al., 2009, 2011; Lv et al., 2016; Wei et al., 2016), we found that romantic love and addiction have the significant differences in resting-state brain network. Therefore, systematic comparison between romantic love and addiction may be helpful to understand the similarities and differences of them, and may inspire a new possible treatment to addiction.

In general, romantic love usually undergoes two phases. The first phase of romantic love is falling in love which has more a character of excitation and stress (Marazziti and Canale, 2004; Aron et al., 2005). After a few months (about 6 months) the relationship develops into second phase which has a character of calm, safety and balance (Stárka, 2007).

For the development of addiction, researchers suggest that the neuroplasticity of addiction consists of two phases, too. During initiation drug use is completely deliberate and voluntary (regulated relapse), and the transient changes in neural functioning continued for hours up to weeks during abstinence (Kalivas and O'Brien, 2008). While during the second phase, drug use is compulsive, and the changes in neuroplasticity become "stable" which last for weeks up to permanency, and turn to be fundamental for the maintenance of the addiction, and are responsible for relapse after a period of abstinence (Kalivas and O'Brien, 2008).

From the perspective of the development stage of romantic love, the early stage of romantic love shows more addictive characteristics. Therefore, the early stage of romantic love is often regarded as a type of behavioral addiction. Although romantic love and **drug addiction** are similar in the early stages, they are different in subsequent stages, as the addictive characteristics of love gradually disappear as the romantic relationships progresses. However, the addictive characteristics are gradually magnified with repeated use of drugs of abuse. Finally, romantic love and drug addiction develop into different behaviors and have different effects on human development.

> **KEY CONCEPT 2 | Drug addiction**
> Drug addiction is a state of compulsive drug use; despite treatment and other attempts to control drug use, addiction is likely to persist.

As romantic love displays some addictive behaviors, and there are many concordances and discordances in development progression of romantic love and drug addiction. Therefore, in this article our hypothesis are that: romantic love and drug addiction may have many concordances and discordances in brain cortical functioning and neuroendocrine factors; and (1) these concordances may be the neurophysiological basis of romantic love as a behavioral addiction, and (2) these discordances may be the neurophysiological basis of romantic love as a prosocial behavior; and (3) these discordances may be the critical factors for the development of drug addiction and further study about these critical factors may help to find a new treatment for drug addiction. In order to verify our hypothesis, we compare romantic love and drug addiction from three relevant aspects: behavioral characteristics, brain functioning and neuroendocrine factors.

The comparisons between romantic love and drug addiction indicate that romantic love and drug addiction both display the functional enhancement in reward and emotion regulation network. Except the similar neural changes, romantic love display special function enhancement in social cognition network, while drug addiction display special dysfunction in cognitive control network. The comparisons of neurochemical alterations show that there are many similarities in DA system, while significant differences in OT system for romantic love and drug addiction. These indicate that the functional alterations in reward and emotion regulation network and the DA system may be the neurophysiological basis of romantic love as a behavioral addiction, and the functional alterations in social cognition network and the OT system may be the neurophysiological basis of romantic love as a prosocial behavior. It seems that the OT system is a critical factor for the development of addiction. Further, study the OT system may help to find a new treatment for drug addiction.

COMPARISONS OF ROMANTIC LOVE AND DRUG ADDICTION: THE BEHAVIORAL CHARACTERISTICS

Fisher (1998) proposed that mammals typically exhibit three primary categories of mating- and reproduction-related emotions: lust, attraction, and attachment. Lust is characterized by cravings for sexual gratification, and it motivates individuals to seek sexual union with specific individuals. Attraction is characterized by increased energy and focused attention in mammals, thereby facilitating mate choice and enabling individuals to focus on a partner. Attachment is characterized by maintenance of close social contact in mammals, and is described as feelings of calm, comfort, and emotional union between human partners. Lust and attraction are the primary emotional categories that correspond to the core characteristic "longing for union" during early romantic love. This core characteristic is very similar to addictive symptoms, including the induction of intense drug-seeking behavior by either the drug itself or drug-related cues. Additionally, the negative emotions induced by love disruption are also similar to the acute withdrawal symptoms following drug discontinuation. From the perspective of considering love to be an attachment process, romantic love and drug addiction may have additional similarities. Furthermore, DSM-5 criteria describe some more detailed comparisons between drug addiction and romantic love (see **Table 1**).

While romantic love is rarely considered a pathological disorder (Burkett and Young, 2012), early phase romantic love ("falling in love") is characterized by euphoria, intensely focused attention on the preferred individual, obsessive thinking about the person, increased energy, as well as emotional dependency on and craving for emotional union with the beloved (Aron et al., 2005).The early phase of romantic love lasts ~6 months (Marazziti and Canale, 2004). After a few months, the stress-liking features, such as obsessive thinking, emotional dependency, and craving, subside and are replaced by feelings of calm, safety, and balance (Stárka, 2007). Additionally, for the long-term relationship, the feelings of closeness and the decision making about the commitment to a relationship play relatively large parts (Sternberg, 1986).

However, for people with drug addiction, behaviors progress from initial self-administration to impulsive drug use, and finally develop into compulsive drug use. With repeated drug use, the stress-liking features, and the detrimental effects become progressively more serious. Moreover, for the repeated drug abuse, the obsessive drug-seeking and craving for abused drug play the key roles (Volkow et al., 2006).

Generally, in the early stage of romantic love, lovers display some addictive characteristics, primarily the stress-liking features. However, the stress-liking features changes differently over time in people with drug addiction, becoming progressively worse with repeated drug use. Understanding these differences may contribute to discovering treatments for preventing and curing addiction.

COMPARISON OF ROMANTIC LOVE AND DRUG ADDICTION: BRAIN FUNCTIONING

Comparison of neuroimaging studies regarding romantic love and drug addiction must consider two primary outcomes: (a) the response to direct effects of the partner or drug-related cues, and (b) spontaneous neural activity without effects induced by known external stimulation. Responses to directly related cues reflect state neural activity and spontaneous neural activity primarily reflects trait neural activity (Fox and Raichle, 2007).

Exposure to Partner or Drug-Related Cues

When viewing pictures of their partner, lovers show significant activation in some brain regions which include the ventral tegmental area (VTA), nucleus accumbens (NAC), caudate, insula, dorsal anterior cingulate cortex (dACC), dorsolateral prefrontal cortex (dlPFC), hippocampus, posterior cingulate cortex (PCC), precuneus, temporo-parietal junction (TPJ), and hypothalamus (Bartels and Zeki, 2000; Aron et al., 2005; Ortigue et al., 2007; Xu et al., 2011; Acevedo et al., 2012). In our recent study, we found that the NAC and medial prefrontal cortex (mPFC) show activation while lovers were exposed to their partner related cue (Wang et al., 2016).

For addicts, while exposed to drug cues, they show significant activation in many brain regions which include the VTA, NAC, caudate, insula, dACC, dlPFC, mPFC, ventral anterior cingulate cortex (vACC), medial orbitofrontal cortex (mOFC), inferior frontal gyrus (IFG), and amygdale (Volkow et al., 2003; Baler and Volkow, 2006). Moreover, our earlier study found that when exposed to smoke-related cue the dlPFC, mPFC, vACC, occipital cortex, insula, right amygdala and dACC showed significant activity in smokers (Zhang et al., 2009, 2011). More recently, we reviewed the addiction-related cue-induced neural changes, addicts showed that right orbitofrontal cortex (OFC), right NAC, bilateral anterior cingulated (ACC), mPFC, right dlPFC, right caudate nucleus, left parahippocampus ware activated by addiction-related cues (Zhang et al., 2016).

It is obvious that the brain regions of romantic love overlap with drug addiction include VTA, NAC, caudate, insula, dACC, mPFC, and dlPFC (see **Figure 1**). Other than the overlapping regions, there are additional brain regions that are activated only during romantic love or drug addiction (see **Figure 1**). Specifically, activated brain regions for romantic love include the hippocampus, PCC, precuneus, TPJ, and hypothalamus. Regions uniquely activated in drug addicts include the mPFC, vACC, mOFC, IFG, and amygdala.

The VTA, NAC, and caudate comprise the mesolimbic system, and are primarily associated with pleasure, general arousal, focused attention and motivation to pursue and acquire rewards and mediated primarily by dopamine system activity (Delgado et al., 2000; Schultz, 2000; Elliott et al., 2003). These regions of the reward system are directly associated with addiction in many studies of addiction (Breiter et al., 1997; Panksepp et al., 2002; Melis et al., 2005; Volkow et al., 2007; Frascella et al., 2010) and romantic love (Bartels and Zeki, 2000; Aron et al., 2005; Ortigue et al., 2007; Xu et al., 2011; Acevedo et al., 2012).

The dACC contributes to monitoring conflict via information processing, and facilitates compensatory adjustments to cognitive control (Botvinick et al., 2004). The PCC contributes to social cognition, and social trustworthiness (Maddock, 1999; Winston et al., 2002). During romantic love, increased activation in the dACC is associated with suppressed obsessive thinking (Aron et al., 2005), and altered activation in the PCC indicates that social cognition and social trustworthiness significantly increase with increased duration of the love relationship. For example,

TABLE 1 | DSM-5 criteria and other characteristics of substance use disorders as compared to love.

Substance use disorders criteria and other symptoms	Similarities in love	Differences in love
IMPAIRED CONTROL		
Substance is taken in larger amounts or over a longer period than originally intended	Sensation of "time flying" when with the partner	
Persistent desire or repeated to cut down or regulate substance use and unsuccessful attempt to decrease or discontinue use	Sensation of not being able to stay away from the partner; failed attempt (s) to break up	
Spending a great deal of time to obtain, use, recover	Dating	
The craving for drug easily induced by drug and drug-associated cues	The longing for reciprocity easily induced by partner and partner-associated stimuli	
SOCIAL IMPAIRMENT		
Result in a failure to fulfill major role obligations at work, school, or home		The romantic relationship may improve the social cognition
Continued substance use despite having persistent or recurrent social or interpersonal problems caused or exacerbated by the effects of the substance		Do not cause social or interpersonal problems
Important social, occupational, or recreational activities are given up or reduced	Less of time with friends	
RISKY USE OF THE SUBSTANCE		
Continued use despite knowledge of a persistent or recurrent physical or psychological problem that is likely to have been caused or exacerbated by use	(a very few case) Physically or emotionally abusive relationships; staying with someone who "isn't right for you"	In most cases, especially female, when clear know someone who "isn't right for you," individual will end the relationship
PHARMACOLOGICAL CRITERIA		
Tolerance (marked increase in amount; marked decrease in effect)	Transition from early euphoria to contentment	
Characteristic withdrawal symptoms; substance taken to relieve withdrawal	Grief (from loss); separation anxiety when apart	
OTHER SYMPTOMS		
Stress-induced reinstatement	Consolation-seeking	
Drug and drug-associated stimuli induce the intense physiological arousal	In early romantic love, partner and partner-associated stimuli induce the intense physiological arousal	A few months after initially fall in love, the intense physiological arousal gradually reduce
Chronic drug abuse induce the impairment of decision-making		Individuals display a better decision-making, such as commitment, to establish the healthy long-term relationship
Compulsive drug-seeking behavior; obsessive thinking for drug	In early romantic love, intrusive thinking or preoccupation with the partner; obsessive thinking for partner	A few months after initially fall in love, the obsessive thinking gradually reduce and is replaced by calm, safety and balance
Chronic drug abuse induce the impairment of inhibitory control; higher impulsivity		Lovers do not display the impairment of inhibitory control and the changes of impulsivity

when viewing pictures of a romantic partner, activation of the dACC and PCC indicates a significant positive correlation with the duration of the love relationship. Additionally, scatter plots of dACC or PCC activity and duration of the relationship indicate that lovers in longer relationships (8–17 months) respond differently than those in relatively short relationships (1–7 months). Furthermore, the dACC and the PCC are negatively activated during short relationships (1–7 months), but positively activated during longer relationships (8–17 months) (Aron et al., 2005). The addictive characteristics (e.g., stress-liking) disappear ~6 months after initially falling in love, therefore, alterations in dACC and PCC activation are potential neural bases for the disappearance of addictive characteristics.

Activation of the ventral prefrontal cortex, especially the mPFC, mOFC, and vACC, is correlated with the strength of cravings in people with drug addiction (Goldstein and Volkow, 2011). However, activation of the dorsal prefrontal cortex, especially the dlPFC, dACC, and IFG, is correlated with suppression of drug cravings. For example, instructions to resist cravings while viewing smoking-related videos resulted in increased activity in the dlPFC, dACC, and IFG in smokers, as well as decreased activity in the mOFC and vACC (Goldstein and Volkow, 2011).

Taken together, the overlapping brain regions activity during romantic love and drug addiction indicate that both lovers and people with addiction display activated basic stimulus detection functions (such as reward prediction and reward experience), as well as activated primary emotional reactions (strong urges for drug/partner) when exposed to partner-or drug-related cues (see **Figure 2**). However, romantic love and drug addiction can be differentiated based on other cognitive functions (see **Figure 2**). People with addiction experience strong drug

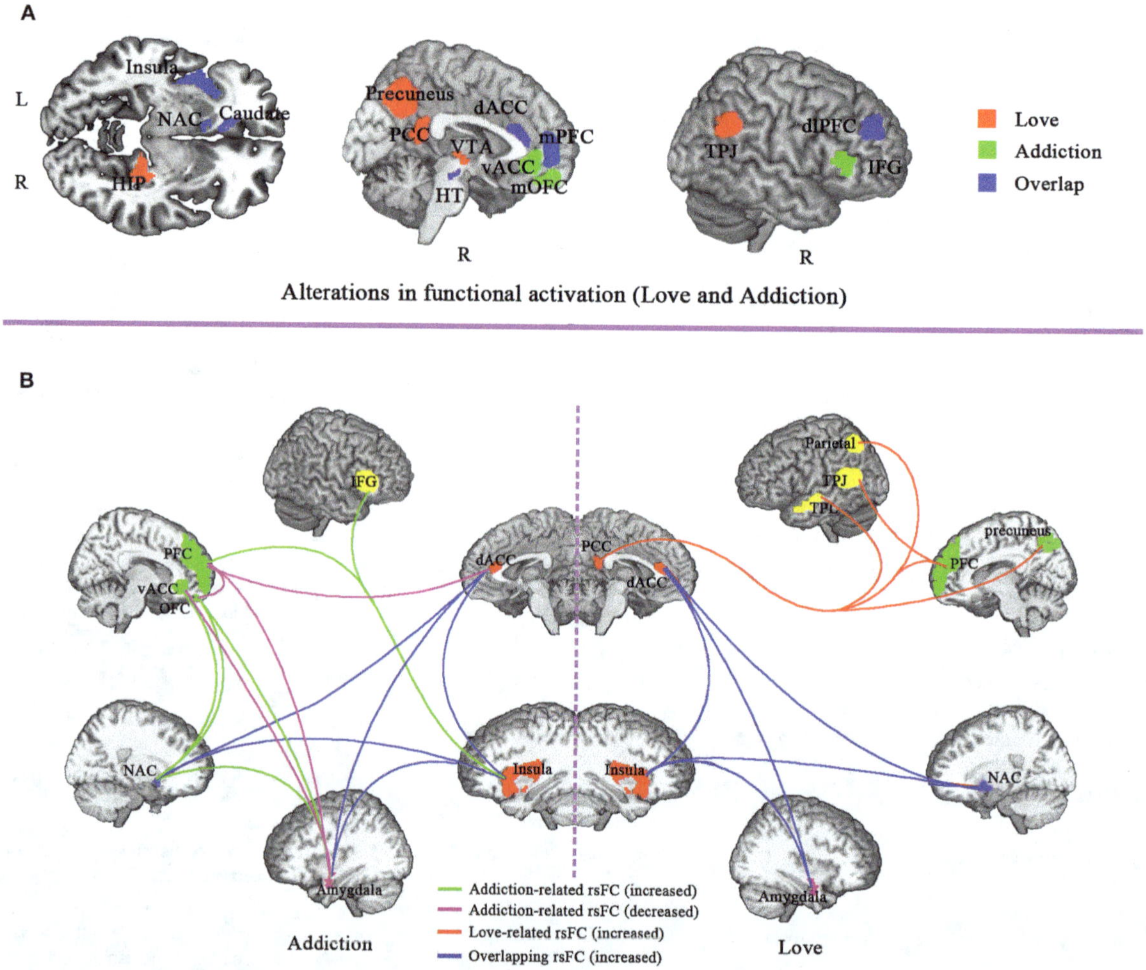

FIGURE 1 | Comparison of brain functional alteration between drug addiction and romantic love. (A) Alterations in functional activation in brain regions involved in love and addiction. Red, love-related functional activation; green, addiction-related functional activation; blue, overlap of functional activation for love and addiction. **(B)** Alterations in resting-state functional connectivity (rsFC) for love and addiction. Green, addiction-related functional connectivity increase; Red, love-related functional connectivity increase; blue, overlap functional connectivity increase for love and addiction; purple, addiction-related functional connectivity decrease. ACC, anterior cingulated cortex; vACC, ventral anterior cingulate; dACC, dorsal anterior cingulate cortex; PCC, posterior cingulate cortex; OFC, orbitofrontal cortex; IFG, inferior frontal gyrus; dlPFC, dorsolateral prefrontal cortex; PFC, prefrontal cortex; VTA, ventral tegmental area; NAC, nucleus accumbens; TPJ, temporo-parietal junction, HIP, hippocampus; HT, hypothalamus; TEP, temporal cortex.

cravings and obsessive thinking. However, in lovers, the obsessive thinking and stress-liking features gradually disappear, and conflict monitoring and social cognition are gradually enhanced as the love relationship progresses, and the dACC and PCC may be involved in these changes. Additionally, the neural changes may alter the relationship progression, and the love relationship eventually does not develop into addiction.

Spontaneous Neural Activation during Love and Addiction

In this section, we will use the evidences that we have provided previously to compare the romantic love related and addiction-related resting-state functional connectivity (rsFC). rsFC is an important index for measuring spontaneous neural activity, reflecting functional communication between brain regions. In general, rsFC is defined as the temporal dependency between spatially remote neurophysiological events (Van Den Heuvel and Pol, 2010). Compared with task-activation rsFC has a better signal to noise ratio, and can be used to study multiple cortical systems (Fox and Greicius, 2010). Most of the previous neuroimaging studies of romantic love only focused on the specific external stimuli induced functional changes of brain regions (Bartels and Zeki, 2000; Aron et al., 2005; Ortigue et al., 2007; Xu et al., 2011; Acevedo et al., 2012), and did not provide evidences about romantic love related functional alteration of brain network. In our previous original research study (Song et al., 2015), which was published on *frontiers in human neuroscience*, we used resting state functional magnetic resonance imaging (fMRI) to study love-related changes in

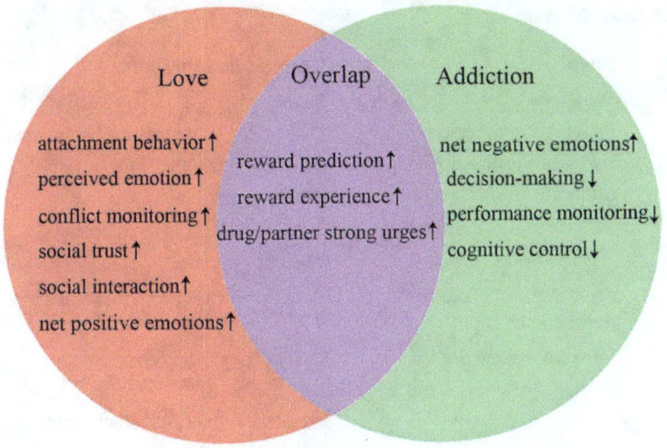

FIGURE 2 | Comparison of cognitive functions. ↑, function increases; ↓, function decreases.

resting state functional connectivity. Our study provided new and important evidences of romantic love related functional alteration of brain network, which suggested that the love-related functional alterations was also observed at the brain network level.

Specifically, in our previous original research study (Song et al., 2015), we used rsfMRI data to compare the functional connectivity (FC) across an "in-love" group (LG, currently intensely in love), an "ended-love" group (ELG, ended romantic relationship recently), and a "single" group (SG, never fallen in love). Results showed that rsFC within the reward and emotion regulation network (dACC, insula, caudate, amygdala, and NAC) as well as rsFC in the social cognition network (TPJ, PCC, MPFC, inferior parietal, precuneus, and temporal lobe) was significantly increased in the LG (in comparison to the ELG and SG).

The addiction related studies showed that addicts displayed increased rsFC within the reward and emotion regulation network (dACC, insula, amygdala, and NAC); between the reward circuit and the motivation circuit (NAC-vACC, NAC-OFC), as well as between the memory/learning circuit and the motivation circuit (amygdala-OFC; Gu et al., 2010; Ma et al., 2010; Sutherland et al., 2012). Moreover, our previous studies showed that rsFC between mPFC and insula, and between dACC and insual displayed significant increased in smoker (Zhang et al., 2011; Wei et al., 2016).

It is obvious that the increased rsFC of romantic love overlaps with that of drug addiction include rsFC between the insula and dACC, between the insula and NAC, between dACC and NAC, between dACC and amygdala, and between the insula and amgdala. While other rsFC indices are specific to love or addiction (Gu et al., 2010; Ma et al., 2010; Sutherland et al., 2012; Song et al., 2015; see **Figure 1**).

The ACC, NAC, insula, and amygdala are core components of the brain systems that play an important role in the processing of sensory and emotional information, reward, and motivational processes (Mogenson et al., 1980). These increased rsFC indicated that the reward signal processed in NAC and the emotion signals processed in amygdala are transmitted to the insula more effectively. The control of a goal-directed behavior will involve both the insula, representing awareness, and the ACC, representing the control of directed effort (Craig, 2009). Thus, these increased rsFC are consistent with more integration of conscious awareness within conflict monitoring processes, and may be responsible for promoting individuals to detect drug- or partner-related cues with greater sensitivity. Moreover, this may be the neural basis of incentive-sensitization theory of addiction, which suggested that repeated exposure to potentially addictive drugs can persistently change brain cells and circuits that normally regulate the attribution of incentive salience to stimuli, a psychological process involved in motivated behavior, and the nature of these "neuroadaptations" is to render these brain circuits hypersensitive in a way that results in pathological levels of incentive salience being attributed to drugs and drug-related cues (Robinson and Berridge, 1993).

Similarly to task-related activation of brain regions, overlapping rsFC demonstrates that both lovers and people with addiction experience activated basic conscious awareness and more integration of partner- or drug-related conscious awareness within conflict monitoring processes (see **Figure 2**). Furthermore, lovers demonstrate more effective awareness of emotional states, enhanced conflict monitoring, increased social trustworthiness, and improved social interaction abilities. These skills may mitigate stress-liking features, thereby facilitating progression of the romantic relationship.

Except for the overlapping, lovers display specifically increased rsFC within the social cognition network (e.g., the temporo-parietal junction (TPJ), PCC, medial prefrontal cortex (mPFC), inferior parietal cortex, precuneus, and temporal lobe; Song et al., 2015). These alterations in functional connectivity may indicate that lovers have more social trust, and have better social interaction abilities. These skills may mitigate stress-liking features and contribute to maintaining the romantic relationship.

Except for the overlapping, people with addiction display specifically increased rsFC between the reward circuit and the motivation circuit (NAC-vACC, NAC-OFC), as well as between the memory/learning circuit and the motivation circuit (amygdala-OFC). Specifically, decreased rsFC indices are observed between the control circuit and the motivation circuit (PFC-OFC), between the cognitive circuit and the memory/learning circuit (PFC-amygdala, and vACC-amygdala), and within the control circuit (PFC-ACC; Gu et al., 2010; Ma et al., 2010). These alterations in functional connectivity support the addiction model proposed by Volkow et al. (2003), and indicate enhanced salience for an addictive drug and its related cues, combined with reduced cognitive control during addiction (Ma et al., 2010). The rsFC between the insula and the control circuit is also altered in people with addiction. Specifically, the ventral and dorsal anterior insula have significantly increased functional connectivity with the dACC, dorsal mPFC, and lateral PFC. Furthermore, the posterior insula displays significantly decreased functional connectivity with the dACC, dorsal mPFC, lateral PFC, and anterior insula (Cisler et al., 2013). Posterior insula cortex activity is associated with changes in bodily states, and the anterior insula cortex mediates subjective awareness of bodily states. Increased functional connectivity between the anterior insula and prefrontal networks indicates enhanced awareness or detection of drug cues or internal craving-related bodily states, and may contribute to biased decision-making processes. Decreased functional connectivity between the posterior insula and prefrontal networks, as well as between the posterior insula and anterior insula, indicate that the influence of somatic states on performance monitoring and attention is diminished (Cisler et al., 2013).

These different alterations of rsFC indicate that people with addiction also experience reduced cognitive control, performance monitoring lacking regulation of the somatic states, and over-valuation of the salience of the drug and its related cues. These alterations may result in subsequent impulsive and compulsive repeated drug consumption, or relapse after protracted periods of abstinence. In general, the results of comparisons of rsFC between romantic love and drug addiction display some similarities to the results of comparisons of task-induced brain activation. Although there are some differences between romantic love and drug addiction (see **Figure 2**), the reduced cognitive control and the weakened social cognition may be the most important differences between romantic love and drug addiction. Developing strategies to improve cognitive control and social cognition may therefore be useful for treating drug addiction.

COMPARISON OF ROMANTIC LOVE AND DRUG ADDICTION: NEUROENDOCRINE FACTORS

Pair bonding and romantic love have previously been conceptualized as attachment processes (Hazan and Shaver, 1987; Fraley and Shaver, 2000). In order to distinguish animal and human studies, we describe this process as pair bonding in animals and as romantic love in humans. However, most neuroendocrine studies of pair bonding and drug addiction are conducted in animals. Therefore, we compare neuroendocrine alterations between pair bonding and drug addiction (see **Table 2**) by reviewing several animal models. Neurotransmitters and neuropeptides involved in pair bonding and drug addiction include primarily dopamine (DA), corticotropin-releasing factor (CRF), oxytocin (OT), and arginine vasopressin (AVP). DA, CRF, OT, AVP, and their receptors (including DA receptors: D1R and D2R, CRF receptors: CRF-R1 and CRF-R1, the OT receptor: OTR, and AVP receptors:V1aR, V1bR, and V2R) contribute significantly to pair bonding and drug addiction. DA is generally regarded as a crucial contributor to the biological reward and motivational processes (Esch and Stefano, 2005). CRF is involved in the neurobiology underlying stress, fear, and anxiety (Bale and Vale, 2004). Additionally, OT and AVP are associated with processing and retention of social information (Hollander et al., 2007).

In this section, neurochemical alterations during both maintenance and disruption of pair bonding and drug addiction will be discussed.

TABLE 2 | Function and alterations of neurochemical systems involved in love and addiction.

	Love	Drug addiction
MAINTENANCE		
DA	D1R promotes maintenance	D1R and D2R promote maintenance
	Plasticity in striatalD1R promotes maintenance	Plasticity in striatal D2R promotes maintenance
CRF	CRF promotes maintenance	CRF-R1 promotes maintenance
		CRF-R2 may inhibit maintenance
	Plasticity in CRF promotes maintenance	Plasticity in CRF promotes maintenance
OT	OT is not necessary for maintenance	OTR inhibits maintenance
		Plasticity in the OT system promotes maintenance
DISRUPTION		
DA		D2R promotes relapse
CRF	Released after disruption	Released after disruption
	Plasticity in hypothalamic CRF promotes return to partner	Plasticity in hypothalamic CRF-R1 promotes relapse, CRF-R2 may inhibit relapse
OT	Released after disruption	Released after disruption
	OT inhibits return to partner	Endogenous plasticity in the OT system promotes relapse
		Exogenous OT inhibits relapse

DA, dopamine; CRF, corticotropin-releasing factor; OT, oxytocin; AVP, arginine vasopressin.

Maintenance of Pair Bonding and Drug Addiction

Neurotransmitters and neuropeptides are important contributors to the maintenance of both pair bonding and drug addiction. Activation of D1R promotes maintenance of pair bonding and drug abuse, and CRF increases in the NAC also promote pair bonding maintenance (Aragona et al., 2006; Grippo et al., 2007; Burkett and Young, 2012). Additionally, D2R and CRF-R1 activation in the central nervous system also promote maintenance of drug use; however, activation of OTR and CRF-R2 inhibit drug addiction maintenance (Carson et al., 2010; Koob, 2010; Zanos et al., 2014). Pair bonding and chronic exposure to drugs of abuse induce plasticity in DA and CRF receptors, which promotes the maintenances of pair bonding and drug addiction (Nakajima and McKenzie, 1986; Zorrilla et al., 2001; Bosch et al., 2009; Burkett and Young, 2012).

However, there are also some significant differences between neuroendocrine factors that facilitate the maintenance of pair bonding and drug addiction. Chronic administration of an abused drug produces a decrease in D2R in the NAC (Grieder et al., 2012), as well as decreases in endogenous OT and OTR density in the central nervous system (Johns et al., 1997; Light et al., 2004; Jarrett et al., 2006). These changes in D2R expression in the NAC are associated with decreased baseline metabolic activity in the OFC, ACC, and dlPFC, and these changes may promote compulsive drug intake and reinstatement of drug-seeking behavior (Narendran et al., 2005; Volkow et al.,

2008; Asensio et al., 2010). Alterations in endogenous OT indicate that the endogenous OT system may be not sufficient to affect drug-induced consequences, although the exogenous OT is a potential treatment for drug addiction. Similar changes do not occur during pair bonding. As pair bonding continues, D2R do not display plastic changes combined with functional enhancement of the OT system (Burkett and Young, 2012; Schneiderman et al., 2012). These plastic changes are potential neural mechanisms underlying the differences between the development of addiction and love. As described above, lovers display addictive characteristics during early romantic love, but these characteristics gradually disappear as the romantic relationship progresses. Functional changes to the OT system may be the neural basis of this process. Other than reduced functioning of the OT system, people with addiction also experience D2R functional damage and decreased baseline metabolic activity in the OFC, ACC, and dlPFC. These findings suggest that stress-liking features become more intense, and also that cognitive control is impaired with repeated drug abuse.

Disruption of Pair Bonding and Drug Addiction

Similarly to drug addiction withdrawal, a disruption to pair bonding often induces profound grieving, anxiety, stress, and depressive-like behaviors (Bosch et al., 2009). In conjunction with these symptoms, CRF and OT increase significantly in the central nervous system (Bartz and Hollander, 2006; Grippo et al., 2007). Furthermore, disruption of pair bonding induces plastic changes in the hypothalamic CRF system, and these changes are associated with individuals returning to their former partner (Grippo et al., 2007). Although disruption of drug use also induces plastic changes in the hypothalamic CRF system, the changes to CRF-R1 and CRF-R2 have different effects on subsequent relapse, with promoting and inhibiting effects, respectively (Koob, 1999). OT has similar effects on the disruption of both pair bonding and drug use, including inhibiting return to the previous partner or addiction relapse. This effect likely occurs via relieving disruption-induced anxiety, stress, and depressive-like behaviors (Kovács et al., 1981; Gibbs, 1984; Cui et al., 2001; Pedersen et al., 2013). During drug addiction, however, the endogenous OT system may be not sufficient to affect drug-induced consequences, as chronic administration of the abused drug results in lower endogenous OT baseline activity (Light et al., 2004). Therefore, the combination of reduced activity of the endogenous OT system and a dysfunctional prefrontal cortex, described in the previous section, contribute to a high risk for relapse even after protracted periods of abstinence. During pair bonding, functional enhancement of the OT system facilitates maintenance of the relationship, whereas after disruption of pair bonding, functional enhancement of the OT system inhibits return to the partner. These findings indicate that individuals who have experienced love demonstrate improved social adaptation abilities, and enhanced function of the OT system may be the neural basis for this strength. In general, differences occur between romantic love and drug addiction in the maintenance and disruption stages, and changes to the OT system may be the neural basis of these differences.

A NEW POSSIBLE TREATMENT TO ADDICTION BASED ON THE OXYTOCIN

As described above, comparison of romantic love and drug addiction progression indicates that there are some similarities between the early stage romantic love and drug addiction, and romantic love are considered as a behavioral addiction, while there are many significant differences between the later stage romantic love and drug addiction, and romantic love eventually developed into a prosocial behavior. Moreover, comparison of romantic love and drug addiction using neuroimaging studies indicates that the function enhancement of reward and emotion regulate system may be the neural basis of the similarities between the early stage of romantic love and drug addiction. However, the difference of functional alteration of social cognition system and the cognitive control related brain regions may be the neural basis of the differences between the later stage romantic love and drug addiction. e.g., addicts display the impairment of cognitive control and social cognition. Furthermore, romantic love and chronic administration of abused drug both induce the plastic changes of the DA and OT systems. The previous studies suggested that functional changes in DA system were associated with the dysfunction in reward network (Henry and White, 1995; Aragona et al., 2006; Anderson et al., 2008; Bertran-Gonzalez et al., 2008) and emotion regulation network (Davidson et al., 2000). Moreover, previous study suggested that oxytocin could induce functional connectivity changes within social cognition network (Riem et al., 2013). It seems that the dysfunction of OT system may be the neurochemical basis of the impairment of cognitive control and social cognition in addicts. Therefore, to study how to improve abused drug induced the impairment of the OT system, cognitive control, and social cognition may be help to find the treatment of drug addiction.

Exogenous administration of OT can attenuate the development of tolerance for drugs of abuse, as well as mitigate withdrawal symptoms and minimize reinstatement of drug use (Kovács et al., 1998). For example, repeated administration of cocaine produces behavioral tolerance to the sniffing-induced effects of cocaine. OT pretreatment in cocaine-tolerant rats reduced tolerance for cocaine and produced effects similar to those in non-tolerant control rats (Sarnyai et al., 1992). Additionally, exogenous administration of OT, such as by intranasal administration, increases activity in brain regions associated with cognitive control and social cognition, including the striatum, middle frontal gyrus, dlPFC, IFG, mPFC, OFC, ACC, PCC, and superior temporal sulcus (Riem et al., 2011; Bethlehem et al., 2013; Gordon et al., 2013; Liu et al., 2015). Furthermore, functional connectivity between brain regions (between the amygdala and ACC, between the amygdala and anterior insula) is also enhanced (Bethlehem et al., 2013). These findings indicate that exogenous administration of OT may improve or reverse addictive drug use by reversing D2R-related decreases in baseline metabolic activity in the OFC and ACC, and may partially improve the abnormal functional connectivity between brain regions that occurs during addiction. A recent study suggests that there are also D2R-OTR heteromers with facilitatory receptor–receptor interactions in the striatum, and that these heteromers are associated with changes in social and emotional behavior (Romero-Fernandez et al., 2013). These functional improvements may facilitate cognitive control and performance monitoring in people with addiction, decrease impulsive and compulsive repeated drug consumption, and reduce relapse rates after protracted periods of abstinence. Additionally, the improvement of social cognition by exogenous administration of OT can break the object-orientated rewards and execution of habitual behavioral loops to mitigate the compulsive repeated drug consumption (McGregor and Bowen, 2012).

Although some researchers regard OT administration as a potential treatment for drug addiction (McGregor and Bowen, 2012; Tops et al., 2014), most studies are currently in the preclinical stage (McGregor and Bowen, 2012). Additionally, the mechanisms of OT effects have not yet been elucidated. Through comparing romantic love and drug addiction, we discovered a potential mechanism for the ability of OT to mitigate or reverse the development of drug addiction. These two mechanisms include: (a) mitigation of stress and anxiety, (b) facilitation of social interactions, and (c) the improvement of cognitive control. Activation of stress systems is critical to motivating drug-seeking, which may then develop into drug addiction (Koob, 2008). OT exerts an anti-stress effect and attenuates the stress and anxiety responses (Neumann and Landgraf, 2012). For example, exogenous administration of OT reduces stress-induced corticosterone release and also reduces adrenocorticotropic hormone and CRF mRNA expression (Windle et al., 1997, 2004; Parker et al., 2005). Social interaction may influence drug addiction, and a recent study proposes that activation of OT by facilitating social interaction may attenuate drug addiction (McGregor and Bowen, 2012). Repeated administration of abused drugs induces neuroplasticity of the DA and OT systems that may bias behavior toward object-orientated rewards and execution of habitual behavioral loops (Everitt and Robbins, 2013). Social attachment and exogenous administration of OT may reverse this bias toward social stimuli, which may be associated with termination of object-orientated behaviors and attenuation of the compulsive drug-seeking behaviors (McGregor and Bowen, 2012; Tops et al., 2014). For drug addiction, the tolerance, compulsive drug-seeking, withdrawal symptoms and relapse are the core symptoms. To attenuate the development of tolerance of abused drug and mitigate the withdrawal symptoms may attenuate the development of addiction or partially reverse the the corrosive effects of long-term drugs abuse. However, the relapse and compulsive drug-seeking are the most critical obstacle to treat drug addiction, and the improvement of cognitive control and social attachment may be the key for overcoming relapse and mitigate compulsive drug-seeking (Amaro et al., 1999; Volkow et al., 2006). Exogenous administration of OT can effectively improve the function of cognitive control and social cognition related brain regions and this imply that improving cognitive control and social cognition may be the most important reasons for OT as a potential treatment of drug addiction.

SUMMARY AND FUTURE DIRECTIONS

In early romantic relationships, lovers display some characteristics of addiction, but these characteristics disappear after several months. Alterations of functioning in brain regions (especially the dACC and PCC) and neuroendocrine activities (especially the OT system) may be the potential neural bases for the changes in associated behaviors and emotions. During drug addiction, the relapse and compulsive drug-seeking are the most critical obstacle to treat drug addiction (Amaro et al., 1999), and the drug craving is a key contributor to relapse (Volkow et al., 2006). When resisting cravings while viewing drug-related cues, people with addiction experienced increased activity in the dlPFC, dACC, and IFG (Goldstein and Volkow, 2011). These brain regions are primarily involved in cognitive control, and the dACC is critical to monitoring control (Botvinick et al., 2004). The IFG is primarily involved in inhibition and attentional control (Hampshire et al., 2010), whereas the dlPFC contributes to executive control (Wagner et al., 2001). Previous studies suggest that exogenous administration of OT increases activity in these regions (Riem et al., 2011; Gordon et al., 2013; Liu et al., 2015). Exogenous administration of OT can also increase the activity of PCC that is mainly involving in social cognition (Gordon et al., 2013). These findings imply that exogenous administration of OT can improve the cognitive control function and social cognition to inhibit the drug craving and compulsive drug-seeking.

Additionally, we do not compare the brain structure of romantic love and drug addiction. The reason is lack of study that investigates the brain structure of romantic relationship. For romantic love we also do not discuss the resting state brain functioning changes in long period of romantic relationship (the length of relationship more than 18 months). Future research should investigate these questions in order to learn more about the neural mechanism of romantic love.

Most studies addressing treatment of addiction with OT emphasize the effects of OT on attenuating the development of tolerance, as well as on mitigating the withdrawal symptoms of addiction. However, these studies do not comprehensively discuss the therapeutic effects of OT as an addiction treatment. We suggest that OT administration may improve cognitive control in people with drug addiction, thereby inhibiting drug cravings and reducing the probability of relapse. The OT administration can also improve social cognition in people with drug addiction, thereby breaking the object-orientated rewards and execution of habitual behavioral loops to mitigate the compulsive drug-seeking. Therefore, future research should further investigate this possibility and elucidate the mechanisms for OT as a potential treatment for drug addiction.

AUTHOR CONTRIBUTIONS

Conceive and writing frame design: HS and XZ. Wrote the paper: ZZ and HS. Revise the manuscript: HS, XZ, YZ, and ZZ.

ACKNOWLEDGMENTS

This work was supported by grants from the National Natural Science Foundation of China (31230032, 31171083, and 31471071), the Fundamental Research Funds for the Central Universities of China (SWU 1509134 and WK2070000033), the 100 Talents Program of the Chinese Academy of Sciences (KJ2070000018), and Hefei Science Center, CAS "User with Potential" (2015HSC-UP017).

REFERENCES

1. Acevedo, B. P., Aron, A., Fisher, H. E., and Brown, L. L. (2012). Neural correlates of long-term intense romantic love. *Soc. Cogn. Affect. Neurosci.* 7, 145–159. doi: 10.1093/scan/nsq092
2. Amaro, H., Nieves, R., Johannes, S. W., and Cabeza, N. M. L. (1999). Substance abuse treatment: critical issues and challenges in the treatment of Latina women. *Hisp. J. Behav. Sci.* 21, 266–282. doi: 10.1177/0739986399213005
3. Anderson, S. M., Famous, K. R., Sadri-Vakili, G., Kumaresan, V., Schmidt, H. D., Bass, C. E., et al. (2008). CaMKII: a biochemical bridge linking accumbens dopamine and glutamate systems in cocaine seeking. *Nat. Neurosci.* 11, 344–353. doi: 10.1038/nn2054
4. Aragona, B. J., Liu, Y., Yu, Y. J., Curtis, J. T., Detwiler, J. M., Insel, T. R., et al. (2006). Nucleus accumbens dopamine differentially mediates the formation and maintenance of monogamous pair bonds. *Nat. Neurosci.* 9, 133–139. doi: 10.1038/nn1613
5. Aron, A., Fisher, H., Mashek, D. J., Strong, G., Li, H., and Brown, L. L. (2005). Reward, motivation, and emotion systems associated with early-stage intense romantic love. *J. Neurophysiol.* 94, 327–337. doi: 10.1152/jn.00838.2004
6. Asensio, S., Romero, M. J., Romero, F. J., Wong, C., Alia-Klein, N., Tomasi, D., et al. (2010). Striatal dopamine D2 receptor availability predicts the thalamic and medial prefrontal responses to reward in cocaine abusers three years later. *Synapse* 64, 397–402. doi: 10.1002/syn.20741
7. Association, A. P. (2013). *Diagnostic and Statistical Manual of Mental Disorders (DSM- 5®)*. Washington, DC; London: American Psychiatric Pub.
9. Bale, T. L., and Vale, W. W. (2004). CRF and CRF receptors: role in stress responsivity and other behaviors. *Annu. Rev. Pharmacol. Toxicol.* 44, 525–557. doi: 10.1146/annurev.pharmtox.44.101802.121410
10. Baler, R. D., and Volkow, N. D. (2006). Drug addiction: the neurobiology of disrupted self-control. *Trends Mol. Med.* 12, 559–566. doi: 10.1016/j.molmed.2006.10.005
11. Bartels, A., and Zeki, S. (2000). The neural basis of romantic love. *Neuroreport* 11, 3829–3834. doi: 10.1097/00001756-200011270-00046
12. Bartz, J. A., and Hollander, E. (2006). The neuroscience of affiliation: forging links between basic and clinical research on neuropeptides and social behavior. *Horm. Behav.* 50, 518–528. doi: 10.1016/j.yhbeh.2006.06.018
13. Bertran-Gonzalez, J., Bosch, C., Maroteaux, M., Matamales, M., Hervé, D., Valjent, E., et al. (2008). Opposing patterns of signaling activation in dopamine D1 and D2 receptor-expressing striatal neurons in response to cocaine and haloperidol. *J. Neurosci.* 28, 5671–5685. doi: 10.1523/JNEUROSCI.1039-08.2008
14. Bethlehem, R. A., van Honk, J., Auyeung, B., and Baron-Cohen, S. (2013). Oxytocin, brain physiology, and functional connectivity: a review of intranasal oxytocin fMRI studies. *Psychoneuroendocrinology* 38, 962–974. doi: 10.1016/j.psyneuen.2012.10.011
15. Bosch, O. J., Nair, H. P., Ahern, T. H., Neumann, I. D., and Young, L. J. (2009). The CRF system mediates increased passive stress-coping behavior following the loss of a bonded partner in a monogamous rodent. *Neuropsychopharmacology* 34, 1406–1415. doi: 10.1038/npp.2008.154
16. Botvinick, M. M., Cohen, J. D., and Carter, C. S. (2004). Conflict monitoring and anterior cingulate cortex: an update. *Trends Cogn. Sci.* 8, 539–546. doi: 10.1016/j.tics.2004.10.003
17. Breiter, H. C., Gollub, R. L., Weisskoff, R. M., Kennedy, D. N., Makris, N., Berke, J. D., et al. (1997). Acute effects of cocaine on human brain activity and emotion. *Neuron* 19, 591–611. doi: 10.1016/S0896-6273(00)80374-8
18. Burkett, J. P., and Young, L. J. (2012). The behavioral, anatomical and pharmacological parallels between social attachment, love and addiction. *Psychopharmacology* 224, 1–26. doi: 10.1007/s00213-012-2794-x
19. Carson, D. S., Cornish, J. L., Guastella, A. J., Hunt, G. E., and McGregor, I. S. (2010). Oxytocin decreases methamphetamine self-administration, methamphetamine hyperactivity, and relapse to methamphetamine-seeking behaviour in rats. *Neuropharmacology* 58, 38–43. doi: 10.1016/j.neuropharm.2009.06.018
20. Cisler, J. M., Elton, A., Kennedy, A. P., Young, J., Smitherman, S., James, G. A., et al. (2013). Altered functional connectivity of the insular cortex across prefrontal networks in cocaine addiction. *Psychiatry Res. Neuroimag.* 213, 39–46. doi: 10.1016/j.pscychresns.2013.02.007
21. Craig, A. (2009). How do you feel–now? The anterior insula and human awareness. *Nat. Rev. Neurosci.* 10, 59–70. doi: 10.1038/nrn2555
22. Cui, S.-S., Bowen, R. C., Gu, G.-B., Hannesson, D. K., Peter, H. Y., and Zhang, X. (2001). Prevention of cannabinoid withdrawal syndrome by lithium: involvement of oxytocinergic neuronal activation. *J. Neurosci.* 21, 9867–9876.
23. Davidson, R. J., Putnam, K. M., and Larson, C. L. (2000). Dysfunction in the neural circuitry of emotion regulation–a possible prelude to violence. *Science* 289, 591–594. doi: 10.1126/science.289.5479.591
24. Delgado, M. R., Nystrom, L. E., Fissell, C., Noll, D., and Fiez, J. A. (2000). Tracking the hemodynamic responses to reward and punishment in the striatum. *J. Neurophysiol.* 84, 3072–3077.
25. Elliott, R., Newman, J. L., Longe, O. A., and Deakin, J. W. (2003). Differential response patterns in the striatum and orbitofrontal cortex to financial reward in humans: a parametric functional magnetic resonance imaging study. *J. Neurosci.* 23, 303–307.
26. Esch, T., and Stefano, G. B. (2005). The neurobiology of love. *Neuro Endocrinol. Lett.* 26, 175–192.
27. Everitt, B. J., and Robbins, T. W. (2013). From the ventral to the dorsal striatum: devolving views of their roles in drug addiction. *Neurosci. Biobehav. Rev.* 37, 1946–1954. doi: 10.1016/j.neubiorev.2013.02.010
28. Fisher, H. E. (1998). Lust, attraction, and attachment in mammalian reproduction. *Hum. Nat.* 9, 23–52. doi: 10.1007/s12110-998-1010-5
29. Fisher, H. E., Xu, X., Aron, A., and Brown, L. L. (2016). Intense, passionate, romantic love: a natural addiction? How the fields that investigate romance and substance abuse can inform each other. *Front. Psychol.* 7:687. doi: 10.3389/fpsyg.2016.00687
30. Fox, M. D., and Greicius, M. (2010). Clinical applications of resting state functional connectivity. *Front. Syst. Neurosci.* 4:19. doi: 10.3389/fnsys.2010.00019
31. Fox, M. D., and Raichle, M. E. (2007). Spontaneous fluctuations in brain activity observed with functional magnetic resonance imaging. *Nat. Rev. Neurosci.* 8, 700–711. doi: 10.1038/nrn2201
32. Fraley, R. C., and Shaver, P. R. (2000). Adult romantic attachment: theoretical developments, emerging controversies, and unanswered questions. *Rev. Gen. Psychol.* 4, 132–154. doi: 10.1037/1089-2680.4.2.132
33. Frascella, J., Potenza, M. N., Brown, L. L., and Childress, A. R. (2010). Shared brain vulnerabilities open the way for nonsubstance addictions: carving addiction at a new joint? *Ann. N.Y. Acad. Sci.* 1187, 294–315. doi: 10.1111/j.1749- 6632.2009.05420.x
34. Gibbs, D. M. (1984). Dissociation of oxytocin, vasopressin and corticotropin secretion during different types of stress. *Life Sci.* 35, 487–491. doi: 10.1016/0024-3205(84)90241-8
35. Goldstein, R. Z., and Volkow, N. D. (2011). Dysfunction of the prefrontal cortex in addiction: neuroimaging findings and clinical implications. *Nat. Rev. Neurosci.* 12, 652–669. doi: 10.1038/nrn3119
36. Gordon, I., Vander Wyk, B. C., Bennett, R. H., Cordeaux, C., Lucas, M. V., Eilbott, J. A., et al. (2013). Oxytocin enhances brain function in children with autism. *Proc. Natl. Acad. Sci. U.S.A.* 110, 20953–20958. doi: 10.1073/pnas.1312857110
37. Grieder, T. E., George, O., Tan, H., George, S. R., Le Foll, B., Laviolette, S. R., et al. (2012). Phasic D1 and tonic D2 dopamine receptor signaling double dissociate the motivational effects of acute nicotine and chronic nicotine withdrawal. *Proc. Natl. Acad. Sci. U.S.A.* 109, 3101–3106. doi: 10.1073/pnas.1114422109
38. Grippo, A. J., Cushing, B. S., and Carter, C. S. (2007). Depression-like behavior and stressor-induced neuroendocrine activation in female prairie
39. voles exposed to chronic social isolation. *Psychosom. Med.* 69, 149–157. doi: 10.1097/PSY.0b013e31802f054b
40. Gu, H., Salmeron, B. J., Ross, T. J., Geng, X., Zhan, W., Stein, E. A., et al. (2010). Mesocorticolimbic circuits are impaired in chronic cocaine users as demonstrated by resting-state functional connectivity. *Neuroimage* 53, 593–601. doi: 10.1016/j.neuroimage.2010.06.066
41. Hampshire, A., Chamberlain, S. R., Monti, M. M., Duncan, J., and Owen, A. M.

(2010). The role of the right inferior frontal gyrus: inhibition and attentional control. *Neuroimage* 50, 1313–1319. doi: 10.1016/j.neuroimage.2009.12.109

42. Hatfield, E., and Rapson, R. L. (1987). Passionate love/sexual desire: can the same paradigm explain both? *Arch. Sex. Behav.* 16, 259–278. doi: 10.1007/BF01541613
43. Hatfield, E., and Sprecher, S. (1986). Measuring passionate love in intimate relationships. *J. Adolesc.* 9, 383–410. doi: 10.1016/S0140-1971(86)80043-4
44. Hazan, C., and Shaver, P. (1987). Romantic love conceptualized as an attachment process. *J. Pers. Soc. Psychol.* 52, 511–524. doi: 10.1037/0022-3514.52.3.511
45. Henry, D. J., and White, F. J. (1995). The persistence of behavioral sensitization to cocaine parallels enhanced inhibition of nucleus accumbens neurons. *J. Neurosci.* 15, 6287–6299.
46. Hollander, E., Bartz, J., Chaplin, W., Phillips, A., Sumner, J., Soorya, L., et al. (2007). Oxytocin increases retention of social cognition in autism. *Biol. Psychiatry* 61, 498–503. doi: 10.1016/j.biopsych.2006.05.030
47. Jarrett, T., McMurray, M., Walker, C., and Johns, J. (2006). Cocaine treatment alters oxytocin receptor binding but not mRNA production in postpartum rat dams. *Neuropeptides* 40, 161–167. doi: 10.1016/j.npep.2006.03.002
48. Johns, J. M., Lubin, D., Walker, C., Meter, K., and Mason, G. (1997). Chronic gestational cocaine treatment decreases oxytocin levels in the medial preoptic area, ventral tegmental area and hippocampus in Sprague-Dawley rats. *Neuropeptides* 31, 439–443. doi: 10.1016/S0143-4179(97)90037-8
49. Kalivas, P. W., and O'Brien, C. (2008). Drug addiction as a pathology of staged neuroplasticity. *Neuropsychopharmacology* 33, 166–180. doi: 10.1038/sj.npp.1301564
50. Koob, G. F. (1999). Corticotropin-releasing factor, norepinephrine, and stress. *Biol. Psychiatry* 46, 1167–1180. doi: 10.1016/S0006-3223(99)00164-X
51. Koob, G. F. (2008). A role for brain stress systems in addiction. *Neuron* 59, 11–34. doi: 10.1016/j.neuron.2008.06.012
52. Koob, G. F. (2010). The role of CRF and CRF-related peptides in the dark side of addiction. *Brain Res.* 1314, 3–14. doi: 10.1016/j.brainres.2009.11.008
53. Kovács, G. L., Sarnyai, Z., and Szabó, G. (1998). Oxytocin and addiction: a review. *Psychoneuroendocrinology* 23, 945–962. doi: 10.1016/S0306-4530(98)00064-X
54. Kovács, G. L., Szontágh, L., Baláspiri, L., Hódi, K., Bohus, P., and Telegdy, G. (1981). On the mode of action of an oxytocin derivative (Z-Pro-D-Leu) on morphine-dependence in mice. *Neuropharmacology* 20, 647–651. doi: 10.1016/0028-3908(81)90111-8
55. Liebowitz, M. R. (1983). *The Chemistry of Love.* Little: Brown.
56. Light, K. C., Grewen, K. M., Amico, J. A., Boccia, M., Brownley, K. A., and Johns, J. M. (2004). Deficits in plasma oxytocin responses and increased negative affect, stress, and blood pressure in mothers with cocaine exposure during pregnancy. *Addict. Behav.* 8, 1541–1564. doi: 10.1016/j.addbeh.2004.02.062
57. Liu, N., Hadj-Bouziane, F., Jones, K. B., Turchi, J. N., Averbeck, B. B., and Ungerleider, L. G. (2015). Oxytocin modulates fMRI responses to facial expression in macaques. *Proc. Natl. Acad. Sci. U.S.A.* 112, E3123–E3130. doi: 10.1073/pnas.1508097112
58. Lv, W., Wu, Q., Liu, X., Chen, Y., Song, H., Yang, L., et al. (2016). Cue reactivity in nicotine and alcohol addiction: a cross-cultural view. *Front. Psychol.* 7:1335. doi: 10.3389/fpsyg.2016.01335
59. Ma, N., Liu, Y., Li, N., Wang, C.-X., Zhang, H., Jiang, X.-F., et al. (2010). Addiction related alteration in resting-state brain connectivity. *Neuroimage* 49, 738–744. doi: 10.1016/j.neuroimage.2009.08.037
60. Maddock, R. J. (1999). The retrosplenial cortex and emotion: new insights from functional neuroimaging of the human brain. *Trends Neurosci.* 22, 310–316. doi: 10.1016/S0166-2236(98)01374-5
61. Marazziti, D., and Canale, D. (2004). Hormonal changes when falling in love. *Psychoneuroendocrinology* 29, 931–936. doi: 10.1016/j.psyneuen.2003.08.006
62. McGregor, I. S., and Bowen, M. T. (2012). Breaking the loop: oxytocin as a potential treatment for drug addiction. *Horm. Behav.* 61, 331–339. doi: 10.1016/j.yhbeh.2011.12.001
63. Melis, M., Spiga, S., and Diana, M. (2005). The dopamine hypothesis of drug addiction: hypodopaminergic state. *Int. Rev. Neurobiol.* 63, 101–154. doi: 10.1016/S0074-7742(05)63005-X
64. Meloy, J. R., and Fisher, H. (2005). Some thoughts on the neurobiology of stalking. *J. Forensic Sci.* 50, 1472–1480. doi: 10.1520/JFS2004508
65. Mogenson, G. J., Jones, D. L., and Yim, C. Y. (1980). From motivation to action: functional interface between the limbic system and the motor system. *Prog. Neurobiol.* 14, 69–97. doi: 10.1016/0301-0082(80)90018-0
66. Nakajima, S., and McKenzie, G. M. (1986). Reduction of the rewarding effect of brain stimulation by a blockade of dopamine D1 receptor with SCH 23390. *Pharmacol. Biochem. Behav.* 24, 919–923. doi: 10.1016/0091-3057(86)90437-5
67. Narendran, R., Frankle, W. G., Keefe, R., Gil, R., Martinez, D., Slifstein, M., et al. (2005). Altered prefrontal dopaminergic function in chronic recreational ketamine users. *Am. J. Psychiatry* 162, 2352–2359. doi: 10.1176/appi.ajp.162.12.2352
68. Neumann, I. D., and Landgraf, R. (2012). Balance of brain oxytocin and vasopressin: implications for anxiety, depression, and social behaviors. *Trends Neurosci.* 35, 649–659. doi: 10.1016/j.tins.2012.08.004
69. Ortigue, S., Bianchi-Demicheli, F., Hamilton, A. D. C., and Grafton, S. T. (2007). The neural basis of love as a subliminal prime: an event-related functional magnetic resonance imaging study. *J. Cogn. Neurosci.* 19, 1218–1230. doi: 10.1162/jocn.2007.19.7.1218
70. Panksepp, J., Knutson, B., and Burgdorf, J. (2002). The role of brain emotional systems in addictions: a neuro-evolutionary perspective and new 'self-report' animal model. *Addiction* 97, 459–469. doi: 10.1046/j.1360-0443.2002.00025.x
71. Parker, K. J., Buckmaster, C. L., Schatzberg, A. F., and Lyons, D. M. (2005). Intranasal oxytocin administration attenuates the ACTH stress response in monkeys. *Psychoneuroendocrinology* 30, 924–929. doi: 10.1016/j.psyneuen.2005.04.002
72. Pedersen, C. A., Smedley, K. L., Leserman, J., Jarskog, L. F., Rau, S. W., Kampov-Polevoi, A., et al. (2013). Intranasal oxytocin blocks alcohol withdrawal in human subjects. *Alcoholism Clin. Exp. Res.* 37, 484–489. doi: 10.1111/j.1530-0277.2012.01958.x
73. Riem, M. M. E., Bakermans-Kranenburg, M. J., Pieper, S., Tops, M., Boksem, M. A. S., Vermeiren, R. R. J. M., et al. (2011). Oxytocin modulates amygdala, insula, and inferior frontal gyrus responses to infant crying: a randomized controlled trial. *Biol. psychiatry* 70, 291–297. doi: 10.1016/j.biopsych.2011.02.006
74. Riem, M. M., van IJzendoorn, M. H., Tops, M., Boksem, M. A., Rombouts, S. A., and Bakermans-Kranenburg, M. J. (2013). Oxytocin effects on complex brain networks are moderated by experiences of maternal love withdrawal. *Eur. Neuropsychopharm.* 23, 1288–1295. doi: 10.1016/j.euroneuro.2013. 01.011
75. Robinson, T. E., and Berridge, K. C. (1993). The neural basis of drug craving: an incentive-sensitization theory of addiction. *Brain Res. Rev.* 18, 247–291.
76. Romero-Fernandez, W., Borroto-Escuela, D., Agnati, L., and Fuxe, K. (2013). Evidence for the existence of dopamine d2-oxytocin receptor heteromers in the ventral and dorsal striatum with facilitatory receptor-receptor interactions. *Mol. Psychiatry* 18, 849–850. doi: 10.1038/mp.2012.103
77. Sarnyai, Z., Bíró, É., Babarczy, E., Vecsernyes, M., Laczi, F., Szabó, G., et al. (1992). Oxytocin modulates behavioural adaptation to repeated treatment with cocaine in rats. *Neuropharmacology* 31, 593–598. doi: 10.1016/0028-3908(92)90192-R
78. Schneiderman, I., Zagoory-Sharon, O., Leckman, J. F., and Feldman, R. (2012). Oxytocin during the initial stages of romantic attachment: relations to couples' interactive reciprocity. *Psychoneuroendocrinology* 37, 1277–1285. doi: 10.1016/j.psyneuen.2011.12.021
79. Schultz, W. (2000). Multiple reward signals in the brain. *Nat. Rev. Neurosci.* 1, 199–207. doi: 10.1038/35044563
80. Song, H., Zou, Z., Kou, J., Liu, Y., Yang, L., Zilverstand, A., et al. (2015). Love-related changes in the brain: a resting-state functional magnetic resonance imaging study. *Front. Hum. Neurosci.* 9:71. doi: 10.3389/fnhum.2015.00071
81. Stárka, L. (2007). Endocrine factors of pair bonding. *Prague Med. Rep.* 108, 297–305.
82. Sternberg, R. J. (1986). A triangular theory of love. *Psychol. Rev.* 93, 119–135.
83. Sutherland, M. T., McHugh, M. J., Pariyadath, V., and Stein, E. A. (2012). Resting state functional connectivity in addiction: lessons learned and a road ahead. *Neuroimage* 62, 2281–2295. doi: 10.1016/j.neuroimage.2012.01.117
84. Tops, M., Koole, S. L., IJzerman, H., and Buisman-Pijlman, F. T. (2014). Why social attachment and oxytocin protect against addiction and stress: insights from the dynamics between ventral and dorsal corticostriatal systems. *Pharmacol. Biochem. Behav.* 119, 39–48. doi: 10.1016/j.pbb.2013.07.015
85. Van Den Heuvel, M. P., and Pol, H. E. H. (2010). Exploring the brain network: a review on resting-state fMRI functional connectivity. *Eur. Neuropsychopharmacol.* 20, 519–534. doi: 10.1016/j.euroneuro.2010.03.008
86. Volkow, N. D., Fowler, J. S., and Wang, G.-J. (2003). The addicted human brain: insights from imaging studies. *J. Clin. Invest.* 111, 1444–1451. doi: 10.1172/JCI18533
87. Volkow, N. D., Fowler, J. S., Wang, G.-J., Swanson, J. M., and Telang, F. (2007). Dopamine in drug abuse and addiction: results of imaging studies and treatment implications. *Arch. Neurol. Chicago* 64, 1575–1579. doi: 10.1001/archneur.64.11.1575
88. Volkow, N. D., Wang, G.-J., Telang, F., Fowler, J. S., Logan, J., Childress, A.-R., et al. (2006). Cocaine cues and dopamine in dorsal striatum: mechanism of craving in cocaine addiction. *J. Neurosci.* 26, 6583–6588. doi: 10.1523/JNEUROSCI.1544-06.2006

89. Volkow, N. D., Wang, G.-J., Telang, F., Fowler, J. S., Thanos, P. K., Logan, J., et al. (2008). Low dopamine striatal D2 receptors are associated with prefrontal metabolism in obese subjects: possible contributing factors. *Neuroimage* 42, 1537–1543. doi: 10.1016/j.neuroimage.2008.06.002
90. Wang, Y., Zhang, Y., Chen, Y., Jing, F., Wang, Z., Hao, Y., et al. (2016). Modulatory effect of romantic love on value estimation and its neural mechanism. *Neuroreport* 27, 323–328. doi: 10.1097/wnr.0000000000000541
91. Wagner, A. D., Maril, A., Bjork, R. A., and Schacter, D. L. (2001). Prefrontal contributions to executive control: fMRI evidence for functional distinctions within lateral prefrontal cortex. *Neuroimage* 14, 1337–1347.
92. Wei, Z., Yang, N., Liu, Y., Yang, L., Wang, Y., Han, L., et al. (2016). Resting-state functional connectivity between the dorsal anterior cingulate cortex and thalamus is associated with risky decision-making in nicotine addicts. *Sci. Rep.* 6:21778. doi: 10.1038/srep21778
93. Windle, R. J., Kershaw, Y. M., Shanks, N., Wood, S. A., Lightman, S. L., and Ingram, C. D. (2004). Oxytocin attenuates stress-induced c-fos mRNA expression in specific forebrain regions associated with modulation of hypothalamo–pituitary–adrenal activity. *J. Neurosci.* 24, 2974–2982. doi: 10.1523/JNEUROSCI.3432-03.2004
94. Windle, R., Shanks, N., Lightman, S. L., and Ingram, C. D. (1997). Central oxytocin administration reduces stress-induced corticosterone release and anxiety behavior in rats 1. *Endocrinology* 138, 2829–2834. doi: 10.1210/en.138.7.2829
95. Winston, J. S., Strange, B. A., O'Doherty, J., and Dolan, R. J. (2002). Automatic and intentional brain responses during evaluation of trustworthiness of faces. *Nat. Neurosci.* 5, 277–283. doi: 10.1038/nn816
96. Xu, X., Aron, A., Brown, L., Cao, G., Feng, T., and Weng, X. (2011). Reward and motivation systems: a brain mapping study of early-stage intense romantic love in Chinese participants. *Hum. Brain Mapp.* 32, 249–257. doi: 10.1002/hbm.21017
97. Zanos, P., Georgiou, P., Wright, S. R., Hourani, S. M., Kitchen, I., Winsky-Sommerer, R., et al. (2014). The oxytocin analogue carbetocin prevents emotional impairment and stress-induced reinstatement of opioid-seeking in morphine-abstinent mice. *Neuropsychopharmacology* 39, 855–865. doi: 10.1038/npp.2013.285
98. Zhang, X., Chen, X., Yu, Y., Sun, D., Ma, N., He, S., et al. (2009). Masked smoking-related images modulate brain activity in smokers. *Hum. Brain Mapp.* 30, 896–907. doi: 10.1002/hbm.20552
99. Zhang, X., Salmeron, B. J., Ross, T. J., Gu, H., Geng, X., Yang, Y., et al. (2011). Anatomical differences and network characteristics underlying smoking cue reactivity. *Neuroimage* 54, 131–141. doi: 10.1016/j.neuroimage.2010.07.063
100. Zhang, Y., Ndasauka, Y., Hou, J., Chen, J., zhuang Yang, L., Wang, Y., et al. (2016). Cue-induced behavioral and neural changes among excessive internet gamers and possible application of cue exposure therapy to internet gaming disorder. *Front. Psychol.* 7:675. doi: 10.3389/fpsyg.2016.00675
101. Zorrilla, E. P., Valdez, G. R., and Weiss, F. (2001). Changes in levels of regional CRF-like-immunoreactivity and plasma corticosterone during protracted drug withdrawal in dependent rats. *Psychopharmacology* 158, 374–381. doi: 10.1007/s002130100773

Permissions

All chapters in this book were first published by Frontiers; hereby published with permission under the Creative Commons Attribution License or equivalent. Every chapter published in this book has been scrutinized by our experts. Their significance has been extensively debated. The topics covered herein carry significant findings which will fuel the growth of the discipline. They may even be implemented as practical applications or may be referred to as a beginning point for another development.

The contributors of this book come from diverse backgrounds, making this book a truly international effort. This book will bring forth new frontiers with its revolutionizing research information and detailed analysis of the nascent developments around the world.

We would like to thank all the contributing authors for lending their expertise to make the book truly unique. They have played a crucial role in the development of this book. Without their invaluable contributions this book wouldn't have been possible. They have made vital efforts to compile up to date information on the varied aspects of this subject to make this book a valuable addition to the collection of many professionals and students.

This book was conceptualized with the vision of imparting up-to-date information and advanced data in this field. To ensure the same, a matchless editorial board was set up. Every individual on the board went through rigorous rounds of assessment to prove their worth. After which they invested a large part of their time researching and compiling the most relevant data for our readers.

The editorial board has been involved in producing this book since its inception. They have spent rigorous hours researching and exploring the diverse topics which have resulted in the successful publishing of this book. They have passed on their knowledge of decades through this book. To expedite this challenging task, the publisher supported the team at every step. A small team of assistant editors was also appointed to further simplify the editing procedure and attain best results for the readers.

Apart from the editorial board, the designing team has also invested a significant amount of their time in understanding the subject and creating the most relevant covers. They scrutinized every image to scout for the most suitable representation of the subject and create an appropriate cover for the book.

The publishing team has been an ardent support to the editorial, designing and production team. Their endless efforts to recruit the best for this project, has resulted in the accomplishment of this book. They are a veteran in the field of academics and their pool of knowledge is as vast as their experience in printing. Their expertise and guidance has proved useful at every step. Their uncompromising quality standards have made this book an exceptional effort. Their encouragement from time to time has been an inspiration for everyone.

The publisher and the editorial board hope that this book will prove to be a valuable piece of knowledge for researchers, students, practitioners and scholars across the globe.

List of Contributors

Jennifer L. Stewart and Robin L. Aupperle
Laureate Institute for Brain Research, Tulsa, OK, United States
Department of Community Medicine, University of Tulsa, Tulsa, OK, United States

Jerzy Bodurka
Laureate Institute for Brain Research, Tulsa, OK, United States

April C. May
Joint Doctoral Program in Clinical Psychology, San Diego State University, University of California, San Diego, San Diego, CA, United States

Jochem M. Jansen
Department of Psychiatry, Amsterdam Institute for Addiction Research, Amsterdam UMC, University of Amsterdam, Amsterdam, Netherlands
Institute for Criminal Law and Criminology, Faculty of Law, Leiden University, Leiden, Netherlands

Wim van den Brink
Department of Psychiatry, Amsterdam Institute for Addiction Research, Amsterdam UMC, University of Amsterdam, Amsterdam, Netherlands

Odile A. van den Heuvel, Stella J. de Wit and Dick J. Veltman
Department of Psychiatry, Amsterdam UMC, Vrije Universiteit Amsterdam, Amsterdam, Netherlands
Department of Anatomy and Neurosciences, Amsterdam Neuroscience, Amsterdam UMC, Vrije Universiteit Amsterdam, Amsterdam, Netherlands

Ysbrand D. van der Werf
Department of Anatomy and Neurosciences, Amsterdam Neuroscience, Amsterdam UMC, Vrije Universiteit Amsterdam, Amsterdam, Netherlands

Anna E. Goudriaan
Department of Psychiatry, Amsterdam Institute for Addiction Research, Amsterdam UMC, University of Amsterdam, Amsterdam, Netherlands
Department of Research and Quality of Care, Arkin, Amsterdam, Netherlands

Rachel F. Smallwood
National Institute of Neurological Disorders and Stroke, National Institutes of Health, Bethesda, MD, United States

Larry R. Price
Metholology, Measurement and Statistical Analysis, Texas State University, San Marcos, TX, United States

Jenna L. Campbell
Department of Communication Sciences and Disorders, University of New Hampshire, Durham, NH, United States

Jennifer S. Potter and Amy S. Garrett
Department of Psychiatry, University of Texas Health Science Center San Antonio, San Antonio, TX, United States

Sebastian W. Atalla and Todd B. Monroe
College of Nursing, The Ohio State University, Columbus, OH, United States

Semra A. Aytur
Department of Health Management and Policy, University of New Hampshire, Durham, NH, United States

Donald A. Robin
Department of Communication Sciences and Disorders, University of New Hampshire, Durham, NH, United States
Interdisciplinary Program in Neuroscience and Behavior, University of New Hampshire, Durham, NH, United States

Jane E. Joseph, Brandon K. Vaughan and Christopher C. Camp
Department of Neuroscience, Medical University of South Carolina, Charleston, SC, United States

Nathaniel L. Baker
Department of Public Health Sciences, Medical University of South Carolina, Charleston, SC, United States

Brian J. Sherman and Megan Moran-Santa Maria
Department of Psychiatry and Behavioral Sciences, Medical University of South Carolina, Charleston, SC, United States

Aimee McRae-Clark and Kathleen T. Brady
Department of Psychiatry and Behavioral Sciences, Medical University of South Carolina, Charleston, SC, United States
Ralph H. Johnson VA Medical Center, Charleston, SC, United States

Marsha E. Bates and Jennifer F. Buckman
Cardiac Neuroscience Laboratory, Department of Kinesiology and Health, Rutgers University-New Brunswick, Piscataway, NJ, United States
Center of Alcohol Studies, Rutgers University-New Brunswick, Piscataway, NJ, United States

Laura M. Lesnewich and Sarah Grace Uhouse
Center of Alcohol Studies, Rutgers University-New Brunswick, Piscataway, NJ, United States
Cardiac Neuroscience Laboratory, Department of Psychology, Rutgers University-New Brunswick, Piscataway, NJ, United States

Suril Gohel
Department of Health Informatics, School of Health Professions, Rutgers University-Newark, Newark, NJ, United States

Antonio Verdejo-Garcia
Turner Institute for Brain and Mental Health, Monash University, Melbourne, VIC, Australia

Valentina Lorenzetti
School of Psychology, Faculty of Health Sciences, Australian Catholic University, Canberra, ACT, Australia

Dan I. Lubman
Eastern Health Clinical School Turning Point, Eastern Health, Richmond, VIC, Australia

Victoria Manning, Hugh Piercy and Shalini Arunogiri
Eastern Health Clinical School Turning Point, Eastern Health, Richmond, VIC, Australia
Eastern Health Clinical School, Monash University, Melbourne, VIC, Australia

Raimondo Bruno
School of Medicine, University of Tasmania, Hobart, TAS, Australia

Rob Hester
School of Psychological Sciences, University of Melbourne, Melbourne, VIC, Australia

Alex Baldacchino
Department of Psychiatry, University of California, San Francisco, San Francisco, CA, United States

David Pennington
San Francisco Veterans Affairs Health Care System (SFVAHCS), San Francisco, CA, United States
Department of Psychiatry, University of California, San Francisco, San Francisco, CA, United States

Serenella Tolomeo
School of Medicine, University of St Andrews, Medical and Biological Science Building, North Haugh, St Andrews, United Kingdom
Department of Psychology, National University of Singapore, Singapore, Singapore

Salvatore Campanella
Laboratoire de Psychologie Médicale et d'Addictologie, ULB Neuroscience Institute (UNI), CHU Brugmann-Université Libre de Bruxelles (U.L.B.), Brussels, Belgium

Stacey B. Daughters
Department of Psychology and Neuroscience, University of North Carolina at Chapel Hill, Chapel Hill, NC, United States

Christos Kouimtsidis
Department of Psychiatry, Surrey and Borders Partnership NHS Foundation Trust, Leatherhead, United Kingdom

Dieter J. Meyerhoff
DVA Medical Center and Department of Radiology and Biomedical Imaging, University of California San Francisco, School of Medicine, San Francisco, CA, United States

Annaketurah Ralph
School of Psychology, University of Queensland, Brisbane, QLD, Australia

Tara Rezapour
Department of Cognitive Psychology, Institute for Cognitive Sciences Studies, Tehran, Iran

Hosna Tavakoli
Department of Cognitive Psychology, Institute for Cognitive Sciences Studies, Tehran, Iran
Iranian National Center for Addiction Studies, Tehran University of Medical Sciences, Tehran, Iran

Mehran Zare-Bidoky
Iranian National Center for Addiction Studies, Tehran University of Medical Sciences, Tehran, Iran
School of Medicine, Shahid-Sadoughi University of Medical Sciences, Yazd, Iran

Anna Zilverstand
Department of Psychiatry, University of Minnesota, Minneapolis, MN, United States

Douglas Steele
Medical School, University of Dundee, Ninewells Hospital, Scotland, United Kingdom

Scott J. Moeller
Department of Psychiatry, Renaissance School of Medicine at Stony Brook University, Stony Brook, NY, United States

Martin Paulus
Laureate Institute for Brain Research, University of Tulsa, Tulsa, OK, United States

Hamed Ekhtiari
Laureate Institute for Brain Research, University of Tulsa, Tulsa, OK, United States
Institute for Cognitive Science Studies, Tehran, Iran
Iranian National Center for Addiction Studies, Tehran University of Medical Sciences, Tehran, Iran

Yann Chye, Erynn Christensen and Murat Yücel
Brain and Mental Health Research Hub, Monash Institute of Cognitive and Clinical Neurosciences, School of Psychological Sciences, Monash University, Melbourne, VIC, Australia

Nadia Solowij
School of Psychology and Illawarra Health and Medical Research Institute, University of Wollongong, Wollongong, NSW, Australia
The Australian Centre for Cannabinoid Clinical and Research Excellence, New Lambton Heights, NSW, Australia

Marianne Destoop and Geert Dom
Collaborative Antwerp Psychiatric Research Institute (CAPRI), Faculty of Medicine and Health Sciences, University of Antwerp, Antwerp, Belgium
Department of Addiction, Psychiatric Hospital Multiversum, Boechout, Belgium

Violette Coppens and Manuel Morrens
Faculty of Medicine and Health Sciences, Collaborative Antwerp Psychiatric Research Institute (CAPRI), University of Antwerp, Antwerp, Belgium
Scientific Initiative of Neuropsychiatric and Psychopharmacological Studies (SINAPS), University Department of Psychiatry, Duffel, Belgium

Emma Jane Rose and Giorgia Picci
Program for Translational Research on Adversity and Neurodevelopment (P-TRAN), The Edna Bennett Pierce Prevention Research Center, The Pennsylvania State University, University Park, PA, USA

Diana H. Fishbein
Program for Translational Research on Adversity and Neurodevelopment (P-TRAN), The Edna Bennett Pierce Prevention Research Center, The Pennsylvania State University, University Park, PA, USA
Department of Human Development and Family Studies, The Pennsylvania State University, University Park, PA, USA

Steve Sharman
School of Psychology, College of Applied Health and Communities, University of East London, London, United Kingdom
Department of Psychology, University of Cambridge, Cambridge, United Kingdom

Luke Clark
Department of Psychology, University of Cambridge, Cambridge, United Kingdom
Centre for Gambling Research at UBC, Department of Psychology, University of British Columbia, Vancouver, BC, Canada

Amanda Roberts
School of Psychology, College of Social Science, University of Lincoln, Lincoln, United Kingdom

Rosanna Michalczuk
Department of Psychology, University of Cambridge, Cambridge, United Kingdom
South London and Maudsley Trust, Bethlem Royal Hospital, London, United Kingdom

Rachel Cocks
Department of Psychology, University of Cambridge, Cambridge, United Kingdom
Royal Holloway, University of London, London, United Kingdom

Henrietta Bowden-Jones
National Problem Gambling Clinic, London, United Kingdom
Faculty of Medicine, Faculty of Medicine Centre, Imperial College London, London, United Kingdom

Zoha Deldar
Institute for Cognitive Science Studies, Tehran, Iran

Hamid Reza Pouretemad
Institute for Cognitive and Brain Sciences (ICBS), Shahid Beheshti University, Tehran, Iran

Ali Khatibi
Department of Neurology and Neurosurgery, McGill University, Montreal, QC, Canada
Centre of Precision Rehabilitation for Spinal Pain (CPR Spine), School of Sport, Exercise and Rehabilitation Sciences, University of Birmingham, Birmingham, AL, United States

Erica N. Grodin and Lara A. Ray
Department of Psychology, University of California, Los Angeles, Los Angeles, CA, United States
Department of Psychiatry and Biobehavioral Sciences, UCLA School of Medicine, University of California, Los Angeles, Los Angeles, CA, United States

Aaron C. Lim
Department of Psychology, University of California, Los Angeles, Los Angeles, CA, United States

Mitchell P. Karno
Department of Psychiatry and Biobehavioral Sciences, UCLA School of Medicine, University of California, Los Angeles, Los Angeles, CA, United States

James MacKillop
Department of Psychiatry and Behavioral Neurosciences, McMaster University, Hamilton, ON, Canada

Natalia Albein-Urios
Cognitive Neuroscience Unit, School of Psychology, Deakin University, Geelong, VIC, Australia

Jose M. Martinez-Gonzalez
Centro Provincial de Drogodependencias, Diputación de Granada, Granada, Spain

Oscar Lozano-Rojas
Departamento de Psicología Clínica, Experimental y Social, Universidad de Huelva, Huelva, Spain
Research Center on Natural Resources, Health and Environment, University of Huelva, Huelva, Spain

Simasadat Noorbakhsh, Mohammad H. Afzali, Elroy Boers and Patricia J. Conrod
Département de Psychiatrie, Université de Montréal, Centre de Recherche du CHU Sainte-Justine, Montréal, QC, Canada

Lee Hogarth, Lorna Hardy and Alexandra Bakou
School of Psychology, University of Exeter, Exeter, United Kingdom

Justin Mahlberg and Sharon Cashel
School of Social Sciences and Psychology, Western Sydney University, Sydney, NSW, Australia

Gabrielle Weidemann and Ahmed A. Moustafa
School of Social Sciences and Psychology, Western Sydney University, Sydney, NSW, Australia
MARCS Institute for Brain, Behaviour and Development, Western Sydney University, Sydney, NSW, Australia

Salman Shahzad and Nasreen Bano
Institute of Clinical Psychology, University of Karachi, Karachi, Pakistan

Nasreen Begum
Department of Applied Psychology, Virtual University of Pakistan, Lahore, Pakistan

Hendrée E. Jones
Department of Obstetrics & Gynecology, University of North Carolina at Chapel Hill, Chapel Hill, NC, United States

Yu Tian, Yanli Zhao, Fengling Lv and Ningbo Qin
Department of Marxism, Qingdao University of Science and Technology, Qingdao, China

Peipei Chen
Department of Psychology, Shandong Normal University, Jinan, China

Zhiling Zou
Faculty of Psychology, Southwest University, Chongqing, China

Hongwen Song
Faculty of Psychology, Southwest University, Chongqing, China
Center of Medical Physics and Technology, Hefei Institutes of Physical Science, CAS, Hefei, China

Yuting Zhang
Chinese Academy of Sciences Key Laboratory of Brain Function and Disease, School of Life Sciences, University of Science and Technology of China, Hefei, China

Xiaochu Zhang
Center of Medical Physics and Technology, Hefei Institutes of Physical Science, CAS, Hefei, China
Chinese Academy of Sciences Key Laboratory of Brain Function and Disease, School of Life Sciences, University of Science and Technology of China, Hefei, China
School of Humanities and Social Science, University of Science and Technology of China, Hefei, China
Centers for Biomedical Engineering, University of Science and Technology of China, Hefei, China

Index

www.ingramcontent.com/pod-product-compliance
Lightning Source LLC
LaVergne TN
LVHW081015210926
848485LV00004B/866

9781646475490